Pseudomonas aeruginosa as an Opportunistic Pathogen

INFECTIOUS AGENTS AND PATHOGENESIS

Series Editors: Mauro Bendinelli, *University of Pisa*
Herman Friedman, *University of South Florida*

COXSACKIEVIRUSES
A General Update
　Edited by Mauro Bendinelli and Herman Friedman

FUNGAL INFECTIONS AND IMMUNE RESPONSES
　Edited by Juneann W. Murphy, Herman Friedman, and Mauro Bendinelli

MYCOBACTERIUM TUBERCULOSIS
Interactions with the Immune System
　Edited by Mauro Bendinelli and Herman Friedman

NEUROPATHOGENIC VIRUSES AND IMMUNITY
　Edited by Steven Specter, Mauro Bendinelli, and Herman Friedman

PSEUDOMONAS AERUGINOSA AS AN OPPORTUNISTIC PATHOGEN
　Edited by Mario Campa, Mauro Bendinelli, and Herman Friedman

VIRUS-INDUCED IMMUNOSUPPRESSION
　Edited by Steven Specter, Mauro Bendinelli, and Herman Friedman

Pseudomonas aeruginosa as an Opportunistic Pathogen

Edited by

Mario Campa
University of Pisa
Pisa, Italy

Mauro Bendinelli
University of Pisa
Pisa, Italy

and

Herman Friedman
University of South Florida
Tampa, Florida

Plenum Press • New York and London

Library of Congress Cataloging-in-Publication Data

Pseudomonas aeruginosa as an opportunistic pathogen / edited by Mario
  Campa, Mauro Bendinelli, and Herman Friedman.
       p.   cm. -- (Infectious agents and pathogenesis)
    Includes bibliographical references and index.
    ISBN 0-306-44265-5
    1. Pseudomonas aeruginosa infections. 2. Opportunistic
  infections.   I. Campa, Mario. II. Bendinelli, Mauro.
  III. Friedman, Herman. IV. Series.
    [DNLM: 1. Pseudomonas Aeruginosa. 2. Pseudomonas Infections.   QW
  131 P9735]
  QR201.P74P7 1992
  616'.0145--dc20
  DNLM/DLC
  for Library of Congress   92-48759
                                                                     CIP

ISBN 0-306-44265-5

©1993 Plenum Press, New York
A Division of Plenum Publishing Corporation
233 Spring Street, New York, N.Y. 10013

All rights reserved

No part of this book may be reproduced, stored in a retrieval system, or transmitted
in any form or by any means, electronic, mechanical, photocopying, microfilming,
recording, or otherwise, without written permission from the Publisher

Printed in the United States of America

Contributors

DALE R. ABRAHAMSON • Department of Cell Biology, University of Alabama at Birmingham, UAB Station, Birmingham, Alabama 35294

ANDREW W. ARTENSTEIN • Infectious Disease Service, Department of Medicine, Walter Reed Army Medical Center, and Department of Bacterial Diseases, Walter Reed Army Institute of Research, Washington, D.C. 20307-5001

ALI AZGHANI • Department of Biochemistry, University of Texas Health Science Center at Tyler, Tyler, Texas 75710

FRANCIS BELLIDO • Eli Lilly, 1214 Geneva, Switzerland

RICHARD S. BERK • Department of Immunology and Microbiology, Wayne State University School of Medicine, Detroit, Michigan 48201

KONRAD BOTZENHART • Department of General Hygiene and Environmental Hygiene, Hygiene-Institut, University of Tübingen, D-7400 Tübingen, Germany

MARIO CAMPA • Department of Biomedicine, Clinical Microbiology Section, University of Pisa, 56127 Pisa, Italy

MICHAEL S. COLLINS • Miles Pharmaceutical Division, Miles Inc., West Haven, Connecticut 06516-4175

ALAN S. CROSS • Infectious Disease Service, Department of Medicine, Walter Reed Army Medical Center, and Department of Bacterial Diseases, Walter Reed Army Institute of Research, Washington, D.C. 20307-5001

STANLEY J. CRYZ, JR. • Swiss Serum and Vaccine Institute, CH-3001 Berne, Switzerland

GERD DÖRING • Department of General Hygiene and Environmental Hygiene, Hygiene-Institut, University of Tübingen, D-7400 Tübingen, Germany

DARRELL R. GALLOWAY • Department of Microbiology, The Ohio State University, Columbus, Ohio 43210-1292

ROBERT E. W. HANCOCK • Department of Microbiology, University of British Columbia, Vancouver, British Columbia, Canada V6T 1W5

LOUIS W. HECK • Department of Medicine, Veterans Administration Medical Center, University of Alabama at Birmingham, UAB Station, Birmingham, Alabama 35294

JANEL HECTOR • Department of Biochemistry, University of Texas Health Science Center at Tyler, Tyler, Texas 75710

IAN ALAN HOLDER • Shriners Burns Institute, Cincinnati, Ohio 45229-3095

RANDALL T. IRVIN • Department of Medical Microbiology and Infectious Diseases, University of Alberta, Edmonton, Alberta, Canada T6G 2H7

ALICE JOHNSON • Department of Biochemistry, University of Texas Health Science Center at Tyler, Tyler, Texas 75710

FRED JOSEPH, JR. • Department of Pediatrics, Louisiana State University Medical Center, New Orleans, Louisiana 70112

ANTONELLA LUPETTI • Department of Biomedicine, Clinical Microbiology Section, University of Pisa, 56127 Pisa, Italy

PAOLA MARELLI • Department of Biomedicine, Clinical Microbiology Section, University of Pisa, 56127 Pisa, Italy

RANDAL E. MORRIS • Department of Anatomy and Cell Biology, University of Cincinnati College of Medicine, Cincinnati, Ohio 45267-0521

GERALD B. PIER • Channing Laboratory, Department of Medicine, Brigham and Women's Hospital, Harvard Medical School, Boston, Massachusetts 02115-5899

CATHARINE B. SAELINGER • Department of Molecular Genetics, Biochemistry, and Microbiology, University of Cincinnati College of Medicine, Cincinnati, Ohio 45267-0524

CHRISTINE M. SHUMARD • Diagnostics Division, Abbott Laboratories, Abbott Park, Illinois 60064

RICARDO U. SORENSEN • Department of Pediatrics, Louisiana State University Medical Center, New Orleans, Louisiana 70112

DAVID P. SPEERT • Departments of Pediatrics and Microbiology and the Canadian Bacterial Diseases Network, University of British Columbia, and Division of Infectious and Immunological Diseases, British Columbia's Children's Hospital, Research Centre, Vancouver, British Columbia, Canada V5Z 4H4

ROBERT STEADMAN • Institute of Nephrology, Cardiff Royal Infirmary, Cardiff, Wales CF2 1SZ

DONALD E. WOODS • Department of Microbiology and Infectious Diseases, University of Calgary Health Sciences Centre, Calgary, Alberta, Canada T2N 4N1

DANIEL J. WOZNIAK • Department of Microbiology and Immunology, University of Tennessee, Memphis, Tennessee 38163

Preface

This volume is devoted to *Pseudomonas aeruginosa* as an "opportunistic" pathogen in humans. We have attempted to provide balanced coverage of epidemiology, pathogenesis, clinical features, and control measures. All the chapters have been contributed by outstanding authorities on specific aspects of *P. aeruginosa* research. This book should prove useful to physicians and surgeons who have in their care patients infected, or at risk of becoming infected, with *P. aeruginosa* and who want to gain a greater understanding of this elusive microorganism, the diseases it produces, and means of control. We also hope that the book will stimulate further studies on the mechanisms whereby *P. aeruginosa* establishes itself and causes disease in compromised patients.

The opportunistic behavior of this bacterium was recognized a long time ago. Since then, the extent of our knowledge about *P. aeruginosa* and microbes in general has burgeoned. Nevertheless, there are still few real clues as to why *P. aeruginosa* infection is much less common than one would expect considering the wide distribution of this bacterium in nature and why it mainly infects individuals whose local or systemic antibacterial defenses are compromised.

Because of its minimal growth requirements and nutritional flexibility, *P. aeruginosa* is particularly able to adapt to changing ecological conditions. It is also capable of surviving for long periods, especially in moist environments. In addition, the poor permeability of its outer membrane makes it intrinsically resistant to many disinfectants and antimicrobial agents, and it is therefore well adapted to compete with antibiotic-secreting microorganisms in its natural ecosystem, the soil, and to exploit the selective advantages provided by hospital environments.

Understanding why in healthy humans—in spite of the large variety of virulent factors produced by the microorganism—the carrier state is generally rare and unstable and, in contrast, infection of the immunocompromised is common and severe is not only a challenge per se but may also help shed light on opportunistic microorganisms in general. The number of immunocompromised individuals has exploded worldwide as a consequence of progresses in modern medicine and, more recently, the epidemic of acquired immunodeficiency syndrome. There is a consensus that this population "class" will increase considerably in the next few decades. This will not only expand the number of potential victims of opportunistic infections but may also provide new opportunities for pseudomonads and other agents to gradually adapt better to the human host. New knowledge may help reduce such risks.

We are grateful to the excellent scientists who provided enthusiastic support for the preparation of this volume, and we are confident that their collective effort will be appreciated by the reader.

Mario Campa
Mauro Bendinelli
Herman Friedman

Contents

1. Ecology and Epidemiology of *Pseudomonas aeruginosa*
   KONRAD BOTZENHART and GERD DÖRING

   1. Introduction 1
   2. Ecology 2
      2.1. Adaptability 2
      2.2. Inanimate Environment 3
      2.3. Healthy Humans 6
   3. Epidemiology 7
      3.1. Incidence of Infections 7
      3.2. Routes of Transmission 7
   4. Résumé 12
      References 13

2. Attachment and Colonization of *Pseudomonas aeruginosa*: Role of the Surface Structures
   RANDALL T. IRVIN

   1. Introduction 19
   2. Role of Adherence in Pathogenesis 20
      2.1. Morphology of Adherence to Human Respiratory Cells .. 21
      2.2. Effect of Epithelial Cell Type on Adherence 21
   3. Adhesins 22
      3.1. Structure and Function of the Capsule 23
      3.2. Exoenzyme S 28
      3.3. Structure of Pili 29

	3.4. Synthesis and Assembly of Pili	29
	3.5. Structural Variability in Pilins	30
	3.6. Pilin-Pilin Interactions	30
	3.7. Function of Pili	31
	3.8. The Pilus and Exoenzyme S Receptor(s)	32
	3.9. Structural Organization of Pili	33
4.	Summary and Conclusion	33
	References	36

3. Phenazine Pigments in *Pseudomonas aeruginosa* Infection

RICARDO U. SORENSON and FRED JOSEPH, JR.

1.	Introduction	43
2.	Structure and Chemical Properties	44
3.	Purification, Synthesis, and Methods of Detection	46
4.	Regulation of Phenazine Production and Possible Function	47
5.	Biological Effects of Phenazine Pigments	48
	5.1. Effect on Bacteria	48
	5.2. Effect on Mitochondrial Respiration	49
	5.3. Effect on Neutrophil Function	49
	5.4. Effect on Cell Proliferation and Cytokine Secretion	50
	5.5. Effect on Ciliary Beating	51
	5.6. Intratracheal Instillation of Pyocyanine *in Vivo*	52
	5.7. Effect on Vascular Reactivity	52
6.	Phenazine Pigments in *Pseudomonas* Infections	52
	6.1. Presence of Phenazine Pigments at Sites of Infection	52
	6.2. Role of Phenazines in Chronic *P. aeruginosa* Infections	53
7.	Concluding Remarks	53
	References	54

4. Regulation of Toxin A Synthesis in *Pseudomonas aeruginosa*

CHRISTINE M. SHUMARD, DANIEL J. WOZNIAK, and DARRELL R. GALLOWAY

1.	Introduction	59
	1.1. Historical Perspectives Regarding the Regulation of Toxin A Synthesis	60
2.	Influence of Environmental Factors on Toxin A Synthesis	61
	2.1. Regulation of Toxin A Production by Iron	62
3.	Genetic Regulation of Toxin A Synthesis	64
	3.1. Evidence for an Activator	64

	3.2. Characterization of *toxR*: A Gene Involved in the Positive Regulation of Toxin A Synthesis	66
	3.3. Transcriptional Analysis of the *toxR* Gene	67
	3.4. Report on a Second Gene Involved in Regulation of Toxin A Production: *regB*	68
	3.5. Mutational Analysis of Genes Involved in Toxin A Regulation	68
	3.6. The Role of *toxR* in the Regulation of Toxin A Expression	69
	3.7. Evidence for Additional Factors Regulating Toxin A Synthesis	72
4.	Summary and Conclusions	73
	References	74

5. Susceptibility of Mammalian Cells to *Pseudomonas* Exotoxin A
RANDAL E. MORRIS and CATHARINE B. SAELINGER

1.	Introduction	79
2.	Structure-Function Relationship	81
3.	Receptor-Mediated Endocytosis	83
	3.1. Role of Acidic Compartments	86
	3.2. Temperature Dependence	86
4.	Similarities with Viral Entry	87
5.	Experimental Data	88
	5.1. The Binding Event	88
	5.2. Endocytic Uptake of *Pseudomonas* and Diphtheria Toxins by Mouse LM Fibroblasts	89
	5.3. Activation and Escape of *Pseudomonas* Toxin in LM Fibroblasts	93
	5.4. Isolation of the Receptor for *Pseudomonas* Exotoxin A from Mouse LM Fibroblasts	97
6.	A Cell Line Resistant to *Pseudomonas* Exotoxin A—Ovcar Cells	98
7.	Chimeric Toxins	98
8.	Conclusions	99
	References	100

6. Role of Exotoxins in the Pathogenesis of *P. aeruginosa* Infections
DARRELL R. GALLOWAY

1.	Introduction and Historical Perspectives	107
	1.1. *Pseudomonas aeruginosa*—The Opportunistic Pathogen	108
2.	Exotoxin A	110

3.	Exoenzyme S	113
4.	Elastase	115
5.	Phospholipases	119
6.	In Conclusion	120
	References	121

7. The Role of Proteases in the Pathogenesis of *Pseudomonas aeruginosa* Infections

ROBERT STEADMAN, LOUIS W. HECK, and DALE R. ABRAHAMSON

1.	Introduction	129
2.	The Control of Protease Secretion	130
3.	Protease Involvement in Pathogenicity	131
4.	Tissue Damage Induced by Proteases	132
5.	Effects of Proteases on the Immune System	135
6.	Inhibition of Proteases	139
7.	Summary	139
	References	140

8. Genetic Regulation and Expression of Elastase in *Pseudomonas aeruginosa*

JANEL HECTOR, ALI AZGHANI, and ALICE JOHNSON

1.	Introduction	145
	1.1. *Pseudomonas* Elastase	146
	1.2. Chemistry	146
	1.3. Biological Effects	147
	1.4. Bacterial Adherence	149
2.	Environmental Effects on Elastase Production	149
	2.1. Source	150
	2.2. Antibiotics	150
	2.3. Culture Conditions	150
	2.4. Media Composition	150
	2.5. Duration of Culture	151
3.	Molecular Biology Studies	152
	3.1. Elastase-Deficient Mutants	152
	3.2. Elastase Genes	154
	3.3. Processing of Elastase	155
	3.4. Secretion	157

4. Conclusions 159
   References 159

9. *Pseudomonas aeruginosa*—Phagocytic Cell Interactions
   DAVID P. SPEERT

1. Introduction 163
2. Mechanisms of Phagocytosis 164
   2.1. Professional Phagocytic Cells: In Defense against Infection 164
   2.2. The Process of Phagocytosis 164
   2.3. Opsonic and Nonopsonic Phagocytosis 165
3. Phagocytosis of *Pseudomonas aeruginosa* 166
   3.1. Opsonic Phagocytosis 166
   3.2. Nonopsonic Phagocytosis 167
4. Phagocytic Killing of *Pseudomonas aeruginosa* 168
   4.1. Bactericidal Mechanisms of Phagocytic Cells 168
   4.2. Mechanism of *Pseudomonas aeruginosa* Killing 169
5. *Pseudomonas aeruginosa* Products with Effects on Phagocytosis 169
   5.1. Cytotoxins 170
   5.2. Elastase 171
   5.3. Exotoxin A 171
   5.4. Mucoid Exopolysaccharide 172
   5.5. Slime Glycolipoprotein 172
   5.6. Pyocyanine 173
6. Disease States in which Phagocytic Dysfunction May Predispose to Infections with *Pseudomonas aeruginosa* 173
   6.1. Neutropenia 173
   6.2. Thermal Burns 174
   6.3. Cystic Fibrosis 174
   References 176

10. Genetic Regulation of the Murine Corneal and Non-Corneal Response to *Pseudomonas aeruginosa*
    RICHARD S. BERK

1. Introduction 183
2. Non-Ocular Studies 185
   2.1. Systemic Infections—Genetic Studies 185
   2.2 T-cell Immunity—Genetic Studies 185
3. Corneal Infections 188

	3.1. Genetic Studies	188
	3.2. Humoral Response of Resistant and Susceptible Mice	197
	3.3. Role of Complement in Corneal Resistance	199
	3.4. Role of Age in Resistance	199
	3.5. Immunization Studies	200
4.	Discussion	200
	References	202

11. Effects of *Pseudomonas aeruginosa* on Immune Functions
MARIO CAMPA, PAOLA MARELLI, and ANTONELLA LUPETTI

1.	Introduction	207
2.	Interference with Nonspecific Immune Defense Mechanisms	208
3.	Interference with Specific Immune Defense Mechanisms	212
4.	Concluding Remarks	216
	References	216

12. Local and Disseminated Diseases Caused by *Pseudomonas aeruginosa*
ANDREW W. ARTENSTEIN and ALAN S. CROSS

1.	Introduction	223
2.	Bacteremia	224
	2.1. Epidemiology	224
	2.2. Clinical Presentation	225
	2.3. Dermatologic Features	225
	2.4. Therapy	225
	2.5. Prognosis	226
3.	Endocarditis	226
	3.1. Epidemiology	226
	3.2. Clinical Presentation	227
	3.3. Therapy	227
4.	Respiratory Infections	227
	4.1. Epidemiology	227
	4.2. Clinical Presentation	228
	4.3. Radiology	228
	4.4. Therapy	228
	4.5. Cystic Fibrosis	229
5.	Urinary Tract Infections	229
	5.1. Epidemiology	229

	5.2.	Clinical Presentation	229
	5.3.	Therapy	229
6.	Bone and Joint Infections		230
	6.1.	Epidemiology	230
	6.2.	Addict-associated Infection	230
	6.3.	Osteochondritis	230
7.	Central Nervous System Infections		231
	7.1.	Meningitis	231
	7.2.	Brain Abscess	231
8.	Wound Infections		232
9.	Skin Infections		232
	9.1.	General Considerations	232
	9.2.	Clinical Syndromes	232
10.	Ocular Infections		233
	10.1.	General Considerations	233
	10.2.	Keratitis	234
	10.3.	Endophthalmitis	234
11.	Otolaryngologic Infections		235
	11.1.	General Considerations	235
	11.2.	External Otitis	235
	11.3.	Malignant External Otitis	235
	11.4.	Other Syndromes	236
12.	Dialysis Infections		237
	12.1.	General Considerations	237
	12.2.	Clinical Features	237
13.	Gastrointestinal Infections		237
	13.1.	General Considerations	237
	13.2.	Typhlitis	238
	13.3.	Perirectal Disease	238
14.	Miscellaneous Infections		239
	References		239

13. Chronic *Pseudomonas aeruginosa* Lung Infection in Cystic Fibrosis Patients

GERD DÖRING

1.	Introduction		245
2.	Acquisition		246
	2.1.	In Hospitals	246
	2.2.	Outside of Hospitals	247
	2.3.	Intestinal Colonization	248
3.	Virulence and Host Defense		248

	3.1.	Adhesion	248
	3.2.	Virulence Determinants	250
	3.3.	Persistence: The Surface Enlargement Strategy	256
	3.4.	Tissue Damage: A Neutrophil Enzyme Effect	257
4.	New Strategies for Therapy and Prevention		258
	4.1.	Antibiotics	258
	4.2.	Anti-Inflammatory Therapy	258
	4.3.	Immunoprophylaxis and Immunotherapy	259
	4.4.	Disinfection and Hygiene	260
	References		260

14. *P. aeruginosa* Burn Infections: Pathogenesis and Treatment
IAN ALAN HOLDER

1.	Introduction and Brief History	275
2.	Antimicrobial Treatment: Parenteral and Topical	276
3.	Immunotherapy	277
4.	*Pseudomonas* Virulence-associated Factors: Their Role in Pathogenesis in Burned Hosts	277
	4.1. Exotoxin A	279
	4.2. Proteolytic Enzymes	281
	4.3. Pili	283
	4.4. Flagella, Motility, and Chemotaxis	284
5.	Speculations on the Role(s) of *Pseudomonas* Virulence-associated Factors on the Pathogenic Process of Burn Wound Infections and Novel Treatment Approaches	285
	References	290

15. Acquired Resistance to *P. aeruginosa*
GERALD B. PIER

1.	Introduction	297
2.	Immunity to Infection	298
3.	Acquired Resistance to Infection in Non-CF Humans	299
	3.1. Naturally Acquired Active Immunity to Non-CF-Associated *P. aeruginosa* Infections	299
	3.2. Vaccine-Induced Immunity to Non-CF-Associated *P. aeruginosa* Isolates	300
	3.3. Antibody Isotype, Complement, and Phagocytes in Acquired Resistance to Non-CF-Associated *P. aeruginosa* Infection	303

    3.4. T-cell Immunity to Non-CF-Associated Isolates of
         P. aeruginosa 304
 4. Acquired Resistance to Infection in CF Patients 305
    4.1. Naturally Acquired Resistance Among CF Patients to
         P. aeruginosa Infection 306
    4.2. Vaccine-Induced Immunity and Prospective
         Immunotherapeutic Strategies 306
    4.3. Antibody Isotype, Complement, and Phagocytes in
         Acquired Resistance to Infection in CF Patients 308
 5. Summary 311
    References 311

16. Susceptibility and Resistance of *Pseudomonas aeruginosa* to
    Antimicrobial Agents

    FRANCIS BELLIDO and ROBERT E. W. HANCOCK

 1. Introduction 321
 2. β-Lactams 322
    2.1. Antipseudomonal β-Lactams 322
    2.2. Determinants of Efficacy 324
    2.3. Resistance 330
 3. Aminoglycosides 331
    3.1. Determinants of Efficacy 331
    3.2. Outer Membrane Permeation 334
    3.3. Cytoplasmic Membrane Penetration 335
    3.4. Plasmid-Mediated Resistance 336
    3.5. Clinical Resistance Development 336
 4. Quinolones 338
    4.1. Determinants of Efficacy 338
    4.2. Uptake Across the Outer Membrane 338
    4.3. Assays of Quinolone Uptake 341
    4.4. Mechanisms of Resistance 341
    References 342

17. Immunochemical Prophylaxis against *Pseudomonas aeruginosa*

    MICHAEL S. COLLINS

 1. Introduction 349
 2. Active Immunotherapy 350
    2.1. Complex Vaccines, LPS-based 351
    2.2. Defined Vaccines, LPS-based 351
    2.3. Defined LPS-based Vaccines of Low Toxicity 352

		2.4.	Cross-protective Vaccines	352
3.	Passive Immunotherapy			353
		3.1.	Immune Serum Globulin	354
		3.2.	Immune Serum Globulin for Intravenous Infusion	354
		3.3.	Hyperimmune Immunoglobulin	356
4.	Monoclonal Antibodies			363
		4.1.	Core Glycolipid Immunity	363
		4.2.	Immunotherapy with *P. aeruginosa*-Specific Monoclonal Antibodies	365
		4.3.	Safety and Efficacy Considerations for Monoclonal Antibody Therapy	369
	References			369

18. The State of the Art in the Development of *Pseudomonas aeruginosa* Vaccines

STANLEY J. CRYZ, JR.

1.	Clinical Significance	383
2.	Human Immunity to *P. aeruginosa*	384
3.	Development and Clinical Evaluation of Immunological Agents against *P. aeruginosa*	387
	3.1. Background	387
	3.2. *P. aeruginosa* Vaccines	387
4.	Passive Immunotherapy	390
	4.1. Human Monoclonal Antibodies against *P. aeruginosa*	391
	References	392

19. Perspectives for the Control of Chronic *Pseudomonas aeruginosa* Lung Infections of Cystic Fibrosis Patients

DONALD E. WOODS

1.	Introduction	397
2.	Animal Studies	398
3.	Regulation of Virulence	400
4.	Direct versus Indirect Lung Injury	400
5.	Effects of Antibiotics on Virulence	401
6.	Patient Studies	403
7.	Role of *P. aeruginosa* in Exacerbations of Lung Disease	406
8.	Conclusion	407
	References	409

Index 411

Ecology and Epidemiology of *Pseudomonas aeruginosa*

KONRAD BOTZENHART and GERD DÖRING

1. INTRODUCTION

The first description of *Pseudomonas aeruginosa* as a distinct bacterial species was made at the end of the nineteenth century, after Pasteur's development of sterile culture media. Screening for dyes provided the stimulus for the first scientific study on *P. aeruginosa* published by pharmacist Carle Gessard in 1882 and entitled "On the blue and green coloration of bandages."[1] This characteristic pigmentation, later attributed to a phenazine derivative, pyocyanine, is reflected in the old names *Bacillus pyocyaneus*, *Pseudomonas polycolor*, *Bakterium aeruginosa* and *Pseudomonas pyocyaneus*. Although the ability of *P. aeruginosa* to produce infections was noticed by 1889,[2] its pathogenicity was doubted,[3] and *P. aeruginosa* was regarded mainly as a source of potent antimicrobial substances.[4] Before 1947 only 91 cases of septicemia attributable to *P. aeruginosa* were reported in the literature.[5] Its importance as a human pathogen, especially in hospitalized patients, did not emerge until the second half of the twentieth century,[6] although the organism was certainly present in the inanimate and human environment before then. Because *P. aeruginosa* is easy to culture and identify it is unlikely that it was missed by clinical microbiologists. Thus, the considerable change in the significance of

---

KONRAD BOTZENHART and GERD DÖRING • Department of General Hygiene and Environmental Hygiene, Hygiene-Institut, University of Tübingen, D-7400 Tübingen, Germany.

Pseudomonas aeruginosa as an Opportunistic Pathogen, edited by Mario Campa *et al.* Plenum Press, New York, 1993.

P. aeruginosa as a nosocomial pathogen probably reflects advances made in the life sciences as well as changes in the susceptibility of patients.

The development of antibiotics and immunosuppressive agents, improvements in intensive care, surgery, and treatment regimes for many diseases have increased life expectancies for many patient groups. Patients with severe burns, cystic fibrosis (CF), cancer, and paraplegia, for example, existed at the beginning of our century, but usually succumbed early after the disease onset. Additionally, the number of premature infants has increased in children's hospitals, and the number of elderly is growing in many developed countries of the world due to improved living conditions. These patient groups have in common an impaired defense system resulting from underlying disease, its specific treatment, or their age. It is this trait that accompanies infections with *P. aeruginosa* and has prompted the characterization of this organism as "opportunistic." The increasing use of catheterization and other invasive techniques further facilitates infections with *P. aeruginosa*, which currently is responsible for 10–11% of all nosocomial infections.

Although antibiotic therapy has considerably improved the management of infectious diseases, many *P. aeruginosa* infections do not respond to the application of anti-pseudomonal drugs and become chronic. Others, such as *P. aeruginosa* corneal infections, develop too fast for appropriate chemotherapy. Under these circumstances, prevention of *P. aeruginosa* infections by precautionary measures is an appropriate alternative. Knowledge of *P. aeruginosa* ecology is a prerequisite for the study of its epidemiology. Because the tools of molecular biology now allow us to type *P. aeruginosa* strains more accurately than in the past, it may be possible to better identify the routes of transmission that lead to infection and ultimately to apply hygienic means to disinfect the relevant reservoirs.

An excellent review by Rhame[7] summarizes the findings of *P. aeruginosa* ecology and epidemiology up to 1979. Since that time, *P. aeruginosa* has not changed its "ecological niches" and may be isolated from the same reservoirs in the environment. Also, the incidence of nosocomial infections due to *P. aeruginosa* has not changed dramatically since one of us reviewed the literature in 1986.[8] Therefore, this chapter will emphasize more recent results elucidating transmission routes inside and outside of hospitals in different high-risk patient groups using molecular epidemiology.

2. ECOLOGY

2.1. Adaptability

Microbial ecology describes the complex relationships between microorganisms and the external world, *i.e.*, the inanimate and the animate environment, inorganic and organic compounds, friends and enemies. The ability to adapt to a mostly hostile environment largely determines the success of a microbial life form. The mode of adaptability determines where we might find a certain microorganism in the environment. We are only beginning to understand how microorganisms adapt. Molecular biology defines adaptability as gene regulation. The bacteria, constantly sensing their environment, may turn genes on or off or merely adjust their levels of expression[9–11] in response to signals such as osmolarity, temperature, pH, Ca^{2+}, iron or anaerobicity. Gene regulation will finally result in phenotypic changes. Adaptable microorganisms may therefore appear in different guises, depending on the environment. Assumptions made from experiments involving a given bacterial phenotype cannot be extrapolated to another phenotype. The sensitivity of bacteria grown *in vitro* to DNA-affecting antibiotics, and their insensitivity to the same drugs *in vivo*, is a well-known example.

P. aeruginosa is tremendously versatile. The long list of reports of *P. aeruginosa* in the inanimate and human environment[7,8] has led to its description as a "ubiquitous" microorganism. The basis for this versatility is a huge arsenal of enzymes that enables the organism to use a large variety of substances as nutrients and to change its appearance like a chameleon.

The most impressive phenotypic change is the reversible switch from nonmucoid to mucoid variant, which is accompanied by the production of large amounts of exopolysaccharide (alginate). Mucoid *P. aeruginosa* strains emerge in moist environments. Some scientists have speculated, teleologically, that the mucoid state facilitates bacterial adhesion by bridging the electrostatic repulsion barrier between the bacterial and the environmental surface, to prevent *P. aeruginosa* from being swept away by respiratory tract cilia or by turbulence in a fluid environment and to protect the organisms from phagocytes and other enemies.[12,13] Furthermore, the glycocalyx or macrocolony represents a trap for nutrients in aquatic environments.[13] The macrocolony growth mode of *P. aeruginosa* makes this organism an ideal water microbe. However, it is not ubiquitous in all water samples.

2.2. Inanimate Environment

P. aeruginosa is probably not a marine organism, because the high salt concentration in seawater restricts its growth. It may be recovered, however, from seawater near sewage outfalls and polluted river outlets.[7,14,15] Furthermore, *P. aeruginosa* is seldom isolated from unpolluted water.[15–17] It has never been described as a member of the groundwater microflora. It is present in low concentrations in samples from private homes and schools, creeks, and other unpolluted water sources such as drinking water.[7,8] Water reservoirs polluted by humans or animals, such as with sewage, are the most frequent sources of *P. aeruginosa*. It has been isolated from sink drains, toilets and showers, and other bathroom fixtures, air humidifiers, sanitary plumbing, and all kinds of medical devices and equipment that work with water.[8] A comparison of sinks inside and outside of hospitals showed that hospitals are generally more highly contaminated with *P. aeruginosa* than are private homes.[18] Sinks in new hospital settings are mostly free of *P. aeruginosa*, but rapidly become contaminated,[19] indicating the crucial role of contaminated or infected human individuals in strain transmission.

P. aeruginosa is also detected in swimming pools and whirlpools, where higher temperatures are conducive to its growth.[7] There, *P. aeruginosa* grows primarily in the recirculation system and on the filters.[20] Water tubes in dentists' chairs are often contaminated with *P. aeruginosa*,[21] and electron microscope analysis of the tubes reveals attached microcolonies that resist normal hydrogen peroxide disinfection (Fig. 1).[21,22] Single organisms may be shed from the macrocolonies attached to the walls. In contrast with the cells in macrocolonies these "swarmers" are equipped with flagella for directed motility, appear nonmucoid, and do differ phenotypically in other respects.[13] In toilet or sink drains, swarmer cells may exceed 10^9 organisms per ml after undisturbed overnight growth. The first opening of the water tap or flushing of the toilet will reduce their numbers by several orders of magnitude (G. Döring, unpublished data). In suitable aquatic environments, *P. aeruginosa* may colonize many different kinds of surfaces, including stainless steel.[23,24]

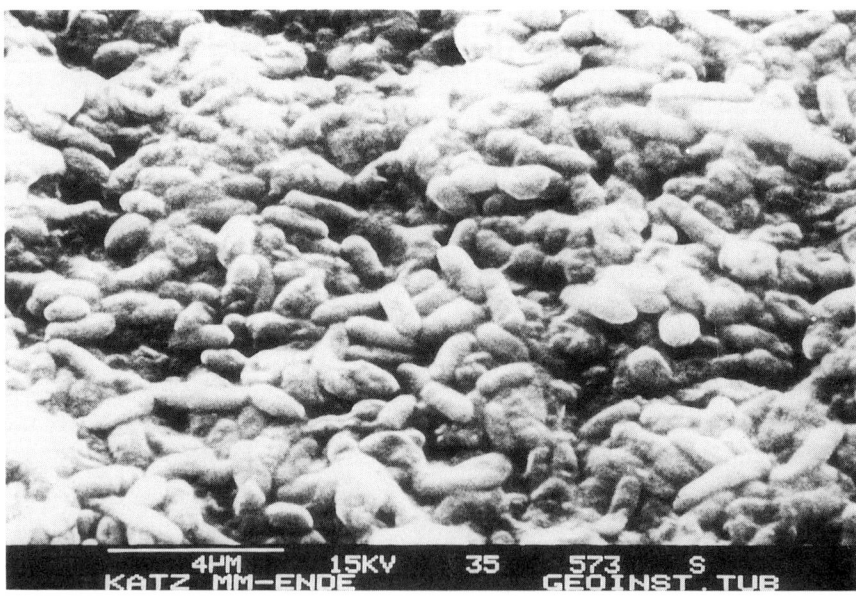

FIGURE 1. Scanning electron micrograph of gram-negative bacteria on the inner surface of a silicon tube from a dentist's chair.

Whereas the frequent isolation of *P. aeruginosa* from nutrient-rich water reservoirs is understandable, its multiplication in distilled water of a purity of more than 71,000 ohms[25] has always puzzled scientists.[7] The suggestion that the organisms use gaseous nutrients that dissolve in water[25] does not seem convincing. Apparently it is difficult to purify water to an extent that does not allow growth of *P. aeruginosa*.

P. aeruginosa has also been isolated from soil, especially from the rhizosphere,[26,27] and from a number of plants and vegetables.[27] When a suspension of *P. aeruginosa* was sprayed on soil or grass, *P. aeruginosa* was recovered for up to 130 days.[28] Its survival time in aerosols and on dry surfaces is relatively short and clearly dependent on relative humidity (rh) and light (Fig. 2).[29] The half-life $t_{1/2}$ survival of strain PAO1 was 51.8 min at 80% rh and 10.2 min at 36% rh. At 36% rh, light reduced the $t_{1/2}$ of the nonmucoid strain WT20 from 25.5 min to 13.3 min. Interestingly, the mucoid strain MUC20 revealed a $t_{1/2}$ of 10.9 min without and 3.5 min with light.[29] In contrast to

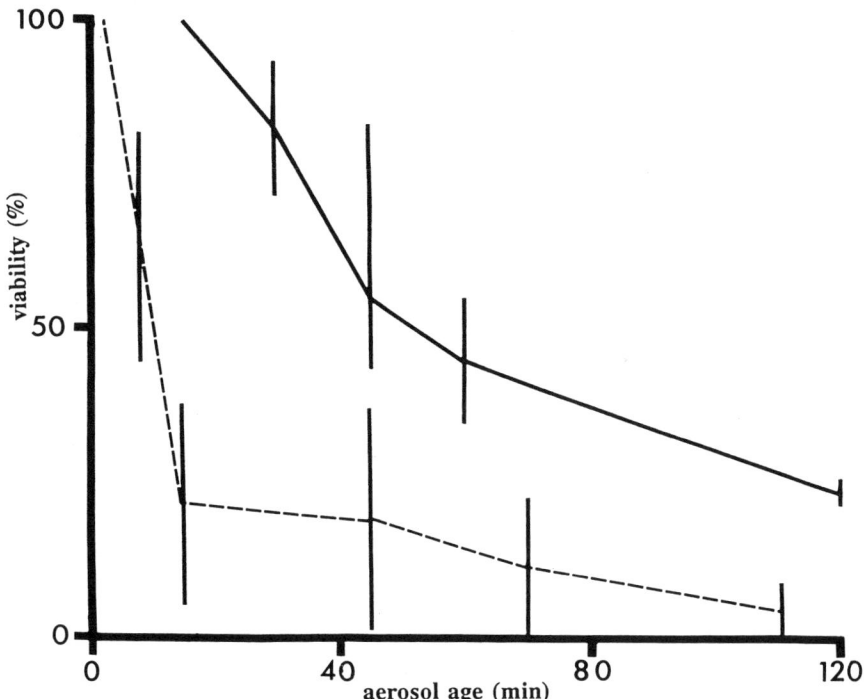

FIGURE 2. Survival of aerosolized *Pseudomonas aeruginosa* PAO1 in a rotating aerosol chamber at 80% relative humidity (rh) (—), and 36% rh (---) without light. Means of three independent determinations ± SD are given. (With kind permission of Gustav Fischer Verlag, Stuttgart, from ref. 29.)

other bacterial species, most gram-negative bacteria including *P. aeruginosa* are short-lived in dry environments.[27,29–31]

Most *P. aeruginosa*–plant interactions are thought to be detrimental for the plant.[32] As in other plant-pathogenic fluorescent pseudomonads,[33] the alginate-like exopolysaccharide may represent an important virulence factor in these interactions. Recently, however, a *P. aeruginosa* strain that promotes plant growth was described.[26] This characteristic, as well as its ability to degrade a variety of organic compounds,[34–38] suggests the potential of *P. aeruginosa* strains for industrial purposes and for the environmental detoxification of pesticides and other synthetic chemicals. (With regard to the release of genetically engineered microorganisms into the environment, it is important to note the reported environmental gene transfer between *P. aeruginosa* strains in freshwater habitats[39,40] and methods for recovering released strains.[41]) The degradation of organic compounds by *P. aeruginosa* strains may also explain their high resistance to disinfectants including quaternary ammonium compounds and chlorinated phenols.[42–45] Contaminated disinfectants have repeatedly caused infections in the past.[46,47]

2.3. Healthy Humans

P. aeruginosa is seldom isolated from healthy humans. Feces of from 1.2 to 2.3% of healthy individuals outside of hospitals are contaminated with the organism,[27,48–50] although the source may be ingestion of food contaminated with this opportunistic pathogen.[51] Gastric acidity and substances produced by a variety of anaerobic and facultative anaerobic bacteria, particularly the volatile fatty acids from *Bacteroides spp.*, are thought to be involved in protection against intestinal colonization by *P. aeruginosa*.[52] Only when more than 10^6 organisms were ingested was *P. aeruginosa* regularly recovered from the stool of healthy individuals.[53] However, the use of antibiotics significantly decreased the number of bacteria that had to be ingested before a positive recovery was made in the stools.[54] This is similar to findings in animal experiments, where the addition of penicillin to drinking water led to intestinal colonization by *P. aeruginosa*.[54] The authors speculate that the normal flora of the intestine is disrupted by the antibiotics, leaving space for *P. aeruginosa* to adhere. The use of antibiotics in hospitalized patients may increase considerably the incidence of *P. aeruginosa*-positive stools.[55] Nevertheless, a number of patients with CF who are treated over the course of years with oral antibiotics against *Staphylococcus aureus* do not seem to carry *P. aeruginosa* in their intestines (see Chapter 13).[18] Skin carriage is also rare; survival curves of *P. aeruginosa* reveal the detrimental effect on the organism of normal human skin.[56] Any impairment of normal host defenses may lead eventually to increased colonization of human epithelial surfaces by *P. aeruginosa*. Additionally, the colonization rate of *P. aeruginosa* is dependent on host age in some cases. An investigation of the frequency of *P. aeruginosa* in the oral cavity of healthy adults showed the highest isolation rate in the age group of 54–63 years.[57]

3. EPIDEMIOLOGY

3.1. Incidence of Infections

Because *P. aeruginosa* causes infections only in compromised patients, most of the recorded infections occur in hospitals. However, due to the frequent isolation of *P. aeruginosa* from sewage and other reservoirs outside hospitals, patients with CF, for example, may also acquire the pathogen outside the hospital (see also Chapter 13). From 1980 to 1990, *P. aeruginosa* remained the second most frequent gram-negative bacterium causing infections in hospitalized patients.[7] Data from the National Nosocomial Infections Surveillance System (NNIS) instituted by the U.S. Centers for Disease Control in Atlanta reveal that *P. aeruginosa* caused 11.4% of nosocomial infections of all sites, 12.7% of urinary tract infections, 16.9% of lower respiratory infections, and 8.9% of surgical wound infections.[58] Similar rates are seen in an epidemiological study carried out from 1980 to 1984 in the North Carolina Memorial Hospital.[59] From 1984 to 1988 the NNIS reported that *P. aeruginosa* rose in rank from fourth to first as the most frequent pathogen of nosocomial septicemia.[60] Responsible for this trend is increased drug resistance to various antibiotics including aminoglycosides,[61] cephalosporins,[62] and quinolones.[63] *P. aeruginosa* was also the most common organism causing bacteremia in a U.S. burn center between 1953 and 1983, representing 10.3%.[64] A significant reduction in the frequency of *P. aeruginosa* bacteremia was achieved when patients were isolated in the following years in a new burn unit,[64] reflecting the beneficial application of improved hygiene. Isolation of hospitalized CF patients also led to a decrease in the number of *P. aeruginosa* pulmonary infections.[65,66] Both the less frequent isolation of *P. aeruginosa* in new hospital settings as well as improved aseptic techniques may explain the significant drop in the percentage of intubated patients colonized with *P. aeruginosa* (14% to 6.5%; $p < 0.001$) in the first year after an intensive therapy unit moved into a new building (Döring, G., unpublished data). However, no such trend was noticed in a similar study done elsewhere.[67] Furthermore, nosocomial cross-colonization has not been regarded as an important mode of dissemination of *P. aeruginosa* strains.[68]

3.2. Routes of Transmission

The elucidation of bacterial transmission routes in general and especially within the hospital is a difficult task, because we must distinguish among contacts between patients, between patients and healthy carriers (*e.g.*, hospital personnel), and between patients and environmental sources. A reliable and highly discriminatory typing method is crucial to any investigation of transmission routes. Such methods have been developed for *P. aeruginosa*.

3.2.1. Typing Methods

Because they are based on strain differences in chromosomal DNA rather than on phenotypical differences, genotyping methods[69–75] represent more stable strain markers than the older typing methods for *P. aeruginosa* such as serotyping[76–79] and pyocin[80] or phage typing,[81] especially in light of rapid phenotypic changes resulting from gene regulation. Thus, *P. aeruginosa* strains from CF patients are mostly polyagglutinable due to the loss of major parts of the polysaccharide chains of the lipopolysaccharide,[82] in turn possibly due to the effect of bacteriophages,[83] and mostly immotile due to the loss of flagella. Such strains are less sensitive to lysis by typing phages.[84] Also, changes in bacterial metabolism due to antibiotic therapy may alter pyocin production patterns.[85] Nevertheless, the older methods have also been effective in many cases and have elucidated epidemics and routes of infection. Furthermore, any typing method has theoretical and technical limitations, especially with regard to the "identity" of two strains.[73,74]

Our laboratory used the exotoxin A (ETA) probe to investigate routes of transmission of *P. aeruginosa* inside and outside of hospitals.[69,70] The probe contains a hypervariable region upstream of the ETA gene and is therefore discriminatory. We applied this method to evaluate patients with CF,[18,71] paraplegia[87] or episodes of acute leukemia,[86] a mixed patient group in a children's hospital ward,[29] and intubated patients at an intensive therapy unit. The usefulness of this probe is underlined by the findings that CF patients who have had no contact with each other and have not been hospitalized usually harbor different strains of *P. aeruginosa* and that PAO1, the well-known *P. aeruginosa* test strain cultivated in different laboratories in the world, is genotypically identical.

3.2.2. Transmission via Hospital Personnel

When *P. aeruginosa* strains from 46 CF patients were typed, four episodes of cross-infection were detected.[71] Whether cross-infection was due to a direct patient-to-patient contact or whether transmission occurred via contaminated environmental reservoirs was not investigated in this study. The latter possibility is supported by the finding that the majority of newly acquired *P. aeruginosa* strains was not derived from other infected CF patients.[71] To investigate such an environment–patient transmission route of *P. aeruginosa*, we sampled and typed *P. aeruginosa* strains from patients who had minimal or no contact at all with each other, such as patients with acute leukemia receiving cytostatic therapy, paraplegic patients, and intubated patients. Of 119 patients with leukemia, 18 were found to be colonized or infected during

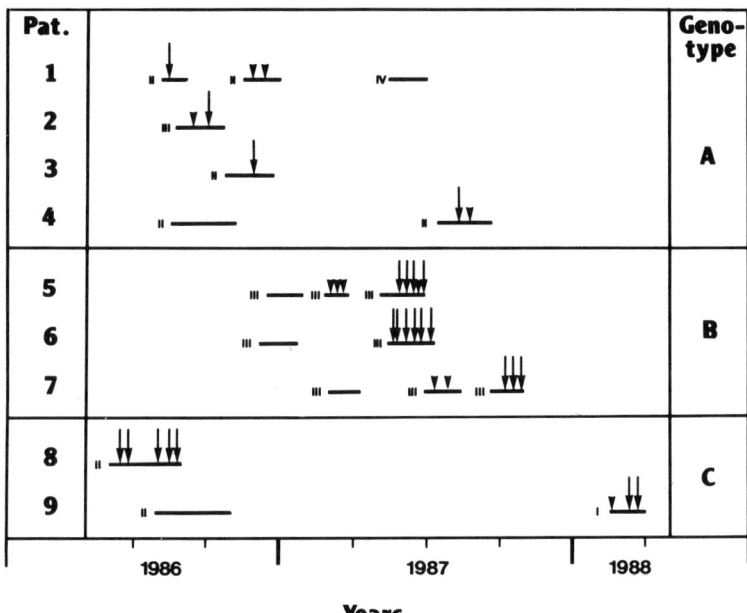

FIGURE 3. Genotypically identical isolates of *Pseudomonas aeruginosa* (strain A, patients no. 1–4; strain B, patients no. 5–7; strain C, patients no. 8–9) recovered from more than one patient with acute leukemia. Arrows indicate isolation of strains that are genotypically identical (↓) or for which the genotype was not determined (▼). Solid bars indicate periods of hospital admission, Roman numerals the ward numbers (I–IV). (With kind permission of Vieweg Publishers, Wiesbaden, from ref. 86.)

a 2 year study period. Twelve different *P. aeruginosa* genotypes were detected. Groups of up to three patients were colonized by identical genotypes,[86] suggesting nosocomial transmission (Fig. 3). In another epidemiological study of *P. aeruginosa* in oncology patients, 12% of the patients were colonized at admission and 10% acquired *P. aeruginosa*.[88] A considerable incidence of nosocomial infection was also found in hospitalized paraplegic patients.[87] Up to four patients were infected by single *P. aeruginosa* genotypes that could also be isolated from the environment of the ward. *P. aeruginosa* strains were present in 51% of all accessible water reservoirs of the paraplegic wards. The finding that identical *P. aeruginosa* genotypes were isolated from a male paraplegic patient and from the toilet of the female personnel strongly suggests transmission by hospital personnel.[87]

This notion was further substantiated in a longitudinal investigation of intubated patients receiving mechanical ventilation in an intensive therapy unit. In at least eight of the 15 immobile patients colonized or infected with *P. aeruginosa*, the respective *P. aeruginosa* genotype was hospital-acquired and most probably transmitted by hospital personnel, because the strains were isolated from the hospital environment or from other patients who were already colonized (Döring, G., unpublished data). Furthermore, such a transmission route from the sinks to hands was also found in the mixed infectious disease ward of a children's hospital,[29] where *P. aeruginosa* was sampled longitudinally from patients, hospital personnel and the hospital environment (Fig. 4). In total, 46% of the personnel had *P. aeruginosa*-positive hand cultures. Colonization of personnel hands occurred after the personnel had entered the hospital; hand cultures were negative in all samples taken at entrance. This suggests that *P. aeruginosa* colonization of hospital personnel and subsequently of patients derives at least in part from the widespread

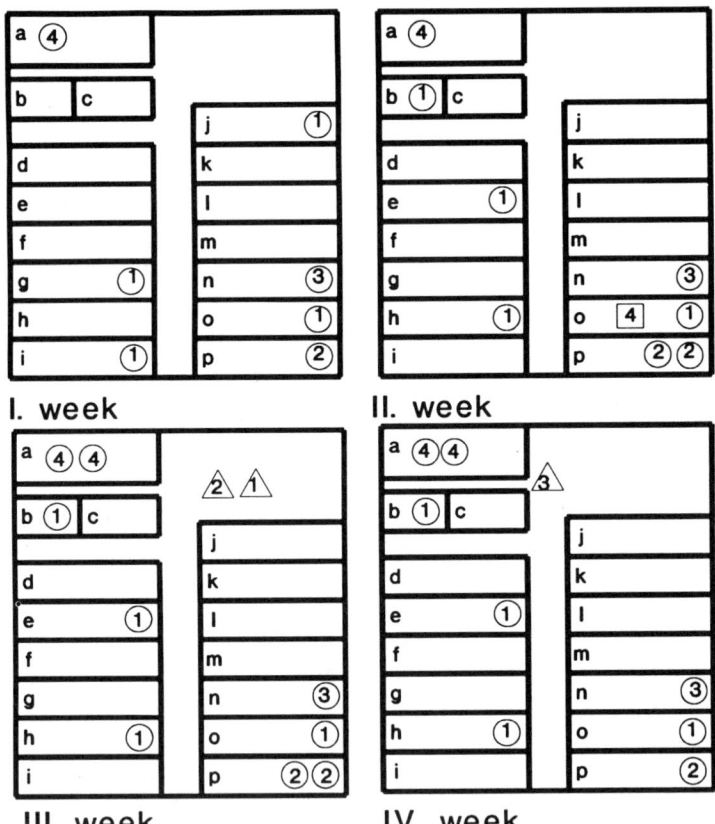

FIGURE 4. Distribution of *Pseudomonas aeruginosa* genotypes P1–P4 in environmental water reservoirs (○), and occurrence on hands of the personnel (△) and in the stool of one patient (□) in the mixed infectious disease ward of a children's hospital. *P. aeruginosa* was sampled for 4 weeks and the distribution of the genotypes on the schematic ground-plan of the ward is given for each week I–IV: (a) toilet with washbasin; (b) kitchen; (c) bath; (d) personnel room; (e–i) and (n–p) patient rooms; (j) endoscopy room; (k) waste room; (l) toilet; (m) doctor's room. (Courtesy of C. Wolz, adapted from ref. 29.)

contamination of sanitary installations and other hospital equipment where the organism multiplies and persists for long periods of time. This theory is also substantiated by studies carried out 20 years ago by several investigators on *P. aeruginosa* strain transmission in hospitals.[89-92]

3.2.3. Aerosol Transmission from Sink Drains

Because the transmission of sink drain organisms to patients is difficult to understand at first glance, the role of waste-traps as reservoirs from which infection may start in hospitals has been questioned in the past.[93] Nevertheless, backsplash and aerosol production has been shown to occur during handwashing and toilet flushing[29,89,94-96] and *P. aeruginosa* was detected on agar plates placed up to 10 feet away from a washbasin while the faucet was activated for three 10-sec intervals.[89] When a toilet was contaminated with *Escherichia coli*, and agar plates were exposed throughout the room, flushing of the toilet resulted in detectable bacteria in a limited area around the toilet within the first 2 hr and for up to 6 hr in a more random distribution of *E. coli* in the room.[90] When hand washing was performed in a *P. aeruginosa*-contaminated washbasin without soap, 2400 colony forming units (CFU) of PAO1 were grown on the filter membrane after the hands were dried and immersed in a sterile plastic bag containing 100 ml of physiological saline. Hand washing with soap yielded 1200 PAO1 CFU per 100 ml saline.[29] Thus, normal handwashing without appropriate disinfection afterwards may lead to contamination with microorganisms persisting in the sink drains rather than to decontamination. If patients with a high risk of acquiring *P. aeruginosa* or other bacteria (*i.e.*, patients with CF) wash their hands or brush their teeth in contaminated washbasins, colonization and infection may occur. Close contact with contaminated reservoirs seems to be important for the contraction of pathogens via aerosols, because survival of *P. aeruginosa* in aerosols is relatively short and comparable to the survival times of other gram-negative rods (see section 2.2). Microbial hazard is highest the first time water is run or when toilets are flushed in the morning, when planktonic *P. aeruginosa* organisms have multiplied considerably from the wall-attached glycocalyx. Therefore, hygienic measures to decontaminate sinks and toilets are recommended, as well as improved hygienic measures for hand disinfection.

3.2.4. Prevention

The high *P. aeruginosa* contamination rates in sinks has led to several attempts to eradicate *P. aeruginosa* in hospital sink drains.[29,93,94,96-98] However, the heating devices proposed by several authors[93,96-98] have not found general acceptance and currently are little-known. The cost of such devices, the increasing use of plastic sink drains which do not allow heating, and the general lack of credence in the mechanism by which *P. aeruginosa* or other pathogenic bacteria in the sink drain may contaminate hands during handwashing may explain this situation. An improved heating device has recently been developed[29] and is currently under clinical investigation. However, improvements in the dispensing and use of disinfectants, the isolation of infected patients, and improvements in aseptic techniques, most notably the use of gloves for many nursing procedures, also have proved to be successful in reducing *P. aeruginosa* infections in hospitals.

3.2.5. Endogenous Infection Routes

The question is difficult to answer whether *P. aeruginosa* infections in hospitals originate from contaminated environmental reservoirs or are a consequence of endogenous bacterial carriage prior to admission to a special unit of the hospital. Both possibilities have to be considered. Patients pre-colonized at the time of admission to intensive care units seem to be responsible for a considerable percentage of subsequent *P. aeruginosa* infections.[55,99] Intestinal carriage of *P. aeruginosa*, which is enhanced after antibiotic therapy, may lead to oropharyngeal colonization via retrograde migration of the organisms, especially in patients treated with antacids.[102] In a recent study in an intensive therapy unit, *P. aeruginosa* colonization of the gastrointestinal tract preceded colonization of the oropharynx with identical genotypes in two colonized cases. An external transmission route involving hospital personnel cannot be ruled out (Döring, G., unpublished data). Another possible infection route for *P. aeruginosa*, especially in neutropenic patients, is translocation from the gastrointestinal tract to the bloodstream. Eighty-one percent of 16 such patients with bacteremia caused by *P. aeruginosa* were intestinal carriers of the same strain.[101]

4. RÉSUMÉ

In the last decade, considerable progress has been made in understanding the ecology and epidemiology of *P. aeruginosa*. In particular, Costerton's biofilm concept of *P. aeruginosa* has greatly contributed to our understanding of the reasons for its survival and persistence in nature and disease.[13] Molecular microbiology can explain the genetic basis for the considerable adaptability of this aquatic organism. In the future its huge enzymatic arsenal may be used to detoxify polluted soil and for other environmental purposes. Molecular epidemiology techniques have been used successfully to type *P. aeruginosa* strains and, hence, to define transmission routes from environmental reservoirs to high-risk patient groups. These findings should lead to the application of hygienic measures to prevent *P. aeruginosa* infections, because antibiotics have been only partially successful in the treatment of infections with *P. aeruginosa*, which is the second most frequent gram-negative nosocomial pathogen.

ACKNOWLEDGMENTS. The authors are very grateful to M. L. Vasil and J. W. Ogle for providing the DNA probe for *P. aeruginosa* typing and to C. Wolz for *P. aeruginosa* typing and the supervision of many environmental studies. We are further indebted to J. W. Costerton, N. Høiby, and E. Thofern for fruitful and stimulating discussions and D. Blaurock for language corrections.

REFERENCES

1. Gessard, C., 1982, Sur les colorations bleue et verte des lignes à pansements, *C. R. Acad. Sci. Serie D* **94:**536–538.
2. Bouchard, C., 1889, Influence qu'exerce sur la maladie charbonneuse l'inoculation du *Bacille pyocyanique*, *C. R. Acad. Sci. Serie D* **108:**713–714.
3. Fraenkel, E., 1917, Über die Menschenpathogenität des *Bacillus pyocyaneus*. Weitere 13 Fälle, *Z. Hyg.* **84:**367–424.
4. Schoenthal, B., 1941, The nature of the antibacterial agents present in *Pseudomonas pyocyanea* cultures, *Br. J. Exp. Pathol.* **22:**137–147.
5. Stanley, M. M., 1947, *Bacillus pyocyaneus* infections: A review of cases and discussion of newer therapy including streptomycin, *Am. J. Med.* **2:**253–277, 347–367.
6. Finland, M., 1980, Experiences with *Pseudomonas aeruginosa* at Boston City Hospital over the last half-century, in: *Pseudomonas aeruginosa, the Organism, Diseases It Causes, and Their Treatment* (L. D. Sabath, ed.), Hans Huber Publishers, Bern, pp. 244–264.
7. Rhame, F. S., 1980, The ecology and epidemiology of *Pseudomonas aeruginosa*, in: *Pseudomonas aeruginosa, the Organism, Diseases It Causes, and Their Treatment* (L. D. Sabath, ed.), Hans Huber Publishers, Bern, pp. 31–51.
8. Botzenhart, K., and Rüden, H., 1987, Hospital infections caused by *Pseudomonas aeruginosa*, *Antibiot. Chemother.* **39:**1–15.
9. Finlay, B. B., and Falkow, S., 1989, Common themes in microbial pathogenicity, *Microbiol. Rev.* **53:**210–230.
10. Higgins, C. F., Hinton, J. C. D., Hulton, C. S. J., Owen-Hughes, T., Pavitt, G. D., and Seirafi, A., 1990, Protein H1: A role for chromatin structure in the regulation of bacterial gene expression and virulence?, *Mol. Microbiol.* **4:**2007–2012.
11. Miller, J. F., Mekalanos, J. J., and Falkow, S., 1989, Coordinate regulation and sensory transduction in the control of bacterial virulence, *Science* **243:**916–922.
12. Fletscher, M., and Floodgate, G. D., 1973, An electron-microscopic demonstration of an acidic polysaccharide involved in the adhesion of a marine bacterium to solid surfaces, *J. Gen. Microbiol.* **74:**325–334.
13. Costerton, J. W., Cheng, K.-J., Geesey, G. G., Ladd, T. I., Nickel, J. C., Dasgupta, M., and Marrie, T. J., 1987, Bacterial biofilms in nature and disease, *Ann. Rev. Microbiol.* **41:** 435–464.
14. Cheung, W. H. S., Chang, K. C. K., and Hung, R. P. S., 1991, Variations in microbial indicator densities in beach water and health-related assessment of bathing water quality, *Epidemiol. Infect.* **106:**329–344.
15. Botzenhart, K., Wolf, R., and Thofern, E., 1975, Das Verhalten von *Pseudomonas aeruginosa* in Oberflächenwasser, Kühlwasser und Abwasser, *Zentralbl. Bakteriol, Hyg. I. Abt. Orig. B*, **161:**72–83.

16. Hoadley, A. W., McCoy, E., and Rohlich, G. A., 1968, Untersuchungen über *Pseudomonas aeruginosa* in Oberflächengewässern. I. Quellen, *Arch. Hyg.* **152**:328–338.
17. Hoadley, A. W., McCoy, E., and Rohlich, G. A., 1968, Untersuchungen über *Pseudomonas aeruginosa* in Oberflächengewässern. II. Auftreten und Verhalten, *Arch. Hyg.* **152**: 339–345.
18. Döring, G., Bareth, H., Gairing, A., Wolz, C., and Botzenhart, K., 1989, Genotyping of *Pseudomonas aeruginosa* sputum and stool isolates from cystic fibrosis patients: Evidence for intestinal colonization and spreading into toilets. *Epidem. Infect.* **103**:555–564.
19. Van Saene, H. K. F., Van Putte, J. C., Van Saene, J. J. M., Van de Gromde, T. W., and Van Warmerdam, E. G. A., 1989, Sink flora in a long-stay hospital is determined by the patients' oral and rectal flora, *Epidemiol. Infect.* **102**:231–238.
20. Botzenhart, K., Thofern, E., and Külpmann, W. R., 1974, Schwimmbadfilter und bakteriologische Qualität des Badewassers, *Öff. Gesundh.-Wesen* **36**:326–331.
21. Exner, M., Tuschewitzki, G. J., and Haun, F., 1982, Rasterelektronenoptische Darstellung der Wandbesiedlung wasserführender Kunststoffschläuche, *Zentralbl. Bakteriol. Hyg. I. Abt. Orig. B* **176**:425–434.
22. Katz, T., Hahn, T., Netuschil, L., and Botzenhart, K., 1990, Keimbesiedlung von zahnärztlichen Behandlungseinheiten ohne und mit Desinfektionseinrichtung, *Quintessenz* **8**:1345–1355.
23. Botzenhart, K., and Thofern, E., 1967, Bakteriologische Untersuchungen an Reihenwaschmaschinen, *Das Krankenhaus* **59**:322–330.
24. Vanhaecke, E., Remon, J.-P., Moors, M., Raes, F., De Rudder, D., and van Peteghem, A., 1990, Kinetics of *Pseudomonas aeruginosa* adhesion to 304 and 316-L stainless steel: Role of cell surface hydrophobicity, *Appl. Environ. Microbiol.* **56**:788–795.
25. Favero, M. S., Carson, L. A., Bond, W. W., and Petersen, N. J., 1971, *Pseudomonas aeruginosa*: Growth in distilled water from hospitals, *Science* **173**:836–838.
26. Höfte, M., Mergeay, M., and Verstraete, W., 1990, Marking the rhizopseudomonas strain 7NSK$_2$ with a Mu d(lac) element for ecological studies, *Appl. Environ. Microbiol.* **56**:1046–1052.
27. Mitcherlich, E., and Marth, E. H., 1984, *Microbial survival in the environment*, Springer, Berlin.
28. Botzenhart, K., Egler, W., Attar, Y., Ernst, G., Fischer, P., Krizek, L., and Wurz, D., 1979, Microbial emission, immision and changes in the germ count in the cooling water during operation of wet cooling towers. IV. Communication: Microbial immision in the vicinity of wet cooling towers, *Zentralbl. Bacteriol. Hyg. I. Abt. Orig. B* **169**:164–205.
29. Döring, G., Ulrich, M., Müller, W., Bitzer, J., Schmidt-Koenig, L., Münst, L., Grupp, H., Wolz, C., Stern, M., and Botzenhart, K., 1991, Generation of *Pseudomonas aeruginosa* aerosols during handwashing from contaminated sink drains, transmission to hands of hospital personnel, and its prevention by use of a new heating device. *Zentralbl. Hyg.* **191**: 494–505.
30. Hambleton, P., Dennis, P. J., and Fitzgeorge R., 1984, Survival of airborne *Legionella pneumophila*, in: *Legionella. Proceedings of the 2nd International Symposium* (C. Thornesberry, A. Balows, J. C. Feeley, and W. Jakuboski, eds.), American Society for Microbiology, pp. 301–302, Washington, D.C.
31. Müller, W., Gröning, K., and Hartmann, F., 1981, De Tenazität von Bakterien im luftgetragenen Zustand I. Mitteilung: Experimentelle Untersuchungen zur Bestimmung der Absterbekonstante ß$_{biol}$ für *E. coli*, *Salmonella spp.* und *P. mutocida*, *Zentralbl. Bakteriol. Hyg. I. Abt. Orig. B* **172**:367–376.
32. Lebeda, A., Kudela, V., and Jedlickova, Z., 1984, Pathogenicity of *Pseudomonas aeruginosa* for plants and animals, *Acta Phytophathol. Acad. Sci. Hung.* **19**:271–284.
33. Fett, W. F., Osman, S. F., Fishman, M. L., and Siebles III, T. S., 1986, Alginate production by plant-pathogenic pseudomonads, *Appl. Environ. Microbiol.* **52**:466–473.

34. Golovleva, L. A., Pertsova, R. N., Boronin, A. M., Travkin, V. M., and Kozlovsky, S. A., 1988, Kelthane degradation by genetically engineered *Pseudomonas aeruginosa* BS827 in a soil ecosystem, *Appl. Environ. Microbiol.* **54:**1587–1590.
35. Higson, F. K., and Focht, D. D., 1990, Degradation of 2-bromobenzoic acid by a strain of *Pseudomonas aeruginosa*, *Appl. Environ. Microbiol.* **56:**1615–1619.
36. Hickey, W. J., and Focht, D. D., 1990, Degradation of mono-, di, and trihalogenated benzoid acids by *Pseudomonas aeruginosa* JB2, *Appl. Environ. Microbiol.* **56:**3842–3850.
37. Leathen, W. W., and Kinsel, N. A., 1963, The identification of microorganisms that utilize jet fuel, *Rev. Ind. Microbiol.* **4:**9–16.
38. Ribbons, D. W., 1970, Specificity of monohydric phenol oxidations by meta cleavage pathways in *Pseudomonas aeruginosa* T 1, *Arch. Microbiol.* **74:**103–115.
39. O'Morchoe, S. B., Ogunseitan, O., Sayler, G. S., and Miller, R. V., 1988, Conjugal transfer of R68.45 and FP5 between *Pseudomonas aeruginosa* strains in a freshwater environment, *Appl. Environ. Microbiol.* **54:**1923–1929.
40. Saye, D. J., Ogusseitan, O. A., Sayler, G. S., and Miller, R. V., 1990, Transduction of linked chromosomal genes between *Pseudomonas aeruginosa* strains during incubation in situ in a freshwater habitat, *Appl. Environ. Microbiol.* **56:**140–145.
41. Morgan, J. A. W., Winstanley, C., Pickup, R. W., and Saunders, J. R., 1991, Rapid immunocapture of *Pseudomonas putida* cells from lake water by using bacterial flagella, *Appl. Environ. Microbiol.* **57:**503–509.
42. Adair, F. W., Geftic, S. G., and Gelzer, J., 1969, Resistance of *Pseudomonas* to quaternary ammonium compounds, *Appl. Microbiol.* **18:**299–302.
43. Bean, H. S., and Farrell, R. C., 1967, The persistence of *Pseudomonas aeruginosa* in aqueous solutions of phenols, *J. Pharm. Pharmacol.* **19:**183–188.
44. Carlson, L. A., Favero, M. S., Bond, W. W., Petersen, N. J., 1972, Factors affecting comparative resistance of naturally occurring and subcultured *Pseudomonas aeruginosa* to disinfectants, *Appl. Microbiol.* **23:**863–869.
45. Lowbury, E. J. L., 1951, Contamination of cetrimide and other fluids with *Pseudomonas pyocyanea*, *Br. J. Ind. Med.* **8:**22–25.
46. Botzenhart, K., and Thofern, E., 1969, *Pseudomonas aeruginosa* an ärztlichem Instrumentarium, *Der Chirurg* **40:**40–43.
47. Fierer, J., Taylor, P. M., and Gezon, H. M., 1967, *Pseudomonas aeruginosa* epidemic traced to delivery-room resuscitators, *New Engl. J. Med.* **276:**991–996.
48. Lányi, B., Gregács, M., and Adám, M. M., 1966, Incidence of *Pseudomonas aeruginosa* serogroups in water and human faeces. *Acta Microbiol. Acad. Sci. Hung.* **13:**319–326.
49. Linde, K., and Kittlick, M., 1963, Zum Nachweis von *Bacterium pyocyaneum* in menschlichem Untersuchungsmaterial. *Arch. Hyg.* **146:**126–138.
50. Botzenhart, K., 1974, Zur Ökologie fakultativ-pathogener Bakterien mit geringen Nährstoffansprüchen im Krankenhaus, *Immun. Infekt.* **2:**110–113.
51. Remington, J. S., and Schimpff, S. C., 1981, Please don't eat the salads. *New Engl. J. Med.* **304:**433–435.
52. Levison, M. E., 1977, Factors influencing colonization of the gastrointestinal tract with *Pseudomonas aeruginosa*, in: *Pseudomonas aeruginosa: Ecological Aspects and Patient Colonization* (V. M. Young, ed.), Raven Press, New York, pp. 97–109.
53. Buck, A. C., and Cooke, E. M., 1969, The fate of ingested *Pseudomonas aeruginosa* in normal persons, *J. Med. Microbiol.* **2:**521–525.
54. Hentges, D. J., Stein, A. J., Casey, S. W., and Que, J. U., 1985, Protective role of intestinal flora against infection with *Pseudomonas aeruginosa* in mice: Influence of antibiotics on colonization resistance, *Infect. Immun.* **47:**118–122.
55. Murthy, S. K., Baltch, A. L., Smith, R. P., Desjardins, E. K., Hammer, M. C., Conroy, J. V., and Michelsen, P. B., 1989, Oropharyngeal and fecal carriage of *Pseudomonas aeruginosa* in hospital patients, *J. Clin. Microbiol.* **27:**35–40.

56. McBride, M. E., Duncan, W. C., and Knox, J. M., 1975, Physiological and environmental control of gram-negative bacteria on skin, *Br. J. Dermatol.* **93**:191–199.
57. Botzenhart, K., Puhr, O. F., and Döring, G., 1985, *Pseudomonas aeruginosa* in the oral cavity of healthy adults: Frequency and age distribution, *Zentralbl. Bakteriol. Hyg. I. Abt. Orig. B* **180**:471–479.
58. Horan, T. C., White, J. W., Jarvis, W. R., Emori, T. G., Culver, D. H., Munn, V. P., Thornsberry, C., Olson, D. R., and Hughes, D. F., 1986, Nosocomial infections surveillance, *Morbid. Mortal. Wkly. Rep.* **35**:17–29.
59. Brawley, R. L., Weber, D. J., Samsa, G. P., and Rutala, W. A., 1989, Multiple nosocomial infections, an incidence study, *Am. J. Epidemiol.* **130**:769–780.
60. Horan, T. C., Culver, D., Jarvis, W. R., Emori, G., Banerjee, S., Martone, W., and Saunsberry, C., 1988, Pathogens causing nosocomial infections, *Antimicrobic Newsletter* **5**:65–67.
61. Olson, B., Weinstein, R. A., Nathan, C., Chamberlin, W., and Kabins, S. A., 1985, Occult aminoglycoside resistance in *Pseudomonas aeruginosa*: Epidemiology and implications for therapy and control, *J. Infect. Dis.* **152**:769–774.
62. Mulgrave, L., 1991, The changing ecology of hospital bacteria and the selective role of cephalosporins, *Epidemiol. Infect.* **106**:121–132.
63. Iyobe, S., Hirai, K., and Hashimoto, H., 1991, Drug resistance of *Pseudomonas aeruginosa* with special reference to new quinolones, *Antibiot. Chemother.* **44**:209–214.
64. McManus, A. T., 1989, *Pseudomonas aeruginosa*: A controlled burn pathogen? *Antibiot. Chemother.* **42**:103–108.
65. Tümmler, B., Koopmann, U., Grothues, D., Weissbrodt, H., Steinkamp, G., and von der Hardt, H., 1991, Nosocomial acquisition of *Pseudomonas aeruginosa* by cystic fibrosis patients, *J. Clin. Microbiol.* **29**:1265–1267.
66. Høiby, N., and Pedersen, S. S., 1989, Cross-infection with *Pseudomonas aeruginosa* in Danish cystic fibrosis patients, *Antibiot. Chemother.* **42**:124–129.
67. Maki, D. G., Alvarado, C. J., Hassemer, C. A., Zilz, M. A., 1982, Relation of the inanimate hospital environment to endemic nosocomial infection, *New Engl. J. Med.* **307**:1562–1566.
68. MacArthur, R. D., Lehman, M. H., Currie-McCumber, C. A., and Shlaes, D. M., 1988, The epidemiology of gentamicin-resistant *Pseudomonas aeruginosa* on an intermediate care unit, *Am. J. Epidemiol.* **128**:821–827.
69. Ogle, J. W., Janda, J. M., Woods, D. E., and Vasil, M. L., 1987, Characterization and use of a DNA probe as an epidemiological marker for *Pseudomonas aeruginosa. J. Infect. Dis.* **155**:119–126.
70. Vasil, M., Chamberlain, C., and Grant, C. R., 1986, Molecular studies of Pseudomonas exotoxin A gene, *Infect. Immun.* **52**:538–548.
71. Wolz, C., Kiosz, G., Ogle, J. W., Vasil, M. L., Schaad, U., Botzenhart, K. and Döring, G., 1989, *Pseudomonas aeruginosa* cross-colonization and persistence in patients with cystic fibrosis. Use of a DNA probe. *Epidemiol. Infect.* **102**:205–214.
72. Römling, U., Grothes, D., and Tümmler, B., 1991, Whole DNA genome typing, *Antibiot. Chemother.* **44**:1–7.
73. Ojeniyi, B., Wolz, C., Döring, G., Lam, J. S., Rosdahl, V. T., and Høiby, N., 1990, Typing of polyagglutinable *Pseudomonas aeruginosa* isolates from cystic fibrosis patients. *Acta Pathol. Microbiol. Immunol. Scand.* **98**:423–431.
74. Ojeniyi, B., and Høiby, N., 1991, Comparison of different typing methods of *Pseudomonas aeruginosa, Antibiot. Chemother.* **44**:13–22.
75. Speert, D. P., Campbell, M. E., Farmer, S. W., Volpel, K., Joffe, A. M., and Paranchych, W., 1989, Use of a pilin gene probe to study molecular epidemiology of *Pseudomonas aeruginosa, J. Clin. Microbiol.* **27**:2589–2593.
76. Habs, J., 1957, Untersuchungen über O-Antigene von *Pseudomonas aeruginosa, Z. Hyg. Infektionskr.* **144**:218–228.
77. Lanyi, B., and Bergan, T., 1978, Serological characterization of *Pseudomonas aeruginosa*, in:

Methods of Microbiology (T. Bergan, and J. R. Norris, eds.), Academic Press, London, vol. 10, pp. 93–168.
78. Ansorg, R., 1978, Flagella-spezifisches H-Antigenschema von *Pseudomonas aeruginosa*, *Zentralbl. Bakteriol. Microbiol. Hyg. A*, **242:**228–238.
79. Lam, J. S., MacDonald, L. A., Kropinski, A. M., and Speert, D. P., 1988, Characterization of non-typable strains of *Pseudomonas aeruginosa* from cystic fibrosis patients by means of monoclonal antibodies and SDS-polyacrylamide gel electrophoresis, *Serodiag. Immunother. Infect. Dis.* **2:**365–374.
80. Govan, J. W. R., 1978, Pyocin typing of *Pseudomonas aeruginosa*, in: *Methods of Microbiology* (T. Bergan, and J. R. Norris, eds.), Academic Press, London, Vol. 10, pp. 61–91.
81. Bergan, T., 1978, Phage typing of *Pseudomonas aeruginosa*, in: *Methods of Microbiology* (T. Bergan, and J. R. Norris, eds.), Academic Press, London, vol. 10, pp. 169–199.
82. Ojeniyi, B., Baek, L., and Høiby, N., 1985, Polyagglutinability due to loss of O-antigenic determinants in *Pseudomonas aeruginosa* strains isolated from cystic fibrosis patients, *Acta Pathol. Microbiol. Scand. [B]* **93:**7–13.
83. Ojeniyi, B., 1988, Bacteriophages in sputum of cystic fibrosis patients as a possible cause of in vivo changes in serotypes of *Pseudomonas aeruginosa*, *Acta Pathol. Microbiol. Immunol. Scand.* **96:**294–298.
84. Pitt, T. L., Epidemiological typing of *Pseudomonas aeruginosa*, *Eur. J. Clin. Microbiol. Infect. Dis.* **7:**238–247.
85. Thomassen, M. J., Demko, C. A., Doershuk, C. F., and Root, J. M., 1985, *Pseudomonas aeruginosa* isolates: Comparison of isolates from campers and from sibling pairs with cystic fibrosis, *Pediat. Pulmonol.* **1:**40–45.
86. Kern, W., Wolz, C., and Döring, G., 1990, Molecular epidemiological study of *Pseudomonas aeruginosa* isolates from patients with acute leukemia, *Eur. J. Clin. Microbiol. Infect. Dis.* **9:**257–261.
87. Worlitzsch, D., Wolz, C., Botzenhart, K., Hansis, M., Burgdörfer, H., Ogle, J. W., and Döring, G., 1989, Molecular epidemiology of *Pseudomonas aeruginosa* urinary tract infections in paraplegic patients. *Zentralbl. Hyg.* **189:**175–184.
88. Griffith, S. J., Nathan, C., Selander, R. K., Chamberlin, W., Gordon, S., Kabins, S., and Weinstein, R. A., 1989, The epidemiology of *Pseudomonas aeruginosa* in oncology patients in a general hospital, *J. Infect. Dis.* **160:**1030–1036.
89. Brown, D. G., and Baublis, J., 1977, Reservoirs of *Pseudomonas* in an intensive care unit for newborn infants: mechanisms of control, *J. Pediatr.* **90:**453–457.
90. Chadwick, P., 1973, Relative importance of airborne and other routes in the infection of tracheostomised patients with *Pseudomonas aeruginosa*, in: *Airborne Transmission and Airborne Infection*, 6th Intern. Symp. on Aerobiology, (J. F. Hers and K. C. Winkler, eds.), Oosthock Publ. Co., Utrecht, The Netherlands, pp. 481–489.
91. Noone, M. R., Pitt, T. L., Bedder, M., Hewlett, A. M., and Rogers, K. B., 1983, *Pseudomonas aeruginosa* colonization in an intensive therapy unit: Role of cross infection and host factors, *Br. Med. J.* **286:**341–344.
92. Levin, M. H., Olson, B., Nathan, C., Kabins, S. A., and Weinstein, R. A., 1984, *Pseudomonas* in the sinks in an intensive care unit in relation to patients, *J. Clin. Pathol.* **37:**424–427.
93. Ayliffe, G. A., Babb, J. R., Collins, B. J., Lowbury, E. J. L., and Newsom, S. W. B., 1974, *Pseudomonas aeruginosa* in hospital sinks, *Lancet* **i:**578–581.
94. Gerba, C. P., Wallis, C., and Melnick, J. L., 1975, Microbiological hazards of household toilets: Droplet production and the fate of residual organisms, *Appl. Microbiol.* **30:**229–237.
95. Darlow, H. M., and Bale, W. R., 1959, Infective hazards of water-closets. *Lancet* **i:**1196–1200.
96. Kohn, J. A., 1970, A waste-trap-sterilizing method. *Lancet* **ii:**550–551.
97. Teres, D., Schweers, P., Bushnell, L. S., Hedley-Whyte, P., and Feingold, D. S., 1973, Sources of *Pseudomonas aeruginosa* infection in a respiratory/surgical intensive-therapy unit, *Lancet* **i:**415–417.

98. Mäkelä, P., Ojajärvi, J., and Salminen, E., 1972, Decontaminating waste-trap, *Lancet* **ii:** 1216–1217.
99. Olson, B., Weinstein, R. A., Nathan, C., and Kabius, S. A., 1984, Epidemiology of endemic *Pseudomonas aeruginosa*: why infection control efforts have failed, *J. Infect. Dis.* **150:** 808–816.
100. Craven, D. E., and Daschner, F. D., 1989, Nosocomial pneumonia in the intubated patient: Role of gastric colonization, *Eur. J. Clin. Microbiol. Infect. Dis.* **8:**40–50.
101. Tancrede, C. H., and Andremont, A. O., 1985, Bacterial translocation and gram-negative bacteremia in patients with hematological malignancies, *J. Infect. Dis.* **152:**99–103.

Attachment and Colonization of *Pseudomonas aeruginosa*: Role of the Surface Structures

RANDALL T. IRVIN

1. INTRODUCTION

Cystic fibrosis (CF) patients frequently suffer from chronic *Pseudomonas aeruginosa* pulmonary infections.[1-3] These pulmonary infections are thought to be initiated by the attachment to and subsequent colonization of the mucosal epithelium of the upper respiratory tract by *P. aeruginosa* and followed by a descending infection mechanism.[2,4-6] The initial pulmonary infection is generally due to nonmucoid strains of *P. aeruginosa*,[7-10] but following the initial infection mucoid strains predominate and are isolated in 50%[11] to 90%[12] of all CF patients. Increasing severity of the pulmonary infection appears to be correlated with the appearance and predominance of mucoid strains of *P. aeruginosa* in the sputum of CF patients.[1,7,8,10] Significantly, phenotypic switching of a nonmucoid to mucoid phenotype has been noted in an *in vivo* chronic lung infection model without antibiotic selection,[13] which suggests that the mucoid phenotype is not selected for by antibiotic utilization.

2. ROLE OF ADHERENCE IN PATHOGENESIS

Adherence of *P. aeruginosa* to the mucosal epithelial surface of the oropharynx is thought to be the initial step of *P. aeruginosa* respiratory infections. The initial studies of Johanson *et al.*[4-6] established that gram-negative oropharyngeal colonization precedes the onset of clinical infection. Our studies have extended these observations and have indicated that increased *P. aeruginosa* adherence to human tracheal epithelial cells (TEC) is correlated with the acquisition of clinical pneumonia in intubated intensive care unit (ICU) patients and that, when the pneumonitis resolves, *P. aeruginosa* adherence to TEC decreases.[14] The change in *P. aeruginosa* adherence to a patient's TEC is due to TEC cell surface changes that influence the ease with which *P. aeruginosa* binds to receptor sites; the affinity constant for *P. aeruginosa* binding to TEC is elevated in patients who have clinical disease and decreases as a patient's status improves (Table I). These observations suggest that *P. aeruginosa* may be an opportunistic pathogen as a result of low binding affinity to the respiratory mucosa of healthy individuals. The observations of Niederman *et al.*,[15-17] who have suggested that alterations of the respiratory mucosal environment (in terms of pH, nutrition status, and mucosal IgA levels) play a significant role in the initiation of infection, tend to support this hypothesis.

P. aeruginosa is a common cause of serious corneal infections[18] and the pivotal role of *P. aeruginosa* adherence to the corneal epithelium has been established.[19] *P. aeruginosa* only binds to and colonizes cornea where there has been tissue damage[20] or exposed stroma.[21] It also colonizes immature cornea.[22] Pili have been demonstrated to mediate *Pseudomonas fluorescens* adherence to human cornea.[23] We have recently been able to demonstrate that pili have specific glycoprotein receptors in the mouse corneal epithelium that are developmentally regulated.[24] The poor affinity of *P. aeruginosa* for normal tissue appears to be a basic feature of the *P. aeruginosa* pathogenic mechanism.

TABLE I
Equilibrium Analysis of the Maximum Number of Receptor Sites per Epithelial Cell and the Apparent Association Constant of Binding of *Pseudomonas aeruginosa* Strain K to TEC.[a]

Day	N CFU/cell	Ka ml/CFU
20	239	1.03×10^{-8}
30	261	3.70×10^{-9}

[a]Obtained by bronchoscopy of an intubated patient who was admitted to a surgical intensive care unit following a total esophagectomy because of carcinoma. The patient was ventilated until extubation. TEC were obtained on days 20 and 30. On day 20 the patient was diagnosed as having pneumonitis and presented with diffuse right-sided pulmonary infiltrates which was confirmed by culture of a bronchoscopy specimen obtained with protected specimen brush. On day 30 the patient's pneumonia began to resolve; by day 34 the patient had cleared the pneumonia and on day 36 was extubated.

Pili have been established as a critical virulence factor in corneal scratch infection models where the scratch exposes previously cryptic receptors and induces susceptibility to infection.[23] Unfortunately, a comparable model system has not been established where a specific lesion can induce susceptibility to *P. aeruginosa* respiratory infections. Several animal infection models suggest that the adherence characteristics of a *P. aeruginosa* strain are correlated with the strain's virulence, and antibodies that inhibit *P. aeruginosa* adherence are protective. The critical role of adherence in the initiation of an infection is clear but unambiguous experimental evidence has not been readily obtained.

2.1. Morphology of Adherence to Human Respiratory Cells

The interaction of *P. aeruginosa* with human respiratory epithelial cells is a dynamic process that is readily observed microscopically. There is no apparent chemotactic response of *P. aeruginosa* to either human buccal epithelial cells (BEC) or TEC and the initial interaction of a bacterium with the eucaryotic cell appears to be a random collision event. Following the initial collision (which generally involves the end or pole of the bacterium), the motion of the bacterium is rapidly and significantly altered and frequently results in at least transitory binding of the bacterium to the epithelial cell (generally by the pole of the cell accompanied by significant bacterial rotation around the long axis of the cell). Following the initial interaction of a bacterium with an epithelial cell, there is generally significant flagellar activity and bacterial motion for 15–60 sec (during which time the bacterium frequently dissociates from the epithelial cell surface and resumes normal swimming), which is then followed by a period of senescence. At apparently random intervals, flagellar activity apparently is re-initiated and some bacteria subsequently dissociate from the epithelial cells. The binding to and desorption of *P. aeruginosa* from epithelial cells readily attains an equilibrium that can be demonstrated by the concentration-dependent displacement of bound bacteria by free bacteria.[25–29] The adherence of nonmucoid cells generally only involves the poles of the bacterium, whereas mucoid cells generally interact with epithelial cells with their entire cell surface.

2.2. Effect of Epithelial Cell Type on Adherence

P. aeruginosa adherence studies have employed a variety of tissues and cell types as substrates and there is no consensus as to what system is optimal. Human BEC collected from healthy, nonsmoking, male volunteers have been used widely as a convenient, plentiful substrate for examining *P. aeruginosa* adherence. There are serious concerns that the largely nonviable BEC that are in the process of being shed from the oral mucosal surface may not be an appropriate substrate,[17] although they possess receptors for all known *P. aeruginosa* adhesins. We have examined *P. aeruginosa* adherence to human ciliated TEC obtained by bronchoscopic brushing of the trachea of volunteers, surgical patients, and ICU patients and have found that they yield results mostly equivalent to those obtained with BEC. Human TEC obtained by bronchoscopy have functional cilia, are polarized and exclude trypan blue, but they may represent a disturbed or somewhat damaged cell because they have been physically removed from the respiratory mucosal membrane. The receptor activity of TEC accurately reflects the physiological status of the individual that they were obtained from.[14] Zoutman et al.[30] have demonstrated, at least for canine TEC, that damaged TEC have a far greater affinity for P. aeruginosa than do undamaged TEC. Employing a primary source of human respiratory epithelial cells as a substrate rather than cultured human cell lines or epithelial cells of other species offers the advantage of employing receptors that are likely closer to the receptors recognized in situ.

P. aeruginosa binds preferentially to the cilia of TEC aligning with the major axis of the cilia if the P. aeruginosa strain uses both pili and alginate as adhesins,[31] and by a pole of the bacterium if the strain does not utilize an alginate adhesin. A kinetic analysis of the nonmucoid PAK isolate binding to TEC indicates that the maximum number of receptor sites/TEC is equivalent to the number of receptor sites found of BEC but that the apparent association (K_a) of binding is somewhat different[27] likely due more to better steric access to receptor sites rather than to significant structural differences in the receptors found on TEC compared with BEC. P. aeruginosa uses alginate, pili, and presumably exoenzyme S (exo-S)[32] as adhesins for binding to TEC.[25,27] The level of P. aeruginosa adherence to a patient's TEC is not affected by intubation or the duration of intubation, but does accurately reflect the risk of acquisition of clinical pneumonia in intubated ICU patients.[16] The change in the adhesion index for P. aeruginosa binding to TEC of a patient is due to a change in the apparent K_a (the K_a increases when a patient is susceptible to infection and decreases as the physiological status of the patient improves) of binding rather than a change in the number of bacterial binding sites (Table I).

We feel that examining the adherence of P. aeruginosa to BEC is a reasonable alternative to using TEC to facilitate experimental progress (obtaining TEC is difficult and sporadic at best, given the difficulties in obtaining informed consents and coordinating clinical and laboratory schedules) as the same adhesins are used. However, we feel that it is imperative to verify the results obtained by utilizing BEC with TEC, given the observed morphological evidence of receptor localization for TEC.

3. ADHESINS

While the critical role of P. aeruginosa adherence to the respiratory mucosal surface has been recognized for some time, the mechanisms that mediate P. aeruginosa adherence have not been as readily established. Equilibrium analysis of *P. aeruginosa* binding to BEC is relatively complex and two classes of adhesin–receptor interactions can be resolved (Fig. 1), one of high affinity and the other of low affinity. Only one class of adhesin–receptor interactions can generally be resolved for nonmucoid isolates (Fig. 2), although for most strains microcolony formation (due to induction of alginate synthesis) occasionally occurs in nonmucoid isolates and subsequently two classes of adhesin–receptor interactions can be resolved by equilibrium analysis of binding.[26]

The role of alginate and pili as *P. aeruginosa* adhesins was readily demonstrated. The principal component of the *P. aeruginosa* capsule, alginate, can mediate binding to respiratory epithelial cells.[25,33,34] The role of pili in mediating *P. aeruginosa* adherence to respiratory epithelial cells is also well-established.[27,33,35,36] The role of exo-S as a *P. aeruginosa* adhesin has been demonstrated only recently[32] although the existence of a third adhesin was anticipated, as the adherence of the nonmucoid isolate PAK to BEC could not be completely inhibited by antibodies specific for pili even when complete inhibition of pilus binding to BEC could be demonstrated.[37]

The relative contribution of the three separate *P. aeruginosa* adhesins to virulence and the initiation of infection is difficult to assess. The affinity of an adhesin for its receptor accurately describes the outcome of any competition for receptors[38] and provides an objective assessment of the effectiveness of a particular adhesin. The relative affinities thus indicate which adhesins play more significant roles in the initiation of an infection. Based on the affinities of adhesins for their appropriate receptors, alginate does not play a significant role in the initiation of an infection,[28,38] given low numbers of pathogen and the relatively inefficient binding process (Table II). It appears likely that the alginate adhesin plays a substantial role in the descending infection model as, once sufficient numbers of *P. aeruginosa* are present (due to colonization and growth on the mucosal surface), there is a significant level of alginate-mediated binding to mucosal epithelial cells. Alginate-mediated binding allows for intact microcolonies to bind to the epithelium at a single receptor site, which significantly increases the number of bacteria that can be bound to a single cell.[26] Biofilm formation can thus proceed rapidly, effectively limiting the host response. The relative significance of exo-S and pili as adhesins for initiating an infection remains to be clarified.

3.1. Structure and Function of the Capsule

The mucoid colony type of *P. aeruginosa* is associated with presence of alginic acid, an extracellular polysaccharide composed of L-guluronic and D-mannuronic acid.[39–41] The alginic acid or mucoid substance of Høiby[8–10] following synthesis and excretion remains loosely associated with the *P. aeruginosa* cell envelope in what has been termed a "slime layer"[41] or perhaps what more appropriately may be termed a peripheral capsule.[42–44]

The presence of an alginic acid peripheral capsule appears to decrease

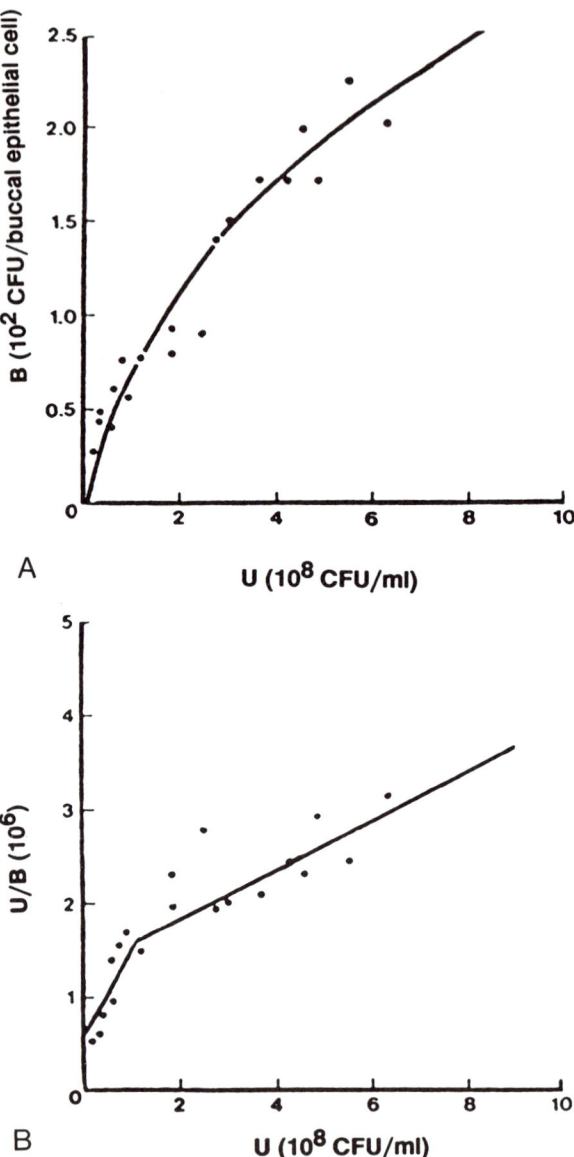

FIGURE 1. (A) Binding isotherm of the adherence of the mucoid *P. aeruginosa* strain K311-1 to human buccal epithelial cells. B = bound bacteria and U = unbound bacterial concentration at equilibrium. (B) Langmuir adsorption transformation of the data in (A). Note that two classes of receptor-adhesin are resolvable. Maximum number of receptor sites and apparent affinity constant are given in Table II for the alginate and pilus adhesins of strain K311-1.

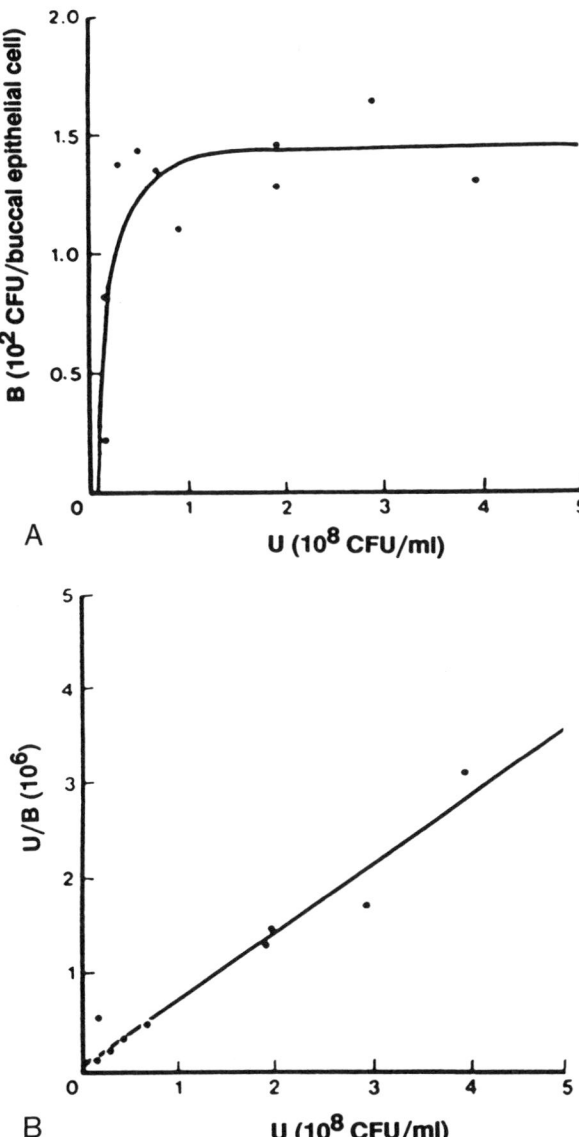

FIGURE 2. (A) Binding isotherm of the adherence of the nonmucoid *P. aeruginosa* strain K91-2 to human BEC. B = bound bacteria and U = unbound bacterial concentration at equilibrium. (B) Langmuir adsorption transformation of the data in (A). Maximum number of receptor sites and apparent affinity constant given in Table II.

TABLE II
Equilibrium Analysis of the Adherence of a Number
of Nonmucoid and Mucoid *Pseudomonas aeruginosa*
Clinical Isolates to Human BEC.

Strain	Phenotype	Adhesin	N CFU/cell	Ka ml/CFU
K91-2	Nonmucoid	Pilus	138	9.4×10^{-7}
2898	Nonmucoid	Pilus	45	2.8×10^{-8}
492a	Mucoid[a]	Pilus	33	5.3×10^{-9}
K311-1	Mucoid[b]	Pilus	112	1.6×10^{-8}
		Alginate	391	1.9×10^{-9}

[a]Strain 492a produces an alginate that does not bind to human respiratory epithelial cells.
[b]Strain 311-1 produces an alginate that functions as an adhesin.

susceptibility of the organism to antibiotics and to surface-active agents such as deoxycholate.[45] The peripheral capsule also inhibits phagocytosis of *P. aeruginosa* by macrophages *in vitro*,[46–51] increases survival times in rat lungs,[52] and appears to enhance the survival of the organism in high oxygen tension environments,[53] possibly by the scavenging of free radicals.[54]

The presence of a capsule is not always advantageous to *P. aeruginosa*, because energy and export requirements for the production of the capsule result in a slightly slower growth rate for mucoid strains compared with nonmucoid or acapsular strains.[45] Thus, unless there is a selective advantage for the presence of a capsule (such as the presence of a surfactant or an antibiotic), nonmucoid strains or revertants of mucoid strains rapidly predominate in a culture to the exclusion of mucoid strains.[65] Mucoid isolates are not overgrown in the cystic fibrosis (CF) lung.[2,10] The capsule of the mucoid strains of *P. aeruginosa* is apparently of advantage *in situ* in the chronically infected lung of the CF patient. In a chronic lung infection model, nonmucoid isolates convert to phenotypically mucoid isolates without antibiotic selective pressure.[13]

The expression of the peripheral capsule or mucoid phenotype is highly regulated, with expression dependent upon several regulatory loci that are separated from the structural genes for the synthesis and export of alginate.[55–60] It is now evident that even nonmucoid *P. aeruginosa* strains have some cell surface-localized alginate present in the form of a partial microcapsule.[61] The microalginate capsule is considerably smaller in dimension that the capsule found on mucoid strains, which appear to have lost the ability to regulate the synthesis of alginate and thus the size of their capsule.

Elucidation of the role of the *P. aeruginosa* capsule has been complicated by the realization that mucoid strains and their alginate varies considerably.[62] Alginate has been shown to vary tremendously in the ratio of guluronic to mannuronic acid and in degree of acetylation.[63–66] Structural variation in alginates from various strains is also reflected immunologically; several discrete alginate epitopes have been identified.[67-69] In addition, various lectins (rat lung, human fetal lung and human placental) also bind to specific structural forms of *P. aeruginosa* alginates.[65-70] Several authors have suggested that alginate may be involved in the adhesion of the pathogen to epithelial surfaces.[25,26,28,29,34,71-74] We have confirmed that certain alginate epitopes act as *P. aeruginosa* adhesins and bind specifically to human epithelial cells, whereas others do not.[25] Interestingly, cell-free alginate can bind to a surface and then promote the subsequent binding of *P. aeruginosa* to the cell through an epitope-specific alginate–outer membrane interaction (Fig. 3). This alginate-promoted adherence mechanism may facilitate the colonization of the lower airway following upper airway colonization.

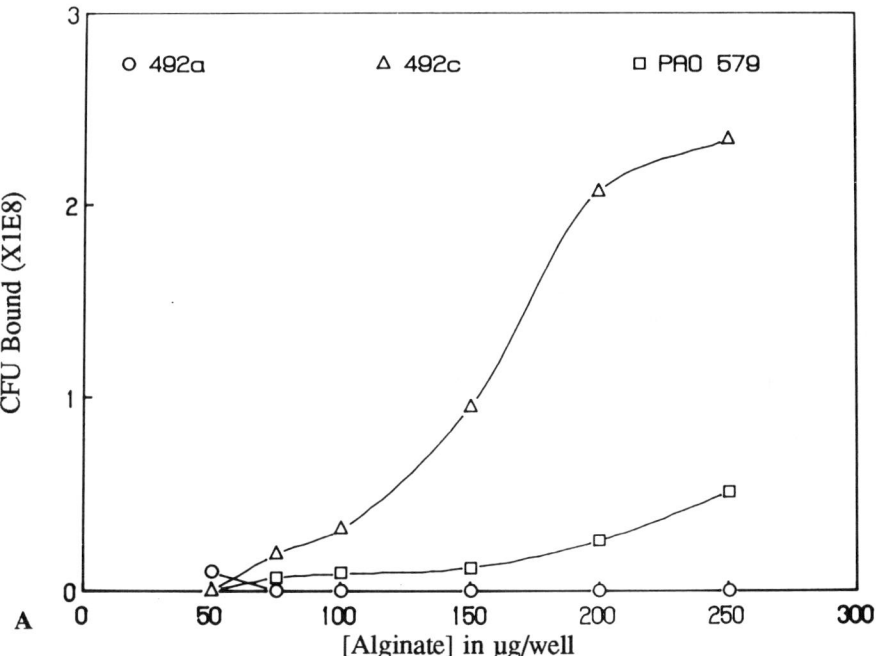

FIGURE 3. (A) Binding of whole cells of *P. aeruginosa* mucoid isolates 492c, PAO 579, and 492a to purified strain 492c alginate immobilized in microtiter wells. Strains 492c and PAO 579 produce alginate that binds to human respiratory epithelial cells whereas the alginate produced by strain 492a does not function as an adhesin. (B) Binding of outer membrane prepared from *P. aeruginosa* strains 492c, PAO 579, and 492a to purified alginate from strain 492c that is immobilized in microtiter wells.

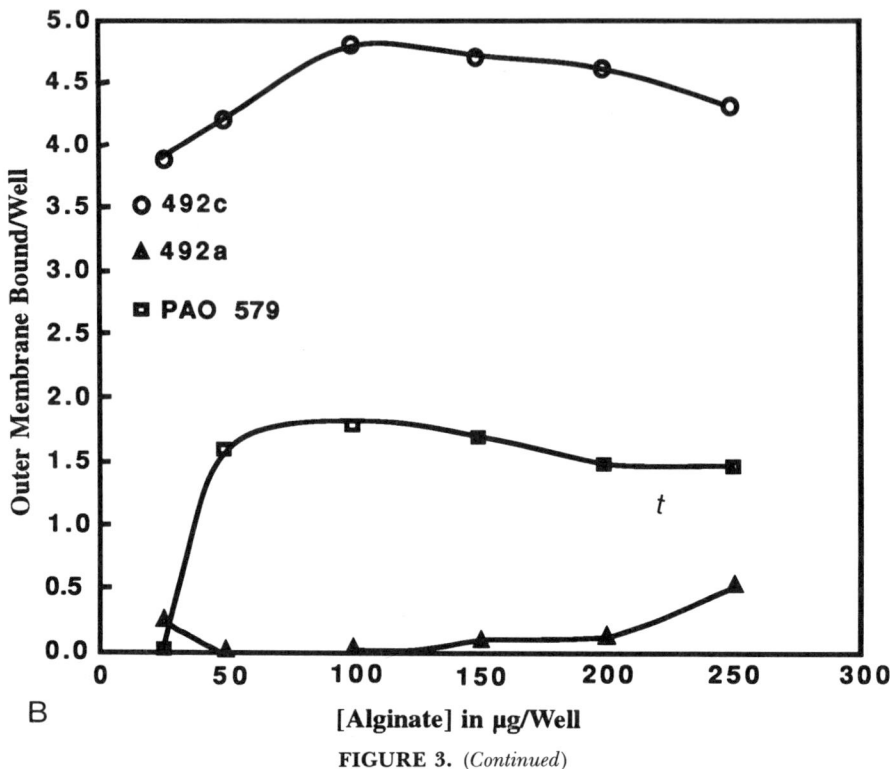

FIGURE 3. (*Continued*)

3.2. Exoenzyme S

Exo-S is a significant *P. aeruginosa* virulence factor.[75,76] Exo-S functions as a toxin by ADP-ribosylating a number of eucaryotic cellular proteins.[77] Exo-S can be purified in two separate forms,[78] one that is enzymatically active (has active ADP-ribosylating activity) and one that constitutes an active cytotoxin, is normally found associated with the outer surface of the outer membrane, and constitutes a functional adhesin.[32] Exo-S appears to bind specifically to the glycolipid asialo-GM_1.[32,79] Recently, we have established the existence of considerable homology between the C-terminal region of *P. aeruginosa* strain KB-7 pilin and exo-S (Woods, personal communication). Exo-S was also found to react with monoclonal and polyclonal antibodies specific for the C-terminal region of *P. aeruginosa* pilin, and the reciprocal interactions were also observed. The degree of similarity between exo-S and *P. aeruginosa* pilin is under active investigation; clearly exo-S and pili use similar or identical molecular adhesion mechanisms.

3.3. Structure of Pili

The majority of *P. aeruginosa* strains possess somatic, retractable, polar pili. The pili are characterized by having an N-terminal residue that consists of N-methyl Phenylalanine (MePhe),[80–84] and are considered to be the prototype of what have been termed type 4 pili.[85] The polar pili of *P. aeruginosa* are long linear filaments with a mean diameter of 5.2 nm and an average length of 2500 nm[86–88] and are composed of a single protein termed pilin that generally has a size of ~15 KDa.[83,89–95]

Pilin is initially synthesized as a larger precursor that is proteolytically modified in the membrane and then reversibly assembled into a functional pilus in the outer membrane.[83,91,94–101] The primary amino acid sequences of the PAK and PAO pilins have been determined biochemically,[90,92,93] and the sequences obtained agree with those deduced by sequencing the structural gene.[91,94,95,99] Mature PAK pilin is a single polypeptide of 144 amino acids with an N-terminal of N-methyl Phenylalanine[80] and an intra-chain disulfide bridge between residues 129 and 142. PAK pilin may be cleaved proteolytically with trypsin to produce four polypeptide fragments (cT-I, cT-II, cT-III, and cT-IV). The immunodominant antigenic determinant of pilin resides in the cT-III fragment (residues 54–120).[93,102]

Several *P. aeruginosa* pilins have now been cloned and sequenced and these results, along with restriction polymorphism studies, indicate that virtually all clinical isolates carry one of ~7 different pilin structural genes (W. Paranchych, personal communication). The N-terminal end of pilin is highly conserved whereas the C-terminal end may be considered semi-conserved.[83,84,95,103] The pilin structural gene is found in virtually all clinical isolates, but the gene appears to be transcriptionally regulated[60,83,94,99,101] and thus may not be expressed under all environmental conditions.

3.4. Synthesis and Assembly of Pili

P. aeruginosa pili are assembled from a pre-pilin that is processed during protein export to produce the final pilin.[91,94,96,99,100] The synthesized pilin appears to be stored in the outer membrane of the cell before assembly into an intact pilus.[104] Growth or assembly of pili occurs from the base of the pilus[105,106] and this is consistent with the presence of pilin monomer pools in the outer membrane.[104]

Pilin proteins may assemble into pili that present unique antigenic epitopes associated with the shaft and tip regions of the pilus.[83–107] Similarly, bacteriophage receptor sites reside in specific regions of the pilus. The *P. aeruginosa* pilus is capable of retraction or extension,[108–111] similar to the retraction ability of conjugative pili.[83]

3.5. Structural Variability in Pilins

Frequently, bacterial cells express multiple types of pili simultaneously and there is mounting evidence that several pathogens use phase variation or equivalent genetic manipulations to alter the pilus structures that are surface-expressed at any one time.[83,112] The variation of pilus structure in pathogenic bacteria appears to be due to selective pressure. The immunologically dominant region of *P. aeruginosa* pilin is found in the central region of the protein,[93,102] whereas the N-terminal and C-terminal portions of the protein are reasonably conserved in the different *P. aeruginosa* pilins. The N-terminal region is thought to be highly conserved due to processing and assembly constraints.[83,103]

3.6. Pilin-Pilin Interactions

In a number of species a single bacterium can simultaneously possess more than one type of pili; however, a single pilus (with a limited number of exceptions) consists of a single type of pilin. Pilus-associated adhesins must be assembled into a functional pilus and this requires substantial homology with pilin structural proteins, as has been noted for both the tip-associated papG adhesin[106,113,114] and the type 1 adhesin that is laterally associated with the filament of the type 1 pili.[115–117]

Considerable conservation exists, in terms of both amino acid sequences and DNA sequences, among the various MePhe pili.[83,103] Conservation in the MePhe pili allows for the synthesis and assembly of intact pili from MePhe pilins of various species in *P. aeruginosa*.[81,82,84,103,118] MePhe pilins have been cloned and expressed in *Escherichia coli*, but assembly of pilin into functional pili has not been observed, likely because of a basic difference in the processing and assembly of pili in *Escherichia coli*.[91,94]

When the gene for *Bacteroides nodosus* pilin is cloned and expressed in *P. aeruginosa*, the pili produced are functional and immunologically indistinguishable from those synthesized by *Bacteroides nodosus*.[81,82] An immunocytochemical study of *P. aeruginosa* cells that contained both the *P. aeruginosa* and *B. nodosus* pilin genes revealed cells with both types of pili. Elleman and Peterson[82] observed hybrid pili (~0.1% of the pili) with *Pseudomonas* and *Bacteroides* pilin subunits in homogeneous but discrete segments of a single pilus. These authors suggested that only one pilin gene may be expressed at a time. A cell that contains two pilin structural genes thus produces Fimbria containing only a single pilin type or rare hybrid Fimbriae that contain two types of pilin subunits where each subunit is found in a discrete homogenous region. Beard *et al.*[84] examined the expression of *Moraxella bovis* pilin in *P. aeruginosa* and observed very rare pili that were heterologous in terms of their subunits (the pilin monomers were not always observed in homogeneous segments of the pili), likely due to retraction and growth of pili utilizing heterologous pilin monomer pools in the outer membrane. The subunit–interfacial regions of the MePhe pilins exhibit significant homology, suggesting that severe structural restraints may be imposed on the protein to insure pilus processing and assembly.

3.7. Function of Pili

Woods et al.[36,119–121] initially suggested that *P. aeruginosa* uses pili to bind to proteolytically modified BEC in which cell surface fibronectin had been removed, creating new bacterial cell-surface receptor sites. Ramphal et al.[33–35,73,122] examined the adherence of *P. aeruginosa* to mouse TEC and observed that intubation or HCl injury facilitated *P. aeruginosa* adherence, and that both pili and alginate functioned as adhesins.

P. aeruginosa pili have also been implicated as adhesins for the attachment of *P. aeruginosa* to healthy and thermally damaged murine epidermal cells.[123] The role of pili and alginate in mediating attachment to hamster tracheal epithelium has also been established.[71,72,74] We confirmed that both pili and alginate are used by *P. aeruginosa* as adhesins to mediate attachment to both human BEC and human TEC.[25,27] Thus a number of systems have been used to examine *P. aeruginosa* adherence, and a clear role for both pili and alginate as adhesins has been established. Equilibrium analysis of *P. aeruginosa* binding to BEC in the presence of purified pili indicates that pili inhibit the adherence of whole cells by a competitive inhibition mechanism and thus bind to the same receptors as do whole bacteria.[27]

Whereas it is clear that the *P. aeruginosa* pilus functions as an adhesin, the actual nature of the adhesin has not been determined irrefutably. Elegant studies with *E. coli* have established that the P pilus and the type I pilus both have low copy number tip-associated proteins that function as the adhesin, rather than the pilin structural protein.[106,113,114,116] While there is currently no evidence to suggest a distinct *P. aeruginosa* pilus-associated adhesin, there is no irrefutable evidence to the contrary.

The *P. aeruginosa* pilin structural protein does contain a functional adhesin. We have established that the C-terminal fragment of PAK pilin and synthetic peptides of an identical sequence bind specifically to both BEC and TEC. The binding of PAK pili and a synthetic peptide (with the same sequence as the C-terminal region of PAK pilin) to TEC is identical when examined by immunofluorescence. We have also demonstrated that this synthetic peptide effectively competes with purified PAK pili for binding sites on BEC.[124]

Monoclonal antibodies (MAb) directed against the cT-I or cT-II regions of PAK pilin do not inhibit the adherence of PAK to BEC,[125] but all the MAb directed against the cT-IV region of pilin (the specificity of the monoclonal antibodies was confirmed by competition enzyme-linked immunoabsorbent assays [ELISA] employing synthetic peptides) that we have examined inhibit the adherence of PAK to BECs.[37,125] MAb produced against P pili by de Ree et al.[108] included antibodies that were specific for the minor Pap components that constitute the adhesin. We have not found any similar types of MAb.

Schmidt et al.[126] found considerable homology between linear sections of the pilin structural protein and accessory pilus-associated proteins that function as the adhesin for the *E. coli* digalactoside-binding pilin. Further, Schmidt et al.[126] found that synthetic peptides of these sequences induced the synthesis of protective antibody that prevented colonization and infection in an animal model. Abraham et al.[116] also observed considerable structural homology between type I pilin and the type I accessory proteins. Considerable effort will be required to establish unambiguously whether the *P. aeruginosa* pilus adhesin is actually pilin or a pilus accessory protein (which has a high degree of homology with the C-terminal region of pilin) that is located at the tip of the pilus. Antibodies specific for the C-terminal region of pilin are protective in passive immunization studies, and active immunization with PAK $(128-144)_{ox}$ coupled to a protein carrier also results in protection against *P. aeruginosa* infection (W. Paranchych, personal communication).

Variability in the sequence of *P. aeruginosa* pilins accounts for significant variation in pilus affinity for respiratory epithelial cells (Table II), and may allow for a degree of variation in the structure required for pilus receptor activity. The affinity and the number of receptors present on a BEC cell surface varies substantially from strain to strain (Table II). A given strain's virulence may thus directly depend upon the pilin produced.

3.8. The Pilus and Exoenzyme S Receptor(s)

The nature of the pilus receptor(s) is still unclear. *P. aeruginosa* pili have been reported to bind to a sialic acid-containing component found on the epithelial cell surface[74] and a carbohydrate-containing component of respiratory mucin.[33,127–129] We have observed pilus receptor activity in several blotted cell-surface BEC glycopeptides and noted that receptor activity is dependent upon the presence of carbohydrate.[130] Monosaccharide inhibition and enzymatic modification studies on blotted putative receptors suggest that L-fucose and sialic acid are components of the pilus receptor.

Krivan et al.[131] reported that *P. aeruginosa* binds specifically to asialo-GM_1, requiring β-D-N-acetyl-galactosamine β(1,4) D-galactose as a minimal carbohydrate component, although the nature of the adhesin that mediated binding to the glycolipid was not tested. Lingwood et al.[79] and Baker et al.[32] subsequently reported that exo-S binds to asialo-GM_1. A similar glycolipid-binding specificity has ben noted for a large number of respiratory pathogens.[131–135] Suggestions of potential cross-contamination of exo-S and pili preparations led to a careful examination of the antigenicity of exo-S and *P. aeruginosa* pili. The monoclonal antibody PK 99H, specific for PAK pilin (and the linear epitope DEQFIPK in particular[136]) was found to bind specifically to exo-S even in the absence of a directly homologous sequence. PK 99H was found to bind specifically to purified exo-S and to inhibit exo-S activity. Subsequent DNA homology searches revealed a region of exo-S with considerable homology to the epithelial-cell-binding domain region of some *P. aeruginosa*. The immunological cross-reactivity of exo-S and *P. aeruginosa* pili has been confirmed by competitive ELISA employing a number of authentic *P. aeruginosa* pili.

Current literature on the nature of the pilus receptor is confusing and contradictory. Recently we have obtained data that may clarify the situation to a certain extent. Ramphal *et al.*[127–129] have reported that *P. aeruginosa* pili bind specifically to human respiratory mucin; however, we have been able to observe only non-specific, hydrophobically mediated interaction of *P. aeruginosa* pili with highly purified human respiratory or gastric mucin.[137] However, we have confirmed that *P. aeruginosa* pili bind to several glycopeptides, which appear to contain β-D-N-acetyl-galactosamine β(1,4) D-galactose as a portion of their structural carbohydrate component, in the corneal epithelia of the mouse.[24] The unexpected sequence and immunological homology of exo-S and *P. aeruginosa* pilin subsequently led to the exploration of the ability of exo-S and *P. aeruginosa* pili to bind to asialo-GM_1 and the synthetic disaccharide β-D-N-acetyl-galactosamine β(1,4) D-galactose. Both *P. aeruginosa* pili and exo-S were found to bind specifically to asialo-GM_1 and the synthetic disaccharide β-D-N-acetyl-galactosamine β(1,4) D-galactose. It is likely that Ramphal *et al.*[127–129] observed binding of *P. aeruginosa* to human mucins due to low-level contamination of their mucin preparations with glycolipids that can function as receptors for both exo-S and *P. aeruginosa* pili.

3.9. Structural Organization of Pili

Whereas *P. aeruginosa* pili are composed of a single monomer, the structure is asymmetrical, with the tip and the basal portion of the pilus expressing unique antigens. MAb PK 3B binds only to the basal portion of the pilus[138] and does not inhibit *P. aeruginosa* pilus adhesin function (Fig. 4a,b).[37] MAb PK 99H, which binds to the C-terminal region of pilin[37,136] and inhibits *P. aeruginosa* pilus adhesin function, binds to the tip of the pilus (Fig. 4c).[137] The synthetic disaccharide β-D-N-acetyl-galactosamine β(1,4) D-galactose was also found to bind only to the tip of *P. aeruginosa* pili (Fig. 4d). The structural organization of the *P. aeruginosa* pilus is diagramed in Fig. 5.

4. SUMMARY AND CONCLUSION

P. aeruginosa pulmonary infections continue to constitute a major source of morbidity and mortality despite novel and aggressive antimicrobial ther-

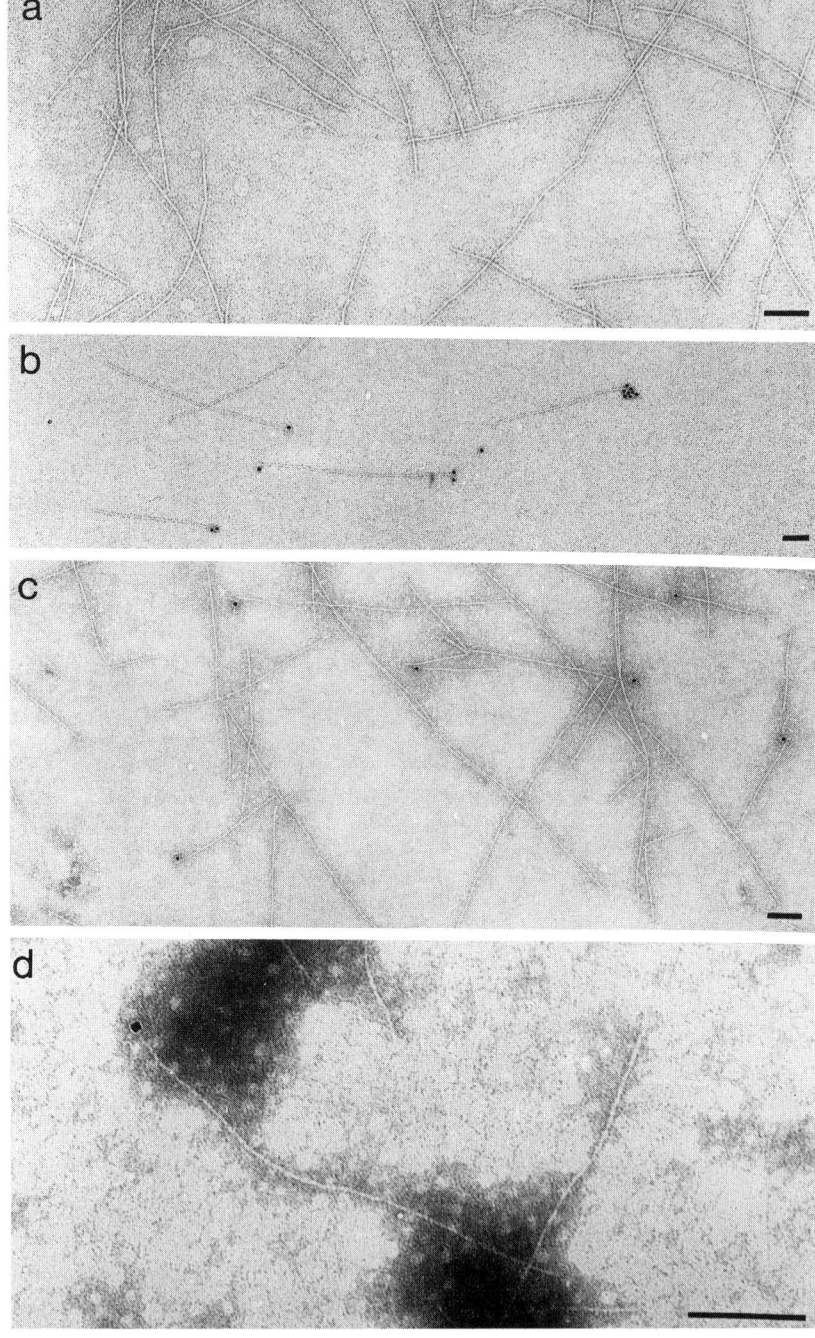

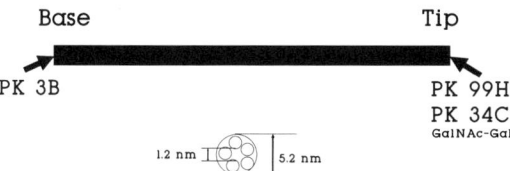

FIGURE 5. Schematic drawing of PAK pili indicating the assembly of pilin monomers into an asymmetrical pilus where monoclonal antibody PK 3B binds to pilin subunits exposed on the basal portion of pili fragments, whereas GalNAc-Gal and the monoclonal antibodies PK 99H and PK 34C bind to the tip of the pilus. The pilus is assembled from pilin monomers with five subunits per helical turn, and each turn of the helix gives 0.41 nm pitch.

apy. The initial stage of *P. aeruginosa* pulmonary infections is the adherence of the pathogen to an epithelial surface (likely the oropharyngeal epithelium) followed by colonization of that surface. Following initial colonization, *P. aeruginosa* uses a descending infection model to colonize and infect the lower airway.

P. aeruginosa uses at least three separate adhesins (alginate, exo-S and pili) to bind to a patient's respiratory epithelial cells. The two adhesins that appear to be responsible for initiating *P. aeruginosa* colonization are pili and exo-S, which have the highest apparent affinity constants for respiratory epithelial cells. The lower affinity adhesin, alginate, likely contributes significantly in the colonization of the lower airway when there are significantly higher populations of *Pseudomonas* in the airway.

Whereas exo-S and pili are distinct structurally and biochemically, they both bind to the same respiratory epithelial cell surface receptors. Significant similarity has been detected between a defined region of exo-S and pilin (Woods, personal communication), and this region appears to mediate the binding of the toxin and pili to epithelial cells.

Currently, relatively little is known concerning the nature or structure of the cell surface receptors to which *P. aeruginosa* binds. The role of glycolipids

FIGURE 4. (a) Negative stain preparation of purified pili obtained from *P. aeruginosa* strain K (PAK pili). The bar in this and subsequent micrographs represents 0.1 μm. (b) Colloidal gold localization of monoclonal antibody PK 3B binding to the base of PAK pili. (c) Colloidal gold localization of monoclonal antibody PK 99H binding to the tip of PAK pili. (d) Colloidal gold localization of the binding of biotinylated β-N-acetyl-galactosamine-β(1.4)-galactose to the tip of PAK pili.

and specific glycoproteins as receptors for *P. aeruginosa* cells and purified adhesins remains to be clarified. The role of the adhesins in *P. aeruginosa* pathogenesis is critical; a number of animal studies have demonstrated that both alginate and pili can induce homologous protective immunity[36,51,123,139] and antibodies directed against the binding domain of pilin are protective in animal infection models. The future looks promising for the development of an efficacious vaccine that would function by preventing *P. aeruginosa* adherence and colonization.

REFERENCES

1. Doggett, R. G., 1979, *Pseudomonas aeruginosa: Clinical Manifestations of Infection and Current Therapy*, Academic Press, New York.
2. Gilligan, P. H., 1991, Microbiology of airway disease in patients with cystic fibrosis, *Clin. Microbiol. Rev.* **4**:35–51.
3. Wood, R. E., Boat, T. F., and Doershuk, C. F., 1976, Cystic fibrosis, *Am. Rev. Respir. Dis.* **113**:833–878.
4. Johanson, W. G., Jr., Higuchi, J. H., Chaudhuri, T. Woods, D. E., 1980, Bacterial adherence to epithelial cells in the bacillary colonization of the respiratory tract, *Am. Rev. Resp. Dis.* **121**:55–63.
5. Johanson, W. G., Jr., Pierce, A. K., Sanford, J. P., and Thomas, G. D., 1972, Nosocomial respiratory infections with gram-negative bacilli. The significance of colonization of the respiratory tract, *Ann. Intern. Med.* **77**:701–706.
6. Johanson, W. G., Jr., Woods, D. E., and Chaudhuri, T., 1979, Association of respiratory tract colonization with adherence of gram-negative bacilli to epithelial cells, *J. Infect. Dis.* **139**:667–673.
7. Doggett, R. G., 1969, Incidence of mucoid *Pseudomonas aeruginosa* from clinical sources, *Appl. Microbiol.* **18**:936–937.
8. Høiby, N., 1974, *Pseudomonas aeruginosa* infection in cystic fibrosis. Relationship between mucoid strains of *Pseudomonas aeruginosa* and humoral immune response, *Acta Pathol. Microbiol. Scand. Sect. B* **82**:551–558.
9. Høiby, N., 1975, Prevalence of mucoid strains of *Pseudomonas aeruginosa* in bacteriological specimens from patients with cystic fibrosis and patients without cystic fibrosis, *Acta Pathol. Microbiol. Scand. Sect. B* **83**:321–327.
10. Høiby, N., 1982, Microbiology of lung infections in cystic fibrosis patients, *Acta Paediatr. Scand.* **301** (Suppl.):33–54.
11. Kulczycki, L. L., Murphy, T. M., and Bellanti, J. A., 1978, *Pseudomonas aeruginosa* colonization in cystic fibrosis. A study of 160 patients, *J. Am. Med. Assoc.* **240**:30–34.
12. Luraya-Cussay, L. R., Cundy, K. R., and Huang, N. N., 1976, *Pseudomonas* carrier rates of patients with cystic fibrosis and members of their families, *J. Pediatr.* **89**:23–26.
13. Woods, D. E., Sokol, P. A., Bryan, L. E., Storey, D. G., Mattingly, J., Vogel, H. J., and Ceri, H., 1991, *In vivo* regulation of virulence in *Pseudomonas aeruginosa* associated with genetic rearrangement, *J. Infect. Dis.* **163**:143–149.
14. Todd, T., Franklin, A. L., Gurman, G., Mankinen-Irvin, P. M., and Irvin, R. T., 1989, Augmented bacterial adherence to ciliated tracheal epithelial cells in an intensive care unit population, *Am. Rev. Respir. Dis.* **140**:1585–1589.
15. Niederman, M. S., Merrill, W. W., Ferranti, R. D., Pagano, K. W., Palmer, L. B., and Reynolds, H. Y., 1984, Nutritional status and bacterial binding in the lower respiratory tract in patients with chronic tracheostomy, *Ann. Int. Med.* **100**:795–800.

16. Niederman, M. S., Merrill, W. W., Polomski, L. M., Reynolds, H. Y., and Gee, J. B. L., 1986, Influence of sputum IgA and elastase on tracheal cell bacterial adherence, *Am. Rev. Resp. Dis.* **144:**255–260.
17. Niederman, M. S., Rafferty, T. D., Sasaki, C. T., Merrill, W. W., Matthay, R. A., and Reynolds, H. Y., 1983, Comparison of bacterial adherence to ciliated and squamous epithelial cells obtained from the human respiratory tract, *Am. Rev. Respir. Dis.* **127:**85–90.
18. Laibson, P. R., 1972, Annual review: Cornea and sclera, *Arch. Ophthalmol.* **88:**553–574.
19. Ramphal, R., McNiece, M. T., and Polack, F. M., 1981, Adherence of *Pseudomonas aeruginosa* to the injured cornea: A step in the pathogenesis of corneal infections, *Ann. Ophthalmol.* **13:** 421–425.
20. Hazlet, L. D., Moon, M., and Berk, R. S., 1986, *In vivo* identification of Hazlet, L. D., Moon, M., and Berk, R. S., 1986, *In vivo* identification of sialic acid as the ocular receptor for *Pseudomonas aeruginosa*, *Infect. Immun.* **51:**687–689.
21. Stern, G. A., Weitzenkorn, D., and Valenti, J., 1982, Adherence of *Pseudomonas aeruginosa* to the mouse cornea: Epithelial vs stromal adherence, *Arch. Ophthalmol* **100:**1956.
22. Hazlet, L. D., Rosen, D. D., and Berk, R. S., 1978, Age-related susceptibility to *Pseudomonas aeruginosa* ocular infections in mice, *Infect. Immun.* **20:**25–29.
23. Reichert, R. W., Das, N. D., and Zam, Z. S., 1983, Adherence properties of *Pseudomonas* pili to epithelial cells of the human cornea, *Curr. Eye Res.* **2:**289–293.
24. Rudner, X. L., Zheng, Z., Berk, R. S., Irvin, R. T., and Hazlett, L. D., 1991, Corneal epithelial glycoproteins exhibit *P. aeruginosa* pilus binding activity, submitted.
25. Doig, P., Smith, N. R., Todd, T., and Irvin, R. T., 1987, Characterization of the binding of *Pseudomonas aeruginosa* alginate to human epithelial cells, *Infect. Immun.* **55:**1517–1522.
26. Doig, P., Tapping, R., Mankinen-Irvin, P., and Irvin, R. T., 1989, Effect of microcolony formation on the adherence of *Pseudomonas aeruginosa* to human buccal epithelial cells, *Microb. Ecol. Health Dis.* **2:**203–209.
27. Doig, P., Todd, T., Sastry, P. A., Lee, K. K., Hodges, R. S., Paranchych, W., and Irvin, R. T., 1988, Role of pili in the adhesion of *Pseudomonas aeruginosa* to human respiratory epithelial cells, *Infect. Immun.* **56:**1641–1646.
28. McEachran, D. W., and Irvin, R. T., 1985, Adhesion of *Pseudomonas aeruginosa* to human buccal epithelial cells: Evidence for two classes of receptors, *Can. J. Microbiol.* **31:**563–569.
29. McEachran, D. W., and Irvin, R. T., 1986, A new method for the irreversible attachment of cells or proteins to polystyrene tissue culture plates for use in the study of bacterial adhesion, *J. Microbiol. Methods* **5:**99–111.
30. Zoutman, D. E., Hulbert, W. C., Pasloske, B. L., Joffe, A. M., Volpel, K., Trebilock, M. K., and Paranchych, W., 1991, The role of polar pili in the adherence of *Pseudomonas aeruginosa* to injured canine tracheal epithelial cells: A semiquantitative morphologic study, *Scanning Electron Microsc.* **5:**109–126.
31. Franklin, A. L., Todd, T., Gurman, G., Black, D., Mankinen-Irvin, P. M., and Irvin, R. T., 1987, Adherence of *Pseudomonas aeruginosa* to cilia of human tracheal epithelial cells, *Infect. Immun.* **55:**1523–1525.
32. Baker, N. R., Minor, V., Deal, C., Sahhrabadi, M. S., Simpson, D. A., and Woods, D. E., 1991, *Pseudomonas aeruginosa* exoenzyme S is an adhesin, *Infect. Immun.* **59:**2859–2863.
33. Ramphal, R., and Pyle, M., 1983, Evidence for mucins and sialic acid as receptors for *Pseudomonas aeruginosa* in the lower respiratory tract, *Infect. Immun.* **41:**339–344.
34. Ramphal, R., and Pier, G. B., 1985, Role of *Pseudomonas aeruginosa* mucoid exopolysaccharide in adherence of tracheal cells, *Infect. Immun.* **47:**1–4.
35. Ramphal, R., Sadoff, J. C., Pyle, M., and Silipigni, J. D., 1984, Role of pili in the adherence of *Pseudomonas aeruginosa* to injured tracheal epithelium, *Infect. Immun.* **44:**38–40.
36. Woods, D. E., Straus, D. C., Johanson, W. G., Jr., Berry, V. K., and Bass, J. A., 1980, Role of pili in adherence of *Pseudomonas aeruginosa* to mammalian buccal epithelial cells, *Infect. Immun.* **29:**1146–1151.

37. Doig, P., Sastry, P. A., Hodges, R. S., Lee, K. K., Paranchych, W., and Irvin, R. T., 1990, Inhibition of pilus-mediated adhesion of *Pseudomonas aeruginosa* to human buccal epithelial cells by monoclonal antibodies directed against pili, *Infect. Immun.* **58**:124–130.
38. Irvin, R. T., Doig, P. C., Sastry, P. A., Heller, B., and Paranchych, W., 1989, Competition for bacterial receptor sites on respiratory epithelial cells by *Pseudomonas aeruginosa* strains of heterologous pilus type: Usefulness of kinetic parameters in predicting the outcome, *Microb. Ecol. Health Dis.* **3**:39–47.
39. Linker, A., and Jones, R. S., 1966, A new polysaccharide resembling alginic acid isolated from *Pseudomonas*, *J. Biol. Chem.* **241**:3845–3851.
40. Evans, L.R., and Linker, A., 1973, Production and characterization of the slime polysaccharide of *Pseudomonas aeruginosa*, *J. Bacteriol.* **116**:915–924.
41. Sutherland, I. W., 1977, Bacterial exopolysaccharides. Their nature and production. In: *Surface Carbohydrates of the Prokaryotic Cell* (I. W. Sutherland, ed.), Academic Press, London, pp. 27–96.
42. Cheng, K-J., Irvin, R. T., and Costerton, J. W., 1981, Autochthonous and pathogenic colonization of animal tissues by bacteria, *Can. J. Microbiol.* **27**:461–490.
43. Costerton, J. W., Irvin, R. T., and Cheng, K-J., 1981, The bacteria glycocalyx in nature and disease, *Ann. Rev. Microbiol.* **35**:299–324.
44. Costeron, J. W., Irvin, R. T., and Cheng, K-J., 1981, The role of bacterial surface structures in pathogenesis, *CRC Crit. Rev. Microbiol.* **8**:303–338.
45. Govan, J. R. W., and Fyfe, J. A. M., 1978, Mucoid *Pseudomonas aeruginosa* and cystic fibrosis: Resistance of the mucoid form to carbenicillin, flucloxacillin and tobramycin and the isolation of mucoid variants *in vitro*, *J. Antimicrob. Chemother.* **4**:233–240.
46. Schwarzmann, S., and Boring, J. R., III, 1971, Antiphagocytic effect of slime from a mucoid strain of *Pseudomonas aeruginosa*, *Infect. Immun.* **3**:762–767.
47. Baltimore, R. S., and Mitchell, M., 1980, Immunologic investigations of mucoid strains of *Pseudomonas aeruginosa*: Comparison of susceptibility to opsonic antibody in mucoid and nonmucoid strains, *J. Infect. Dis.* **141**:238–247.
48. Ruhen, R. W., Holt, P. G., and Padadimitriou, J. M., 1980, Antiphagocytic effect of *Pseudomonas aeruginosa* exopolysaccharide, *J. Clin. Pathol.* **33**:1221–1222.
49. Meshulam, T., Obedeanu, N., Merzbach, D., and Sobel, J. D., 1984, Phagocytosis of mucoid and nonmucoid strains of *Pseudomonas aeruginosa*, *Clin. Immun. Immunopathol.* **32**:151–165.
50. Ames, P., DesJardins, D., and Pier, G. B., 1985, Opsonophagocytic killing activity of rabbit antibody to *Pseudomonas aeruginosa* mucoid exopolysaccharide, *Infect. Immun.* **49**:281–285.
51. Woods, D. E., and Bryan, L. E., 1985, Studies on the ability of alginate to act as a protective immunogen against infection with *Pseudomonas aeruginosa* in animals, **151**:581–588.
52. Govan, J. R. W., Fyfe, J. A. M., and Baker, N. R., 1983, Heterogeneity and reduction in pulmonary clearance of mucoid *Pseudomonas aeruginosa*, *Rev. Infect. Dis.* **5**:S874–S875.
53. Krieg, D. P., Bass, J. A., and Mattingly, S. J., 1986, Aeration selects for mucoid phenotype of *Pseudomonas aeruginosa*, *J. Clin. Microbiol.* **24**:986–990.
54. Learn, D. B., Brestel, E. P., and Seetharama, S., 1987, Hypochlorite scavenging by *Pseudomonas aeruginosa* alginate, *Infect. Immun.* **55**:1813–1818.
55. Darzins, A., and Chakrabarty, A. M., 1984, Cloning of genes controlling alginate biosynthesis from a mucoid cystic fibrosis isolate of *Pseudomonas aeruginosa*, *J. Bacteriol.* **159**:9–18.
56. Deretic, V., and Konyecsni, W. M., 1990, A procaryotic regulatory factor with a histone H1-like carboxy-terminal domain: Clonal variation of repeats within algP, a gene involved in regulation of mucoidy in *Pseudomonas aeruginosa*, *J. Bacteriol.* **172**:5544–5554.
57. Kato, J., Misra, T. K., and Chakrabarty, A. M., 1990, AlgR3, a protein resembling eukaryotic histone H1, regulates alginate synthesis in *Pseudomonas aeruginosa*, *Proc. Natl. Acad. Sci. USA* **87**:2887–2891.
58. Konyecsni, W. M., and Deretic, V., 1990, DNA sequence and expression analysis of algP and

algQ, components of the multigene system transcriptionally regulating mucoidy in *Pseudomonas aeruginosa:* algP contains multiple direct repeats, *J. Bacteriol.* **172:**2511–2520.
59. Mohr, C. D., and Deretic, V., 1990, Gene-scrambling mutagenesis: generation and analysis of insertional mutations in the alginate regulatory region of *Pseudomonas aeruginosa, J. Bacteriol.* **172:**6252–6260.
60. Mohr, C. D., Martin, D. W., Konyecsni, W. M., Govan, J. R. W., Lory, S., and Deretic, V., 1990, Role of the far-upstream sites of the *alg*D promoter and the *alg*R and *rpo*N genes in environmental modulation of mucoidy in *Pseudomonas aeruginosa, J. Bacteriol.* **172:**6576–6580.
61. Pier, G. B., DesJardin, D., Aguilar, T., Barnard, M., and Speert, D., 1986, Polysaccharide surface antigens expressed by nonmucoid isolates of *Pseudomonas aeruginosa* from cystic fibrosis patients, *J. Clin. Microbiol.* **24:**189–196.
62. Pugashetti, K. B., Metzger, H. M., Jr., Vadas, L., and Feingold, D. S., 1982, Phenotypic differences among clinically isolated mucoid *Pseudomonas aeruginosa* strains, *J. Clin. Microbiol.* **16:**686–691.
63. Piggott, N. H., Sutherland, I. W., and Jarman, T. R., 1982, Alginate synthesis by mucoid strains of *Pseudomonas aeruginosa* PAO, *Eur. J. Appl. Microbiol. Biotechnol.* **16:**131–135.
64. Piggott, N. H., Sutherland, I. W., and Jarman, T. R., 1982, Enzymes involved in the biosynthesis of alginate by *Pseudomonas aeruginosa, Eur. J. Appl. Microbiol. Biotechnol.* **13:**179–183.
65. McArthur, H. A. I., and Ceri, H., 1983, Interaction of a rat lung lectin with the exopolysaccharides of *Pseudomonas aeruginosa, Infect. Immun.* **42:**574–578.
66. Sherbrock-Cox, V., Russell, N. J., and Gacesa, P., 1984, The purification and chemical characterization of the alginate present in the extracellular material produced by mucoid strains of *Pseudomonas aeruginosa, Carbohydr. Res.* **135:**147–154.
67. Pier, G. B., Matthews, W. J., and Eardley, D. D., 1983, Immunochemical characterization of the mucoid exopolysaccharide of *Pseudomonas aeruginosa, J. Infect. Dis.* **147:**494–503.
68. Daley, L., Pier, G. B., Liporace, J. D., and Eardley, D. D., 1985, Polyclonal B cell stimulation and interleukin 1 induction by the mucoid exopolysaccharide of *Pseudomonas aeruginosa* associated with cystic fibrosis, *J. Immunol.* **134:**3089–3093.
69. Irvin, R. T., and Ceri, H., 1985, Immunochemical examination of the *Pseudomonas aeruginosa* glycocalyx: A monoclonal antibody which recognizes L-guluronic acid residues of alginic acid, *Can. J. Microbiol.* **31:**268–275.
70. Ceri, H., McArthur, H. A. I., and Whitfield, C., 1986, Association of alginate from *Pseudomonas aeruginosa* with two forms of heparin-binding lectin isolated from rat lung, *Infect. Immun.* **51:**1–5.
71. Baker, N. R., and Marcus, H., 1982, Adherence of clinical isolates of *Pseudomonas aeruginosa* to hamster tracheal epithelium *in vitro, Curr. Microbiol.* **7:**35–40.
72. Baker, N. R., and Tao, Y., 1982, A tracheal culture model of respiratory tract infection with *Pseudomonas aeruginosa, In Vitro,* **18:**369–376.
73. Ramphal, R., and Pyle, M., 1983, Adherence of mucoid and nonmucoid *Pseudomonas aeruginosa* to acid-injured tracheal epithelium, *Infect. Immun.* **41:**345–351.
74. Marcus, H., and Baker, N. R., 1985, Quantitation of adherence of mucoid and nonmucoid *Pseudomonas aeruginosa* to hamster tracheal epithelium, *Infect. Immun.* **47:**723–729.
75. Woods, D. E., and Sokol, P. A., 1985, Use of transposon mutants to assess the role of exoenzyme S in chronic pulmonary disease due to *Pseudomonas aeruginosa, Eur. J. Clin. Microbiol.* **4:**163–169.
76. Woods, D. E., To, M., and Sokol, P. A., 1989, *Pseudomonas aeruginosa* exoenzyme S as a pathogenic determinant in respiratory tract infections, *Antibiot. Chemother.* **42:**27–35.
77. Coburn, J., Yatt, R. T., Iglewski, B. H., and Gill, D. M., 1989, Several GTP-binding proteins, including p21$^{c-h-ras}$, are preferred substrates of *Pseudomonas aeruginosa* exoenzyme S, *J. Biol. Chem.* **264:**9004–9008.

78. Woods, D. E., and Que, J. U., 1987, Purification of *Pseudomonas aeruginosa* exoenzyme S, *Infect. Immun.* **55**:579–586.
79. Lingwood, C. A., Cheng, M., Krivan, H. C., and Woods, D. E., 1991, Glycolipid receptor binding specificity of exoenzyme S from *Pseudomonas aeruginosa*, *Biochem. Biophys. Res. Comm.* **175**:1076–1081.
80. Frost, L. S., Carpenter, M., and Paranchych, W., 1978, N-methyphenylalaline at the N-terminus of pilin isolated from *Pseudomonas aeruginosa* K, *Nature* **271**:87–89.
81. Elleman, T. C., Hoyne, P. A., Stewart, D. J., McKern, N. M., and Peterson, J. E., 1986, Expression of pili from *Bacteroides nodosus* in *Pseudomonas aeruginosa*, *J. Bacteriol.* **168**:574–580.
82. Elleman, T. C., and Peterson, J. E., 1987, Expression of multiple types of N-methyl Phe pili in *Pseudomonas aeruginosa*, *Mol. Microbiol.* **1**:377–380.
83. Paranchych, W., and Frost, L. S., 1988, The physiology and biochemistry of pili, *Adv. Microbiol. Phys.* **29**:53–114.
84. Beard, M. K. M., Mattick, J. S., Moore, L. J., Mott, M. R., Marrs, C. F., and Egerton, J. R., 1990, Morphogenetic expression of *Moraxella bovis* fimbriae (pili) in *Pseudomonas aeruginosa*, *J. Bacteriol.* **172**:2601–2607.
85. Ottow, J. C. G., 1975, Ecology, physiology, and genetics of fimbriae and pili, *Ann. Rev. Microbiol.* **29**:79–108.
86. Folkhard, W., Leonard, K. R., Malsey, S., Marvin, D. A., Dubochet, J., Engel, A., Achtman, M., and Helmuth, R., 1979, X-ray diffraction and electron microscopic studies on the structure of bacterial F-pili, *J. Mol. Biol.* **130**:145–160.
87. Folkhard, W., Marvin, D.A., Watts, T. H., and Paranchych, W., 1981, Structure of polar pili from *Pseudomonas aeruginosa* strains K and O, *J. Mol. Biol.* **149**:79–93.
88. Marvin, D. A., and Folkhard, W., 1986, Structure of F-pili: Reassessment of the symmetry. *J. Mol. Biol.* **191**:299–300.
89. Frost, L. S., and Paranchych, W., 1977, Composition and molecular weight of pili purified from *Pseudomonas aeruginosa* K, *J. Bacteriol.* **131**:259–269.
90. Paranchych, W., Sastry, P. A., Frost, L. S., Carpenter, M., Armstrong, G. D., and Watts, T. H., 1979, Biochemical studies on pili isolated from *Pseudomonas aeruginosa* strain PAO, *Can. J. Microbiol.* **26**:1175–1181.
91. Pasloske, B. L., Finlay, B. B., and Paranchych, W., 1985, Cloning and sequencing of *Pseudomonas aeruginosa* PAK pilin gene, *FEBS Lett.* **183**:408–412.
92. Sastry, P. A., Finlay, B. B., Pasloske, B. L., Paranchych, W., Pearlstone, J. R., and Smillie, L. B., 1985, Comparative studies on the amino acid and nucleotide sequences of pilin derived from *Pseudomonas aeruginosa* PAK and PAO, *J. Bacteriol.* **164**:571–577.
93. Sastry, P. A., Pearlstone, J. R., Smillie, L. B., and Paranchych, W., 1985, Studies on the primary structure and antigenic determinants of pilin isolated from *Pseudomonas aeruginosa* K, *Can. J. Biochem. Cell Biol.* **63**:284–291.
94. Johnson, K., Parker, M. L., and Lory, S., 1986, Nucleotide sequence and transcriptional initiation site of two *Pseudomonas aeruginosa* pilin genes, *J. Biol. Chem.* **261**:15703–15708.
95. Pasloske, B. L, Sastry, P. A., Finlay, B. B., and Paranchych, W., 1988, Two unusual pilin sequences from different isolates of *Pseudomonas aeruginosa*, *J. Bacteriol.* **170**:3738–3741.
96. Finlay, B. B., Pasloske, B. L., and Paranchych, W., 1986, Expression of the *Pseudomonas aeruginosa* PAK pilin gene in *Escherichia coli*, *J. Bacteriol.* **165**:625–630.
97. Strom, M. S., and Lory, S., 1986, Cloning and expression of the pilin gene of *Pseudomonas aeruginosa* PAK in *Escherichia coli*, *J. Bacteriol.* **167**:367–372.
98. Johnson, K., and Lory, S., 1987, Characterization of *Pseudomonas aeruginosa* mutants with altered piliation, *J. Bacteriol.* **169**:5663–5667.
99. Strom, M. S., and Lory, S., 1987, Mapping of export signals of *Pseudomonas aeruginosa* pilin with alkaline phosphatase fusions, *J. Bacteriol.* **169**:3181–3188.
100. Pasloske, B. L., and Paranchych, W., 1988, The expression of mutant pilins in *Pseudomonas aeruginosa*: Fifth position glutamate affects pilin methylation, *Mol. Microbiol.* **2**:489–495.

101. Nunn, D., Bergman, S., and Lory, S., 1990, Products of three accessory genes, *pil*B, *pil*C, and *pil*D, are required for biogenesis of *Pseudomonas aeruginosa* pili, *J. Bacteriol.* **172**:2911–2919.
102. Watts, T. H., Sastry, P. A., Hodges, R. S., and Paranchych, W., 1983, Mapping of antigenic determinants of *Pseudomonas aeruginosa* PAK polar pili, *Infect. Immun.* **42**:113–121.
103. Dalrymple, B., and Mattick, J. S., 1987, An analysis of the organization and evolution of the type 4 fimbrial (MePhe) subunit proteins, *J. Mol. Evol.* **25**:261–269.
104. Watts, T. H., Worobec, E. A., and Paranchych, W., 1982, Identification of pilin pools in the membranes of *Pseudomonas aeruginosa*, *J. Bacteriol.* **152**:687–691.
105. Leow, M. A., Holt, S. C., and Eisenstein, B. I., 1987, Immunoelectron microscopic analysis of elongation of type 1 fimbriae in *Escherichia coli*, *J. Bacteriol.* **169**:157–163.
106. Lund, B., Lindberg, F., Marklund, B.-I., and Normark, S., 1987, The PapG protein is the a-D-galactopyranosyl-(1-4)-β-d galactopyranose-binding adhesin of uropathogenic *Escherichia coli*, *Proc. Natl. Acad. Sci. USA* **84**:5898–5902.
107. Worobec, E. A., Frost, L. S., Pieroni, P., Armstrong, G. D., Hodges, R. S., Parker, J. M. R., Finlay, B. B., and Paranchych, W., 1986, Location of the antigenic determinants of conjunctive F-like pili, *J. Bacteriol.* **167**:660–665.
108. Bradley, D. E., 1972, A study of pili on *Pseudomonas aeruginosa*, *Genet. Res.* **19**:39–51.
109. Bradley, D. E., 1974, The adsorption of *Pseudomonas aeruginosa* pilus-dependent bacteriophages to a host mutant with nonretractile pili, *Virology* **58**:149–163.
110. Bradley, D. E., and Pitt, T. L., 1974, Pilus-dependence of four *Pseudomonas aeruginosa* bacteriophages with non-contractile tails, *J. Gen. Virol.* **24**:1–15.
111. Bradley, D. E., 1980, A function of *Pseudomonas aeruginosa* PAO polar pili: Twitching motility, *Can. J. Microbiol.* **26**:146–154.
112. Fulks, K .A., Marrs, C. F., Stevens, S. P., and Green, M. R., 1990, Sequence analysis of the inversion region containing the pilin genes of *Moraxella bovis*, *J. Bacteriol.* **172**:310–316.
113. De Ree, J. M., Schwillens, P., and van den Boscht, J. F., 1987, Monoclonal antibodies raised against Pap fimbriae recognize minor component(s) involved in receptor binding, *Microb. Pathogen.* **2**:113–121.
114. Lund, B., Lindberg, F., and Normark, S., 1988, Structure and antigenic properties of the tip-located P pilus proteins of uropathogenic *Escherichia coli*, *J. Bacteriol.* **170**:1887–1894.
115. Mirelman, D., and Ofek, I., 1986, Introduction to microbial lectins and agglutinins. In: *Microbial Lectins and Agglutinins: Properties and Biological Activity* (D. Mirelman, ed.), John Wiley & Sons, Inc., New York, pp. 1–19.
116. Abraham, S. N., Goguen, J. D., Sun, D., Klemm, P. and Beachey, E. H., 1987, Identification of two ancillary subunits of *Escherichia coli* type 1 fimbriae by using antibodies against synthetic oligopeptides of *fim* gene products, *J. Bacteriol.* **169**:5530–5536.
117. Hanson, M. S., Hempel, J., and Brinton, C. C., Jr., 1988, Purification of the *Escherichia coli* type 1 pilin and minor pilus proteins and partial characterization of the adhesin protein, *J. Bacteriol.* **170**:3350–3358.
118. Mattick, J. S., Bills, M. M., Anderson, B. J., Dalrymple, B., Mott, M. R., and Egerton, J. R., 1987, Morphogenetic expression of *Bacteroides nodosus* fimbriae in *Pseudomonas aeruginosa*, *J. Bacteriol.* **169**:33–41.
119. Woods, D. E., Bass, J. A., Johanson, W.G., Jr., and Straus, D.C., 1980, Role of adherence in the pathogenesis of *Pseudomonas aeruginosa* lung infection in cystic fibrosis patients, *Infect. Immun.* **30**:694–699.
120. Woods, D. E., Straus, D. C., Johanson, W. G., Jr., and Bass, J. A., 1981, Role of salivary protease activity in adherence of gram-negative bacilli to mammalian buccal epithelial cells in vivo, *J. Clin. Invest.* **68**:1435–1440.
121. Woods, D.E., Straus, D.C., Johanson, W.G., Jr., and Bass, J.A., 1983, Factors influencing the adherence of *Pseudomonas aeruginosa* to mammalian buccal epithelial cells, *Rev. Infect. Dis.* **5**:S847–S851.

122. Ramphal, R., Small, P. M., Shands, J. W., Jr., Fischlschweiger, W., and Small, P. A., Jr., 1980, Adherence of *Pseudomonas aeruginosa* to tracheal cells injured by influenza infection or by endotracheal intubation, *Infect. Immun.* **27**:614–619.
123. Sato, H., Okinaga, K., and Saito, H., 1988, Role of pili in the pathogenesis of *Pseudomonas aeruginosa* burn infection, *Microbiol. Immunol.* **32**:131–139.
124. Irvin, R. T., Doig, P., Lee, K. K., Sastry, P. A., Paranchych, W., Todd, T., and Hodges, R. S., 1989, Characterization of the *Pseudomonas aeruginosa* pilus adhesin: Confirmation that the pilin structural protein subunit contains a human epithelial cell binding domain, *Infect. Immun.* **57**:3720–3726.
125. Lee, K. K., Doig, P., Irvin, R. T., Paranchych, W., and Hodges, R. S., 1989, Mapping the surface regions of *Pseudomonas aeruginosa* PAK pilin: The importance of the C-terminal region for adherence to human buccal epithelial cells, *Molec. Microbiol.* **3**:1493–1499.
126. Schmidt, M. A., and O'Hanley, P., 1988, Synthetic peptides corresponding to protective epitopes of *Escherichia coli* digalactoside-binding pilin prevent infection in a murine pyelonephritis model, *Proc. Natl. Acad. Sci. USA* **85**:1247–1251.
127. Ramphal, R., and Pyle, M., 1985, Further characterization of the tracheal receptor for *Pseudomonas aeruginosa, Eur. J. Clin. Microbiol.* **4**:160–162.
128. Vishwanath, S., and Ramphal, R., 1985, Adherence of *Pseudomonas aeruginosa* to human tracheobronchial mucin, *Infect. Immun.* **45**:197–202.
129. Ramphal, R., Carnoy, C., Fievre, S., Michalski, J.-C., Houdret, N., Lamblin, G., Strecker, G., and Roussel, P., 1991, *Pseudomonas aeruginosa* recognizes carbohydrate chains containing type 1 (Galβ1-3GlcNAc) or type 2 (Galβ1-4GlcNAc) disaccharide units, *Infect. Immun.* **59**: 700–704.
130. Doig, P., Paranchych, W., Sastry, P. A., and Irvin, R. T., 1989, Human buccal epithelial cell receptors of *Pseudomonas aeruginosa*: Identification of glycoproteins with pilus binding activity, *Can. J. Microbiol.* **35**:1141–1145.
131. Krivan, H. C., Roberts, D. D., and Ginsburg, V., 1988, Many pulmonary pathogenic bacteria bind specifically to the carbohydrate sequence GalNAcβ1-4Gal found in some glycolipids, *Proc. Natl. Acad. Sci. USA* **85**:6157–6161.
132. Stromberg, N., Deal, C., Nyberg, G., Normark, S., So, M., and Karlsson, K.-A., '988, Identification of carbohydrate structures that are possible receptors for *Neisseria gonorrhoeae, Proc. Natl. Acad. Sci. USA* **85**:4902–4906.
133. Karlsson, K.-A., 1989, Animal glycosphingolipids as membrane attachment sites for bacteria, *Ann. Rev. Biochem.* **58**:309–350.
134. Jimenez-Lucho, V., Ginsburg, V., and Krivan, H. C., 1990, *Cryptococcus neoformans, Candida albicans,* and other fungi bind specifically to the glycosphingolipid lactosylceramide (Galβ1-4Glcβ1-1Cer), a possible adhesion receptor for yeasts, *Infect. Immun.* **58**:2085–2090.
135. Nyberg, G., Stromberg, N., Johnsson, A., Karlsson, K.-A., and Normark, S., 1990, Erythrocyte gangliosides act as receptors for *Neisseria subflava:* Identification of the Sia-1 adhesin, *Infect. Immun.* **58**:2555–2563.
136. Wong, W. Y., Irvin, R. T., Paranchych, W., and Hodges, R. S., 1991, Antigen-antibody interactions: Elucidation of the epitope and strain-specificity of a monoclonal antibody directed against the pilin adherence domain of *Pseudomonas aeruginosa* strain K, submitted.
137. Sajjan, U., Reisman, J., Doig, P., Irvin, R. T., Forstner, G., and Forstner, J., 1991, Interaction of nonmucoid *Pseudomonas aeruginosa* with normal human intestinal mucin and respiratory mucin from patients with cystic fibrosis, *J. Clin. Invest.*, in press.
138. Irvin, R. T., 1990, Hydrophobicity of proteins and bacterial fimbriae. In: *Microbial Cell Surface Hydrophobicity* (Doyle, R. J., and Rosenberg, M., eds.), American Society for Microbiology, Washington, D.C., pp. 137–178.
139. Garner, C. V., DesJardins, D., and Pier, G. B., 1990, Immunogenic properties of *Pseudomonas aeruginosa* mucoid exopolysaccharide, *Infect. Immun.* **58**:1835–1842.

Phenazine Pigments in *Pseudomonas aeruginosa* Infection

RICARDO U. SORENSEN and FRED JOSEPH, JR.

1. INTRODUCTION

The phenazines constitute one group of chemical species among a number of groups referred to collectively as secondary metabolites of fluorescent pseudomonads. The other groups include lipids, pyrroles, indoles, amino acids and peptides, pterines, and miscellaneous compounds.[1] Phenazines are low molecular weight compounds containing a three-ringed, heterocyclic nucleus with nitrogen substitution at the center positions of 5 and 10. More than 50 naturally occurring phenazines, representing every color of the visible light spectrum, are produced by 32 bacterial species. However, among clinically significant bacteria, the production of phenazine pigments is a distinctive feature of *Pseudomonas aeruginosa*.[2] We have postulated that these small, nonantigenic metabolites may escape neutralization by antibodies and alter lung defense mechanisms in chronic *P. aeruginosa* infections.[3,4] In this chapter we will review the chemical structure and properties of phenazine pigments, their known biological effects, and their possible role in chronic *P. aeruginosa* infections.

RICARDO U. SORENSEN and FRED JOSEPH, JR. • Department of Pediatrics, Louisiana State University Medical Center, New Orleans, Louisiana 70112.

Pseudomonas aeruginosa as an Opportunistic Pathogen, edited by Mario Campa *et al.* Plenum Press, New York, 1993.

2. STRUCTURE AND CHEMICAL PROPERTIES

The phenazines may be classified into three groups according to the number of carbon substituents (0, 1, and 2) on the heterocyclic ring system. Within each group, each chemical species is identified by the position and type of end grouping attached to the phenazine nucleus. Phenazines produced by *P. aeruginosa* include pyocyanine (5-methyl-1-hydroxy phenazinium betaine), oxychlororaphine (phenazine-1-carboxamide), phenazine-1-carboxylic acid, chlororaphine (oxychlororaphine 5, 10-dihydro derivative), aeruginosin A (5-methyl-7-amino-1-carboxyphenazinium betaine), and aeruginosin B (5-methyl-7-amino-1-carboxy-3-sulphophenazinium betaine).[2] Pyocyanine (pyo) is a blue-green pigment responsible for the distinctive discoloration observed in the pus of some patients; its presence led to the original designation of *P. aeruginosa* as *Bacillus pyocyaneus*. 1-hydroxyphenazine (1-hp), a compound likely to be a decomposition product of pyo through the loss of the 5-methyl group, is found in supernatants of aged *P. aeruginosa* cultures. The structures of the parent phenazine compound, with substituent and end grouping numbering system, as well as the structures of pyo and 1-hp are shown in Fig. 1.[2] A description of the parent phenazine compound and the representative phenazines pyo and 1-hp is important to an understanding of the chemistry and biological effects of these compounds.

The parent phenazine compound has no end groupings and is uncharged. The molecular weight of phenazine is 180.2. It is insoluble in water, but is moderately soluble in alcohol and benzene. A large excess of acid protonates the compound completely, according to UV spectral studies.

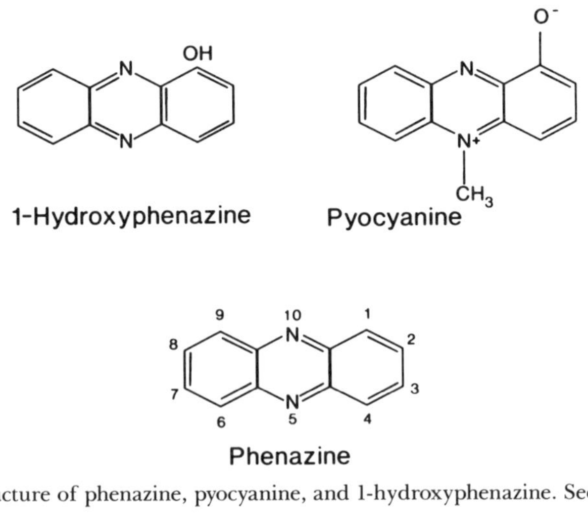

FIGURE 1. Structure of phenazine, pyocyanine, and 1-hydroxyphenazine. See text for discussion.

Using electrochemical techniques, it has been demonstrated that phenazine is reduced in both aqueous and nonaqueous media. The reduction occurs in two one-electron steps at low pH and in one two-electron step at a higher pH in an aqueous system. Phenazine does not interact with molecular oxygen or with superoxide anion in neutral, non-aqueous media. However, phenazine becomes reduced under increasing oxygen concentrations.[5] Because the relatively inactive phenazine is the parent compound for many biologically active derivatives, it points out the importance of end groupings for the chemical and biological properties of these compounds.

The molecular weight of pyo is 210.2. It forms dark blue needles in water. In solid form, pyo is stable for weeks in a dry and dark environment but decomposes on long storage. This redox dye is zwitterionic in nature, conferring solubility in aqueous and organic solvents. It is very soluble in chloroform and soluble in hot water, hot ethanol, acetone, glacial acetic acid, pyridine, phenol, and ethyl acetate. Pyo is an electron acceptor and carrier. In oxidized form, it is blue; in reduced form, it is colorless (leucopyocyanine). The reduced leucopyocyanine is oxidized rapidly by oxygen. The oxidized form of pyo resonates between two forms. A double-bonded oxygen is present in position 1 in one form. The other active, zwitterionic form has a positive charge at position 5 and a negative charge on the single-bonded oxygen at position 1 (Fig. 1). Leucopyocyanine has an ordinary hydroxyl group at position 1 with no resonance.[6]

Zaugg studied the absorption curves that result during progressive oxidation of the reduced forms of pyo and its parent compound phenazine methosulfate. He found that in water buffered to pH 7 to 8 a significant amount of free radical forms of these compounds existed. Based on these observations he concluded that oxidation or reduction through electron transfer was possible at physiological pH values.[7] In solutions of pH 7 to 8, pyo has maximum light absorption peaks at 239, 312, 379, and 690 nm.[8] Absorption spectra in acidic and basic solutions will vary. Pyo in 0.1M HCl has an absorption maximum at 520 nm and in methanol at 690 nm.[9]

The molecule 1-hp is also referred to as hemipyocyanine and 1-phenazinol in the literature. Its molecular weight is 196.2. It does not carry a charge in its structural formula. It is soluble in aqueous alkaline solutions with a purplish-red color that turns yellow on neutralization (*Merck Index*, 1989). It is slightly soluble in hot water and freely soluble in the usual organic solvents except petroleum ether. The compound has maximum absorption peaks of 210, 239, 291, 372, and 519 nm in water (Joseph and Sorensen, unpublished observations). At a pH of 1, 1-hp has maximum absorption at 273 nm and at a pH of 12, maximum absorption is at 373 nm.[10]

When acid (protons) is added to either pyo or 1-hp, these compounds exhibit the chemical characteristics of a positively charged (cationic) species. Upon addition of base (electrons), the compounds become negatively charged (anionic). The charges of the two phenazines secreted by *P.*

aeruginosa in biological fluids have not been characterized. But one may hypothesize that in neutral body fluids, pyo has an equal distribution of positive and negative charges and that 1-hp may carry no charge or a slight negative charge if a hydrogen is lost from the hydroxyl end grouping.

Cyclic volt-ammeter studies of eight phenazines and phenazine-N-oxides have shown that the more positive the reduction potential of the position 5 cationic moiety, the higher the reactive potency.[11] Pyo and other charged phenazines could function as charge transfer catalysts during aerobic oxidations of substrates. Some of the biological effects of pyo could be due to its ability to first abstract an electron from a substrate such as a protein (reduction), and then donate the electron to an acceptor such as oxygen (oxidation). Subsequently, toxic oxygen radicals could alter various cell functions.

3. PURIFICATION, SYNTHESIS, AND METHODS OF DETECTION

Pyo may be derived from cultures of *P. aeruginosa* and *Streptococcus cyanoflavus*; 1-hp has been isolated from cultures of *S. thioluteus* and *P. aureofaciens*,[2] and from aged *P. aeruginosa* cultures.[12] The most common method of extracting pyo is by chloroform.[6]

Pyo may be prepared through photooxidation of phenazine methosulfate (PMS), followed by subsequent purification steps.[13] 1-hp may be prepared from 1-methoxyphenazine[14] or by incubating pyo in 0.2M NaOH for 18 hr at 20°C.[9] The molecule 1-hp may appear as a by-product in the preparation of pyo.

Several methods are available to detect pyo. Direct detection in bacterial cultures is facilitated by a pyo-fluorescein agar that is a specific indicator for pyo and pyoverdin, detected as a yellow pigment.[15] In culture supernatants and biological fluids, pyo may be detected by thin-layer chromatography (TLC), gas chromatography (GC)–mass spectrometry, and high-performance liquid chromatography (HPLC). TLC is a quick, accurate, and inexpensive method for separating and identifying different phenazines. Using long-wave and short-wave ultraviolet light and staining with iodine vapors, pyo, 1-hp, and many small molecular weight compounds of less than 10,000 Da can be detected and separated from *P. aeruginosa* culture supernatant filtrates using Whatman LK6F silica gel plates and a solvent system of chloroform: methanol(9:2). The limit of sensitivity in a sample of 0.1 ml is 0.2 µg (10 µM) for pyo and 1.5 µg (75 µM) for 1-hp.[16]

HPLC is a useful tool to measure some phenazine pigments. However, it also has limitations imposed by the chemical nature of the different phenazines. Some phenazines can be separated using a modification of the method described by Heyes and Salmon for phenothiazines.[17] Using a reversed-phase, C18, 250 × 4.6 mm analytical column with a gradient elution starting at 26% acetonitrile:74% H2O:0.2% acetic acid and ending at a concentration of 90% acetonitrile with a 3% per min rise, it has been possible to separate pyocyanine, methoxyphenazine, and dimethoxyphenazine and several as yet unidentified small molecular weight compounds.[16,18] The 1-hp is not resolved in a sharp peak under these conditions.

Watson *et al.* have monitored pyo and 1-hp at 254 and 280 nm on a C18, reverse-phase, HPLC column using a linear gradient starting at 5% v/v aqueous acetic acid and ending at 40% isopropanol in aqueous acetic acid with a flow rate of 2 ml/min.[9] These authors also analyzed pyo and 1-hp using GC/mass spectrometry techniques. A 30-m, 0.25-mm internal diameter, SE54-fused silica capillary column with a temperature ramp from 100° to 280°C was used. Samples were chromatographed directly or as 3,5-bis (trifluoromethyl) benzoyl derivatives. Still, it was not possible to obtain conclusive data on pyo purified from *P. aeruginosa* cultures. The investigators concluded that there were no simple and reliable assays for pyocyanine and phenazines in complex biological matrices.

It is interesting to note that the chromatography techniques (HPLC and GC) used so far have employed column phases usually associated with the analysis of non-polar compounds. Phenazines, having charged moieties or end groupings, usually are polar. This polarity may account for some of the difficulties encountered in their analysis.

No studies have focused on the stability of pure pyo and 1-hp. In a series of experiments in the authors' laboratory, both compounds were no longer detectable by both TLC and HPLC after using aqueous standards but a few times. Pyo has been reported to be stable at pH 9 but to decompose at pH 12 into a compound whose spectral properties are the same as 1-hp and 5-ethylphenazine. In a series of experiments with 5-methylphenazine and its derivatives, it was observed that these compounds are unstable in light and alkaline solutions.[10] Although the causes for this instability were not elucidated, the authors concluded that the spectra of phenazine derivatives varies according to structural characteristics such as cationic charge (alkylation) at position 5, substitution at position 1 and combinations of these. It is possible that some of these compounds could remain biologically active even after undergoing chemical changes that may not allow their detection by TLC and HPLC.

4. REGULATION OF PHENAZINE PRODUCTION AND POSSIBLE FUNCTION

The type and quantity of phenazine pigments secreted vary considerably depending on culture conditions. However, the regulatory mechanisms and the advantages of the secretion of pigments for bacterial growth and survival are largely unknown. Pyo is probably synthesized *in toto* from shikimic acid, which is incorporated into the pyo molecule. Studies with other pigments suggest conversion from one pigment to another.[19]

The production of pyo *in vitro* is heavily regulated by the presence of nutrients in the media[20,21] and also by antibiotics, *e.g.*, chloramphenicol and erythromycin.[22] Phosphate deficiency was proposed as early as 1969 as necessary for pyo synthesis.[23] Pyo production begins when the phosphate level reaches a critical minimal level and terminates when reaching a maximal level. When the phosphate level is increased at the appropriate time, an increase in cell mass is observed.[24] At a high density of bacteria and low oxygen tension, pyo is reduced to leukopyocyanin which in turn can reduce Fe(III) and release Fe from transferrin. This observation led Cox to postulate that pyo may help *P. aeruginosa* obtain the iron needed for persistent and expanding infections.[25] However, it is not clear if iron deficiency stimulates pyo production by *P. aeruginosa*. The antibiotic effect of pyo against protozoans and several other bacteria may allow *P. aeruginosa* to survive in the intensively competitive natural soil environment.[26]

5. BIOLOGICAL EFFECTS OF PHENAZINE PIGMENTS

5.1. Effect on Bacteria

The production by *P. aeruginosa* of bactericidal substances for other bacteria was first noted over a century ago. Pyo was identified as one of the substances responsible for the antibacterial activity in *P. aeruginosa* culture supernatants by Schoental in 1941.[12] Pyo is active against gram-positive bacteria, including several common respiratory pathogens.[18,27] Most gram-negative bacteria and all pseudomonads tested are resistant to pyo. Notably, we found the respiratory pathogen *Hemophilus influenzae* to be sensitive to pyo.[18]

E. coli, a bacterium sensitive only to high concentrations of pyo,[18,27] has been used to study the effect of pyo on bacterial respiration. Hassan and Fridovich concluded that pyo diverts electron flow, increasing the production of superoxide.[28] Thus, sensitivity of bacteria to pyo would be dependent on the presence of oxygen and on the levels of superoxide dismutase and catalase capable of protecting bacteria against the toxic effects of superoxide. Baron and Rowe found that the antibiotic effect of pyo was dependent on active bacterial respiration but not necessarily on the presence of oxygen, suggesting that pyo may be active at several specific points of the respiratory chain.[27]

More recently, it has been demonstrated that oxyradicals are formed in whole cells of *E. coli* in response to pyo and other redox compounds. This was done by observing the signal damping effect exerted by exogenously added superoxide dismutase.[29] Phenazines were shown to become photoreduced intracellularly, then transported across membranes again and to subsequently reduce extracellular cytochrome C.[30]

5.2. Effect on Mitochondrial Respiration

In 1971, Armstrong and Stewart-Tul[1] were the first to identify that 1-hp inhibited uptake of oxygen by mouse liver mitochondria at a site corresponding to cytochrome B.[31] They felt that 1-hp acted as an electron shunt by accepting electrons and transporting them to a "dead end." The following year, the group produced results suggesting that pyo was demethylated by a demethylase, and the product of that demethylation, 1-hp, was responsible for the inhibition of both cytoplasmic and mitochondrial respiration.[32] Their results further showed that the amount of inhibition was controlled by the amount of chemical absorbed by the cells and the duration of exposure.

Recently it was shown that in rat hepatocytes incubated with phenazine methosulfate, the superoxide anion produced caused a substantial decrease in intracellular levels of reduced glutathione, subsequently responsible for a marked loss in protein-free sulfhydryl groups. Intracellular calcium was shown also to accumulate due to inhibition of plasma membrane Ca^{2+}–ATPase.[33]

The effect of phenazines on respiratory enzymes deserves primary consideration because it may explain many of the biological effects of phenazines. The mitochondrial outer membrane is permeable to all molecules of 10,000 Da or less. However, most compounds of this molecular size cannot permeate the impermeable inner membrane where the enzymes of the respiratory chain are imbedded. These enzymes are essential to oxidative phosphorylation responsible for the generation of most of a cell's ATP and 90% of its oxygen uptake. Pyo and other biologically active phenazines may have unique properties that allow them to gain access to the inner membrane and matrix of the mitochondrion.

5.3. Effect on Neutrophil Function

We first reported in 1987 that pyo significantly affected the generation of superoxide by human peripheral blood mononuclear leukocytes (PMN) in a dose-dependent manner.[34] Pyo at 50 μM inhibited phorbol-12-myristate-13-acetate (PMA)-induced superoxide generation by approximately 30%, whereas lower concentrations (less than 5 μM) produced a 200% enhancement of superoxide generation. In these experiments, pyo was not found to induce superoxide generation in absence of PMA. Only a minor effect was noted on the release of neutrophil granule enzymes. Muller et al. subsequently reported that pyo oxidizes NADPH to NADP+ within resting as well as activated PMN. The reduced pyo, leucopyocyanine, then crosses the plasma membrane carrying out reduction equivalents.[35] These authors found that the effect of pyo on NADPH was independent of mitochondria, and that pyo activated the hexose-monophosphate shunt in a dose-dependent manner without generating superoxide. Ras et al. found that pyo, but not hot 1-hp, increased the generation of superoxide and the rate and duration of oxygen consumption by activated PMN. However, 1-hp had a greater effect than pyo on the release of myeloperoxidase and lysozyme by activated PMN.[36] Savage et al. was able to identify 16 rimino phenazines out of 26 dihydrophenazine compounds tested that were responsible for increasing production of superoxide by N-formyl-L-methionyl-L-leucyl-L phenyl-alanine-activated neutrophils.[37] The phenazine nucleus *per se* had no effect on superoxide generation. He concluded that the degree of prooxidative activities of phenazines depended on the nature of the alkylimino group at position 2 of the phenazine core.

5.4. Effect on Cell Proliferation and Cytokine Secretion

In 1983, we first identified pyo as one of the heat-resistant factors responsible for the inhibition of lymphocyte blastogenesis caused by *P. aeruginosa* culture supernatants.[3] The strong inhibitory effect of pyo for lymphocyte blastogenesis was later confirmed by several authors.[38,39] Pyo is also capable of strongly inhibiting the proliferation of malignant cell lines measured both by thymidine incorporation and increases in cell numbers.[40] Interestingly, inhibitory effect of pyo on lymphocyte blastogenesis is not due to cytotoxicity, and normal and malignant cells recover their ability to proliferate after washing and resuspension in fresh culture medium.[3,38,40] Lower doses of pyo consistently produce a small (5–20%) enhancement of lymphocyte proliferative responses.[18,39,40]

At certain concentrations pyo is less inhibitory for cytokine secretion than for DNA replication and cell division. We found that 50 µM pyo inhibited lymphocyte proliferation and also the expression of interleukin 2 (IL-2) receptors and the secretion of IL-2.[41] Muhlradt et al. found that 12.5 µM pyo totally inhibited cell proliferation. However, RNA and protein synthesis was only partially inhibited and IL-2 synthesis was not altered.[38] Ulmer et al. recently reported that lipopolysaccharide-induced IL-1 and tumor necrosis factor α secretion by monocytes was markedly enhanced by pyo.[39] The increase of CR1 and CR2 complement receptor expression on activated monocytes is not altered by pyo.[42] This finding suggests that translocation of surface receptors from intracellular pools that do not require *de novo* protein synthesis is not susceptible to the effects of pyo.

Lymphocyte blastogenesis is also inhibited by 1-hp, but larger concentrations than pyo, e.g. 100 µM, are required to inhibit $\geq$ 95% of thymidine incorporation.[18] Interestingly, the proliferation of malignant cells is largely resistant to inhibition by 1-hp.[40]

Pyo inhibits mitogen-induced lymphocyte blastogenesis at a step past the initial increase in free cytosolic Ca^{2+}, whereas 1-hp inhibits the increase in free cytosolic Ca^{2+}. Not surprisingly, a synergistic effect has been observed when minimally inhibitory doses of pyo and 1-hp are combined (5 µM pyo and 50 µM 1-hp) (Sorensen and Waller, unpublished observations). It is not clear if the difference in activity between pyo and 1-hp reflects different binding sites within the cell, or if the distribution within cells is similar for both pigments, but their activity differs due to their different chemical properties. Synthetic phenazines with side chains that are not water soluble do not inhibit lymphocyte blastogenesis,[18] indicating that a charged moiety on the phenazine molecule is required for inhibition of cell proliferation.

Recent studies with ^{3}H-pyo revealed that 3.5% of the added counts remained bound to cells after centrifugation through silicone oil. Washing of the cell pellet six times decreased the cell-bound fraction to 1% of the original amount, a finding consistent with the reversibility of the inhibitory effect of pyo. Scatchard plot analysis of ^{3}H-pyo binding to lymphocytes suggests the presence of a component of high affinity and low capacity and a "nonspecific" component of much higher capacity and much lower affinity.[40] Further studies are required to determine the exact site(s) of intracellular binding, and to determine if the low and/or high affinity binding sites are responsible for the inhibition of cell proliferation.

Pyo and 1-hp are not the only secondary metabolites responsible for inhibition of cell proliferation in *P. aeruginosa* culture supernatants. Pyo is secreted relatively late in *P. aeruginosa* cultures, and 1-hp is likely to be a breakdown product of pyo. We have detected small molecular weight, heat-resistant inhibitors for lymphocyte proliferation in early *P. aeruginosa* culture supernatants, before inhibitory concentrations of pyo and/or 1-hp are detected.[43] Furthermore, we found that low molecular weight components (≤10,000 Da) from all of 23 broth culture filtrates from *P. aeruginosa* strains inhibited ≥80% of lymphocyte blastogenic responses to mitogens, although only 50% of these culture filtrates contained detectable amounts of pyo.[16] Fractionation of low molecular weight filtrates of these supernatants suggested that the inhibition of lymphocyte proliferation results from the combined effect of several low molecular weight metabolites that have not been identified (Sorensen, unpublished observations).

5.5. Effect on Ciliary Beating

P. aeruginosa culture filtrates obtained after 18 hr have been shown to slow human ciliary beat frequency of nasal ciliated epithelium *in vitro*.[44] Pyo accounted for a significant proportion of this activity. Concentrations ≥ 20 μM pyo caused a gradually increasing ciliostasis over a period of 4 hr. In contrast, 10 to 50 μM 1-hp had a dose dependent, immediate inhibitory effect on ciliary beat frequency, which gradually diminished over the 4-hr observation period.[45] Direct intratracheal instillation of 200 ng pyo into anesthetized guinea pigs caused a 38% inhibition of tracheal mucus velocity at 2 hr, with a decreasing inhibitory effect after 3 hr. A dose of 600 ng produced 60% inhibition without signs of recovery over a 3-hr observation period. Confirming observation *in vitro*, doses ≥100 ng of 1-hp produced an immediate, reversible inhibition of tracheal mucus velocity. Combination of pyo and 1-hp produced an immediate inhibition equivalent to the effect of 1-hp alone, and a late response greater than expected with pyo alone.[46]

5.6. Intratracheal Instillation of Pyocyanine *in Vivo*

The inhibitory effect of pyo on ciliary beating,[46] and the increased secretion of tumor necrosis factor α by activated monocytes in presence of pyo[39] suggested that intratracheal instillation of pyo would produce an inflammatory response and/or enhance colonization with *P. aeruginosa*. When we instilled 0.5 ml of 50 μM pyo or phosphate buffered saline (PBS) into trachea of rats, pyo alone did not induce secretion of tumor necrosis factor measured in bronchoalveolar lavage fluid after 2 hr. Ninety-eight percent of cells obtained after 4 hr were alveolar macrophages, showing that no inflammation and PMN influx had occurred. When aerosolized *P. aeruginosa* was given 30 min after pyo, the percent of PMN and of viable bacteria after 4 hr was almost identical in rats given pyo and in the PBS control group (Nelson and Sorensen, unpublished observations). These results suggested that pyo may be rapidly absorbed *in vivo*, and led to our exploration of possible vascular reactivity of pyo.

5.7. Effect on Vascular Reactivity

Pyo added to isolated pulmonary arterial and venous rings with intact endothelium causes contractions.[47] These findings suggest that during pulmonary infection with *P. aeruginosa*, the release of pyo may markedly alter the distribution of blood flow and the relationship of ventilation to perfusion.

6. PHENAZINE PIGMENTS IN *PSEUDOMONAS* INFECTIONS

6.1. Presence of Phenazine Pigments at Sites of Infection

In the pre-antibiotic era, the dressings of burns that were infected with *P. aeruginosa* were often noted to have a blue-green color due to the presence of pyo. In 1953, Cruickshank and Lowbury noted that pyo was likely to cause local toxicity when soaked wound dressings acted as a reservoir for this pigment. However, he emphasized that intradermal injection of pyo was well tolerated, possibly due to rapid absorption into the circulation.[48]

Presently, chronic *P. aeruginosa* infections are seen almost exclusively in the lung. We detected pyo in supernatant filtrates from six of 11 *P. aeruginosa* isolates from cystic fibrosis (CF) patients, and in seven of the 12 non-CF sputum strains.[16] However, the presence of pyo in *P. aeruginosa* culture supernatants *in vitro* may not reflect its production *in vivo*. For instance, sputa from CF patients tend to be acidic and the composition of different nutrients and presence of antibiotics may contribute to substantial alterations in expression of the *P. aeruginosa* phenotype.[49–51] In most instances, pus produced in *P. aeruginosa* lung infections ranges in color from green to brown, *i.e.*, similar to that observed in *P. aeruginosa* cultures containing mixtures of phenazine pigments with or without pyo. We have examined freshly collected sputum samples from *P. aeruginosa* infected patients for the presence of phenazine pigments. TLC and HPLC analysis revealed the presence of multiple compounds with mobility identical to those compounds present in *P. aeruginosa* culture supernatants.[16] Pyo, at concentrations between 7 and 30 μM, was found in two of the nine CF samples, and in five of the eight non-CF samples. Wilson and coworkers reported finding pyo and 1-hp in the sol phase of sputa from three of five CF patients and six of 13 patients with bronchiectasis.[52] The differences in pyo detection may be explained by different *P. aeruginosa* strains, different antibiotic treatment regimes and/or different sample collection and processing techniques.

6.2. Role of Phenazines in Chronic *P. aeruginosa* Infections

Because the small molecular weight phenazines are unlikely to be antigenic, they are ideal candidates to bypass host defenses in chronic infections and contribute to the persistence of these infections. However, pyo is probably not involved in the initial colonization of the respiratory tract by *P. aeruginosa*. It is found in biologically active concentration only after prolonged culture periods; furthermore, its effect on ciliary beat frequency is delayed. The combined effect of pyo and 1-hp on tracheal mucus velocity, which was found to be most effective in anesthetized guinea pigs, probably does not occur in the early phases of *P. aeruginosa* colonization. Furthermore, as suggested by our experiments with pyo *in vivo*, it is possible that these small metabolites diffuse rapidly from sites of infection.

The concentration of phenazine pigments, as well as that of all other *P. aeruginosa* products, is likely to vary at different lung sites, creating gradients that may cause heterogeneous, sometimes opposing effects on immune cells in the bronchial lumen and bronchial wall. These substances may inhibit cellular immunity and other cellular functions in close proximity to bacterial colonies, and contribute to the acceleration of the inflammatory reaction in the bronchial wall, at a distance from areas of bacterial growth. The full spectrum of biological activities of these compounds needs to be further defined, to determine their role in phagocytic and inflammatory processes.

7. CONCLUDING REMARKS

The regulation and significance of the production of phenazine pigments by *P. aeruginosa* remain poorly understood. Although there is growing information on the various biological effects of some representative phenazines, their role in *P. aeruginosa* infections remains speculative and further research is required for its clarification. Another important area of research is the use of phenazines as tools to understand the susceptibility of different cell activation pathways to enhancement or inhibition by changes in cell respiration.

The difference in activity of different phenazines seems to be linked to their capability of acting as electron carriers and the generation of toxic oxygen radicals. Pyo, due to its zwitterionic structure, seems to be uniquely suited for both enhancing and inhibitory effects on cell function. Although oxygen radicals must be given prime importance in mediating cellular inhibition, we also have discussed evidence for other metabolic activities through which phenazines may alter cell function.

The passage of the phenazines into and out of cellular membranes is an area that has been only lightly explored. In a model that may be relevant for some of the phenazines, it has been shown that positively charged, zwitterionic amino acids have favored entry into voltage negative cells.[53] In addition, the generation of free oxygen radicals by phenazines may alter cell permeability. In red blood cells, it has been shown that nonselective pores may be formed in the membrane as a result of damage caused by oxygen radicals.[54] A remarkable aspect of the effect of phenazines on cell function is the lack of cell cytotoxicity and reversibility. Therefore, the damage caused by these substances must be contained to allow cell survival. A possible mechanism for the containment of damage caused by free radicals is their binding to metallic ions, *e.g.* Mg^{2+}.[55]

All aspects of phenazine production, structure, and biological function discussed in this chapter deserve further investigation. A better understanding of *P. aeruginosa* phenazine pigments is clearly liked to an enhanced understanding of both bacterial and mammalian cell biology.

REFERENCES

1. Leisinger, T., and Margraff, R., 1979, Secondary metabolites of the fluorescent pseudomonads, *Microbiol. Rev.* **43**:422–442.
2. Turner, J., and Messenger, A., 1986, Phenazine pigment production, *Adv. Microb. Physiol.* **27**:211–275.
3. Sorensen, R. U., Klinger, J. D., Cash, H. A., Chase, P. A., and Dearborn, D. G., 1983, In vitro inhibition of lymphocyte proliferation by *Pseudomonas aeruginosa* phenazine pigments, *Infect. Immun.* **41**:321–330.
4. Sorensen, R. U., 1984, Immune responses to pseudomonas and other bacteria in cystic fibrosis patients, in: *Immunological Aspects of Cystic Fibrosis* (E. Shapira, ed.), CRC Press, Boca Raton, Fla., pp. 101–123.
5. Sawyer, R., and Komai, R., 1972, Electrochemistry of phenazine at a platinum electrode in aprotic solvents, *Anal. Chem.* **44**:715–722.
6. Swan, G., and Felton, D., 1972, *The Chemistry of Heterocyclic Compounds, Phenazines*, Wiley (Interscience), New York, N.Y., pp. 174–192.

7. Zaugg, W., 1964, Spectroscopic characteristics and some chemical properties of n-methylphenazinium methyl sulfate (phenazine methosulfate) and pyocyanine at the semiquinoid oxidation level, *J. Biol. Chem.* **239:**3964–3969.
8. Dawson, R., Elliott, D., Elliott, W., and Jones, K., 1989, *Data for Biochemical Research*, Oxford Press, New York, N.Y., pp. 357.
9. Watson, D., MacDermot, J., Wilson, R., Cole, P. J., and Taylor, G. W., 1986, Purification and structural analysis of pyocyanin and 1-hydroxyphenazine, *Eur. J. Biochem.* **159:**309–312.
10. Yomo, T., Sawai, H. Urabe, I., Yamada, Y., and Okada, H., 1989, Synthesis and characterization of 1-substituted 5-alkylphenazine derivatives carrying functional groups, *Eur. J. Biochem.* **179:**293–298.
11. Crawford, P. Scamehorn, R., Hollstein, U., Ryan, M., and Kovacic, P., 1986, Cyclic voltammetry of phenazines and quinoxalines including mono and di-n-oxides. Relation to structure and antimicrobial activity, *Chem. Biol. Interact.* **60:**67–84.
12. Schoental, R., 1941, The nature of the antibacterial agents present in *Pseudomonas pyocyanea* cultures, *Br. J. Exp. Pathol.* **22:**137–147.
13. Knight, M., Hartman, P., Hartman, Z., and Young, V., 1979, A new method of preparation of pyocyanine and demonstration of an unusual bacterial sensitivity, *Anal. Biochem.* **95:** 19–23.
14. Surrey, A., 1946, *Organic Synthesis* **26:**86–87.
15. Gill, V., and Stock, F., 1987, Medium for the simultaneous detection of pyocyanin and fluorescein pigments of *Pseudomonas aeruginosa*, *Am. J. Clin. Pathol.* **88:**110–112.
16. Sorensen, R. U., Waller, R. L., and Klinger, J. D., 1991, Infection and immunity to *Pseudomonas*, *Clin. Rev. Allergy* **9:**47–74.
17. Heyes, W. F., and Salmon, J. R., 1978, Some aspects of the high-performance liquid chromatography of fluophenazine and its esters, *J. Chromatogr.* **156:**309–316.
18. Sorensen, R. U., and Klinger, J. D., 1987, Biological effects of *Pseudomonas aeruginosa* phenazine pigments, *Antibiot. Chemother.* **39:**113–124.
19. Ingledew, W. M., and Campbell, J. J. R., 1969, Evaluation of shikimic acid as a precursor of pyocyanine, *Can. J. Microbiol.* **15:**535–541.
20. Byng, G. S., Eustice, D. C., and Jensen, R. A., 1979, Biosynthesis of phenazine pigments in mutant and wild type cultures of *Pseudomonas aeruginosa*, *J. Bacteriol.* **138:**846–852.
21. Whooley, M. A., and McLoughlin, A.J., 1982, The regulation of pyocyanine production in *Pseudomonas aeruginosa*, *Eur. J. Appl. Microbiol. Biotechnol.* **15:**161–166.
22. Schneierson, S. S., Amsterdam, D., and Perlman, E., 1960, Inhibition of *Pseudomonas aeruginosa* pigment formation by chloramphenicol and erythromycin, *Antibiot. Chemother.* **19:**30–33.
23. Ingledew, W. M., and Campbell, J. J. R., 1969, A new resuspension medium for pyocyanine production, *Can. J. Microbiol.* **15:**595–598.
24. Ingram, J., and Blackwood, A., 1970, Microbial production of phenazines, *Adv. Appl. Microbiol.* **13:**279–280.
25. Cox, C. D., 1986, Role of pyocyanin in the acquisition of iron from transferrin, *Infect. Immun.* **52:**263–270.
26. Rhame, F. S., 1980, The ecology and epidemiology of *Pseudomonas aeruginosa*, in: Pseudomonas aeruginiosa (L. D. Sabath, ed.), Hans Huber, Bern., pp. 31–51.
27. Baron, S. S., and Rowe, J. J., 1981, Antibiotic action of pyocyanin, *Antimicrob. Agents Chemother.* **20:**814–820.
28. Hassan, H. M., and Fridovich, I., 1980, Mechanism of the antibiotic action of pyocyanine, *J. Bacteriol.* **141:**156–163.
29. Schellhorn, H., Pou, S., Moody, C., and Hassan, H. H., 1989, An electron spin resonance study of oxyradical generation in superoxide dismutase- and catalase-deficient mutants of *Escherichia coli* K-12, *Arch. Biochem. Biophys.* **271:**323–331.
30. Martin, J., and Logsdon, N., 1987, Oxygen radicals are generated by dye-mediated intra-

cellular photooxidations: A role for superoxide in photodynamic effects, *Arch. Biochem. Biophys.* **256:**39–49.
31. Armstrong, A. V., and Stewart-Tull, D. E. S., 1971, The site of the activity of extracellular products of *Pseudomonas aeruginosa* in the electron-transport chain in mammalian cell respiration, *J. Med. Microbiol.* **4:**263–269.
32. Stewart-Tull, D. E. S., and Armstrong, A. V., 1972, The effect of 1-hydroxyphenazine and pyocyanin from *Pseudomonas aeruginosa* on mammalian cell respiration, *J. Med. Microbiol.* **5:** 67–73.
33. Maridonneau-Parini, I., Mirabelli, F., Richelmi, P., and Bellomo, G., 1986, Cytotoxicity of phenazine methosulfate in isolated rat hepatocytes is associated with superoxide anion production, thiol oxidation, and alterations in intracellular calcium ion homeostatis, *Toxicol. Lett.* **31:**175–181.
34. Miller, K. M., Dearborn, D. G., and Sorensen, R. U., 1987, *In vitro* effect of synthetic pyocyanine on neutrophil superoxide production, *Infect. Immun.* **55:**344–346.
35. Muller, P., Krohn, K., and Muhlradt, P., 1989, Effects of pyocyanine, a phenazine dye from *Pseudomonas aeruginosa*, on oxidative burst and bacterial killing in human neutrophils, *Infect. Immun.* **57:**2591–2596.
36. Ras, G., Anderson, R., Taylor, G. W., Savage, J., Van Niekerk, E., Wilson, R., and Cole, P. J., 1990, Proinflammatory interactions of pyocyanin and 1-hydroxyphenazine with human neutrophils *in vitro*, *J. Infect. Dis.* **162:**178–185.
37. Savage, J., O'Sullivan, J., Zeis, B., and Anderson, R., 1989, Investigation of the structural properties of dihydrophenazines which contribute to their pro-oxidative interactions with human phagocytes, *J. Antimicrob. Chemother.* **23:**691–700.
38. Muhlradt, P. F., Tsai, H., and Conradt, P., 1986, Effects of pyocyanine, a blue pigment from *Psuedomonas aeruginosa*, on separate steps of T cell activation: Interleukin 2 (IL-2) production, IL-2 receptor formation, proliferation and induction of cytolytic activity, *Eur. J. Immunol.* **16:**434–440.
39. Ulmer, A. J., Pryjma, J., Tarnok, Z., Ernst, M., Flad, H.-D., 1990, Inhibitory and stimulatory effects of *Pseudomonas aeruginosa* pyocyanine on human T and B lymphocytes and human monocytes, *Infect. Immun.* **58:**808–815.
40. Sorensen, R. U., Fredricks, D., Waller, R. L., 1991, Inhibition of normal and malignant cell proliferation by pyocyanine and 1-hydroxyphenazine, *Antibiot. Chemother.*, in press.
41. Nutman, J., Berger, M. Chase, P. A., Dearborn, D. G., Miller, K. M., Waller, R. L., and Sorensen, R. U., 1987, Studies of the mechanism of T cell inhibition by the *Pseudomonas aeruginosa* phenazine pigment pyocyanine, *J. Immunol.* **138:**3481–3487.
42. Berger, M., Sorensen, R. U., Tosi, M., Dearborn, D., and Döring, G., 1989, Complement receptor expression on neutrophils at an inflammatory site, the *Pseudomonas*-infected lung in cystic fibrosis, *J. Clin. Invest.* **84:**302–1313.
43. Sorensen, R. U., Bajaksouzian, S. Konstan, E., Ward, E., and Waller, R. L., 1988, Early secretion of lymphocyte inhibitors by *Pseudomonas aeruginosa in vitro*, *Pediatr. Pulmonol.* (Suppl.) **2:**118.
44. Wilson, R., Roberts, D., and Cole, P., 1985, Effect of bacterial products on human ciliary function *in vitro*, *Thorax* **40:**125–131.
45. Wilson, R., Pitt, T., Taylor, G. W., Watson, D., MacDermot, J. Sykes, D. Roberts, D. and Cole, P. J., 1987, Pyocyanin and 1-hydroxyphenazine produced by *Pseudomonas aeruginosa* inhibit the beating of human respiratory cilia *in vitro*, *J. Clin. Invest.* **79:**221–229.
46. Munro, N., Barker, A., Rutman, A., Taylor, G. W., Watson, D., McDonald-Gibson, W., Towart, R., Taylor, W., Wilson, R., and Cole, P. J., 1989, Effect of pyocyanin and 1-hydroxyphenazine on *in vivo* tracheal mucus velocity, *J. Appl. Physiol.* **67:**316–323.
47. Arena, F., Baiqiang, C., Sorensen, R. U., Hyman, A., and Lippton, H., 1990, Pyocyanine: A bacterial product with novel vascular properties, *Circulation* **82:**111–121.

48. Cruickshank, D. N. D., and Lowbury, E. F. L., 1953, The effect of pyocyanin on human skin cells and leucocytes, *Br. J. Exp. Pathol.* **34**:583–587.
49. Ombaka, E. A. M., Cozens, R., and Brown, M. R. W., 1983, Influence of nutrient limitation of growth on stability and production of virulence factors of mucoid and non-mucoid strains of *Pseudomonas aeruginosa*, *Rev. Infect. Dis.* **5**:S880–S888.
50. Sokol, P. A., and Woods, D. E., 1984, Relationship of iron and extracellular virulence factors to *Pseudomonas aeruginosa* lung infections, *J. Med. Microbiol.* **18**:125–133.
51. Brown, M. K. W., Anwar, H., and Lambert, P. A., 1984, Evidence that mucoid *Pseudomonas aeruginosa* in the cystic fibrosis lung grows under iron-restricted conditions, *FEMS Microb. Lett.* **21**:113–117.
52. Wilson, R., Sykes, D. A., Watson, D., Rutman, A., Taylor, G. W., and Cole, P. J., 1988, Measurement of *Pseudomonas aeruginosa* phenazine pigments in sputum and assessment of their contribution to sputum sol toxicity for respiratory epithelium, *Infect. Immun.* **56**:2515–2517.
53. Zelikovic, I., and Chesney, R., 1989, Ionic requirements for amino acid transport, *Am. J. Kidney Dis.* **14**:313–316.
54. Wittmann, I., Past, T., Tapsonyi, Z., Horvath, T., and Javor, T., 1989, In vitro method for measurement of free radical effects: effect of PMS (phenazine methosulfate) on red blood cell membrane, *Acta Physiol. Hung.* **73**:341–345.
55. Past, T., Wittmann, I., Belagyi, J., and Javor, T., 1989, Effect of ionic milieu to the free radicals generated by phenazine methosulfate (PMS), *Acta Physiol. Hung.* **73**:347–349.

4

Regulation of Toxin A Synthesis in *Pseudomonas aeruginosa*

CHRISTINE M. SHUMARD, DANIEL J. WOZNIAK, and DARRELL R. GALLOWAY

1. INTRODUCTION

Pseudomonas aeruginosa is a classic example of an opportunistic pathogen, rarely a problem in persons with intact host-defense systems, but with remarkable ability to cause serious disease in immunocompromised patients.[1] These immunocompromised hosts often include victims with severe burns, cancer patients, and those suffering with the genetic disease cystic fibrosis (CF). Because infections caused by the organism continue to be an important cause of morbidity and mortality, *P. aeruginosa* has received a great deal of attention in the past 30 years. Although *P. aeruginosa* is not the most frequently encountered bacterial pathogen in hospital-acquired bacteremia, its case-fatality rate is routinely the highest.[2] For example, the reported mortality for *P. aeruginosa* pneumonia is as high as 50–80%.[3] Even with the development of newer antibiotics, resistance remains a problem, necessitating combined antibiotic treatment for severe *P. aeruginosa* infections. In

---

CHRISTINE M. SHUMARD • Diagnostics Division, Abbott Laboratories, Abbott Park, Illinois 60064.   DANIEL J. WOZNIAK • Department of Microbiology and Immunology, University of Tennessee, Memphis, Tennessee 38163.   DARRELL R. GALLOWAY • Department of Microbiology, The Ohio State University, Columbus, Ohio 43210-1292.

Pseudomonas aeruginosa as an Opportunistic Pathogen, edited by Mario Campa *et al.* Plenum Press, New York, 1993.

humans, the type of infection produced by *P. aeruginosa* depends on the site of infection and the host's underlying disease or injury.[4] Some infections, such as eye and ear infections, remain highly localized, whereas others, such as infections in burn victims or severely wounded or traumatized patients, frequently become systemic and cause sepsis.

Because of the seriousness of *P. aeruginosa* infections, there has been considerable interest in examining its pathogenesis. In particular, investigators have focused on identifying factors responsible for *P. aeruginosa* virulence with the aim of developing therapeutic strategies for the control of infections. Data indicate that virulence of *P. aeruginosa* is multifactorial. *P. aeruginosa* synthesizes both cellular and extracellular products that ensure its capability to infect most hosts. The former include lipopolysaccharide (LPS), pili, leukocidin, and alginate, a viscous mucopolysaccharide capsular-like product. Extracellular products include neutral and alkaline proteases, elastase, and two hemolysins: phospholipase C and a rhamnolipid hemolysin.[5,6,7] Two proteins, toxin A (ETA) and exoenzyme S (exo-S), which are adenosine diphosphate ribosyl transferases, are also secreted by *P. aeruginosa*. ETA is the most toxic product secreted by *P. aeruginosa*[8] and therefore its role in the virulence of the organism has been the subject of intense investigation. A review describing the role of exotoxins in *P. aeruginosa* infections is presented by D. R. Galloway in Chapter 6.

The role of ETA in virulence has provided the stimulus for investigations into the mechanism of its production. Regulation of ETA synthesis is a complex process involving many environmental as well as genetic factors, of which only a few have been defined precisely. We begin with a discussion of environmental influences on ETA synthesis. This will be followed by a summary of current knowledge concerning the regulation of ETA expression at the molecular level. Finally, we discuss the relationship between the environmental and genetic factors that regulate ETA synthesis.

1.1. Historical Perspectives Regarding the Regulation of Toxin A Synthesis

Before the turn of the century, Charrin[9] and Barker[10] postulated that a toxin was involved in a "bacillus pyocyaneous" disease. This hypothesis remained dormant until the 1960s when Liu and co-workers[11] discovered that the *P. aeruginosa* extracellular fraction was lethal for mice, and following intradermal injection, caused necrotic lesions in rabbits. Injection of this lethal factor into dogs resulted in severe biochemical changes that often led to shock and death. These changes included acidosis, elevated levels of catecholamines, circulatory collapse, and leukopenia. These observations were similar to those seen in animals with *P. aeruginosa* infections, suggesting the involvement of this factor in pathogenesis. In 1973, Liu *et al.*[12] purified this lethal factor from *P. aeruginosa* cultures and called it toxin A (ETA).

Iglewski and co-workers later demonstrated that ETA inhibited protein synthesis in a manner identical to diphtheria toxin fragment A.[13,14] This inhibition requires NAD+ and results in a block at an elongation step of polypeptide assembly. These studies[13,14] demonstrated that ETA catalyzes the transfer of the adenosine-5′-diphosphate-ribosyl (ADPR) moiety of NAD+ onto elongation factor 2 (EF2), resulting in the inactivation of EF2 and inhibition of protein synthesis. Interestingly, several other bacterial toxins, including diphtheria (DT), cholera (CT), and pertussis toxins (PT) and the *E. coli* heat-labile enterotoxin, have been shown to catalyze similar reactions, and constitute a family of bacterial protein toxins known as mono ADP ribosyltransferases.

2. INFLUENCE OF ENVIRONMENTAL FACTORS ON TOXIN A SYNTHESIS

In 1973, Liu *et al.* described some of the initial parameters for maximal ETA production.[15] Biochemical analysis of ETA had been made difficult by the fact that proteases produced *in vivo* during growth of *P. aeruginosa* appeared to degrade the toxin. Liu circumvented this by utilizing the nonproteolytic strain PA103, which synthesizes ETA in quantities 10-fold greater than the prototype strain PA01.[16] For reference purposes, the *P. aeruginosa* strains discussed in this chapter are shown in Table I. The factors described by Liu for efficient ETA synthesis in the hypertoxigenic PA103 strain included culturing at 32°C with vigorous aeration and the inclusion of certain amino acids, such as glutamate. Glycerol appears to be a requirement for ETA production[15,17] and its positive effect cannot be reproduced with other carbohydrates. In contrast, complex media appear to contain inhibitors of ETA synthesis, which Liu proposed to be derivatives of nucleic acids released upon heating the media. The medium eventually adopted by Liu was a dialysate of trypticase soy broth enriched with 1% glycerol and 50 mM monosodium glutamate (TSBD). This medium is still widely used for ETA production by *P. aeruginosa*.

The presence of specific cations in the culture medium also influences ETA production. Addition of calcium increases ETA yields whereas a moder-

TABLE I
Characteristics of Selected *P. aeruginosa* Strains

Strain	Genotype	Phenotype
PA103	toxA+; toxR+;	ToxR+;toxin A+ (hypertoxigenic)
PA01	toxA+; toxR+	ToxR+;toxin A+ (moderately toxigenic)
PA103-29	toxA+; toxR+;	ToxR−;toxin A+ (hypotoxigenic)

ate amount of cobalt, copper, or manganese decreases the amount of ETA produced.[17,18] Significantly, the presence of iron severely reduces ETA production.[20] Iron similarly affects the production of several other *P. aeruginosa* exoproducts, including alkaline protease, elastase, hemagglutinin, pyochelin, and pyoverdin.[19,20]

2.1. Regulation of Toxin A Production by Iron

In general, the presence of excess iron in the culture medium has been shown to inhibit yields of bacterial toxins, including DT,[21] and *Shigella dysenteriae* type I toxin.[22] Like *P. aeruginosa* ETA, these toxins are produced at maximal levels late in the bacterial growth cycle when iron is limiting. In the case of ETA synthesis, Bjorn et al.[19] reported that media supplemented with as little as 1 μg of Fe^{2+} or Fe^{3+} per ml substantially inhibited the synthesis of ETA. However, Bjorn and co-workers noted that in contrast to the deleterious effect of iron on ETA synthesis, the addition of iron to the medium stimulated *P. aeruginosa* growth.

In a later study,[20] the effect of iron on the yields of exoproducts was examined in seven *P. aeruginosa* strains. All strains demonstrated at least an 85% decrease in ETA yields when cultured in a high-iron medium containing 5 μg of iron/ml compared with a low-iron medium of 0.05 μg iron/ml. In addition, iron was shown to reduce extracellular yields of hemagglutinin, protease, and elastase, but the extent of this inhibition was strain-dependent. In high-iron medium, total extracellular protein yields were also decreased by at least 30%, in spite of the fact that the yield of cells doubled. Based on these findings, the authors concluded that yields of extracellular *P. aeruginosa* products other that ETA are also influenced by the concentration of iron in the growth medium.

Because the effect of excess iron in the culture medium on yields of protease and elastase is strain-dependent and the magnitude of inhibition of ETA synthesis in the presence of iron is similar in all *P. aeruginosa* strains tested, Sokol et al.[23] suggested that proteases and ETA are independently regulated by iron. This group isolated mutants of the prototype *P. aeruginosa* strain PA01 that were resistant to the effect of iron on yields of ETA (*toxC* mutants) or elastase (*elaC* mutants). The mutant strains were identified as iron-transport or iron-regulatory mutants. The *toxC* regulatory mutants synthesized ETA in high-iron medium, yet elastase and alkaline protease yields remained sensitive to iron regulation. Furthermore, the *elaC* regulatory mutants were resistant to the inhibitory effect of iron on elastase yields, but ETA and alkaline protease synthesis were decreased, as seen in the parent strain. These data indicate that in PA01, iron independently regulates yields of these extracellular products.

Sokol et al.[23] also suggested a possible mechanism of iron regulation on exoproduct production. According to this mechanism, *P. aeruginosa* synthesizes a series of specific product repressors that, when complexed with iron, become active and bind to the specific gene product operator(s), thereby preventing transcription and synthesis of those extracellular products. Under conditions of iron limitation, however, the repressors remain inactive and the genes are derepressed. This mechanism resembles that proposed for the iron regulation of DT.[24–27] These studies suggest that the inhibitory effect of iron is mediated through an aporepressor. This aporepressor can only function as a negative controlling factor when complexed with iron as a corepressor. In *E. coli*, the product of the *fur* gene can function as an iron-dependent repressor for the DT promoter.[27] A similar repression may also occur in *P. aeruginosa*. Prince *et al.* have recently shown that a Fur protein analogue exists in *P. aeruginosa* and that this analogue may participate in the iron regulation of ETA production.[28,29]

Studies from two independent laboratories have demonstrated that the inhibitory effect of iron is mediated through transcription of the ETA structural gene *toxA*.[30,31] In 1986, Lory published data supporting the notion that inhibition of ETA synthesis occurs at the level of *toxA* transcription. In this study, cells cultured under conditions of iron deprivation synthesized and excreted ETA during the late exponential and stationary phases of the growth cycle. The production of ETA during this period was concomitant with a sharp increase in the *toxA* mRNA pools. However, addition of iron to the medium resulted in a dramatic decrease in the synthesis of *toxA* mRNA. Because this study only measured steady-state levels of *toxA*-specific mRNA, it was not possible to determine whether the regulation by iron was at the level of transcription initiation or mRNA degradation. Since *P. aeruginosa* cultured in the presence of an iron supplement reached the stationary phase later and at higher cell densities, it was concluded that inhibition of ETA synthesis by iron was a specific regulatory effect and was not simply the consequence of an overall slowdown in cellular metabolism. It was further proposed that an iron-sensing mechanism, including iron-binding siderophores and their membrane receptors, as well as additional factors, are involved in regulating expression of the *toxA* gene.

Using an approach designed to investigate the molecular basis of iron regulation, Grant and Vasil[30] revealed that the *toxA* transcript was present only in *P. aeruginosa* cells cultured under iron-limiting conditions but not in those grown in iron-sufficient medium. The spacing of the transcript origin with respect to the initiation codon mapped in this study differed by one nucleotide.[32] The sequences immediately upstream of the proposed initiation sites did not resemble promoters of any other *Pseudomonas* genes nor the consensus sequence of *E. coli* promoters.[32] To investigate possible iron regulation of the ETA promoter, Grant and Vasil used a fusion of the *toxA* promoter to *lacZ*, the gene coding for β-galactosidase, such that β-galactosidase synthesis was under control of *toxA* promoter.[30] In this system, the *toxA* promoter directed low-level synthesis of β-galactosidase in *E. coli*, yet this synthesis was not regulated by iron. The authors therefore proposed that iron regulates the *toxA* gene in *P. aeruginosa* but not in *E. coli* and that *E. coli* either fails to recognize *toxA* transcriptional signals or lacks a factor required for iron regulation. This group also suggested that expression of ETA from the *toxA* promoter requires an activator present in *P. aeruginosa* but missing in *E. coli*.

3. GENETIC REGULATION OF TOXIN A SYNTHESIS

3.1. Evidence for an Activator

Progress has been rapid in elucidating the biochemical and physical properties of ETA; however, details concerning the regulation of its synthesis have remained elusive. Although it has been shown that various environmental factors influence the production of ETA, little is known about how these environmental signals ultimately affect ETA synthesis. In addition, environmental factors are not the sole regulators of ETA synthesis.

Several lines of evidence support the contention that ETA synthesis is regulated by factors in addition to those from the environment. Some evidence arises from the observation that the yields of ETA vary dramatically from strain to strain.[20] For example, the prototype *P. aeruginosa* strain PA01 produces approximately 10-fold less ETA than the hypertoxigenic strain PA103 (refer to Table I).[33] This effect is also observed with CT synthesis, in that varying amounts of CT are produced by different strains of *Vibrio cholerae*. In *V. cholerae*, increased CT expression is due to amplification of the CT genes in hypertoxinogenic strains.[34] However, duplication of the ETA structural gene does not appear to account for the discrepancy in the amount of ETA produced from different *P. aeruginosa* strains. The *toxA* gene, when present, exists as a single chromosomal copy in all strains of *P. aeruginosa* examined to date.[35] Furthermore, an absolute and explicit amount of ETA is produced from each strain under the same conditions of iron regulation,[35] and thus the variation in ETA production among strains appears to be independent of iron regulation. This data supports the hypothesis that a factor or factors other than iron influence ETA yields. Additionally, the iron regulation studies described previously indicate that transcription of *toxA* is specifically reduced under iron-sufficient conditions.[31] Because this effect cannot be reproduced in *E. coli*,[31] alternative factors may regulate toxin production.

When the *toxA* gene was transcribed from its own promoter in *E. coli*, the production of ETA was not observed, even in low-iron medium,[36] likely due to the lack of an *E. coli* consensus promoter in the 5'-untranslated *toxA* gene sequence. This has often been the case in the lack of expression of genes from *P. aeruginosa* in *E. coli* hosts. In eubacteria, different promoter sequences are often suggestive of a requirement for additional factors, including activators and/or repressors, to regulate expression of the gene in question.

The *toxA* gene has been mapped at about 62 min on the PAO linkage map.[37,38] In addition, three gene loci designated as *tox-1*, *tox-2*, and *tox-3* have been mapped on the PAO chromosome at approximately 26, 23, and 62 min, respectively,[39] and are believed to be ETA regulatory loci.[40] The *tox-1* or *tox-2* genes have not been cloned, whereas the *toxA* gene has been cloned and sequenced.[36] Therefore, at least three genetic loci other than *toxA* appear to be involved in ETA synthesis, and it is possible that these other genes encode regulatory factors that ultimately affect toxin A synthesis.

The first reports of a specific genetic factor involved in the regulation of ETA synthesis were provided by Hedstrom *et al.*[41-43] They isolated a chromosomal DNA fragment from the hypertoxigenic *P. aeruginosa* strain PA103 and found that it dramatically stimulated the expression of ETA when transformed into the hypotoxigenic strain PA103-29. In toxigenic *P. aeruginosa* strains transformed with a plasmid containing the cloned DNA fragment, ETA synthesis was increased 10-fold.[44] Using a combination of immunochemical and genetic approaches, Hedstrom and co-workers demonstrated that the cloned DNA fragment did not contain *toxA* and suggested that the DNA fragment encoded a factor(s) not involved in general processing or transport of ETA or other *P. aeruginosa* virulence factors. Provided with a copy of the original plasmid containing the regulatory fragment constructed by Hedstrom *et al.* (pFHK10), Frank *et al.*[44] confirmed the group's original results and designated the regulatory fragment within pFHK10 as *regA*. The regulatory gene contained within the DNA fragment (pFHK10) was subcloned and sequenced by Wozniak *et al.*,[45] thus defining a gene that was designated *toxR*, consistent with standard genetic nomenclature. The same gene was also sequenced by Hindahl *et al.* from the original plasmid[46] and thus at the present time, the *toxR* gene has also been referred to as *regA*. In subsequent studies, Wick *et al.*[47] described the presence of a second open-reading frame (ORF) present in the original plasmid produced by Hedstrom *et al.* (pFHK10), and designated this sequence *regB*. Thus, the regulatory fragment cloned by Hedstrom *et al.* and later designated as *regA* by Frank *et al.*[44] has been reported to consist of two genes, *toxR* (*regA*) and *regB*. In keeping with convention, in this chapter we use the *toxR* and *regB* designations, which refer to defined sequences corresponding to the separate genes. Inspection of the published *regB* sequence[47] shows striking homology with the amino terminus of a presumptive acetyltransferase gene[48] from *Agrobacterium tumefaciens* (W. V. Shaw, personal communication) and even greater sequence identity with the *E. coli* plasmid NR79 transposon Tn2424 chloramphenicol acetyltransferase (*cat*) gene. Significantly, the initiation codon for this presumptive *cat* gene is located 90 base pairs (bp) downstream of the reported initiation codon for *regB* and is in a different reading frame.

Because most bacterial genes do not overlap, it is highly unlikely that the short *regB* sequence codes for a protein. Based on this analysis, it appears unlikely that the published *regB* sequence influences ETA regulation. The possible participation of the acetyltransferase gene downstream of the *toxR* sequence in ETA regulation is currently being investigated.

3.2. Characterization of *toxR*: A Gene Involved in the Positive Regulation of Toxin A Synthesis

Originally, the *toxR* gene was cloned from the hypertoxin-producing strain PA103[41–43] (see section 2 and Table I). The *toxR* gene enhances ETA synthesis in several *P. aeruginosa* strains, including PA103, PA01, and PA103-29. In addition, *toxR* stimulates ETA synthesis in PA01-PR1,[49] a *toxA* mutant that produces CRM-66, an enzymatically inactive ETA.

The *toxR* gene contains a major ORF of 260 codons, which encodes a protein with a predicted molecular weight of 28,825 Da.[47] Sequence analysis indicates that the ToxR protein is composed of 47% hydrophobic and 28% uncharged polar amino acids. The ToxR protein contains clusters of hydrophobic regions, and one region appears to be at amino-acid position 135, which is highly hydrophobic. These results suggest that ToxR may be a membrane-associated protein.

To test this possibility, *toxR* was expressed in *E. coli* by cloning the gene so that its synthesis was under control of an *E. coli* promoter. A ToxR protein fusion, which includes the first 12 residues of the T7 capsid protein, displayed a molecular weight of 31 kDa, in agreement with the predicted molecular weight of ToxR (28.8 kDa) based on the DNA sequence.[50,51] Other groups have also used strategies to express ToxR in *E. coli*.[52]

Anti-ToxR antiserum was generated against the T7 capsid–ToxR protein fusion. This antiserum was used to identify both the 31-kDa fusion protein expressed in *E. coli* and native 28-kDa ToxR in *P. aeruginosa*. In the latter case, ToxR was observed in both cytoplasmic and membrane fractions of *P. aeruginosa* cells harboring a multicopy plasmid containing *toxR*. Similarly, Zimniak et al.[53] overexpressed *toxR* in *E. coli* and used the overexpressed protein to generate anti-ToxR antiserum. This antiserum localized the majority of the native ToxR protein in *P. aeruginosa* strain PA103 to the membrane fraction. However, when multiple copies of *toxR* are present in *P. aeruginosa*, ToxR is found in approximately equal amounts in the membrane and cytoplasmic fractions.

Procaryotic signal peptides generally contain basic residues near their NH_2-termini, which are often followed by stretches of hydrophobic amino acids.[54] The lack of such sequences in the predicted ToxR amino-acid sequence and the identification of the ToxR protein in both cytoplasmic and membrane fractions of *P. aeruginosa* indicate that the ToxR protein is not secreted from *P. aeruginosa*. It is unlikely that proteins involved in gene expression, such as ToxR, would be secreted, because their physiological function is clearly different from that of exported proteins. Because 47% of the amino acids in ToxR are hydrophobic in nature, the ToxR protein may be membrane-associated in *P. aeruginosa*. Although ToxR lacks long stretches of hydrophobic amino acids that could enable the protein to span a membrane, it may associate with other membrane proteins. Identification of ToxR in both cytoplasmic and membrane components supports this hypothesis. The binding affinity of ToxR with membrane proteins may be sufficiently weak for ToxR to dissociate into the cytoplasmic component during cell fractionation.

3.3. Transcriptional Analysis of the *toxR* Gene

Because transcription of *toxA* is regulated by iron, the possibility of iron regulation of *toxR* also has been investigated. An analysis of *toxR* transcript accumulation throughout the PA103 growth cycle detected two distinct *toxR* transcripts[55] and revealed that transcription of *toxR* follows biphasic kinetics.[56] One transcript, T1, occurs early in the growth cycle, followed by a smaller transcript, T2, which occurs later in the cycle. Two *toxR* transcription start sites have been mapped by primer extension analysis of the T1 and T2 transcripts.[55] The two transcripts are also differentially regulated by iron. In one study, investigators noted that the T1 transcript is not iron-regulated, yet the T2 transcript is produced only in cells grown under iron-limiting conditions, even when the *toxR* gene is present in multiple copies.[55] Sequences immediately upstream of the T2 start site are strikingly similar to promoter sequences present in the diphtheria *tox* gene promoter, which is also regulated by iron. These data suggest the presence of multiple *toxR* promoters that respond differently to cellular iron concentration. In a study that fused *toxR* sequences containing the two transcriptional start sites to reporter genes, Storey *et al.*[57] demonstrated that two separate promoters control *toxR* transcription. An upstream promoter, P1, directs the synthesis of the larger T1 transcript, whereas the P2 promoter is responsible for T2 transcription. In a recent study, Prince *et al.* demonstrated that the presence of multiple copies of the *E. coli fur* gene results in the inhibition of both *toxA* and *toxR* transcription when the gene is placed in a *Pseudomonas* host strain.[29] Interestingly, the authors conclude that the *E. coli fur* gene product inhibits *toxR* transcription from the P1 promoter that has previously been described as being immune to iron regulation,[55] and does not affect *toxR* transcription from the P2 promoter. Thus the issue of iron regulation of toxin production remains unclear and will require further study for clarification. This study also provided some evidence for the existence of a Fur homologue in *Pseudomonas*, which may be involved in iron regulation events including protease production. Clearly, cloning and analysis of the Pseudomonas *fur* homologue will provide an important contribution to our understanding of how iron regulates toxin production.

3.4. Report of a Second Gene Involved in Regulation of Toxin A Production: regB

From the data presented here, it is obvious that the product of the *toxR* gene acts as a positive regulator of ETA synthesis. However, *toxR* expression does not completely account for the varying ETA production observed in different strains of *P. aeruginosa*. The original plasmid containing the cloned *toxR* gene derived from strain PA103 and described by Hedstrom *et al*.[43] also contains a second open-reading frame later proposed to encode for a gene product called RegB.[47] Expression of *regB* on a plasmid introduced into strain PA01 was reported to enhance ETA yields fivefold. However, PA01 produces 10-fold less ETA than strain PA103 and, unlike strain PA103, was reported to lack a functional initiation codon for *regB*.[47] Thus, this report stated that introduction of the putative PA103 *regB* gene into PA01 accounts only for a partial restoration of the ability of strain PA01 to produce toxin in yields equivalent to the hypertoxigenic strain PA103. Because the cloned *toxA* genes from strains PA103 and PA01 do not reveal any major promoter differences,[32] it is not clear why the restoration of a functional *regB* gene in PA01 does not result in a greater increase in ETA synthesis. Recent work from our laboratory has questioned the validity of these results, as our results suggest no significant contribution by the *regB* sequence to ETA regulation (Shumard *et al*., unpublished observations).

The role of *regB* in ETA synthesis is not clear. The putative *regB* gene is located immediately downstream from *toxR*. The *toxR* and *regB* genes are believed to form an operon, similar to the structure of *toxR/toxS*, two regulatory genes involved in the expression of CT in *V. cholerae*.[58] *V. cholerae* ToxR is a transmembrane, DNA-binding protein that activates transcription of the CT genes. The proposed function of the ToxS protein in *V. cholerae* is to stabilize the ToxR protein conformation during its synthesis and thereby enhance its activity.[59] However, it is not known if ToxR and the putative RegB protein from *P. aeruginosa* are functionally similar to the ToxR and ToxS proteins from *V. cholerae* (see section 3.5). In addition, recent evidence has shown that the 5' coding region for an acetyltransferase gene is present in the reported *regB* sequence (W. V. Shaw, personal communication). This result, and the fact that our group was unable to repeat the results of Wick *et al*.,[47] calls into question the existence of the *regB* gene.

3.5. Mutational Analysis of Genes Involved in Toxin A Regulation

Studies in gene regulation have been aided greatly by site-specific chromosomal mutations in the genes involved in this regulation. Strains with mutations in specific genes required for ETA synthesis can be used to study ETA regulation and may also prove helpful in discerning the role of ETA in *P. aeruginosa* pathogenesis. Using a method of gene replacement termed excision marker rescue,[60] we have produced *toxA* and *toxR* insertion mutants in several *P. aeruginosa* strains by replacing the wild-type genes with *toxA* and/or *toxR* genes containing an antibiotic resistance marker. Such insertionally inactivated mutants no longer produce ETA or the ToxR protein.[50–51] Supernatants from each of the *toxA* or *toxR* mutants cultured in TSBD were recovered and analyzed for ETA. *P. aeruginosa* strains with *toxA* insertion mutations do not synthesize ETA or truncated toxin A peptides that are detectable by immunoblot or enzyme assays. Strains with an inactivated *toxR* gene produce detectable ETA, and the levels of ETA synthesized by the *toxR* mutants are strain-dependent. Therefore, *toxR* does not appear to be required for the formation of ETA but instead promotes its efficient synthesis. This data has been confirmed independently using a mutant of *P. aeruginosa* strain PA103 in which the *toxR* gene has been deleted from the chromosome. This mutant also synthesizes ETA, although at much lower levels than the parental strain (M. L. Vasil, personal communication).

The insertionally inactivated *toxA* and *toxR* mutants have been used to map the position of these genes on the *P. aeruginosa* chromosome.[51,61] The *toxA* gene locus has been mapped previously at 62 min on the PA01 chromosome[37] and this has been verified by linkage analysis using the relationship of the antibiotic resistance marker on the *toxA* gene mutant to other markers on the *P. aeruginosa* chromosome. The *toxR* gene appears to be located at a later position than *toxA* on the PA01 linkage map, between 62 and 65 min on the *P. aeruginosa* chromosome.[51] These results have been verified recently by physical mapping of the *toxA* and *toxR* genes.[62]

The phenotype of the *toxA* or *toxR* mutants also has been characterized. Both types of mutant appear physiologically identical to their parental strains based on growth rates, colony and cell morphology, susceptibility to antibiotics, and SDA/PAGE protein profile analyses (D. J. Wozniak, unpublished observations). In addition, the *P. aeruginosa toxR* mutants synthesize parental levels of pilin and elastase (D. J. Wozniak, unpublished observations). Therefore, at the present time, the *P. aeruginosa* ToxR protein does not appear to function as a global regulator analogous to the *V. cholerae* ToxR protein. In addition to its role in CT gene expression, the *V. cholerae* ToxR protein is required for synthesis of a pilus colonization factor and production of an outer-membrane protein[63] and therefore plays a central role in the coordinate transcriptional regulation of multiple *V. cholerae* virulence determinants.

3.6. The Role of *toxR* in the Regulation of Toxin A Expression

The studies described here demonstrate that *toxR* is required for efficient *toxA* expression. There are several means by which *toxR* could affect toxin A synthesis. Here we present data that suggest *toxR* acts at the level of *toxA* gene transcription to promote efficient synthesis of ETA.

Initial evidence for the involvement of *toxR* in the transcriptional activation of *toxA* was provided by mRNA dot-blot analysis. RNA isolated from the hypotoxigenic *P. aeruginosa* strain PA103-29 transformed with a plasmid containing the entire *toxR* gene, revealed elevated levels of *toxA* mRNA when compared with RNA from *P. aeruginosa* control cells containing only the vector. However, when transformed with a plasmid containing only a portion of the *toxR* gene or an insertionally inactivated *toxR* gene, the strains synthesized substantially less *toxA*-specific mRNA.[45]

Additional studies by others[28,55-57,64] have verified that ToxR affects *toxA* transcription. For example, Vasil *et al.*[28] generated a gene fusion consisting of the *toxA* promoter and a promoterless reporter gene, *lacZ*, so that the synthesis of β-galactosidase was under control of the *toxA* promoter. This type of gene fusion has been used to quantitatively assess transcriptional activity of promoters by measuring the amount or activity of the reporter protein. The *toxA* promoter–*lacZ* gene fusion was integrated into the *toxA* locus of the chromosome of both wild-type and mutant *P. aeruginosa* strains and was found to be regulated by iron analogous to ETA synthesis in these strains. When *toxR* was introduced on a multicopy plasmid in these strains, there was an increase in levels of β-galactosidase, indicating transcriptional activation from the *toxA* promoter by ToxR.

Similar analysis has been performed of the transcriptional regulation of the *toxR* gene. Investigations into the regulation of the P1 and P2 *toxR* promoters has provided insight into the potential role of *toxR* in the iron-regulated transcription of *toxA*. A summary of this work was published recently[65] and will not be discussed in detail here. From these studies, it appears that iron regulation of *toxR* is mediated through the P2 promoter, which has been associated with the late-phase transcript of *toxR* (see section 3.3). Several studies have suggested that iron regulation of *toxR* is mediated through the P2 promoter and is ultimately responsible for the iron regulation of *toxA* transcription.[57,65] This is supported by data from several laboratories. For example, Vasil *et al.*[28] reported that β-galactosidase synthesis was no longer iron-regulated in a *P. aeruginosa* strain containing a *toxA* promoter–*lacZ* gene fusion when the synthesis of the ToxR protein was under control of a heterologous promoter. A similar loss of iron regulation of ETA synthesis was observed when multiple copies of the *toxR* gene under control of a heterologous promoter were introduced into *P. aeruginosa* strain PA103 containing an inactivated *toxR* gene (C. M. Shumard, unpublished observations).

The *toxA* promoter–reporter gene fusions have also been used to determine if ToxR is necessary and sufficient for ETA synthesis. In *P. aeruginosa* strain PA103 with a functional *toxR* gene but an inactivated *toxA* gene, introduction of a *toxA* promoter–chloramphenicol acetyltransferase (*cat*) gene fusion demonstrated high levels of CAT synthesis. However, CAT synthesis was substantially, albeit not completely, reduced when the *toxA* promoter–*cat* gene fusion was introduced into a mutant PA103 strain in which the *toxR* gene had been insertionally inactivated.[62] A similar result was obtained when the *toxA* promoter–*cat* gene fusion was introduced into a mutant of strain PA01 that contains an insertionally inactivated *toxR* gene.[51,61] Thus, ToxR enhances transcription of ETA, yet, in its absence a low level of ETA is still synthesized. This provides additional evidence that ToxR is not absolutely required for ETA synthesis.

In the *toxA* promoter–reporter gene fusion studies discussed above, CAT synthesis was controlled entirely by a small DNA fragment that contains the *toxA* promoter. Because this fragment is sufficient for full promoter activity, it is reasonable to assume that binding sites are present for both a transcriptional activator and RNA polymerase. This transcriptional activator may be ToxR, a complex containing ToxR, or a protein regulated by ToxR. The existence of a DNA binding site for a regulatory protein in the *toxA* gene promoter is supported by recent data from Tsaur and Clowes,[66] who demonstrated two distinct sites for *toxA* promoter control expression of ETA synthesis. One of these regions was judged to be involved in the binding of an RNA polymerase.[66] In this study, nucleotide substitutions upstream of the proposed RNA polymerase binding site substantially reduced *toxA* expression, suggesting that a second region of the *toxA* promoter apart from the RNA polymerase binding site is required for maximal ETA synthesis. Tsaur and Clowes reasoned that the binding of an activator at the upstream site may be required for the subsequent binding of RNA polymerase. Within the sequence of the proposed activator binding site, there is a direct repeat of the DNA sequence AATCC, which may be involved in the binding of an activator protein. It is noteworthy that these are the only sites in the *toxA* gene where the nucleotide sequence AATCC is found. This direct repeat is present on the DNA fragment that directs transcription of the promoterless *cat* gene in the studies described above, and thus, it is reasonable to assume that ToxR, a complex with which ToxR is associated, or another protein that ToxR regulates, binds at these sequences, thereby facilitating the binding of RNA polymerase and activation of *toxA* transcription.

In the experiments outlined here, it appears that ToxR stimulates *toxA* transcription. Trans-acting DNA binding proteins are known to be involved in the regulation of several *E. coli* genes.[67] Because ToxR clearly is involved in the regulation of ETA synthesis, *in vitro* DNA binding studies have examined the possibility that ToxR binds to the *toxA* promoter, as computer-aided analysis of the predicted ToxR amino acid sequence revealed a helix-turn-helix DNA binding motif. In these studies, the purified T7 capsid–ToxR fusion protein failed to bind to DNA fragments containing the *toxA* promoter.[68] These results and those of others[52] suggest that ToxR is not involved directly in DNA binding at the *toxA* promoter and that ToxR acts via other means to direct the enhancement of *toxA* mRNA synthesis. The lack of DNA binding exhibited by the fusion protein should be considered a preliminary finding, due to the fact that the native ToxR protein was not used.

3.7. Evidence for Additional Factors Regulating Toxin A Synthesis

Currently, the mechanism of action of ToxR has not been elucidated. ToxR may interact with other factors to facilitate its binding to the *toxA* promoter region. Alternatively, ToxR may act indirectly on *toxA* transcription, possibly by regulating the expression of another gene, which in turn acts directly at the *toxA* promoter. In addition, the role of the putative *regB* gene product has not been defined, if the gene exists. Thus, it is reasonable to consider that other genes and gene products are involved in the regulation of ETA synthesis.

This is borne out by the observation that the combination of ToxR and the putative RegB protein does not account entirely for the strain-specific variability in ETA production. In addition, *toxA* is known to lack *E. coli* promoter consensus sequences and, like *toxR*, is poorly expressed from its own promoter in *E. coli*. Comparison of the upstream *toxR* promoter region with the *toxA* promoter reveals a significant degree of sequence similarity. Genes that lack consensus promoter regions often require an additional protein to facilitate RNA polymerase binding. Because both *toxA* and *toxR* genes lack *E. coli* consensus -10 and -35 sequences, it is possible that these similarities in the promoter elements represent binding sites for an accessory protein.

In fact, recent evidence has been demonstrated for other gene products that regulate toxin A synthesis. For example, Prince et al. recently proposed that a Fur protein analogue exists in *P. aeruginosa*.[28,29] In *E. coli*, Fur acts as a repressor of transcription by binding to specific DNA sequences only in the presence of iron.[69] In *P. aeruginosa*, multiple copies of *E. coli fur* have been shown to repress both *toxR* and *toxA* gene transcription.[29] In addition, a protein from *P. aeruginosa* is recognized by antibodies generated against *E. coli* Fur.[29] This protein may be a *P. aeruginosa* analogue of the *E. coli* Fur repressor. Further evidence for additional factors that regulate ETA synthesis is provided by Blumenthals et al.,[17] indicating that calcium and glycerol increase ETA production at the level of transcription. Thus, there is evidence for negative as well as yet undiscovered positive factors that regulate the synthesis of ETA.

We have recently examined the transcriptional activity of the *toxA* and *toxR* genes in *P. aeruginosa* strain PA01-T20, a mutant of PA01 that produces extremely low levels of ETA.[40] The mutation in strain PA01-T20 has been mapped at 23 min on the PA01 chromosome and is associated with the *tox-2* allele.[40] This mutation cannot be complemented by *toxR* or *toxA* and so appears to provide evidence for another gene associated with the production of ETA. Using gene fusions consisting of the *toxA* and/or *toxR* promoters fused to the chloramphenicol acetyltransferase gene (*cat*), we have examined the transcriptional activity from the *toxA* and *toxR* promoters in strain PA01-T20. Our results indicate that transcription from the *toxR* promoter is normal in strain PA01-T20, but there is little or no transcription from the *toxA* promoter. This result suggests that another protein besides ToxR regulates ETA transcription, and that this protein acts in conjunction with ToxR to increase ETA synthesis.[70]

4. SUMMARY AND CONCLUSIONS

The synthesis of ETA by *P. aeruginosa* is highly regulated and involves several environmental factors, genes, and gene products. At least two activator proteins, ToxR and RegB, have been reported to act to increase the synthesis of the ETA structural gene, *toxA*, in some manner not yet understood. We are currently questioning the validity of the *regB* results and the existence of the *regB* gene as reported by Wick *et al.*[47] At the present time, it is not known if ToxR alone binds to the promoter or regulatory regions of the *toxA* gene. This does not rule out the possibility that ToxR requires other factors in order to bind to *toxA*. In fact, ToxR may act indirectly to increase *toxA* transcription. Therefore, ToxR may function by one of several possible mechanisms. For example, ToxR may regulate the expression or activation of another protein that is more directly involved in ETA transcription. In this case, ToxR may function as a sensor molecule, possibly exerting its effect on the target molecule that activates transcription. However, ToxR does not possess sequence similarity to any of the known bacterial sensor proteins, including ToxR from *V. cholerae* (D. J. Wozniak, unpublished observations). Another possibility is that ToxR acts as an alternative sigma factor to activate *toxA* gene transcription. In any case, because ToxR does not appear to function as a global regulator of *P. aeruginosa* virulence factors, its effect is most likely specific with regard to activation of *toxA* gene transcription. The synthesis of ETA is also tightly regulated by iron and this effect is exerted at the transcriptional level. Iron regulation of *toxR* transcription partially accounts for the iron regulation of ETA synthesis. However, in the absence of a functional *toxR* gene, the synthesis of ETA is still inhibited by iron (M. L. Vasil, personal communication). In addition, even in the absence of functional *toxR* or *regB* genes, ETA is expressed in *P. aeruginosa* under low-iron conditions.[51] Therefore, *toxR* does not appear to be essential for the production of ETA but instead promotes its optimal synthesis.

There is also ample evidence that factors in addition to ToxR regulate ETA synthesis. Evidence for a *P. aeruginosa* Fur analogue supports the contention that both positive and negative regulators influence ETA production. Definitive involvement of an additional regulatory factor, suggested by our studies with strain PA01-T20, awaits additional evidence from studies in progress. The possibility that ETA production is controlled by both activators and repressors is not surprising, considering that its synthesis is highly regulated. Optimal synthesis of ETA in the laboratory occurs during the stationary phase of growth, under specified conditions of temperature, aeration, amino acid content, iron and magnesium concentrations, and carbon source. In fact, the ability to detect conditions of nutrient deprivation may be an important sensing mechanism, allowing an opportunistic pathogen to induce a number of virulence factors when growth conditions are suboptimal, such as in the human host. This mechanism of regulation is seen in a number of pathogenic microorganisms. ETA synthesis appears to be independent of the regulation of any other *P. aeruginosa* virulence factors. This observation supports the concept that *P. aeruginosa* pathogenesis is multifactorial and that virulence is not dependent on a single component. Further analysis of the factors involved in ETA synthesis to determine their precise role in ETA regulation will provide a more complete knowledge of the pathogenicity and basic biology of *P. aeruginosa*.

REFERENCES

1. Bodey, G. P., Bolivar, R., Fainstein, V., and Jadeja, L., 1983, Infections caused by *Pseudomonas aeruginosa*, *Rev. Infect. Dis.* **5**:279–313.
2. Bryan, C. S., Reynolds, K. L., and Brenner, E. R., 1983, Analysis of 1,186 episodes of gram negative bacteremia in non-university hospitals: the effect of antimicrobial therapy, *Rev. Infect. Dis.* **5**:629–638.
3. Pennington, J. E., Reynolds, H. Y., and Carbone, P. P., 1973, Pseudomonas pneumonia: a retrospective study of 36 cases, *Am. J. Med.* **55**:155–160.
4. Wood, R. E., 1976, Pseudomonas: The compromised host, *Hosp. Pract.* **11**:91–100.
5. Pier, G. B., 1985, Pulmonary disease associated with *Pseudomonas aeruginosa* in cystic fibrosis: current status of host- bacterium interaction, *J. Infect. Dis.* **151**:575–580.
6. Nicas, T. I., and Iglewski, B. H., (eds.) 1986, Toxins and virulence factors of *Pseudomonas aeruginosa*, in: *The Bacteria*, Vol. X, Academic Press, New York, pp. 195-213.
7. Cross, A. S., 1985, Evolving epidemiology of *Pseudomonas aeruginosa* infections, *Eur. J. Clin. Microbiol.* **4**:156–159.
8. Liu, P. V., 1974, Extracellular toxins of *Pseudomonas aeruginosa*, *J. Infect. Dis.* (Suppl.) **130**: 94–99.
9. Charrin, A., 1889, La maladie pyocyanique, *Paris*.
10. Barker, L. F., 1897, The clinical symptoms, bacteriologic findings and post-mortem appearances in cases of infection of human beings with bacillus pyocyaneus, *J.A.M.A.* **29**:213–216.
11. Liu, P. V., Abe, Y., and Bates, I. J., 1961, The roles of various fractions of *Pseudomonas aeruginosa* in its pathogenesis, *J. Infect. Dis.* **108**:218–228.
12. Liu, P. V., Yoshii, S., and Hsieh, H., 1973, Exotoxins of *Pseudomonas aeruginosa* II. Concentration, purification, and characterization of exotoxin A, *J. Infect. Dis.* **128**:514–519.
13. Iglewski, B. H., and Kabat, D., 1975, NAD-dependent inhibition of protein synthesis by *Pseudomonas aeruginosa* toxin, *Proc. Natl. Acad. Sci. U.S.A.* **72**:2284–2288.
14. Iglewski, B. H., Liu, P. V., and Kabat, D., 1977, Mechanism of action of *Pseudomonas aeruginosa* exotoxin A: adenosine diphosphate-ribosylation of mammalian elongation factor 2 in vitro and in vivo, *Infect. Immun.* **15**:138–144.
15. Liu, P. V., 1973, Exotoxins of *Pseudomonas aeruginosa*. I. Factors that influence the production of exotoxin A, *J. Infect. Dis.* **128**:506–513.
16. Ohman, D. E., Sadoff, J. C., and Iglewski, B. H., 1980, Toxin A-deficient mutants of *Pseudomonas aeruginosa* PA103: Isolation and characterization, *Infect. Immun.* **28**:899–908.

17. Blumentals, I. I., Skaja, A. K., Kelly, R. M., Clem, T. R., and Shiloach, J., 1987, Effect of culturing conditions on the production of exotoxin A by *Pseudomonas aeruginosa*, *Ann. NY Acad. Sci.* **506**:663–668.
18. Blumentals, I. I., Kelly, R. M., Gorziglia, M., Kaufmann, J. B., and Shiloach, J., 1987, Development of a defined medium and two step culturing method for improved exotoxin A yields from *Pseudomonas aeruginosa*, *Appl. Environ. Microbiol.* **53**:2013–2020.
19. Bjorn, M. J., Iglewski, B. H., Ives, S., Sadoff, J. D., and Vasil, M. L., 1978, Effect of iron on yields of exotoxin A in cultures of *Pseudomonas aeruginosa* PA103, *Infect. Immun.* **19**:785–791.
20. Bjorn, M. J., Sokol, P. A., and Iglewski, B. H., 1979, Influence of iron on yields of extracellular products in *Pseudomonas aeruginosa* cultures, *J. Bacteriol.* **138**:193–200.
21. Pappenheimer, A. M., Jr., 1977, Diphtheria toxin, *Annu. Rev. Biochem.* **46**:69–94.
22. VanHeynigen, W. E., and Gladstone, G. P., 1953, The neurotoxin of *Shigella shigae*. 3. The effect of iron on the production of the toxin, *Br. J. Exp. Pathol.* **34**:221–229.
23. Sokol, P. A., Cox, C. D., and Iglewski, B. H., 1982, *Pseudomonas aeruginosa* mutants altered in their sensitivity to the effect of iron on toxin A or elastase yields, *J. Bacteriol.* **151**:783–787.
24. Murphy, J. R., and Bacha, P. (eds.), 1979, Regulation of diphtheria toxin production, in: *Microbiology 1979* (D. Schlesinger, ed.), Am. Soc. Microbiology, Washington, D.C., pp.181–186.
25. Murphy, J. R., Skiver, J., and McBride, G., 1976, Isolation and partial characterization of a corynebacteriophage B, *tox* operator constitutive-like mutant lysogene of *Corynebacterium diphtheriae*, *J. Virol.* **18**:235–244.
26. Leong, D., and Murphy, J. R., 1985, Characterization of the diphtheria *tox* transcript in *Corynebacterium diphtheriae* and *Escherichia coli*, *J. Bacteriol.* **163**:1114–1119.
27. Tai, S. S., and Holmes, R. K., 1988, Iron regulation of the cloned diphtheria toxin promoter in *Escherichia coli*, *Infect. Immun.* **56**:2430–2436.
28. Vasil, M. L., Grant, C. C. R., and Prince, R. W., 1989, Regulation of exotoxin A synthesis in *Pseudomonas aeruginosa*: characterization of *toxA-lacZ* fusions in wild-type and mutant strains, *Mol. Microbiol.* **3**:371–381.
29. Prince, R. W., Storey, D. G., Vasil, A. I., and Vasil, M. L., 1991, Regulation of *toxA* and *regA* by the *Escherichia coli fur* gene and identification of a Fur homologue in *Pseudomonas aeruginosa* PA103 and PA01, *Mol. Microbiol.* **5**:2823–2831.
30. Grant, C. C. R., and Vasil, M. L., 1986, Analysis of transcription of the exotoxin A gene of *Pseudomonas aeruginosa*, *J. Bacteriol.* **168**:1112–1119.
31. Lory, S., 1986, Effect of iron on accumulation of exotoxin A-specific mRNA in *Pseudomonas aeruginosa*, *J. Bacteriol.* **168**:1451–1456.
32. Chen, H.-T., Jordan, E. M., Wilson, R. B., Draper, R. K., and Clowes, R. C., 1987, Transcription and expression of the exotoxin A gene of *Pseudomonas aeruginosa*, *J. Gen. Microbiol.* **133**:3081–3091.
33. Ohman, D. E., Burns, R. P., and Iglewski, B. H., 1980, Corneal infections in mice with toxin A and elastase mutants of *Pseudomonas aeruginosa*, *J. Infect. Dis.* **142**:547–555.
34. Mekalanos, J. J., 1985, Cholera toxin: genetic analysis, regulation and role in pathogenesis in: *General Approaches to Microbial Pathogenicity*, **118**:97–118.
35. Vasil, M. L., Chamberlin, C., and Grant, C. C. R., 1986, Molecular studies of Pseudomonas exotoxin A gene, *Infect. Immun.* **52**:538–548.
36. Gray, G. L., Smith, D. H., Baldridge, J. S., Harkins, R. N., Vasil, M. L., Chen, E. Y., and Heyneker, H. L., 1984, Cloning, nucleotide sequence and expression in *Escherichia coli* of the exotoxin A structural gene of *Pseudomonas aeruginosa*, *Proc. Natl. Acad. Sci. USA* **81**:2645–2649.
37. Hanne, L. F., Howe, T. R., and Iglewski, B. H., 1983, Locus of the *Pseudomonas aeruginosa* toxin A gene, *J. Bacteriol.* **154**:383–386.
38. O'Hoy, K., and Krishnapillai, V., 1987, Recalibration of the *Pseudomonas aeruginosa* strain PAO chromosome map in time units using high-frequency-of-recombination donors, *Genetics* **115**:611–618.

39. Holloway, B. W., and Matsumoto, H., 1984, *Pseudomonas aeruginosa*, in: *Genetic Maps*, Cold Spring Harbor Laboratories, Cold Spring Harbor, NY.
40. Gray, G. L., and Vasil, M. L., 1981, Isolation and genetic characterization of toxin-deficient mutants of *Pseudomonas aeruginosa* PAO, *J. Bacteriol.* **147:**275–281.
41. Hedstrom, 1984, Comparative toxicities of exotoxin A and the CRM protein of *Pseudomonas aeruginosa*, Am. Soc. Microbiol., 42; B151.
42. Hedstrom, R. C., Funk, C. R., Galloway, D. R., and Pavlovskis, O. R., 1985, Cloning of a gene involved in regulation of exotoxin A expression in *Pseudomonas aeruginosa*, Am. Soc. Microbiol., 69; D91.
43. Hedstrom, R. C., Funk, C. R., Kaper, J. B., Pavlovskis, O. R., and Galloway, D. R., 1986, Cloning of a gene involved in regulation of exotoxin A expression in *Pseudomonas aeruginosa*, *Infect Immun.* **51:**37–42.
44. Frank, D. W., Steinbach, S. F., Bradley, J. M., and Iglewski, B. H., 1985, Genetic studies of *Pseudomonas aeruginosa* exotoxin A, in: *Bacterial Protein Toxins*, (P. Falmagne, J. E. Alouf, F. J. Fehrenbach, J. Jeljaszewicz, and M. Thelestam, eds.), Gustav Fischer, Stuttgart/New York, pp. 261–268.
45. Wozniak, D. J., Cram, D. J., Daniels, C. J., and Galloway, D. R., 1987, Nucleotide sequence and characterization of *toxR*: a gene involved in exotoxin A regulation in *Pseudomonas aeruginosa*, *Nucleic. Acids Res.* **15:**2123–2135.
46. Hindahl, M. S., Frank, D. W., Hamood, A., and Iglewski, B. H., 1988, Characterization of a gene that regulates toxin A synthesis in *Pseudomonas aeruginosa*, *Nucleic Acids Res.* **16:**5699.
47. Wick, M. J., Frank, D. W., Storey, D. G., and Iglewski, B. H., 1990, Identification of *regB*, a gene required for optimal exotoxin A yields in *Pseudomonas aeruginosa*, *Mol. Microbiol.* **4:**489–497.
48. Tennigkeit, J., and Matzura, H., 1991, Nucleotide sequence analysis of a chloramphenicol-resistance determinant from *Agrobacterium tumefaciens* and identification of its gene product, *Gene* **98:**113–116.
49. Galloway, D. R., Hedstrom, R. C., McGowan, J. L., Kessler, S. P., and Wozniak, D. J., 1989, Biochemical analysis of CRM 66: A nonfunctional *Pseudomonas aeruginosa* exotoxin A, *J. Biol. Chem.* **264:**14869–14873.
50. Wozniak, D. J., 1989, The use of gene replacement techniques to generate *toxA* and *toxR Pseudomonas aeruginosa* mutants, Am. Soc. Microbiol. 106; D-144.
51. Wozniak, D. J., Darzins, A., Shumard, C. M., and Galloway, D. R., 1992, Construction and analysis of *Pseudomonas aeruginosa* PA01 *toxA* and *toxR* negative mutations and their use in preliminary mapping of the *toxR* gene, submitted.
52. Hamood, A. N., and Iglewski, B. H., 1990, Expression of the *Pseudomonas aeruginosa toxA* positive regulatory gene (*regA*) in *Escherichia coli*, *J. Bacteriol.* **172:**589–594.
53. Zimniak, L., Dayn, A., and Iglewski, B. H., 1989, Identification of *regA* protein from *Pseudomonas aeruginosa* using anti-RegA antibody, *Biochem. Biophys. Res. Commun.* **163:**1312–1318.
54. Michaelis, S., and Beckwith, J., 1982, Mechanisms of incorporation of cell envelope proteins in *Escherichia coli*, *Annu. Rev. Microbiol.* **36:**435–465.
55. Frank, D. W., Storey, D. G., Hindahl, M. S., and Iglewski, B. H., 1989, Differential regulation by iron of *regA* and *toxA* transcript accumulation by *Pseudomonas aeruginosa*, *J. Bacteriol.* **171:**5304–5313.
56. Frank, D. W., and Iglewski, B. H., 1988, Kinetics of *toxA* and *regA* mRNA accumulation in *Pseudomonas aeruginosa*, *J. Bacteriol.* **170:**4477–4483.
57. Storey, D. G., Frank, D. W., Farinha, M. A., Kropinski, A. M., and Iglewski, B. H., 1990, Multiple promoters control the regulation of the *Pseudomonas aeruginosa regA* gene, *Mol. Microbiol.* **4:**499–503.
58. Miller, V. L., DiRita, V. J., and Mekalanos, J. J., 1989, Identification of *toxS*, a regulatory gene whose product enhances ToxR-mediated activation of the cholera toxin promoter, *J. Bacteriol.* **171:**1288–1293.

59. DiRita, V. J., and Mekalanos, J. J., 1991, Periplasmic interaction between two membrane regulatory proteins, ToxR and ToxS, results in signal transduction and transcriptional activation, *Cell* **64**:29–37.
60. Goldberg, J. B., and Ohman, D. E., 1987, Construction and characterization of *Pseudomonas aeruginosa algB* mutants: role of *algB* in high-level production of alginate, *J. Bacteriol.* **169**: 1593–1602.
61. Wozniak, D. J., Darzins, A., and Galloway, D. R., 1990, Molecular genetics studies of *toxR* and the genetic regulation of exotoxin A synthesis in *Pseudomonas aeruginosa*, Am. Soc. Microbiol. Abstr., 57; B184.
62. Romling, U., Duchene, M., Essar, D. W., Galloway, D. R., Guidi-Rontani, C., Hill, D., Lazdunski, A., Miller, R. A., Schleifer, K. H., Smith, D. W., Toschka, H. Y., and Tummler, B., 1992, Localization of *alg*, *opr*, *phn*, *pho*, 4.5S RNA, 6S RNA, *tox*, *trp*, and *xcp* genes, *rrn* operons, and the chromosomal origin on the physical genome map of *Pseudomonas aeruginosa* PAO, *J. Bacteriol.* **174**:327–330.
63. Taylor, R. K., Miller, V. M., Furlong, D. B., and Mekalanos, J. J., 1987, Use of alkaline phosphatase gene fusions to identify a pilus colonization factor of *Vibrio cholerae*, *Proc. Natl. Acad. Sci. USA* **84**:2833–2837.
64. Hindahl, M. S., Frank, D. W., and Iglewski, B. H., 1987, Molecular studies of a positive regulator of toxin A synthesis in *Pseudomonas aeruginosa*, *Antibiot. Chemother.* **39**:279–289.
65. Wick, M. J., Frank, D. W., Storey, D. G., and Iglewski, B. H., 1990, Structure, function, and regulation of *Pseudomonas aeruginosa* exotoxin A, *Annu. Rev. Microbiol.* **44**:335–363.
66. Tsaur, M.-L., and Clowes, R. C., 1989, Localization of the control region for expression of exotoxin A in *Pseudomonas aeruginosa*, *J. Bacteriol.* **171**:2599–2604.
67. Pabo, C. O., and Sauer, R. T., 1984, Protein-DNA recognition, *Annu. Rev. Biochem.* **53**: 293–321.
68. Wozniak, D. J., Kessler, S. P., and Galloway, D. R., 1992, Molecular analysis of *Pseudomonas aeruginosa* ToxR and its role in exotoxin A expression, submitted.
69. Bragg, A., and Neilands, J. B., 1987, Molecular mechanisms of regulation of siderophore-mediated iron assimilation, *Microbiol. Rev.* **51**:509–518.
70. Shumard, C. M., Wozniak, D. J., Darzins, A., and Galloway, D. R., 1992, submitted.

5

Susceptibility of Mammalian Cells to *Pseudomonas* Exotoxin A

RANDAL E. MORRIS and CATHARINE B. SAELINGER

1. INTRODUCTION

Bacterial toxins exhibit a great diversity in host range, mechanisms of action, and routes by which they reach their targets. In spite of these differences, many of the bacterial toxins, as well as several well-characterized plant toxins, share several common features. These include: (1) binding to a sensitive cell; (2) transport to an intracellular site of action; and (3) enzymatic modification of an intracellular substrate with subsequent alteration of cellular function.

In addition to these properties, many of the toxins have a similar molecular organization. The key feature of this organization is the segregation of functional domains. One domain is the binding region responsible for the toxin's host range, and another domain is the enzymatic region responsible for the toxic effects. In the simplest model these two fragments are held together by a disulfide bridge. The best characterized example of this model is diphtheria toxin (DT). Other toxins that share similar structural features include *Pseudomonas* exotoxin A (ETA), and the plant protein toxins abrin,

---

RANDAL E. MORRIS • Department of Anatomy and Cell Biology, University of Cincinnati College of Medicine, Cincinnati, Ohio 45267-0521.   CATHARINE B. SAELINGER • Department of Molecular Genetics, Biochemistry, and Microbiology, University of Cincinnati College of Medicine, Cincinnati, Ohio 45267-0524.

Pseudomonas aeruginosa as an Opportunistic Pathogen, edited by Mario Campa *et al.* Plenum Press, New York, 1993.

ricin, and modeccin. Other toxins show variations on this theme: included are cholera, pertussis, anthrax, shigella, and *Escherichia coli* heat-labile toxins. Thus, this functional organization appears to have been conserved throughout evolution.

Pseudomonas exotoxin A and diphtheria toxin (DT) are members of a family of bacterial toxins that act by covalently modifying specific target proteins within mammalian cells.[1] Specifically, both ETA and DT enzymatically catalyze the transfer of the ADP-ribose moiety of oxidized NAD (NAD$^+$) to elongation factor 2 (EF2); this inactivates EF2, terminates peptide chain elongation in the cell, and leads to inhibition of protein synthesis and eventual cell death. Both toxins are secreted by their parent bacteria in a proenzyme form; they are not able to catalyze ADP-ribosylation without being activated. On the structural level, both toxins conform to the A-B structure-function model described for a variety of bacterial and plant toxins.[2] In the case of DT (Fig. 1), a single polypeptide chain is cleaved proteolytically and reduced to give two chains. One of these (fragment A or light chain; 21,000 Da) possesses enzymatic activity, and the other (fragment B or heavy chain; 37,000 Da) is the binding fragment. Although enzymatically active fragments of *Pseudomonas* ETA have been isolated,[3,4] under natural conditions this molecule apparently needs to undergo only a conformational change to be converted to the active form.[5] A third functional domain for both molecules has been proposed that is involved in the translocation of the active protein into the cell cytoplasm.[6,7] Despite these similarities, the toxins exhibit little or no immunologic cross-reactivity and share no nucleotide or amino acid homology.[8,9]

Middlebrook and Dorland[10] measured the sensitivities of 21 mammalian cell lines to ETA and DT. They reported that each cell line exhibited 1 to 4 log differences in sensitivity to the two toxins. Further, there is no species-specificity for ETA. In contrast, cell lines derived from different origins exhibit a spectrum of sensitivity to DT with monkey cell lines being exquisitely sensitive, while murine cell lines are very resistant. Cell lines derived from human and hamster sources are intermediate in their sensitivity to DT. In spite of the fact that murine cells are resistant to DT, EF2 isolated from murine sources can be ADP-ribosylated by equimolar concentration of ETA or DT.[11] On the basis of their observations, Middlebrook and Dorland[10] suggest that sensitivity to the toxins is due to binding and internalization by mammalian cells.

In this review we will expand on this hypothesis and show that sensitivity is a consequence of binding of ETA by mammalian cells. Following binding, ETA is internalized by receptor-mediated endocytosis and escapes from an acidic, pre-lysosomal organelle. To develop this hypothesis we will compare and contrast the interaction of DT and ETA with mouse LM fibroblasts. In the latter portion of this review we will present new information concerning

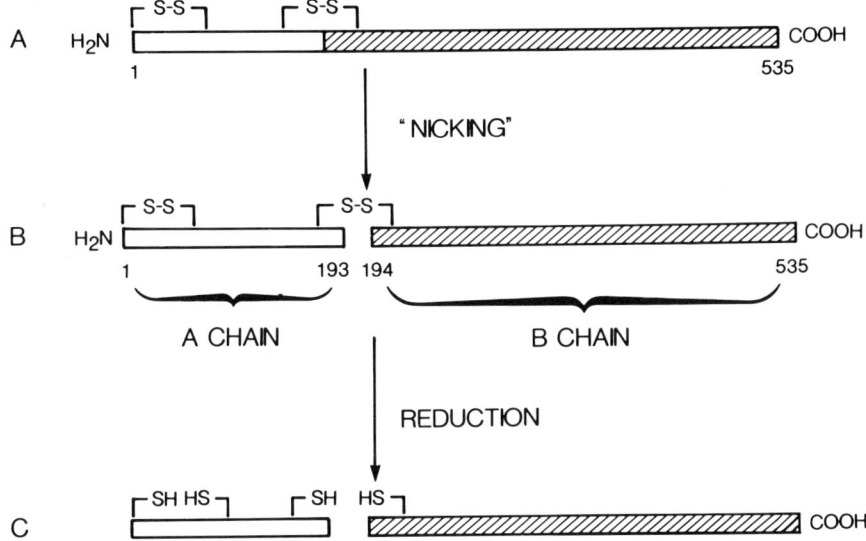

FIGURE 1. Basic structure of diphtheria toxin. (A) Single chain polypeptide toxin, molecular weight ~58,000 Da, as it is excreted from the host bacterium. In this form it is toxic to sensitive cells but has low levels of ADP-ribosyltransferase activity *in vitro*. (B) The toxin is proteolytically nicked to yield a dichain polypeptide held together by a disulfide bridge. This dichain protein is toxic to sensitive cells and shows enzymatic activity *in vitro*. The A chain, M_r ~20,000 Da, has ADP-ribosyltransferase activity. The B chain, M_r ~37,000 Da, has binding activity. The amino-terminal two-thirds of the B chain causes the toxin to insert into artificial lipid bilayers[112,113] under appropriate conditions forming ion-conductive channels. Studies using CRM-45, a 45,000-Da fragment of DT lacking the carboxy terminus of the parent molecule, have established that the binding domain resides in this region. (C) Reduction of the dichain toxin results in the separation of the two chains. Isolated A chains and B chains are non-toxic. (Reproduced from Morris, R. E., and Saelinger, C. B., 1989, in: *Botulinum Neurotoxins and Tetanus Toxin*, [L. L. Simpson, ed.] Academic Press, Inc., San Diego, pp. 121–152, used with permission.)

the isolation of the receptor for ETA and some preliminary information on the interaction of ETA with a resistant cell line.

2. STRUCTURE-FUNCTION RELATIONSHIP

Recent studies by several groups using X-ray crystallography and molecular genetics have elucidated a number of structure–function relationships for PE. Gray *et al.*[9] cloned the structural gene for PE into *E. coli*. Analysis of the cloned gene product revealed that ETA is made up of 638 amino acids from which a 25-amino acid hydrophobic leader peptide is removed during the secretion process. Using cloned fragments, these investigators showed that the ADP-ribosyltransferase activity is associated with the carboxy terminal portion of the molecule. Allured et al.[12] crystallized ETA and examined it by X-ray crystallography at a 3.0-Å resolution. Their data show that PE is composed of three distinct structural domains (Fig. 2). Domain I, which includes residues 1 to 252 (I_a) and 365 to 404 (I_b), is an antiparallel β-structure. Domain II (residues 253 to 364) is composed of six consecutive α-helices with one disulfide linking two of the helices. Domain III (residues 405–613) is less regular than the other two domains. Its most notable feature is an extended cleft.

Hwang et al.[7] characterized the function of each of the domains of ETA by deletion analysis. Their studies show that structural domain I_a is required for binding of the toxin, domain II is required for translocation, and domain III and a portion of domain I_b are required for enzymatic activity. Further analysis of domain I has shown that conversion of Lys 57 to glutamate decreases the toxicity of ETA for 3T3 cells 100-fold, but reduces mouse lethality only fivefold.[13] Toxin that has glutamate instead of Lys in position 57 is not able to compete with binding of wild-type toxin. Thus Lys 57 appears to be required for binding to tissue culture cells. Because mouse lethality was reduced only fivefold by this amino acid substitution, the authors hypothesize that Lys 57 is not essential in the interaction of toxin with liver, the primary target of ETA in vivo. Further studies showed that the region

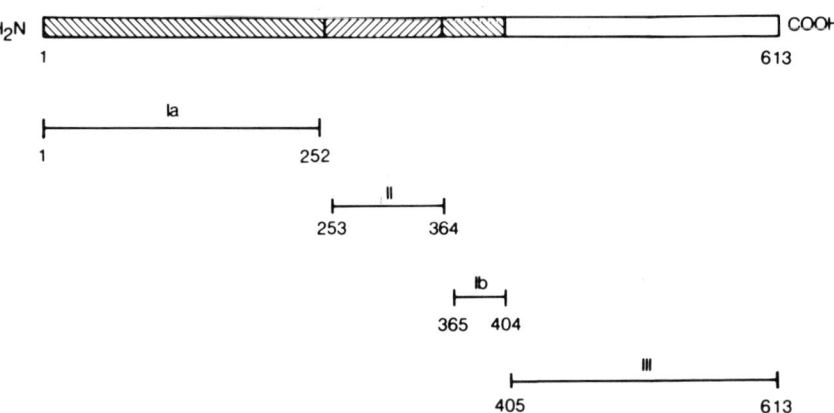

FIGURE 2. Basic structure of *Pseudomonas* ETA. This diagram is based on crystallographic data[12] and genetic analysis.[9] Region III, residues 405 through 613, is the enzymatic domain. Region I, composed of Ia and Ib, has been suggested to be the binding domain. Region II, residues 253 through 365, containing a hydrophobic portion, has been suggested to be the translocation domain. Intramolecular disulfide bonds are formed between the following Cys residues: 11 and 15, 197 and 214, 265 and 287, and 372 and 379. (Reproduced from Morris, R. E., and Saelinger, C. B., 1989, in: *Botulinum Neurotoxins and Tetanus Toxin*, [L. L. Simpson, ed.] Academic Press, Inc., San Diego, pp. 121–152, used with permission.)

responsible for liver toxicity was between amino acids 225 and 252, still part of domain I.

The role of domain II in translocation has been characterized by examining its contribution to secretion from a bacterial cell.[14] When the toxin gene is cloned into *E. coli*, the gene product normally is retained in the cytoplasm. Removal of domain I results in secretion of toxin into the periplasm. When domain II alone, or domains II and III are fused to the gene for a protein which normally is not secreted, the recombinant protein is secreted into the periplasm and into the medium. This suggests that regions of domain II are important for secretion of the toxin molecule across the bacterial cell membrane, and by analogy are required for translocation across the mammalian cell membrane during the intoxication process. The mechanism by which the sequence promotes secretion is not known.

Carroll and Collier[15] used photoaffinity labeling with NAD (a cofactor required for the ADP-ribosylation of EF2) to identify the active site residue of ETA. Using this technique, they identified a Glu residue at position 553 (located in domain III) as the active site for ETA. When this Glu was substituted with Aspartic acid (a conservative substitution), the ADP-ribosyltransferase activity was reduced 1800-fold and the toxicity of the mutagenized protein was reduced by 4 logs when assayed on sensitive LM mouse fibroblasts. Interestingly, a Glu residue in position 148 of DT is the active site of the enzymatic domain of this protein toxin.[16] Recent studies have shown a region of local amino acid homology in the active site of these two toxins.[17] Therefore, the A region of ETA corresponds to domains I_b and III, and the B region corresponds to domains I_a and II.

On a structural level we are able to assign particular functions to discrete regions of the ETA molecule. The interaction of ETA with mammalian cells is less well understood. We postulate that the binding dictates host range specificity and sensitivity to the toxin, once internalized ETA is shuttled by one of the established intracellular trafficking patterns. During its residence in the various intracellular compartments, ETA is converted to the active form and escapes into the cytoplasm. The initial event leading to the expression of toxicity is the receptor-mediated binding, which facilitates the toxin's entry via receptor-mediated endocytosis (RME).

3. RECEPTOR-MEDIATED ENDOCYTOSIS

Since the classical description of RME by Brown, Goldstein and colleagues in the mid-1970s,[18,19] there has been intense interest in the internalization and intracellular routing of various ligands. It is now widely accepted that most growth factors, hormones, and transport proteins enter mammalian cells by RME. The initial event in this process is the binding of the ligand to receptors located on the plasma membrane. In the majority of well-studied systems the receptors are randomly distributed on the cell surface. Following receptor binding, the receptor–ligand complex is seen in thickened regions on the plasma membrane. These thickened regions proceed to invaginate, forming "coated pits." The protein clathrin has been found to impart the coated appearance to the internalization vesicle.[20] During the final stages of the internalization process the clathrin-coated pit seals and is pinched off to become a coated vesicle. The coated vesicle fuses with a noncoated vesicle, the endosome. In this manner, the receptor–ligand complex is transferred from the cell surface to a cytoplasmic compartment.

Endosomes are pleomorphic organelles found in all regions of the cytoplasm. Often they are vacuolar structures associated with tubular elements.[21] They may also resemble multivesicular bodies.[22,23] To date, no specific protein or unique biochemical feature has been described for endosomes. Endosomes are defined as any uncoated vesicles that can be labeled with endocytic tracers prior to their appearance in lysosomes.[24] Their role is to direct the internalized ligand to its proper destination. Although the mechanism determining the route taken by the endosome is unknown, it is probably related to the interaction of the receptor–ligand complex in the endosomal environment. Because endosomal membranes have ATP-dependent proton pumps,[25,26] their intraorganellar pH is between 5 and 6.[27] The acidic pH affects: (1) the internalized ligand's stability of interaction with its receptor, and (2) its conformation.

Four separate intracellular routing patterns have emerged (Fig. 3). All four routes follow RME via clathrin-coated pits as described above. In the first group, exemplified by low-density lipoprotein,[28] ligand and receptor dissociate in the endosomal compartment, owing to the acidic pH of the organelle. Subsequently the ligand (now free in the lumen of the endosome) is routed to the lysosomal compartment for degradation while the receptor is recycled to the cell surface. This process has been demonstrated elegantly with a second ligand, asialoglycoprotein, which enters hepatocytes in an analogous manner.[29] Using double-label immuno-electron microscopy on ultrathin cryosections of rat liver in conjunction with monospecific antibodies and gold–protein A complexes, the authors showed co-localization of asialoglycoprotein and its receptor in coated vesicles near the plasma membrane. As the endocytic process progressed with increased time of warming, the ligand was seen within the lumen of endosomes, while the receptor was seen in tubular extensions emanating from the endosomes. Because this observation suggested dissociation and segregation of asialoglycoprotein and its receptor, the authors termed this compartment CURL (*c*ompartment of *u*ncoupling of *r*eceptor and *l*igand). They have used this technique to show a similar routing pattern for mannose-6-phosphate and its receptor.[30]

In the second trafficking pattern, the receptor–ligand complex remains associated within the endosome and the complex is recycled to the cell surface. The best example of this interaction is the iron-binding protein,

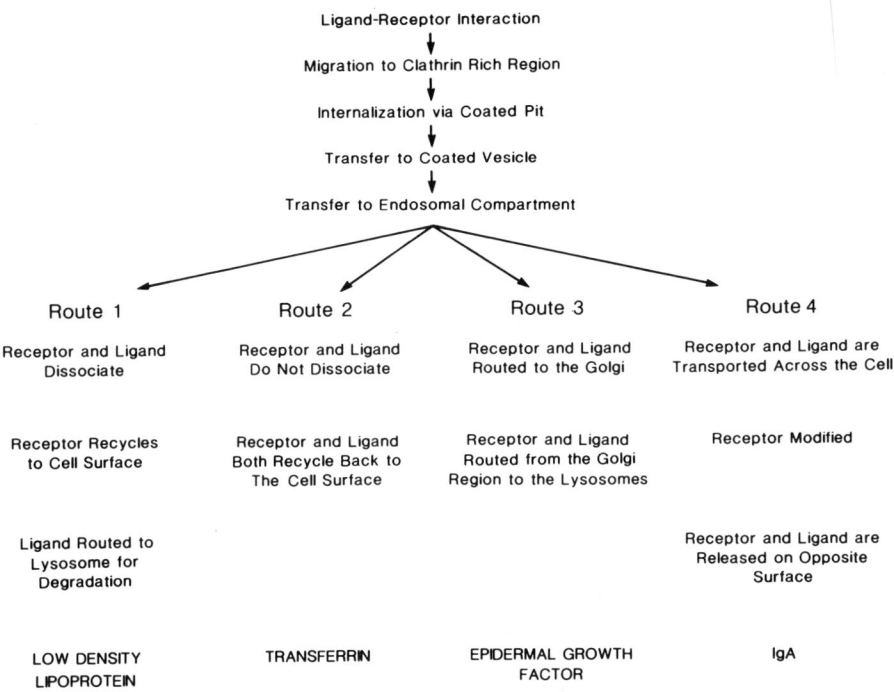

FIGURE 3. Intracellular routing of receptors and ligands after entry by receptor-mediated endocytosis. (Reproduced from Morris, R. E., and Saelinger, C. B., 1989, in: *Botulinum Neurotoxins and Tetanus Toxin*, [L. L. Simpson, ed.] Academic Press, Inc., San Diego, pp. 121–152, used with permission.)

transferrin.[31] A single molecule of apo-transferrin is capable of binding two Fe^{+++} ions, resulting in diferric transferrin or transferrin. Transferrin binds to cell surface receptors that internalize the iron binding protein by RME. Dautry-Varsat *et al.*[32] showed that, while in an acidic environment (pH ≤ 5.5), iron dissociates from the transferrin. They further demonstrated that the transferrin receptor avidly binds apo-transferrin at acidic pH, thereby allowing the ligand to remain attached to its receptor in the endosome. Upon routing to the cell surface, apo-transferrin is released because of the low affinity of the receptor for transferrin at neutral pH. After binding more Fe^{+++}, the apo-transferrin cycle starts anew. These studies clearly demonstrate the acidic nature of the endosomal compartment. This information, taken together with the first routing mechanism (low-density lipoprotein and asialoglycoprotein), establishes the importance of an acidic environment in the intracellular trafficking of internalized ligands.

In the third group, both the ligand and its receptor are routed to the lysosomal compartment for degradation. The best-studied ligands in this category include epidermal growth factor (EGF),[33,34] insulin,[35,36] and altered immunoglobulins, *e.g.* internalized by Fc receptors.[37] Other investigators have reported that a significant fraction of internalized EGF is routed to the Golgi region during its transit to the lysosomal compartment.[38,39] A curious feature of this intracellular trafficking pattern is the observation by DiPaola and Maxfield[40] that EGF and its receptor dissociate at acidic pH. This implies that something in addition to receptor–ligand interaction dictates the intracellular routing. Also, in some cells a small but significant proportion of EGF receptors do recycle.[36,41] Perhaps, as suggested by Beguinot *et al.*[42] this pathway is used to regulate receptor expression, *i.e.* down-regulation.

In the fourth group the ligand and its receptor are transported from one cell surface to another, *e.g.* from the basolateral surface to the apical surface. The best-characterized example in this group is secretory IgA. In the liver dimergic IgA binds to newly synthesized receptor on the sinusoidal surface of the hepatocyte, is internalized, transported to the canalicular surface, and discharged into the bile.[43] The transit, because it is across the cell, is termed transcytosis. Geuze *et al.*[44] have used double-label immuno-electron microscopy to elucidate the transit. By comparison they followed the intracellular routing of receptors for asialoglycoprotein, mannose-6-phosphate, and polymeric IgA. They showed that receptors for the former two ligands colocalized within the tubules of the CURL, whereas Ig-A receptor showed dramatic microheterogeneity. They use this as evidence to support their hypothesis that in addition to its role in uncoupling and sorting recycling receptor from ligand, CURL serves as a compartment to segregate recycling receptors from the receptors involved in transcytosis. During its transit, the IgA receptor is cleaved proteolytically such that a portion of the receptor remains with the dimeric IgA. This receptor fragment is the secretory piece.[45,46] Because transit is a function of the endosomal compartment, this observation suggests that the endosomes may contain proteases. Others also have shown protease activity associated with endosomes.[47,48]

3.1. Role of Acidic Compartments

Acidotropic agents are small lipophilic compounds with an affinity for acidic intracellular compartments, *e.g.* endosomes and lysosomes. After entry into an acidic compartment the acidotropic agent becomes protonated and unable to exit the organelle. The consequence is an increase in intraorganellar pH.[27,49] The net effect of increased pH is the inhibition of intracellular routing; this implies that acidification plays a prominent role in the routing of internalized ligands.[50]

3.2. Temperature Dependence

Normal intracellular trafficking is also influenced by temperature. Weigel and Oka[51] reported that endocytosis of [^{3}H]-asialo-orosomucoid is blocked at temperatures lower than 10°C. Between 10°C and 20°C the rate of endocytosis is directly proportional to the change in temperature. At 20°C there is a sharp increase in the rate of internalization. Dunn et al.[52] have shown that the uptake and catabolism of ^{125}I-asialofetuin increases progressively as the temperature increases from 20°C to 35°C. These investigators showed that at temperatures less than 20°C, lysosomal degradation is blocked. Using both morphological and biochemical assays Dunn et al.[52] showed that endosome–lysosome fusion is greatly reduced. Sleight and Pagano[53] studied the effect of temperature on the internalization of a fluorescent derivative of phosphatidylcholine by hamster lung fibroblasts. They showed that at temperatures lower than 12°C the fluorescent ligand does not enter the cells. Between 12° and 18°C the ligand enters the cell but does not accumulate in the Golgi apparatus; between 18°C and 20°C the fluorescent lipid enters and accumulates in the Golgi apparatus. These results suggest that the phase-transition temperature, *i.e.* the temperature at which membrane lipids become immobile, is 20°C for the lysosomal membranes, and ≃18°C for Golgi membranes.

4. SIMILARITIES WITH VIRAL ENTRY

The intoxication of sensitive mammalian cells by *Pseudomonas* ETA can be viewed as a multistep process involving: (1) binding of the toxin to specific receptors on the cell surface; (2) internalization through clathrin-coated regions of the membrane; (3) intracellular trafficking and activation of the toxin; (4) escape of the enzymatically active polypeptide from membrane-limited cytoplasmic vesicles; and (5) ADP-ribosylation of cytoplasmic EF2. Because there is no reason to believe *a priori* that a cell would possess a receptor for a substance that would kill it, it is reasonable to hypothesize that such a receptor exists for some physiological ligand, *e.g.* a hormone or growth factor. This suggests that microbial toxins have usurped normal cellular machinery to gain entrance into the cytosol. This is analogous to many viruses, which have been shown to enter cells by RME. RME is so efficient in internalizing materials from the extracellular environment that certain viruses have used "opportunistic" receptors on the mammalian cell surface to enter a vulnerable cell. The key events leading to a productive viral infection are binding to cell surface receptors, entry via clathrin-coated pits, transit to the endosomal compartment, and escape of the nucleocapsid by fusion of the viral envelope with the endosomal membrane mediated by a low pH, *i.e.* < 5.5. Three observations by Helenius and colleagues have shown the prominence of the endosome in viral infections. First, infection by enveloped viruses is inhibited by acidotropic agents.[54] Second, infection of BHK-21 cells by Semliki Forest Virus occurs at temperatures between 15° and 20°C, suggesting that the site of escape is the endosomal and not the lysosomal compartment.[22] Third, by infecting BHK-21 cells at 20°C with a SFV mutant that fuses only at pH ≤ 5.5, Kielian *et al.*[55,56] confirmed that the site of nucleocapsid escape is pre-lysosomal and acidic, *i.e.* the endosomal compartment.

Non-enveloped viruses also use RME to enter sensitive cells. Olsnes and colleagues have followed the entry of poliovirus into HeLa cells. Their data show that compounds that dissipate the proton gradient across membranes, and compounds that inhibit acidification, do not inhibit the binding of poliovirus but do prevent infection.[57] They go on to show that at pH ≃ 5.5 the poliovirus capsid undergoes a structural alteration exposing a hydrophobic region of its icosahedral shell. They suggest this conformational change is a prerequisite for infection.[58] These observations are corroborated by the electron microscopic data of Zeichhardt *et al.*,[59] who followed the infection of HEp-2 cells with poliovirus. Their data show entry via clathrin-coated pits and movement to an acidic compartment. Infection but not entry by the virus is blocked by chloroquine, ammonium chloride, or monensin, *i.e.* acidotrophic agents.

Adenovirus is a non-enveloped virus that enters host cells by RME. The initial observations by Chardonnet and Dales[60,61] showed adenovirus entering HeLa cells in membrane-thickened regions by a process termed "viropexis." They observed increasing numbers of free virions in the cytoplasm with time post-internalization. They also reported that at intermediate temperatures of 12° to 20°C, internalization proceeds but release of the virion into the cytoplasm does not occur. More recently FitzGerald and colleagues have shown that adenovirus entry into KB cells is via RME.[62,63] They also have shown that the release of intact virions into the cytoplasm is inhibited by weak bases and monensin.[64] Thus, the disruption of the endosomal membrane appears to require a low pH. They further characterized this low-pH dependence by measuring the interaction of adenovirus capsid proteins with Triton X-114. The penton base protein strongly binds Triton X-114 at pH 5.5 and below, but binds the detergent weakly at pH 7.0 and above. Adenovirus treated with antibody to the penton base proteins is non-infectious. From these data, it is inferred that the penton base protein is required for vesicle disruption.[65] Taken together, data for the enveloped and non-enveloped viruses suggest three common properties for a productive viral infection: (1) binding to a cell surface receptor; (2) internalization via clathrin-coated pits, *i.e.* RME; and (3) escape from the endosomal compartment.

5. EXPERIMENTAL DATA

5.1. The Binding Event

In 1980, using an unlabeled-antibody technique in conjunction with horse spleen ferritin as the electron-dense marker, we followed the binding and internalization of ETA by mouse LM fibroblasts.[66] We showed that ETA binds to the plasma membranes of LM cells and enters via clathrin-coated pits. This was the first demonstration of entry of ETA into a sensitive cell line by RME and suggested the existence of a cell surface receptor for ETA on LM cells.

We next proceeded to characterize the binding event by classical binding techniques using ^{125}I-labeled PE. Numerous attempts to label the toxin by conventional methods resulted in loss of the toxin's biological activity. Eventually we were successful in obtaining ^{125}I-PE by using the Bolton–Hunter reagent (N-succinimide 3-4 hydroxy, 5-[^{125}I] iodophenyl propionate).[67] Using this radio-labeled reagent we characterized the binding of ETA by LM cells. Unfortunately ^{125}I-PE binds to cells at 4°C with high non-specificity. Similar observations have been reported by Moehring and Moehring.[68] To circumvent this problem we measured binding of ^{125}I-PE on paraformaldehyde-fixed LM cells, an approach used by others to quantitate receptor binding.[69,70] Using this system we were able to show specific binding. Saturation is achieved at 5.4 nM toxin, which corresponds to about 100,000 receptors per LM cell. The saturation data are in good agreement with the minimal concentration of ETA required for expression of toxicity, *e.g.* 1 to 2 nM. Further, binding is reversible because 50% of the bound ^{125}I-PE can be displaced by unlabeled PE during a 3-hr incubation period.

We also have used a morphological technique to demonstrate ETA binding to LM cells. In this technique ETA is biotinylated (B-ETA) by incubation with biotinyl-N-hydroxysuccinimide ester at pH 9.2[71] (Fig. 4). B-ETA has been shown to retain biological activity.[72] B-ETA is allowed to bind to LM cells for 30 min at 4°C. After several washes, streptavidin–gold colloids,[73] average diameter 5 nm, are added and monolayers incubated at 4°C for 30 min. Samples are subsequently processed for electron microscopy. We observed saturation at 1.66 nM, corroborating both the biochemical and previous morphological data. Further, we were able to show specific binding by a competition assay in which B-ETA is incubated with LM cells in the presence of a 200-fold excess of native toxin. Incubation in the presence of excess native toxin reduced the amount of gold on the cell surface to that seen in the absence of toxin.[72]

5.2. Endocytic Uptake of *Pseudomonas* and Diphtheria Toxins by Mouse LM Fibroblasts

The intracellular trafficking of *Pseudomonas* exotoxin[66,74,75] and DT,[76] have been studied on the ultrastructural level. Visualization is done using biotinyl–toxin derivatives in conjunction with electron-dense avidin–gold colloids. In both cases, in a sensitive cell (LM or Vero), biotinyl toxin that is bound to the cells at 4°C is distributed randomly on the cell surface. Binding of biotinyl–toxin is totally blocked by native toxins. Within seconds of

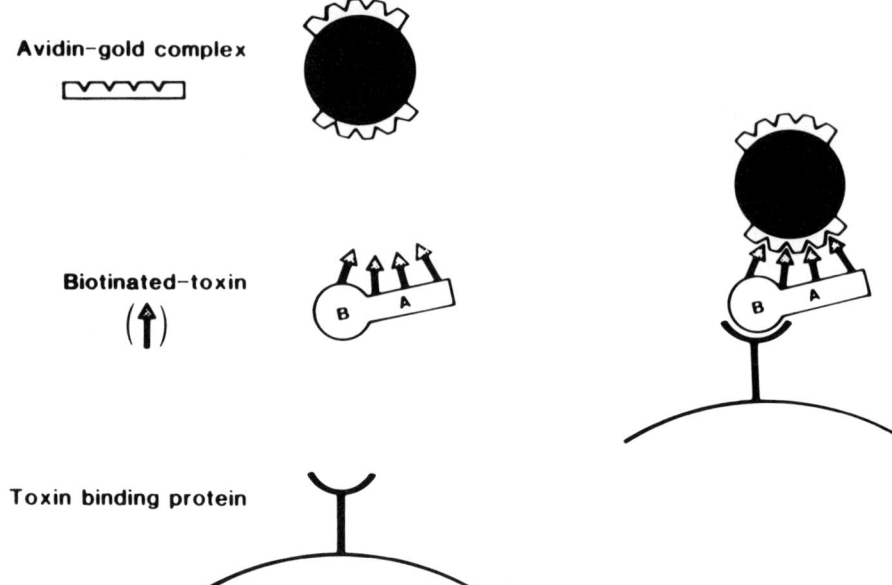

FIGURE 4. The biotinyl-*Pseudomonas* ETA (B-ETA) avidin–gold complex. On the left are the components of complex, on the right is an illustration of the B-ETA avidin–gold complex. All steps shown are done for 30 min. at 4°C on intact mouse LM fibroblasts prior to internalization and subsequent fixation.[71]

warming cells to 37°C, the toxin moves to coated areas of the membrane and within 5 min can be seen intracellularly in noncoated vesicles. Within 12–15 min, toxin is seen in the centrosomal region of the cell, usually in Golgi-associated vesicles or occasionally in Golgi cisternae, and in multivesicular bodies. The toxin is ultimately seen in lysosomes. Representative electron micrographs depicting this movement are given in Fig. 5. Similar kinetics of trafficking are observed via electron microscopy using biotinyl *Pseudomonas* toxin identified with avidin–gold colloids and using biochemical probes.[73] The intracellular path taken by DT in a Vero cell and by *Pseudomonas* exotoxin in an LM cell is similar, if not identical.

In contrast, the movement of DT in a DT-resistant cell (LM) is decidedly different from that in a sensitive cell.[76,77] Binding of biotinyl–DT to an LM cell is only partially blocked by native toxin. Upon warming to 37°C, toxin rapidly enters cells, but not via coated areas. Within 5 min, DT is seen intracellularly in lysosomes. Only rarely is DT seen in the centrosomal region of the LM cell. Thus, DT is routed by one pathway in a toxin-sensitive cell, and by an alternate pathway in a toxin-resistant cell. Presumably, this difference in trafficking results in a difference in toxin processing, and ultimately determines whether or not toxin activity will be expressed.

We postulate that DT binds to the surface of mouse fibroblasts (DT-resistant cells) and enters by a non-specific adsorptive endocytic event. In this manner the routing of DT is similar to the interaction between L cells and cationic ferritin, a ligand known to enter cells by non-specific adsorptive endocytosis.[78,79] Cationic ferritin, like DT, proceeds to the lysosomal compartment after entry. The time frame for intracellular trafficking of both ligands is similar, and in neither instance is there any labeling of the Golgi elements. On the basis of these observations we hypothesize that entry by RME is required for the expression of toxicity.

Other ultrastructural studies lend support to the importance of coated pit-mediated entry for toxicity. In the presence of methylamine, B-ETA enters LM cells through noncoated areas and is sequestered in large electron-lucent vacuoles, usually in association with the vesicle membrane. Toxin remains in these vesicles as long as amine is present, and thus normal protein synthesis is maintained.[74] Upon removal of methylamine, toxin is exocytosed, and is then reinternalized via coated pits (unpublished observations). We hypothesize that the toxin that reenters cells via the typical receptor-mediated pathway is responsible for the inhibition of protein synthesis seen after methylamine removal.

Circumstantial evidence for the role of coated pits in toxin internalization has come from work on depletion of intracellular potassium. Larkin et al.[80] have shown that potassium depletion of human fibroblasts (hypotonic shock followed by incubation in potassium-free medium) stops coated-pit formation and the RME of low-density lipoprotein. Moya et al.[81] used a similar approach to look at the entry of toxins into several mammalian cells. Intracellular potassium depletion fully protected HEp_2 cells from DT, but had no effect on Vero or WI38/SV40 cells. Immunofluorescent studies showed a disappearance of coated pits, subsequent to lowering of intracellular potassium levels, only in HEp_2 cells; a similar loss of clathrin and blocking of coated-pit formation was not seen in Vero or WI38/SV40 cells. Although one has followed internalization of DT on the ultrastructural level in HEp_2 cells, the data strongly support a role for coated pit-mediated entry.

Using similar methods, Sandvig et al.[82] found that potassium depletion protects Vero cells from DT, as well as protecting L cells from ETA. In the case of DT, the authors hypothesized that protection was due to a reduction in the ability of cells to bind DT by an ATP-requiring process. The reduction in binding is time-dependent; that is, depletion of intracellular potassium for 15 min does not alter the amount of DT bound, whereas depletion for 4 hr strongly reduces DT binding. In agreement with the work of Moya et al.[81] there was no reduction in the number of coated pits, as measured by electron microscopy, after potassium depletion.

The Golgi region of the cell also appears to be on the pathway taken by ETA and DT in sensitive cells. Morris and colleagues [73,74,76] consistently see biotinyl–DT or B-ETA (identified by avidin–gold colloids) in the Golgi region of sensitive cells 10 to 20 min after incubation at 37°C. Similar observations are not made in toxin-resistant cells.[77] In experiments in which methylamine is removed, and ETA returns to the cell surface to reenter via coated areas, toxin is also located within the Golgi region of the cell 10 to 20 min after it is seen in coated pits (unpublished observations). The role of the Golgi apparatus in the intoxication process is not clear. We postulate that the Golgi is involved in the processing of toxins to an active form.

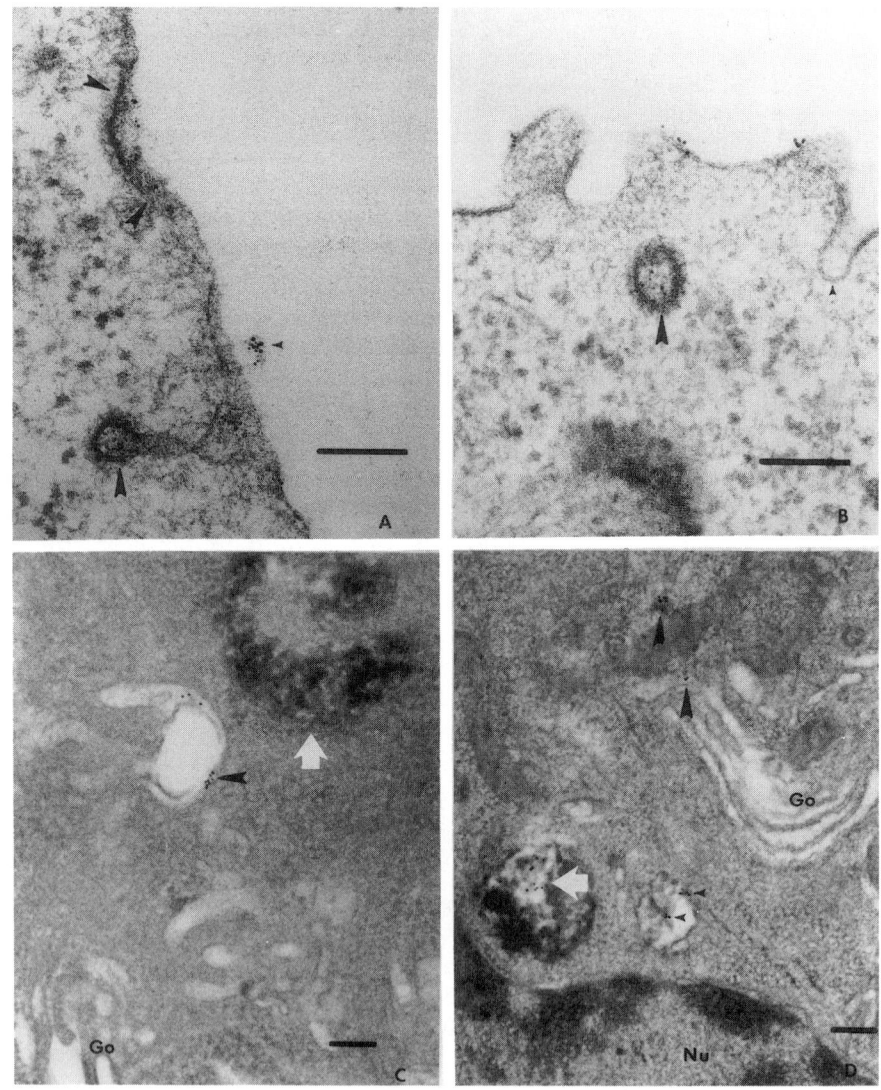

The internalization and intracellular routing of ETA and DT by sensitive cells is similar to that described for EGF,[38,39] that is, entry by RME followed by routing to the lysosomal compartment via the Golgi. The toxins follow the predominant route taken by growth factors and hormones; this observation may explain why cells possess cell surface receptors for substances that are lethal to them. The conclusion is that the toxins fortuitously resemble growth factors or hormones.[83]

5.3. Activation and Escape of *Pseudomonas* Toxin in LM Fibroblasts

Whereas available evidence is convincing that both PE and DT enter toxin-sensitive cells via coated pits and reach an acidic prelysosomal organelle prior to entry into the cell cytoplasm, there is no data as to the site of processing of these toxins from the protoxin form. As described for DT, this process, at least *in vitro*, involves proteolytic cleavage of the toxin molecule and reduction of disulfide bonds to generate fragment A. In contrast, in the case of PE, *in vitro* activation does not necessitate cleavage; rather, a conformational change is sufficient to generate an enzyme-active molecule. These changes may occur: (1) at the plasma membrane, presumably after binding; (2) in the endosome; or (3) in Golgi-associated vesicles.

Little published data address these questions. An acidic pH is required for insertion of either toxin into artificial membranes, and subsequent translocation.[84,85] There is also evidence that an acidic pH alters the conformation of ETA.[86,87] Work in intact tissue culture cells shows that passage through

←

FIGURE 5. Electron micrographs showing binding, internalization, and intracellular trafficking of *Pseudomonas* ETA by mouse LM fibroblasts. Biotinyl-ETA was bound to LM cells at 4°C for 30 min. After three washes with cold Hank's Balanced Salt Solution, avidin–gold colloids (6 nm ave. diam.) were added and incubated at 4°C for 30 min. Samples were washed and warmed to 37°C for the designated time period prior to fixation. (A) Sample that had been warmed for 30 sec; note the occurrence of the toxin–gold conjugates in coated pits (large arrows) and along the plasma membrane (small arrows). (B) 1 min after warming to 37°C; note the toxin–gold conjugates within a coated vesicle (large arrows) and along uncoated regions of the plasma membrane. Compare the appearance of the membrane surrounding the coated vesicle with that of typical unit membrane (small arrows). (C) 5 min after warming to 37°C; the region of the cell shown is identified as near the Golgi (GO) because of the cisternal profiles and associated vesicles. The toxin–gold (large arrows) is seen within an endosome; note the tubular appendages coming off of the luminal body of the organelle (small arrows). A lysosome is also seen (white arrow) and is identified by the presence of dense black precipitate (horseradish peroxidase developed by the diaminobenzidine–H_2O_2 reaction).[73] (D) 20 min after warming to 37°C; toxin–gold conjugates occur in multiple sites in the GO adjacent to the nucleus (Nu). Toxin–gold conjugates are associated with GO-associated vesicles (large arrows), within a multivesicular body (small arrows), and within a lysosome (white arrows). Bars indicate 100 nm. (Reproduced from Morris, R. E., and Saelinger, C. B., 1989, in: *Botulinum Neurotoxins and Tetanus Toxin*, [L. L. Simpson, ed.] Academic Press, Inc., San Diego, pp. 121–152, used with permission.)

an acidic environment is required for expression of toxicity,[73] but details are not known.

We used various combinations of antagonists of toxicity to characterize the temporal relationship of the events leading to toxicity. ETA (at 1 µg per ml) was allowed to bind for 1 hr at 4°C prior to the initiation of the experiment. Cells were then warmed to 37°C. At various times after warming the ability of the antagonists to protect the cells was evaluated. The antagonists used were: (1) trypsin-pronase treatment; (2) antibody; (3) methylamine (20 mM); and (4) incubation at 19°C. The results (Fig. 6) show that trypsin-pronase and antibody protect for only seconds after warming. These treatments, which are used to inactivate surface-bound toxin, suggest that ETA enters LM cells rapidly and efficiently. Methylamine, added 5 to 7 min after ETA entry, still fully protected the cells. This defines the acid-dependent step and correlates well with morphological evidence characterizing the intracellular location of ETA in the endosomal compartment. It is possible to delay shifting cells to 19°C for 14 to 15 min after ETA internalization has begun and still achieve protection. This establishes the temperature-dependent step and correlates with the time ETA is seen in the Golgi region. These results suggest the following series of events leading to ETA escape into the LM cell cytoplasm: (1) binding and entry via RME; (2) acidification and conformational change; and (3) escape. The results do not support the hypothesis that acidification, activation (conversion of the protoxin to the toxin), and escape occur concurrently, because ETA resides in an acidic, pre-lysosomal compartment (methylamine-sensitive step) 7–10 min prior to expression of toxicity (cold-sensitive step).

A similar observation has been reported for intoxication of Vero cells by DT. Marnell et al.[88] showed that DT encounters a pre-lysosomal, low-pH vesicle (i.e., endosome) by 4 min after internalization. Inhibition of protein synthesis, however, was not detected until 20 min after internalization. In a detailed kinetic analysis of intoxication of Vero cells by DT, Hudson and Neville[89] suggest that intracellular acidification affects at least two separate stages of the intoxication process. The first stage corresponds to conformational changes associated with low pH. This is acid-dependent and converts the toxin to the proper conformation for pore formation. The second stage is the translocation event. Although translocation is not acid-dependent, it cannot occur unless the toxin is in the proper conformation (which *is* acid-dependent). The implication of our work and that of others is that about 10 min in an acidic environment is required for the toxins to acquire the conformational change necessary for escape.

Work in our laboratories has shown that subcellular fractionation of LM cells on a Percoll density gradient generates fractions that are enriched in Golgi and plasma membrane-associated enzymes and in light lysosomes (of lighter buoyant density than secondary lysosomes). These fractions are able to stimulate ADP-ribosylation activity when mixed with ETA in a test tube.

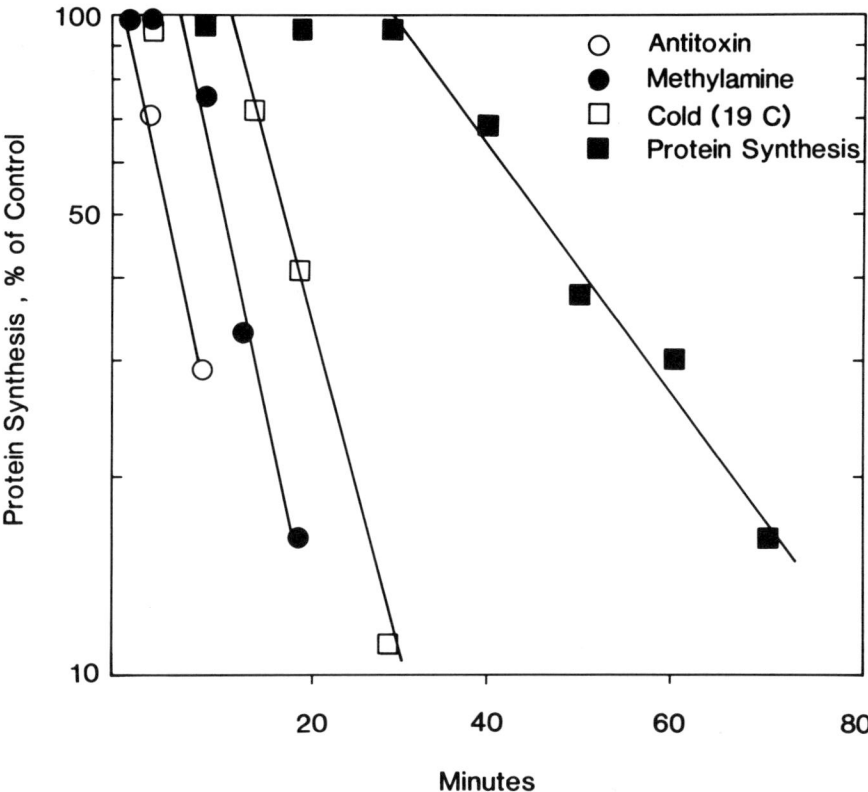

FIGURE 6. Entry of ETA. In all cases, LM monolayers were preincubated with 1 μg of ETA per ml for 1 h at 4°C. (○) Cell culture fluid at 37°C was added and, at indicated times, aspirated, and monolayers were incubated for 30 min at 4°C in medium containing specific antitoxin to neutralize surface ETA. Cells were then washed and incubated at 37°C for 4.5 h, prior to measurement of protein synthesis. Protein synthesis is relative to controls that were treated with antitoxin immediately after 4°C incubation with toxin. (●) Cell culture fluid at 37°C was added; when indicated, medium was replaced with 20 mM methylamine, and cells were incubated at 37°C for 4.5 h until protein synthesis was assayed. Protein synthesis is relative to controls which received 20 mM methylamine 15 min before the cells were put in 37°C medium. (□) Medium at 37°C was added, and when indicated, monolayers were transferred to 19°C medium and incubated for 4.5 h before protein synthesis was measured. Protein synthesis is relative to controls that were placed at 19°C immediately after the preincubation step. (■) Medium at 37°C was added; when indicated, 10 μCi or [^{3}H]leucine per ml was added for 10 min. Data are relative to controls receiving no toxin and are plotted at 5 min after addition of label. (Reproduced from Morris, R. E., and Saelinger, C. B., 1986, *Infect. Immun.* **52**:445–453, used with permission.)

Similar stimulation is also noted at times with endosomal-enriched fractions. Activation is seen only at an acidic pH. These data support the role of a non-lysosomal acidic organelle in the activation of ETA (unpublished observations).

We postulate that transit through the *trans* region of the Golgi is required for conversion of the protoxins to toxins. We propose that the protoxins are nicked and activated at this site. The model we propose for conversion of protoxin to active toxin is analogous to the proteolytic conversion of proproteins to proteins.[90–92] Essentially all peptide hormones and neurotransmitters made by eucaryotic cells are excised from precursor polypeptides (*i.e.*, proproteins) by endoproteolytic scissions at pairs of basic residues that flank the mature hormone (*i.e.*, protein) sequences.[93] The favored sites for the enzymatic cleavage are Arg-Arg and Lys-Arg residues. For example albumin, a non-glycosylated protein produced in hepatocytes, is found as proalbumin within the cisternae of the Golgi apparatus.[94] The processing of the proalbumin to albumin is a late Golgi event probably occurring in the *trans* region.[95]

Both ETA and DT have several paired basic amino acid regions. ETA has an Arg-Arg site at position 182-183, and a Lys-Arg site at position 185 to 186.[9] DT also contains several similar sites: Lys-Arg sites at positions 125 and 172, and Arg-Arg sites at position 192. The latter Arg-rich segment connects the A and B domains and is readily cleaved *in vitro* by trypsin-like enzymes to yield the A and B fragments. A similar cleavage is believed to occur *in vivo* at some stage in the intoxication process.[96] In keeping with the notion that an acidic organelle is required for toxin escape, Anderson and Pathak[97] have shown that the *trans* Golgi cisternae and forming secretory vesicles from human fibroblasts have an acidic pH.

An alternate hypothesis, consistent with the morphological data, is that toxin activation occurs in the endosomal compartment without the need for Golgi involvement. This suggests that a low pH-induced conformational change is sufficient to cause toxin activation or that the endosomal compartment contains proteases. In support of the latter requirement, Diment and Stahl[47] described an endosomal-associated cathepsin D-like protease that is responsible for degradation of ^{125}I-mannose-bovine serum albumin in rabbit alveolar macrophages. Recently, a role has been suggested for endosomal proteases, *i.e.* cathepsin-like proteases, in antigen presentation.[98]

For the following reason, we favor the model implicating the Golgi apparatus as the site for toxin activation. Although it has been shown that EF2 isolated from mouse fibroblasts is sensitive to ADP-ribosylation catalyzed by the A-chain of DT,[11,99] it requires 10^4 to 10^5 more DT molecules to kill mouse fibroblasts (a DT-resistant cell line) than to kill Vero cells (a sensitive cell line). This occurs in spite of the fact that DT binds to mouse fibroblasts.[68,100] Following internalization of DT by mouse LM cells, the toxin is transported directly via endosomes to the lysosomal compartment. In contrast to ETA,

DT is not routed through the Golgi region[80] in this cell line. Based on these observations, our conclusion is that the protoxin is converted to an active toxin in the Golgi.

In a series of recent reports Olsnes and colleagues have presented evidence suggesting a role for the translocation of ricin into the cytosol via the trans Golgi network (TGN). Ricin, a plant toxin, shares structural similarities with ETA. Van Deurs et al.[101] followed the internalization and routing of a monovalent ricin–horseradish peroxidase conjugate (Ri-HRP) in mammalian cells at 18° and 37°C. At the higher temperature Ri-HRP is present within the Golgi elements and toxicity is expressed. At 18°C no Ri-HRP is seen in the Golgi and toxicity is inhibited. This has led them to suggest that ricin may be modified by enzymes present in the Golgi. More recently van Deurs et al.[102] have shown that $\simeq 5\%$ of the ricin internalized by mammalian cells reaches the Golgi after 60 min at 39.5°C, with about 70–80% in the TGN. On the basis of a combined morphological and biochemical approach, they suggest that translocation of the toxic ricin A-chain to the cytosol occurs at a site of convergence between the endocytic and exocytic pathways in the TGN. Similar results were obtained by Youle and Colombatti[103] who studied the ricin intoxication of anti-ricin-producing hybridoma cells.

5.4. Isolation of the Receptor for *Pseudomonas* Exotoxin A from Mouse LM Fibroblasts

We have begun to isolate and characterize a receptor for ETA from mouse LM fibroblasts. We chose this cell line because of data suggesting that there are approximately 100,000 receptors per cell,[67] the fact that toxin enters via coated pits, and evidence that trypsin treatment transiently reduced sensitivity to toxin (unpublished observations). To obtain receptor, cells are homogenized, and receptor is released by detergent treatment. Receptor is purified on a toxin-affinity column, and is characterized by enzyme-linked immunoabsorbent assay (ELISA) and by sodium dodecyl sulfate gel electrophoresis (SDS-PAGE). The solubilized, toxin-binding protein that we have obtained by this method is called receptor, although we have no direct evidence that it is the receptor involved in internalization of those toxin molecules responsible for inhibition of protein synthesis. Receptor isolated by this procedure is approximately 95% homogeneous by silver stain. It has a molecular weight of approximately 325,000 Da, as determined by SDS-PAGE. Treatment with mercaptoethanol does not alter the molecular weight of the molecule, but does reduce its ability to bind toxin. The receptor is stable to freezing and thawing, is stable at 4° to 37°C for several hr, but is destroyed by boiling. We have ELISA evidence that the binding of ETA by the purified receptor is specific and saturable. As little as 25-fold excess native toxin can replace 60% of the B-ETA bound to the receptor.

The receptor molecule is a glycoprotein; treatment with PNGase F, a glycopeptidase that cleaves carbohydrate residues at Asp, causes a reduction in molecular weight, total loss of detectable glycan staining, and a minor loss of toxin binding. Controlled treatment of the affinity-purified receptor with staphylococcal V-8 protease generates several large fragments that bind toxin.

More recently we have identified and begun to characterize a toxin-binding glycoprotein from mouse liver. The liver is the primary target of ETA synthesized when burned mice are infected with *P. aeruginosa*.[104,107] In addition to liver, receptor is found in spleen, kidney, lung and heart. Levels of receptor in these and other tissues will be quantified and contrasted with the level of inhibition of protein synthesis seen in infected animals. At present the only cell in which we have been unable to find a ETA-binding protein is the OVCAR-3 cell line, which is highly resistant to toxin. (See section 6.)

6. A CELL LINE RESISTANT TO *PSEUDOMONAS* EXOTOXIN A— OVCAR CELLS

At the suggestion of Dr. David FitzGerald (NIH/NCI), we evaluated the sensitivity of OVCAR-3 cells to PE. The OVCAR-3 cell line was established by Hamilton *et al.*[105] from malignant ascites from a patient with a progressive adenocarcinoma of the ovary. These authors describe OVCAR-3 cultures as consisting of cells with well-defined, closely approximating margins that grow as monolayers, giving the typical cobblestone-like appearance ascribed to epithelium *in vitro*. At the ultrastructural level the cells showed numerous microvilli, frequent cell–cell attachment sites, and organellar features typical of a non-secretory epithelial cell. We confirmed these observations.

Our initial biochemical assays showed that 150 times more PE was required to stop protein synthesis in OVCAR-3 cells than in LM cells. Short-term binding assays, *i.e.* incubation with ETA at 4°C for 30 min, failed to show binding as measured by immuno-electron microscopy (unpublished observation). Binding could be achieved by a incubation at 4°C for > 18 hr but required high levels of toxin, *i.e.* ≥ 500 ng/ml (unpublished observations). This is reminiscent of the interaction of DT with LM cells.[77]

One explanation for this resistance is the lack of a functional receptor for ETA on OVCAR-3 cells. Supporting this thesis is our observation that when receptor homogenates are prepared from OVCAR-3 cells and run on SDS-PAGE, no receptor is identified by blotting with ETA (unpublished observation). These observations demonstrate that sensitivity to ETA is dependent upon a cell surface receptor for the toxin.

7. CHIMERIC TOXINS

During the past 5 years, FitzGerald, Pastan and colleagues have published numerous papers about using hybrid molecules or chimeric toxins, formed between fragments of ETA and other ligands, as therapeutic agents.[106,107] Their data clearly demonstrate that domain I is essential for binding to cells. A molecular construct lacking domain I is 200-fold less toxic for mouse 3T3 fibroblasts than is native toxin. This truncated molecule (ETA40), which contained domains II, I_b, and III, retained ADP-ribosylation activity.[108] By fusing ETA40 with growth factors such as transforming growth factor 2, interleukin 2, and interleukin 6, FitzGerald and colleagues have created chimeric toxins that are cell-specific cytotoxic agents.[109–111] Taken together these observations support the hypothesis that sensitivity to ETA is a function of RME.

8. CONCLUSIONS

In conclusion, the intoxication of sensitive cells by *Pseudomonas* ETA is a multi-step process mitigated by the interaction of the toxin with cell surface

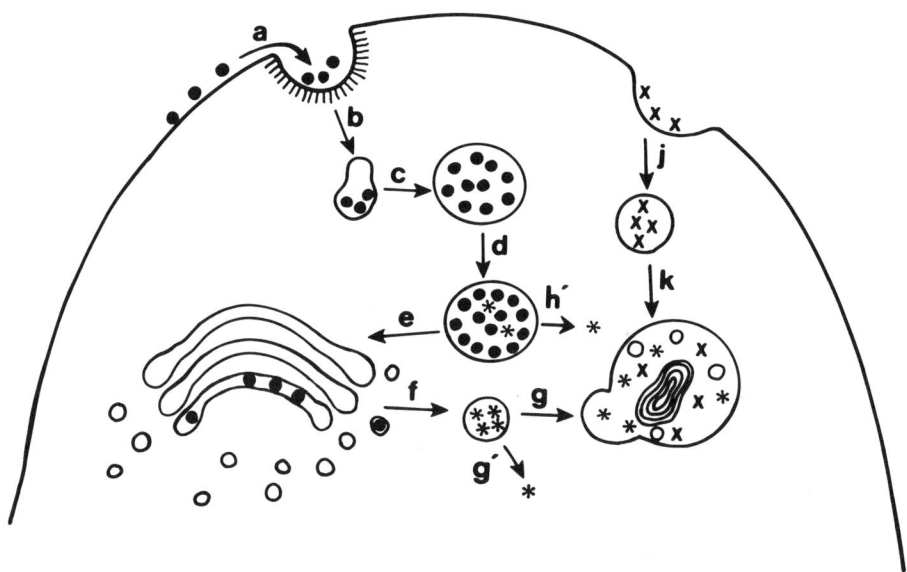

FIGURE 7. Internalization and intracellular trafficking of PE (●) and DT (X) by mouse LM fibroblasts. (a) ETA binds to cell surface receptors and enters by RME via clathrin-coated pits (30 s); (b, c, and d) ETA is progressively routed through the endosomal compartment to the Golgi region (1 min to 10 min); (e and f) ETA is delivered to the Golgi, activated (∗), and exits from the *trans*-Golgi (10 to 20 min); (g) majority of ETA is trafficked to the lysosomal compartment for degradation (≥ 20 min); (g′) some of the activated ETA escapes from a post-Golgi vesicle; (h′) an alternative site of activation and escape is the endosomal compartment; (j) internalization of surface-bound DT through non-clathrin-coated regions; (k) delivery of internalized DT directly to the lysosomal compartment without Golgi involvement (≥ 5 min). (Reproduced from Morris, R. E., 1990, in: *Trafficking of Bacterial Toxins*, [C. B. Saelinger, ed.] CRC Press, Inc., Boca Raton, Florida, pp. 49–70, used with permission.)

receptors. The binding is probably a fortuitous event resulting from the similarity of the toxin to some, as yet unidentified, physiological protein. Following binding, ETA is internalized via clathrin-coated pits and routed to the endosomal compartment. The endosomal compartment serves to transport the ETA to the *trans* Golgi network. It is here that the endocytic and exocytic pathways converge. Both the endosomal and *trans* Golgi compartments are acidic; this, in conjunction with the enzymes housed in the *trans* Golgi, allows for the activation and escape of the ETA. Following escape into the cytosol, ETA acts catalytically to ADP-ribosylate elongation factor, resulting in cessation of protein synthesis and ultimately cell death. A diagram of our model showing the cellular basis for sensitivity to ETA is shown in Fig. 7.

ACKNOWLEDGMENTS. The work presented in this manuscript was supported by funds provided by the National Institutes of Health (AI 17529 and GM 24028). The authors would like to extend their appreciation to the *Journal of Histochemistry and Cytochemistry*, Academic Press, Inc., and CRC Press, Inc., for permitting the use of previously published materials. The final preparation of this manuscript would not have been possible without the assistance of Barbara Burch and Michelle Yee.

REFERENCES

1. Middlebrook, J. L., and Dorland, R. B., 1984, Bacterial toxins: Cellular mechanisms of action, *Microbiol. Rev.* **48:**199–221.
2. Olsnes, S., and Sandvig, K., 1988, How protein toxins enter and kill cells, in: *Immunotoxins*, (A. E. Frankel, ed.), Kluwer, Boston, pp. 39–73.
3. Chung, D. W., and Collier, R. J., 1977, Enzymatically active peptide from the adenosine diphosphate-ribosylating toxin of *Pseudomonas aeruginosa*, *Infect. Immun.* **16:**832–841.
4. Lory, S., and Collier, R. J., 1980, Expression of enzymatic activity by exotoxin from *Pseudomonas aeruginosa*, *Infect. Immun.* **28:**494–501.
5. Leppla, S. H., Martin, O. C., and Muehl, L. A., 1978, The exotoxin of *P. aeruginosa*: A proenzyme having an unusual mode of activation, *Biochem. Biophys. Res. Commun.* **40:**1437–1446.
6. Neville, D. M., Jr., and Hudson, T. H., 1986, Transmembrane transport of diphtheria toxin, related toxins, and colicins, *Annu. Rev. Biochem.* **55:**195–224.
7. Hwang, J., Fitzgerald, D. J., Adhya, S., and Pastan, I., 1987, Functional domains of Pseudomonas exotoxin identified by deletion analysis of the gene expressed in *E. coli*, *Cell* **48:**129–136.
8. Iglewski, B. H., and Kabat, D., 1975, NAD-dependent inhibition of protein synthesis by *Pseudomonas aeruginosa* toxin, *Proc. Natl. Acad. Sci. USA* **72:**2284–2288.
9. Gray, G. L., Smith, D. H., Baldridge, J. S., Harkins, R. N., Vasil, M. L., Chen, E. Y., and Heynecker, H. L., 1984, Cloning, nucleotide sequence, and expression in *Escherichia coli* of the exotoxin A structural gene of *Pseudomonas aeruginosa*, *Proc. Natl. Acad. Sci. USA* **81:**2645–2649.
10. Middlebrook, J. L., and Dorland, L. B., 1977, Response of cultured mammalian cells to the

exotoxins of *Pseudomonas aeruginosa* and *Corynebacterium diphtheriae*: Differential cytotoxicity, *Can. J. Microbiol.* **23**:183–189.

11. Moehring, T. J., and Moehring, J. M., 1977, Selection and characterization of cells resistant to diphtheria toxin and Pseudomonas exotoxin A: Presumptive translational mutants, *Cell* **11**:447–454.
12. Allured, V. S., Collier, R. J., Carroll, S. F., and McKay, D. B., 1986, Structure of exotoxin A of *Pseudomonas aeruginosa* at 3.0-Ångstrom resolution, *Proc. Natl. Acad. Sci. USA* **83**:1320–1324.
13. Jinno, Y., Chaudhary, V. K., Kondo, T., Adhya, S., FitzGerald, D. J., and Pastan, I., 1988, Mutational analysis of domain I of *Pseudomonas* exotoxin, *J. Biol. Chem.* **263**:13203–13207.
14. Chaudhary, V. K., Xu, Y-H., FitzGerald, D., Adhya, S., and Pastan, I., 1988, Role of domain II of *Pseudomonas* exotoxin in the secretion of proteins into the periplasm and medium by *Escherichia coli*, *Proc. Nat. Acad. Sci. USA* **85**:2939–2943.
15. Carroll, S. F., and Collier, R. J., 1987, Active site of *Pseudomonas aeruginosa* exotoxin A. Glutamic acid 553 is photolabeled by NAD and shows functional homology with glutamic acid 148 of diphtheria toxin, *J. Biol. Chem.* **262**:8707–8711.
16. Carroll, S. F., McCloskey, J. A., Crain, P. F., Oppenheimer, N. J., Marschner, T. M., and Collier, R. J., 1985, Photoaffinity labeling of diphtheria toxin fragment A with NAD: Structure of the photoproduct at position 148, *Proc. Nat. Acad. Sci. USA* **82**:7237–7241.
17. Sadoff, J. C., Buck, G. A., Iglewski, B. H., Bjorn, M. J., and Groman, N. B., 1987, Immunological cross-reactivity in the absence of DNA homology between Pseudomonas toxin A and diphtheria toxin, *Infect. Immun.* **37**:250–254.
18. Brown, M. S., Anderson, R. G. W., Basu, S. K., and Goldstein, J. L., 1982, Recycling of cell-surface receptors: Observations from the LDL receptor system, *Cold Spring Harbor Symp. Quant. Biol.* **46**:713–721.
19. Goldstein, J. L., Brown, M. S., Anderson, R. G. W., Russell, D. W., and Schneider, W. J., 1985, Receptor-mediated endocytosis: Concepts emerging from the LDL receptor system, *Annu. Rev. Cell Biol.* **1**:1–39.
20. Pearse, B. M. F., 1987, Clathrin and coated vesicles, *EMBO J.* **6**:2507–2512.
21. Helenius, A., Mellman, I., Wall, D., Hubbard, A., 1983, Endosomes, *Trends in Biochem. Sci.* **8**:245.
22. Marsh, M., Bolzau, E., and Helenius, A., 1983, Penetration of Semliki Forest Virus from acidic prelysosomal vacuoles, *Cell* **32**:931–940.
23. Marsh, M., Griffiths, G., Dean, G. E., Mellman, I., and Helenius, A., 1986, Three dimensional structure of endosomes in BHK-21 cells, *Proc. Natl. Acad. Sci. USA* **83**:2899–2903.
24. Paavola, L. G., Strauss, J. F., Boyd, C. O., Nestler, J. E., 1985, Uptake of gold- and [^{3}H]cholesteryl linoleate-labeled human low density lipoprotein by cultured rat granulosa cells: Cellular mechanisms involved in lipoprotein metabolism and their importance to steroidogenesis, *J. Cell Biol.* **100**:1235–1247.
25. Mellman, I., Fuchs, R., Helenius, A., 1986, Acidification of the endocytic and exocytic pathways, *Ann. Rev. Biochem.* **55**:663–700.
26. Galloway, C. J., Dean, G. E., Marsh, M., Rudnick, G., and Mellman, I., 1983, Acidification of macrophage and fibroblast endocytic vesicles *in vitro*, *Proc. Natl. Acad. Sci. USA* **80**:3334–3338.
27. Tycko, B., and Maxfield, F. R., 1982, Rapid acidification of endocytic vesicles containing α_2-macroglobulin, *Cell* **28**:643–651.
28. Goldstein, J. L., Anderson, R. G. W., and Brown, M. S., 1979, Coated pits, coated vesicles, and receptor mediated endocytosis, *Nature* (London) **279**:679–685.
29. Geuze, H. J., Slot, J. W., and Strous, G. J. A. M., 1983, Intracellular site of asialoglycoprotein receptor-ligand uncoupling: Double-label immunoelectron microscopy during receptor-mediated endocytosis, *Cell* **32**:277–287.
30. Geuze, H. J., Slot, J. W., Strous, G. J. A. M., Hasilik, A., and von Figura, K., 1984,

Ultrastructural localization of the mannose-6-phosphate receptor in rat liver, *J. Cell Biol.* **98**:2047–2054.
31. Ciechanover, A., Schwartz, A. L., and Lodish, H. F., 1983, The asialoglycoprotein receptor internalizes and recycles independently of the transferrin and insulin receptors, *Cell* **32**:267–275.
32. Dautry-Varsat, A., Ciechanover, A., and Lodish, H., 1983, pH and the recycling of transferrin during receptor-mediated endocytosis, *Proc. Natl. Acad. Sci. USA* **80**:2258–2262.
33. Carpenter, G., and Cohen, S., 1976, ^{125}I-labeled human epidermal growth factor. Binding, internalization, and degradation in human fibroblasts, *J. Cell Biol.* **71**:159–171.
34. Carpenter, G., King, L., and Cohen, S., 1978, Epidermal growth factor stimulates phosphorylation in membrane preparations *in vitro*, *Nature* (London) **276**:409–410.
35. Kasuga, M., Karlsson, F. A., and Kahn, C. R., 1981, Insulin stimulates the phosphorylation of the 95,000-dalton subunit of its own receptor, *Science* (Washington D.C.), **215**:185–186.
36. Carpentier, J. L., Gorden, P., Barazzone, P., Freychet, P., LeCam, A., and Orci, L., 1979, Intracellular localization of ^{125}I-labeled insulin in hepatocytes from intact rat liver, *Proc. Nat. Acad. Sci. USA* **76**:2803–2807.
37. Mellman, J., and Plutner, H., 1984, Internalization and degradation of macrophage Fc receptors bound to polyvalent immune complexes, *J. Cell Biol.* **98**:1170–1177.
38. Willingham, M. C., Haigler, H. T., FitzGerald, D. J. P., Gallo, M. G., Rutherford, A. V., and Pastan, I., 1983, The morphologic pathway of binding and internalization of epidermal growth factor in cultured cells. Studies on A431, KB, and 3T3 cells using multiple labelling methods, *Exp. Cell Res.* **146**:163–175.
39. Dunn, W. A., and Hubbard, A. L., 1984, Receptor-mediated endocytosis of epidermal growth factor by hepatocytes in the perfused rat liver: Ligand and receptor dynamics, *J. Cell Biol.* **98**:2148–2159.
40. Di Paola, M., and Maxfield, F. R., 1984, Conformational changes in the receptors for epidermal growth factor and asialoglycoproteins induced by the mildly acidic pH found in endocytic vesicles, *J. Biol. Chem.* **259**:9163–9171.
41. Burwen, S. J., Barker, M. E., Goldman, I. S., Hradek, G. T., Raper, S. E., and Jones, A. L., 1984, Transport of epidermal growth factor by rat liver: Evidence for a non-lysosomal pathway, *J. Cell Biol.* **99**:1259–1265.
42. Beguinot, L., Lyall, R. M., Willingham, M. C., and Pastan, I., 1984, Down-regulation of the epidermal growth factor receptor in KB cells is due to receptor internalization and subsequent degradation in lysosomes, *Proc. Natl. Acad. Sci. USA* **81**:2384–2388.
43. Rensten, R. H., Jones, A. L., Christiansen, W. D., Hradek, G. T., and Underdown, B. J., 1980, Evidence for vesicular transport mechanism in hepatocytes for biliary secretion of immunoglobulin A, *Science* (Washington D.C.) **208**:1276–1278.
44. Geuze, H. J., Slot, J. W., Strous, G. J. A. M., Peppard, J., von Figura, K., Hasilik, A., and Schwartz, A. L., 1984, Intracellular receptor sorting during endocytosis: Comparative immunoelectron microscopy of multiple receptors in rat liver, *Cell* **37**:195–204.
45. Kuhn, L. C., and Kraehenbuhl, J. P., 1979, Role of secretory component, a secreted glycoprotein, in the specific uptake of IgA dimer by epithelial cells, *J. Biol. Chem.* **254**:11072–11081.
46. Mostov, K. E., and Blobel, G., 1982, A transmembrane precursor of secretory component, *J. Biol. Chem.* **257**:11816–11821.
47. Diment, S., and Stahl, P., 1985, Macrophage endosomes contain proteases which degrade endocytosed protein ligands, *J. Biol. Chem.* **260**:15311–15317.
48. Schaudies, R. P., Gorman, R. M., Savage, C. R., Jr., and Poretz, R. O., 1987, Proteolytic processing of epidermal growth factor within endosomes, *Biochem. Biophys. Res. Commun.* **143**:710–713.
49. Ohkuma, S., and Poole, B., 1978, Fluorescence probe measurement of the intralysosomal

pH in living cells and the perturbation of pH by various agents, *Proc. Nat. Acad. Sci. USA* **75:** 3327–3333.
50. Mellman, I., Howe, C., Helenius, A., 1987, The control of membrane traffic on the endocytic pathway, *Curr. Topics Membr. Transp.* **29:**255–288.
51. Weigel, P. H., and Oka, J. A., 1983, The surface content of asialoglycoprotein receptors on isolated hepatocytes is reversibly modulated by changes in temperature, *J. Biol. Chem* **258:** 5089–5093.
52. Dunn, W. A., Hubbard, A. L., and Aronson, N. N., Jr., 1980, Low temperature selectively inhibits fusion between pinocytic vesicles and lysosomes during heterophagy of ^{125}I-asialofetuin by the perfused rat liver, *J. Biol. Chem.* **255:**5971–5978.
53. Sleight, R. G., and Pagano, R. E., 1984, Transport of fluorescent phosphatidylcholine analog from the plasma membrane to the Golgi apparatus, *J. Cell Biol.* **99:**742–751.
54. Helenius, A., and Marsh, M., 1982, Endocytosis of enveloped animal viruses, in: *Membrane Recycling* (D. Evered and G. M. Collins, eds.) Pitman Books Ltd., London, pp. 59–76.
55. Kielian, M. C., Keränen, S., Kääriäinen, L., and Helenius, A., 1984, Membrane fusion mutants of Semliki Forest Virus, *J. Cell Biol.* **98:**139–145.
56. Kielian, M., and Helenius, A., 1984, Role of cholesterol in fusion of Semliki Forest Virus with membranes, *J. Virol.* **52:**281–283.
57. Madshus, I. H., Olsnes, S., and Sandvig, K., 1984, Mechanism of entry into the cytosol of poliovirus type 1: Requirement for low pH, *J. Cell Biol.* **98:**1194–1200.
58. Madshus, I. H., Olsnes, S., and Sandvig, K., 1984, Requirements for entry of poliovirus RNA into cells at low pH, *EMBO J.* **3:**1945–1950.
59. Zeichhardt, H., Wetz, K., Willingmann, P., and Habermehl, K-O., 1985, Entry of poliovirus type 1 and mouse Eberfield (ME) Virus into HEp-2 cells: Receptor-mediated endocytosis and endosomal or lysosomal uncoating, *J. Gen. Virol.* **66:**483–492.
60. Chardonnet, Y., and Dales, S., 1970, Early events in the interaction of adenoviruses with HeLa cells. I. Penetration of type 5 and intracellular release of the DNA genome, *Virology* **40:**462–477.
61. Chardonnet, Y., and Dales, S., 1970, Early events in the interaction of adenoviruses with HeLa cells. II. Comparative observations on the penetration of types 1, 5, 7, and 12, *Virology* **40:**478–485.
62. FitzGerald, D. J. P., Padmanabhan, P., Pastan, I., and Willingham, M. C., 1983, Adenovirus-induced release of epidermal growth factor and *Pseudomonas* toxin into the cytosol of KB cells during receptor-mediated endocytosis, *Cell* **32:**607–617.
63. FitzGerald, D. J. P., Trowbridge, I. S., Pastan, I., and Willingham, M. C., 1983, Enhancement of toxicity of antitransferrin receptor antibody-*Pseudomonas* exotoxin conjugates by adenovirus, *Proc. Nat. Acad. Sci. USA* **80:**4134–4138.
64. Seth, P., FitzGerald, D. J. P., Willingham, M. C., and Pastan, I., 1984, Role of a low pH environment in adenovirus enhancement of the toxicity of a *Pseudomonas* exotoxin-epidermal growth factor conjugate, *J. Virol.* **51:**650–655.
65. Seth, P., FitzGerald, D., Willingham, M., and Pastan, I., 1986, Pathway of adenovirus entry into cells, in: *Virus Attachment and Entry into Cells* (R. L. Crowell and K. Lonberg-Hold, eds.) Am. Soc. Microbiol., Washington, D. C., pp. 191–195.
66. FitzGerald, D., Morris, R. E., and Saelinger, C. B., 1980, Receptor-mediated internalization of *Pseudomonas* toxin by mouse fibroblasts, *Cell* **21:**867–873.
67. Manhart, M. D., Morris, R. E., Bonventre, P. F., Leppla, S., and Saelinger, C. B., 1984, Evidence for *Pseudomonas* exotoxin A receptors on plasma membrane of toxin-sensitive LM fibroblasts, *Infect. Immun.* **45:**596–603.
68. Moehring, J. M., and Moehring, T. J., 1983, Strains of CHO-K1 cells resistant to *Pseudomonas* exotoxin A and cross-resistant to diphtheria toxin and viruses, *Infect. Immun.* **41:** 998–1009.
69. Tietze, C., Schlesinger, P., and Stahl, P., 1980, Chloroquine and ammonium ion inhibit

receptor-mediated endocytosis of mannose-glycoconjugates by macrophages. Apparent inhibition of receptor recycling, *Biochem. Biophys. Res. Commun.* **93:**1–8.
70. Schreiber, A. B., Schlessinger, J., and Edidin, 1984, Interaction between major histocompatibility complex antigens and epidermal growth factor receptors on human cells, *J. Cell Biol.* **98:**725–731.
71. Morris, R. E., and Saelinger, C. B., 1990, Visualization of intracellular trafficking of Proteins, in: *Methods in Enzymology*, Volume 184 (M. Wilchek and E. A. Bayer, eds.), Academic Press, Inc., California, pp. 379–388.
72. Morris, R. E., and Saelinger, C. B., 1984, Visualization of intracellular trafficking. Use of biotinyl ligands in conjunction with avidin-gold colloids, *J. Histochem. Cytochem.* **101:**548–559.
73. Morris, R. E., and Saelinger, C. B., 1986, Reduced temperature alters *Pseudomonas* exotoxin A entry into the mouse LM cell, *Infect. Immun.* **52:**445–453.
74. Morris, R. E., Manhart, M. D., and Saelinger, C. B., 1983, Receptor mediated entry of *Pseudomonas* toxin: Methylamine blocks clustering step, *Infect. Immun.* **40:**806–811.
75. Saelinger, C. B., Morris, R. E., and Foertsch, G., 1985, Trafficking of *Pseudomonas* exotoxin A in mammalian cells, *Eur. J. Clin. Microbiol.* **4:**170–174.
76. Morris, R. E., Gernstein, A. S., Bonventre, P. F., and Saelinger, C. B., 1985, Receptor-mediated entry of diphtheria toxin into monkey kidney (Vero) cells: Electron microscopic evaluation, *Infect. Immun.* **50:**721–727.
77. Morris, R. E., and Saelinger, C. B., 1983, Diphtheria toxin does not enter resistant cells by receptor-mediated endocytosis, *Infect. Immun.* **42:**812–817.
78. van Deurs, B., and Nilausen, K., 1982, Pinocytosis in mouse L-fibroblasts: Ultrastructural evidence for a direct membrane shuttle between the plasma membrane and lysosomal compartment, *J. Cell Biol.* **94:**279–286.
79. van Deurs, B., Nilausen, K., Faergeman, O., and Meinertz, H., 1982, Coated pits and pinocytosis of cationized ferritin in human skin fibroblasts, *Eur. J. Cell. Biol.* **27:**270–278.
80. Larkin, J. M., Brown, M. S., Goldstein, J. L., and Anderson, R. W., 1983, Depletion of intracellular potassium arrests coated pit formation and receptor-mediated endocytosis in fibroblasts, *Cell* **33:**273–285.
81. Moya, M, Dautry-Varsat, A., Goud, B., Louvard, D., and Boquet, P., 1985, Inhibition of coated pit formation in HEp-2 cells blocks the cytotoxicity of diphtheria toxin but not that of ricin toxin, *J. Cell Biol.* **101:**548–559.
82. Sandvig, K., Sundan, A., and Olsnes, S., 1985, Effect of potassium depletion of cells on their sensitivity to diphtheria toxin and *Pseudomonas* toxin, *J. Cell Physiol.* **124:**54–60.
83. Pastan, I., Willingham, M. C., and FitzGerald, D. J. P., 1986, Immunotoxins, *Cell* **47:**641–648.
84. Farahbakhsh, Z. T., Baldwin, R. L., and Wisnieski, B. J., 1986, *Pseudomonas* exotoxin A. Membrane binding, insertion, and traversal, *J. Biol. Chem.* **261:**11404–11408.
85. Donovan, J. J., Simon, M. I., and Montal, M., 1985, Requirements for the translocation of diphtheria toxin fragment A across lipid membranes, *J. Biol. Chem.* **260:**8817–8823.
86. Farahbakhsh, Z. T., Baldwin, R. L., and Wisnieski, B. J., 1987, Effect of low pH on the conformation of *Pseudomonas* exotoxin A, *J. Biol. Chem.* **262:**2256–2261.
87. Idziorek, T., FitzGerald, D., and Pastan, I., 1990, Low pH-induced changes in *Pseudomonas* exotoxin and its domains: Increased binding of Triton X-114, *Infect. Immun.* **58:**1415–1420.
88. Marnell, M. H., Shia, S. P., Stookey, M., and Draper, R. K., 1984, Evidence for penetration of diphtheria toxin to the cytosol through a prelysosomal membrane, *Infect. Immun.* **44:**145–150.
89. Hudson, T. H., and Neville, D. M., 1987, Temporal separation of protein toxin translocation from processing events, *J. Biol. Chem.* **262:**16484–16494.
90. Docherty, K., and Steiner, D. F., 1982, Post-translational proteolysis in polypeptide hormone biosynthesis, *Annu. Rev. Physiol.* **44:**625–638.
91. Steiner, D. F., Docherty, K., and Carroll, R., 1984, Golgi/Granule processing of peptide hormone and neuropeptide precursors: A minireview, *J. Cell Biochem.* **24:**121–130.
92. Marx, J. L., 1987, A new wave of enzymes for clearing prohormones, *Science* (Washington, D.C.), **235:**285–286.

93. Herbert, E., and Uhler, M., 1982, Biosynthesis of polyprotein precursors to regulatory peptides, *Cell* **30**:1–2.
94. Vlasuk, G. P., Ghrayeb, J., and Walz, F. G., Jr., 1980, Proalbumin is bound to the membrane of rat liver smooth microsomes, *Biochem. Biophys. Res. Commun.* **94**:366–372.
95. Judah, J. D., and Nicholls, M. R., 1971, Biosynthesis of rat serum albumin, *Biochem. J.* **123**:649–655.
96. Greenfield, L., Bjorn, M. J., Horn, G., Fong, D., Buck, G. A., Collier, R. J., and Kaplan, D. A., 1983, Nucleotide sequence of the structural gene for diphtheria toxin carried by corynebacteriophage β, *Proc. Natl. Acad. Sci. USA* **80**:6853–6857.
97. Anderson, R. G. W., and Pathak, R. K., 1985, Vesicles of cisternae in the *trans* Golgi apparatus of human fibroblasts are acidic compartments, *Cell* **40**:635–643.
98. Germain, R. N., 1986, The ins and outs of antigen processing and presentation, *Nature* (London) **322**:687–689.
99. Collins, D., and Huang, L., 1987, Cytotoxicity of diphtheria toxin A fragment to toxin-resistant murine cells delivered by pH-sensitive immunoliposomes, *Cancer Res.* **47**:735–739.
100. Heagy, W. E., and Neville, D. M., Jr., 1981, Kinetics of protein synthesis inactivation by diphtheria toxin in toxin resistant L cells, *J. Biol. Chem.* **256**:12788–12792.
101. van Deurs, B., Tónnessen, T. I., Peterson, O. W., Sandvig, K., and Olsnes, S., 1986, Routing of internalized ricin and ricin conjugates to the Golgi complex, *J. Cell Biol.* **102**:37–47.
102. van Deurs, B., Sandvig, K., Peterson, O. W., Olsnes, S., Simon, K., and Griffiths, G., 1988, Estimation of the amount of internalized ricin that reaches the trans-Golgi network, *J. Cell Biol.* **106**:253–267.
103. Youle, R. J., and Colombatti, M., 1987, Hybridoma cells containing intracellular anti-ricin antibodies show ricin meets secretory antibodies before entering the cytosol, *J. Biol. Chem.* **262**:4676–4682.
104. Saelinger, C. B., Snell, K., and Holder, I. A., 1977, Experimental studies on the pathogenesis of infections due to *Pseudomonas aeruginosa*: Direct evidence for toxin production during *Psdudomonas* infection of burned skin tissues, *J. Infect. Dis.* **136**:555–561.
105. Hamilton, T. C., Young, R. C., McKoy, W. M., Grotzinger, K. R., Green, J. A., Chu, E. W., Whang-Peng, J., Rogan, A. M., Green, W. R., and Ozols, R. F., 1983, Characterization of a human ovarian carcinoma cell line (NIH:OVCAR-3) with androgen and estrogen receptors, *Cancer Res.* **43**:5379–5389.
106. FitzGerald, D. J., Willingham, M. C., and Pastan, I., 1988, *Pseudomonas* exotoxin-Immunotoxins, in: *Immunotoxins*, (E. F. Frankel, ed.), Kluwer Academic Publishers, Massachusetts, pp. 161–173.
107. Pastan, I., and FitzGerald, D., 1989, *Pseudomonas* exotoxin: Chimeric toxins, *J. Biol. Chem.* **264**:15157–15160.
108. Kondo, T., FitzGerald, D., Chaudhary, V. K., Adhya, S., and Pastan, I., 1988, Activity of immunotoxins constructed with modified *Pseudomonas* exotoxin A lacking the cell recognition domain, *J. Biol. Chem.* **263**:9470–9475.
109. Chaudhary, V. K., Mizukami, T., Fuerst, T. R., FitzGerald, D. J., Moss, B., Pastan, I., and Berger, E. A., 1988, Selective killing of HIV-infected cells by recombinant human CD4-*Pseudomonas* exotoxin hybrid protein, *Nature* **335**:369–372.
110. Lorberboum-Galski, H., FitzGerald, D., Chaudhary, V., Adhya, S., and Pastan, I., 1988, Cytotoxic activity of an interleukin 2-*Pseudomonas* exotoxin chimeric protein produced in *Escherichia coli*, *Proc. Natl. Acad. Sci. USA* **85**:1922–1926.
111. Siegall, C. B., Chaudhary, V. K., FitzGerald, D. J., and Pastan, I., 1989, Functional analysis of domains II, Ib, and III of *Pseudomonas* exotoxin, *J. Biol. Chem.* **264**:14256–14261.
112. Kagan, B. L., Finkelstein, A., and Colombini, M., 1981, Diphtheria toxin fragment forms large pores in phospholipid bilayer membranes, *Proc. Natl. Acad. Sci. USA* **78**:4950–4954.
113. Donovan, J. J., Simon, M. I., Draper, K. K., and Montal, M., 1981, Diphtheria toxin forms transmembrane channels in planar lipid bilayers, *Proc. Natl. Acad. Sci. USA* **78**:172–176.

6

Role of Exotoxins in the Pathogenesis of *P. aeruginosa* Infections

DARRELL R. GALLOWAY

1. INTRODUCTION AND HISTORICAL PERSPECTIVES

The history of the study of infectious diseases has shown that disease often depends upon the outcome of interactions between the virulence associated-properties of the microbe and the defensive reactions of the host. Our approach to understanding microbial pathogenicity has focused on the identification of virulence factors, shown to be responsible for producing disease when the microbe establishes itself within the host. In some classic examples, such as *clostridium tetani* and *corynebacterium diphtheriae*, a single factor has been shown to be responsible for the disease and vaccines have been developed to prevent such infections or protect against the consequences of these infections.

As encouraging as these examples of the successful application of medical research have proven to be, unfortunately they are not representative of the majority of microbial infections in the human host. Thus, in most infections the invading microbe presents a multitude of virulence-associated factors and in most cases the role of these factors and their precise relationship to the pathology of the infection have not been firmly established. While

---

DARRELL R. GALLOWAY • Department of Microbiology, The Ohio State University, Columbus, Ohio 43210-1292.

Pseudomonas aeruginosa as an Opportunistic Pathogen, edited by Mario Campa *et al.* Plenum Press, New York, 1993.

this realization may be discouraging, there is reason to be more optimistic regarding the study of infectious disease today than ever before. Modern molecular biology has led to the expansion of our abilities to explore disease-causing microorganisms at the molecular and genetic level. The same techniques are being applied to the study of immunology, resulting in a concomitant increase in the information regarding the host response to the infectious agent. Knowledge of the events associated with the interactions between infectious agent and host is accumulating rapidly and leading to innovative approaches to therapeutic intervention.

The study of *Pseudomonas* infections provides a prime example of the complexity of the relationships occurring between potentially pathogenic microbes and the human host. We do not have a complete understanding of the pathogenicity of this opportunistic microorganism. Pathogenicity is clearly multifactoral and dependent upon the immune status of the host; however, research regarding the ability of *Pseudomonas* to cause disease is proceeding rapidly and several recent developments have increased our understanding of its pathogenicity. This review is limited to a consideration of the exoproducts released by *Pseudomonas* and current knowledge about the role of these factors in the pathology associated with *Pseudomonas* infections.

1.1. *Pseudomonas aeruginosa*—The Opportunistic Pathogen

Pseudomonas species constitute a diverse group of microorganisms that are widely distributed in the environment and are part of the normal intestinal flora of many individuals. However, *P. aeruginosa* has become associated with frequent and often serious infections of the immunocompromised host. *P. aeruginosa* is not considered pathogenic, but rather an opportunistic infectious microorganism. This is dramatically evidenced by the frequency with which this organism is associated with nosocomial (hospital-acquired) infections. An estimated seven of every 1000 patients who enter U.S. community hospitals will acquire a *Pseudomonas* infection.[1] *Pseudomonas* infections in immunocompromised patients frequently develop into bacteremias with a high mortality rate in spite of the use of aggressive antibiotic therapy.[2,3,4] In contrast, for reasons that remain obscure, *P. aeruginosa* (as well as *P. cepacia*) appear preferentially to colonize the respiratory tracts of cystic fibrosis patients, with the result of life-threatening chronic infections. *Pseudomonas* infections have often been associated with patients suffering from burn trauma, however the incidence of *Pseudomonas* infections in these patients has receded in recent years due to the implementation of hospital procedures designed to limit the spread of these infections.[5] The high incidence of *Pseudomonas* infections in burn patients may be due in part to the immunosuppression resulting from this type of injury. This possibility is supported by the observation that the overall incidence of *Pseudomonas* infections has been increasing steadily due to the increasing number of immunocompromised patients resulting from increased use of immunosuppressive therapy in the treatment of neoplastic disease and organ transplantation. In addition, *Pseudomonas* has proven to be capable of rapidly developing resistance to antibiotic therapy, which appears to be an important factor in the selection of *P. aeruginosa* as the predominant pathogen emerging from mixed bacterial populations in an infection.

An important consideration in the study of virulence factors and their potential role in the infectious process and associated pathogenicity is the use of an appropriate model system to mimic the disease. Several animal model systems have been developed for the study of *Pseudomonas* infections based upon the immunocompromised status of the host or the site of infection. One commonly used model developed by Stieritz and Holder to study the association between burn trauma and *Pseudomonas* infection, is the burned mouse model.[6] This model has been used widely to show that partial burn trauma dramatically increases susceptibility of a mouse to lethal *Pseudomonas* infection, analogous to the clinical situation observed in burn patients. This model has been used extensively in the study of the pathogenesis of *P. aeruginosa* in burn infections and is described in detail by I. A. Holder in Chapter 14 of this volume.[7] *Pseudomonas* lung infections have been studied using both acute[8,9] and chronic[10] lung infection models in guinea pigs and rats, respectively. The chronic rat lung infection model has been shown to mimic the pathology seen in chronic pulmonary infections in humans.[11] Other models of *Pseudomonas* infection include a neutropenic rabbit model[12] and a neutropenic rat model,[13] designed to reflect the immune-deficient status of the host that is often associated with severe *Pseudomonas* bacteremia. In addition, the rabbit corneal infection model has been used to study the pathology associated with localized *Pseudomonas* infections.[14] The several animal model systems that have been developed to study *Pseudomonas* infections reflect the diversity of this organism's ability to cause a variety of infections in the susceptible host.

Pseudomonas aeruginosa produces a variety of exoproducts, several of which appear to play some role in its pathogenesis. These proposed virulence-associated factors display a variety of biochemical mechanisms and act both individually and in concert to produce infection and disease. The principal exoproducts studied in relation to *Pseudomonas* virulence include exotoxin A (ETA), exoenzyme S (exo-S), elastase, and phospholipase C. Most of the studies that have implicated a role for these exoproducts in pathogenesis have compared the results of infection with wild-type strains and mutant strains that are deficient in the production of the factor being studied. Studies indicate that each of these exoproducts is involved in the infectious process; however, the precise role and relative importance of each remains unclear. Studies designed to discover the function of each of these proteins at the molecular level are currently in progress in several laboratories.

2. EXOTOXIN A

Discovered and purified 30 years ago in the laboratory of P. V. Liu,[15] *P. aeruginosa* exotoxin A (ETA) has been identified as the major virulence-associated factor produced by *P. aeruginosa*. During the past 5 years, ETA has emerged as the best-understood example of all the bacterial protein toxins, largely due to the determination of its three-dimensional structure in 1986.[16] The study of ETA is forming the model upon which other similar bacterial toxins are being studied, and there have been numerous reviews on the subject.[17,18,19] The following is a brief summary of our current understanding of ETA.

ETA is the most toxic product of *P. aeruginosa* and, with rare exceptions, almost every *P. aeruginosa* strain produces ETA.[20,21] ETA is lethal for vertebrates with an experimentally determined LD_{50} for mice in the range of 2.5 μg/kg.[17,22,23] This is approximately 10,000 times the toxicity associated with *Pseudomonas* lipopolysaccharide.[19] ETA is also lethal for rats, rabbits, dogs, and rhesus monkeys, although clinical aspects vary among species.[24–26] In mice, death occurs within 48 hr following toxin injection and appears to be associated with severe liver pathology.[27,28] Pollack reports that intravenous injection of ETA into dogs and monkeys results in decreased cardiac output and lowered systemic arterial blood pressure following an initial delay of some hours. Early hepatocellular necrosis was observed consistently, indicating that liver toxicity appears to be a major factor in the pathology associated with ETA.[19] This has become an important consideration in studies involving the use of ETA or active fragments in the construction of immunotoxin conjugates or chimeric proteins for use in directed cytotoxicity applications. In addition to *in vivo* studies, several *in vitro* studies have shown that ETA is cytotoxic for a variety of cultured cells.[29–31]

ETA is a single-chain polypeptide of 613 amino acids, with a molecular weight of 66,583. ETA has been classified as a member of the adenosine-diphosphate-ribosylating toxins (ADPRT), which include diphtheria toxin (DT), cholera toxin, pertussis toxin, and the *E. coli* heat-labile enterotoxin. All the structural genes encoding these toxins have been cloned and sequenced. All ADPRT toxins bind NAD and covalently link the ADP-ribose moiety to a specified target protein, which results in the impairment of that protein's normal function. In the case of ETA and DT, the target protein is eucaryotic elongation factor 2 (EF2) and the result of ADP-ribosylation of EF2 is the loss of protein synthesis in the target cell. This reaction can be represented as:

$$NAD^+ + EF2 \rightarrow ADPR-EF2 + \text{nicotinamide} + H^+$$

Because these toxins are enzymatic in nature, a single molecule of toxin is probably sufficient to kill the susceptible cell and this has been demonstrated in the case of DT.[32] ETA and DT share the same biochemical mechanism; ETA has been used to reverse the ADP-ribosylation catalyzed by DT.[33] In addition, each toxin possesses the ability to hydrolyze NAD in the absence of EF2, although this represents a minor activity of these toxins. The significance of this NAD glycohydrolase activity is unknown at the present time.

Analysis of the three-dimensional structure of ETA reveals three structural domains.[16,34] Deletion analysis of the ETA structural gene and expression of the resulting ETA fragments has provided evidence correlating ETA functions with these domains.[35] Thus, domain I, which includes residues 1–252 and 365–395, has been associated with receptor binding; domain II, residues 253–364, is believed to be involved in the membrane translocation of ETA once toxin has been incorporated into the cell; and domain III, residues 396–613, is the ADPR-active portion of the molecule. Several studies have shown that the active site of ETA that binds NAD is located within a large cleft in domain III where it has been determined that the Glu 553 residue is required for ADPRT activity.[36] In addition, the His 426 residue, some distance from the NAD site, has also been identified as a critical residue for ADPRT activity, and this residue is thought to be associated with EF2 binding.[37-39]

Although ETA and DT appear to be remarkably similar in terms of biochemical function, early studies indicated that they bear little structural resemblance in DNA sequence homology.[40] It was also discovered that the enzymatic activity (ADP-ribosyltransferase) resided within a N-terminal fragment of DT while the homologous activity in ETA is associated with a C-terminal fragment. However, some degree of structural homology is indicated by studies that demonstrate immunological cross-reactivity between ETA and DT.[40,41] It is noteworthy, however, that neutralizing antisera to one toxin will not result in neutralization of the other toxin. More recently, however, studies conducted in this laboratory using ETA-specific monoclonal antibodies (MAb) have resulted in the discovery of a cross-reactive epitope that exists in several of the ADPRT toxins.[41] Antisera prepared against synthetic peptides, including this epitope, result in the partial inhibition of ADPRT activity in both ETA and DT. MAb that bind to the epitope cross-react with DT, cholera toxin, and pertussis toxin. Results suggest a degree of structural homology between ADPRT toxins despite the apparent lack of homology when the DNA-based sequences of the proteins are compared. This is supported by a recent report comparing the sequence homology between ETA and DT within the NAD-binding region or active site of ETA,[42] which indicates the existence of considerable homology within the active site. Significantly however, the cross-reactive epitope described here does not appear to reside within the active site of ETA (nor presumably that of DT). Collectively, these studies suggest that ETA and DT, and perhaps the other ADPRT, evolved from a common ancestral protein that has undergone major structural rearrangements as well as sequence divergence.

There is considerable current interest in the uptake and processing of the ETA molecule by susceptible cells. Evidence suggests that ETA is incorporated into susceptible cells by receptor-mediated endocytosis (RME).[43] However, a receptor has yet to be identified. Once ETA has been incorporated into the cell, it must leave the endosome and enter the cytoplasmic compartment where it inactivates EF2 and inhibits protein synthesis. This membrane translocation event is critical to an understanding of the toxicity associated with ETA and is the subject of intense investigation. This process is known to be pH-dependent; it has been learned recently that ETA is cleaved within the endocytic vesicle and a 37 kD C-terminal fragment of ETA is translocated to the cytoplasmic compartment.[44] Details of the translocation process, however, remain obscure.

ETA is secreted in a non-active proenzyme form that must undergo modification to become enzymatically active. *In vitro* studies have revealed that partially unfolding the molecule in the presence of urea and reducing agents results in "activation" of toxin,[45,46] presumably by changing the tertiary structure sufficient to expose the active site of the toxin. However, studies in this laboratory have shown that NAD binding occurs in the absence of treatment with urea and dithiothreitol, which suggests that the activation of toxin is not required for NAD binding (unpublished observations). Furthermore, several studies have shown that fragments of ETA produced by limited proteolysis, chemical cleavage, freeze-thawing, or prolonged storage of the purified toxin result in the production of an ADPR-active fragment.[47,48] This has been verified by the production of various ADPR-active fragments of ETA by constructing deletion mutants within the ETA structural gene and expressing the ETA fragments in a suitable host.[35,39,49] Significantly, domain III ADPR-active fragments do not require treatment with urea and dithiothreitol to ADP-ribosylate EF2.[39] Thus it is not clear precisely how the activation process enables ETA to achieve full ADPR capability. One possibility is that the activation process enables ETA to interact with EF2, its target protein.

Several studies, taken together, indicate that ETA contributes to the pathogenesis associated with *P. aeruginosa* infections. The fact that ETA is a potent inhibitor of eucaryotic protein synthesis is a clear indication of its pathogenic potential. It has been established that ETA is lethal when administered to various species.[26,50,51] Furthermore, *in vivo* studies using the burned mouse model (BMM)[52] and the rat chronic lung infection model[11] have shown that ETA is produced during experimental infections. Clinical experience indicates that ETA is produced in human infections[53,54] and that patients recovering from *Pseudomonas* infections exhibit significant anti-ETA titers.[55-57] Analysis of clinical infections indicated that increased chance of survival was associated with high anti-ETA titers.[54] Whereas these results indicate the production of ETA during infections, evidence for a role in pathogenesis comes from several studies. Significantly, Pavlovskis and Shackelford[58] demonstrated *in vivo* in 1974 that ETA inhibits protein synthesis. This study not only established the potential significance of ETA during infection, but was the first work to indicate ETA's mode of action. It was later determined *in vitro*, in direct comparison with the mode of action of DT, that ETA is an ADP-ribosyltransferase that modifies EF2 and inhibits protein synthesis.[59]

Several studies have compared the virulence of nontoxigenic mutants with parent strains in various experimental infection models; the results have been reviewed and are summarized elsewhere.[19,60] In general, it has been shown that nontoxigenic strains are less virulent than strains producing toxin, but this conclusion depends on the animal model system used. For example, in the guinea pig acute lung infection model it has been reported that the nontoxigenic mutant strains were no less virulent than the parental strain.[61] Furthermore, there seems to be no correlation between the level of toxin produced and the degree of virulence. This has been well-documented in the case of strain PA103, which produces high levels of toxin but demonstrates low virulence in the BMM.[12,52,62]

In efforts to determine whether ETA could serve as an effective target antigen for vaccine development, several immunization studies have been conducted designed to protect against infections with tox+ and tox− strains in experimental infection models. In essence, these studies have shown that only partial protection is obtained following active immunization with a toxoid form of ETA.[7] Essentially these collective studies have shown that while ETA is certainly involved in pathogenesis, it is by no means the only virulence factor produced by *Pseudomonas*, and immunization with a suitable ETA toxoid or genetically engineered ETA derivative or fragment will not afford complete protection from *Pseudomonas* infections.

Despite a number of studies the role of ETA in virulence has remained ill-defined. The difficulty associated with the interpretation of these studies is related to the multifactoral nature of *Pseudomonas* virulence and the use of non-related strains and different animal model systems. Taken together, however, the results of many studies make it clear that ETA contributes in several ways to the pathogenesis associated with *Pseudomonas* infections, and it does so in combination with other virulence factors, *e.g.* elastase. For this reason immunization against ETA alone has proven insufficient for protection against *Pseudomonas* infections in any animal model system.

3. EXOENZYME S

In addition to ETA, some strains of *P. aeruginosa* produce another ADP-ribosyltransferase known as exo-S. However, this protein differs from ETA in several respects and progress in exo-S research has been slowed by the apparent difficulty associated with its purification. Exo-S is reported to catalyze the transfer of ADP-ribose from NAD to a number of eucaryotic proteins, yet does not modify EF2. Most recently it has been reported that exo-S mono-ADP-ribosylates the intermediate filament protein vimentin, particularly the disassembled form,[63] as well as several membrane-associated GTP-binding proteins, including the p21 product of the proto-oncogene c-H-*ras*.[64] Although there have been two reports regarding its purification, a description of the properties of exo-S remains confusing. Exo-S has been purified from the spent culture medium of two clinical isolates (DG-1 and 388) that have formed the basis for all the reported work with exo-S. Nicas and Iglewski report two forms of exo-S; a larger 53-kD form that is enzymatically inactive, and a 49-kD form that has ADP-ribosyltransferase activity.[65] Although this report is cited by its authors as the reference for exo-S purification, it lacks details of purification. Exo-S purification from *P. aeruginosa* strain DG-1 has been described by Woods *et al.*[66] in a report that indicated exo-S has an estimated molecular weight of 105,000 (by gel filtration analysis) and appears to consist of a complex of smaller components as revealed by SDS-PAGE analysis. A physical description of exo-S remains unclear. The cloning of the structural gene, and therefore the determination of the gene sequence for exo-S, have not been reported.

Several studies have attempted to determine whether exo-S plays a role in pathogenesis. The most convincing studies have employed a genetic approach using transposon insertional mutagenesis to create mutant strains that have lost the ability to produce exo-S. The virulence of these mutant strains was compared with the wild-type strain in both the chronic lung infection model[67,68] and the BMM.[69] In both model systems evidence indicates that mutants deficient in exo-S are less virulent than the wild-type strain. It is important to note, however, that two studies used a clinical isolate strain (388) reported to lack production of ETA.[70] However, subsequently it has been demonstrated that this strain does produce and secrete some ETA,[71] a fact not taken into account in these studies. This probably accounts for the observation by Bjorn *et al.*[72] that experimental infections using strain 388 resulted in the reduction of EF2 function 48 hr post-infection. Additional studies have reported pathological changes in lung tissue following exposure to purified preparations of exo-S.[73] In addition, it has been reported recently that purified exo-S preparations cause agglutination of rat erythrocytes.[74] However, comparative studies indicate that exo-S is less toxic than ETA, with a reported LD_{50} of 8 μg in mice, as compared to an LD_{50} of 0.3 μg per mouse for ETA.[66]

Exo-S has been studied recently as a potential adhesin, which may be involved in the adherence of *Pseudomonas* to susceptible tissue. Using thin-layer chromatograms to separate various ceramide glycolipid compounds, Baker *et al.*[75] found exo-S binding to gangliotriosyl-(ASMG2, GalNAcB1-4GalB1-4GlcB1-1Cer), gangliotetraosyl-(ASMG1, GalB1-3GalNAcB1-4GalB1-4GlcB1-1Cer), and lactosylceramide (GalB1-4GlcB1-1Cer). Significantly, exo-S does not appear to bind to the sialated derivatives of these compounds, indicating that sialic acid does not play a role in binding. This finding contrasts with an earlier report that indicates sialic acid is required for the binding of exo-S to a 116-kD protein on the surface of rat erythrocytes.[74] Binding of exo-S to these ceramides corresponds to the binding of whole bacteria to the same immobilized glycolipids, leading to the suggestion that exo-S may be a functional adhesin for *Pseudomonas* adherence. This possibility is supported by the demonstration of surface-associated exo-S using immunogold labeling with anti-exo-S antisera.

Whereas these findings are interesting and the implications provocative, they draw into question previous conclusions regarding the nature of exo-S and its location in the cell. Because all previous reports referred to exo-S as a secreted product, it is now important to determine the nature of the implied association of exo-S with the bacterial surface and whether this form differs from the secreted form of the protein. It has never been determined that exo-S is actually secreted from the cell, even though it is purified from the spent culture medium from some *Pseudomonas* strains. It is possible, for example, that exo-S is released into the culture supernatant fraction from dying cells, a possibility supported by the low yield (0.2 µg/ml in culture supernatant) and lengthy culture times (36 hr) reported for the purification of the protein.[66] The fact that exo-S purification involves the use of detergents or organic solvents is suggestive of its association with membrane lipids. Presumably future research will clarify these issues.

Several studies suggest a potential role for exo-S in the pathology associated with *Pseudomonas* infections. However, a precise role for exo-S and its associated ADP-ribosyltransferase activity has yet to be established.

4. ELASTASE

P. aeruginosa produces and secretes two proteolytic enzymes known as elastase and alkaline protease, with elastase the more active and abundant.[76] The first reports describing the purification and initial characterization of *P. aeruginosa* elastase were made by Morihara.[77,78] Elastase was named because of its ability to degrade elastin, which distinguishes it from alkaline protease, but its proteolytic activity far exceeds its elastolytic activity, making the term elastase somewhat inappropriate. The specific elastolytic activity of *P. aeruginosa* elastase was found to be approximately one-half that of the crystalline proteinase of *Bacillus subtilis*, while its proteolytic activity toward casein was four times higher than that of trypsin and about 10 times higher than that of the alkaline proteinase of *P. aeruginosa*.

The three-dimensional structure of *P. aeruginosa* elastase, recently determined at the 1.5 Å level of resolution, is remarkably similar to that of thermolysin from *B. thermoproteolyticus*.[79] *P. aeruginosa* elastase is a neutral metalloproteinase containing one atom each of zinc and calcium. The structural gene for elastase, lasB, recently has been cloned and the amino-acid sequence determined,[80,81] revealing a striking degree of homology with the thermolysin protease. The region of greatest homology (48%) corresponds to a region known to span the active site cleft of thermolysin (residues 138–182 of thermolysin). On the basis of sequence comparison and three-dimensional structural analysis with the placement of known critical residues in the active site of thermolysin, analogous sites have been predicted for elastase.[79,80] These residues include His 140, His 144 and Glu 164 as zinc ligands, Glu 141 as the active center and Tyr 155, His 223 and Asp 221 for substrate binding.

Of particular significance is the fact that elastase is secreted by the cell, although the details have remained elusive. There is considerable interest in the processing and activation of elastase, which is apparently produced in an inactive proenzyme form. The secreted or external form of elastase, which is enzymatically active, has a molecular weight of 33 kD. However, analysis of the open-reading frame corresponding to the lasB structural gene indicates that the gene encodes for a 54-kD precursor form of elastase. In support of the existence of a cytoplasmic precursor of elastase, Kessler and Saffrin have reported the existence of a 60-kD cytoplasmic protein that apparently is cleaved to produce a 56-kD form found in the periplasmic space of P. aeruginosa.[82] The 56-kD protein, termed proelastase I, subsequently is cleaved in the periplasmic space to form products of 20 kD and 36 kD, both of which are enzymatically inactive.[83] In a fashion as yet undescribed, the 36-kD inactive precursor of elastase (proelastase II) secreted from the cell becomes enzymatically active as a 33-kD protein. It has been suggested that the 20-kD fragment cleaved from the 56-kD proelastase I acts to block enzymatic activity of the periplasmic form of elastase (proelastase II). However, this has not been substantiated.

A second gene associated with elastolytic activity recently has been identified. Known as lasA, it encodes for a 40-kD protein postulated to affect the elastolytic activity and/or the secretion and processing of elastase.[84,85] The lasA gene was discovered from a mutant strain of P. aeruginosa (PAO-E64) that is devoid of significant elastolytic activity, yet produces an elastase antigenically indistinguishable from wild-type elastase.[86] E64 was originally described as a temperature-sensitive mutant for the elastase structural gene. It was later determined that this strain causes a mutation in the lasA gene and not in the elastase structural gene, which has been designated lasB.[87] Thus it appeared that the lasA gene product was required for elastolytic activity. In 1987 Goldberg and Ohman successfully cloned the lasA gene from a clinical isolate of P. aeruginosa (FRD2) and demonstrated that lasA complemented the mutation in strain PAO-E64.[88] In a second paper the authors described construction of a lasA mutant strain (FRD2128); because the mutant strain appeared to accumulate a 47-kD protein that reacted with anti-elastase antisera,[84] they postulated that the lasA gene product was involved in processing and activation of an elastase precursor. However, the lasA mutant produced and secreted normal quantities of elastase that was biochemically indistinguishable from the wild-type protein, except that it appeared to have lowered elastolytic activity. It was further proposed that the lasA gene product acted directly upon this "proelastase" form of elastase to activate its elastolytic properties. In 1988 Schad and Iglewski cloned and sequenced the lasA gene from strain PAO1 and used it to express a 40-kD protein in an E. coli host.[85] Their studies indicated that the LasA protein was associated with the outer membranes of E. coli and they proposed similar functions for the LasA protein in P. aeruginosa. However, Peters and Galloway recently reported the purification of an active fragment of the LasA protein from the culture supernatant fraction of strain PAO1 and demonstrated that the purified LasA protein fragment enhanced the elastolytic activities associated with a number of well-described proteolytic enzymes, including P. aeruginosa elastase, thermolysin, proteinase K, and human neutrophil elastase.[89] They postulated that LasA acts directly upon elastin, causing a modification that results in subsequent proteolytic degradation of elastin by a number of proteolytic enzymes and enhancement of the elastolytic activity of elastase. This work indicated that the published lasA sequence was incorrect; the correct sequence has recently been published by Darzins et al.[90] These findings have been confirmed and extended by Wolz et al.[91] who have demonstrated that the LasA protein also enhances the ability of alkaline proteinase to degrade elastin. An elastase-negative mutant was constructed by insertional inactivation of the lasB gene, but this mutant strain still retains the ability to degrade elastin in the absence of elastase production. The elastolytic activity of the lasB mutant is associated with the secretion of the active LasA fragment and this elastolytic activity can be completely inhibited using LasA-specific antisera. These studies indicate that elastolytic activity in Pseudomonas is more complex than previously thought and that further studies must take the LasA protein into account.

Several studies show that elastase is clearly involved in the pathogenicity associated with Pseudomonas infections.[7,92] The precise role elastase plays in the pathogenic process depends upon the type of infection, but it is clear that this proteolytic enzyme is capable of contributing to the destruction of host tissue or defenses in numerous ways. Because approximately 85% of P. aeruginosa strains have been shown to possess elastolytic activity, the probability is great that elastase will be involved in pathogenesis.[93,94]

The toxic and biological properties of purified elastase have been clearly demonstrated. The LD_{50} for mice varies between 60 and 400 μg, depending upon the route of inoculation, indicating that elastase is considerably less toxic than ETA.[95–97] Of particular note is the ability of purified elastase to degrade a number of biologically important molecules that include various complement components,[98] the immunoglobulins IgG, IgA and secretory IgA,[99–101] and laminin,[102] as well as fibrin and human collagens.[102] Elastase has also been reported to inactivate the human alpha-1-proteinase inhibitor[103] and recent evidence suggests that elastase contributes to inactivation of human gamma interferon.[104] In addition, studies using purified elastase have demonstrated that elastase damages pulmonary and corneal tissues[105,106] and has a direct effect on epithelial junctions.[107]

The contribution of elastase during the course of a *Pseudomonas* infection depends on the location of the infection and whether it is chronic or acute. In general, in animal model studies comparing elastolytic strains of *P. aeruginosa* with non-elastolytic strains, it appears that elastase plays a minor role in bacteremic infections.[92] However, in burn infections, elastase appears to contribute directly to the invasiveness of *P. aeruginosa*[62,108,109] In addition to the apparent destruction of anatomic barriers, it has been suggested that elastase-based degradation of protein at the infection site may provide a nutrient base for the bacteria.[110] Several studies have demonstrated the probable involvement of elastase and alkaline protease in lung pathology. Both proteolytic enzymes have been detected in bronchial washings and sputum from cystic fibrosis (CF) patients.[111] Using a hamster tracheal ring explant model, Baker demonstrated that, during infection, elastolytic strains destroy respiratory tract tissue.[112] CF patients with chronic *Pseudomonas* infections produce antisera against elastase and alkaline protease.[55,56,113] In studies using the rat chronic lung infection model[11] and the guinea pig acute lung infection model,[61] elastase-producing strains were shown to be more virulent than strains deficient in elastase production.

Recent findings of Peters and Galloway[89] and Wolz et al.[91] place the findings of the animal model studies into sharper perspective. The elastase-deficient strain (PAO-E64) used in both investigations is not deficient in elastase, but rather is deficient in the production of a functional LasA protein. This means that functional elastase was present, but a functional LasA protein was absent in the E64 mutant strain. The E64 mutation has been mapped to the *las*A gene,[87] which implies that the elastase structural gene (*las*B) in this strain does not carry a mutation and therefore encodes for a normal elastase protein. Therefore, the results of the studies by Woods et al.[11] and Blackwood et al.[61] can be interpreted on the basis of the synergistic effect between the LasA protein and the proteolytic activities of both elastase and alkaline protease, as well as the effects of other proteolytic enzymes present in the infection site. These studies using the E64 *las*A mutant have essentially established that the LasA protein significantly contributes to the virulence of *P. aeruginosa*. This is consistent with the fact that the LasA protein has been shown to enable the enhanced proteolytic degradation of elastin in the presence of elastase and alkaline protease, as well as thermolysin and human neutrophil elastase.[89,91] The validity of this interpretation is strengthened by the finding that the LasA protein acts directly at the level of the elastin substrate, and elastolytic activity can be inhibited in the presence of anti-LasA antisera.[91] These findings indicate that elastase and alkaline protease are important virulence factors in pulmonary infections but the initiating factor for elastolysis (as a special case of proteolysis) appears to be an active fragment of the LasA protein secreted from the cell with elastase and alkaline protease. The LasA protein and/or its active fragment must also be considered for its contribution as a virulence factor.

5. PHOSPHOLIPASES

In recent years an increasing number of reports have concerned the production and secretion of phospholipase enzymes by *P. aeruginosa*. A 78-kD protein with phospholipase and hemolytic activity was described by Kurioka and Liu.[114,115] Designated phospholipase C (PLC), this secreted protein was described as a hemolytic toxin that might be associated with the virulence of *P. aeruginosa*. Liu observed that the production of the PLC hemolysin was phosphate-regulated and proposed that PLC and alkaline phosphatase acted together as a phosphate scavenging system.[114] PLC has the ability to degrade phospholipids commonly found in the membranes of eucaryotic cells but not present in membranes of procaryotic cells. The process of phospholipid degradation also produces diacylglycerol, which can result indirectly in toxic side effects in animals.[116,117]

Many current investigations regarding phospholipase activity in *Pseudomonas* have used a genetic approach. For example, a series of recent papers have described the cloning and expression of the PLC structural gene (*plcS*) in both *E. coli*[118–121] and *P. aeruginosa* host strains. The construction of a mutant strain with a deletion of the entire *plcS* gene led to the discovery of a second, nonhemolytic phospholipase protein, PLC-N.[122,123] The structural gene that encodes for the non-hemolytic phospholipase (*plcN*) has been cloned and sequenced, revealing remarkable sequence homology between the *plcS* and *plcN* gene products.[124,125] The non-hemolytic PLC-N is 73.5 kD, whereas the hemolytic PLC-H has a molecular weight of 78.4 kD.[126] Sequence comparison analysis indicates two domains or regions with high homology: one at the amino terminus (70%) and a middle region that contains 81% homology. Both phospholipases hydrolyze phosphatidylcholine, and each enzyme demonstrates additional specificity. For example, PLC-H will also hydrolyze sphingomyelin, whereas PLC-N will hydrolyze phosphatidylserine. It has been noted that the ability to degrade sphingomyelin may be related to the hemolytic activity of PLC-H. Ostroff *et al.*[125] suggest that PLC-H may hydrolyze the phospholipid substrates present in the outer leaflet of the cell membrane structure (*i.e.* phosphatidylcholine and sphingomyelin), whereas PLC-N degrades phosphatidylserine, which is located primarily within the inner leaflet of the membrane structure. The result is that PLC-H would appear to be hemolytic, whereas PLC-N, which does hydrolyze components of the outer leaflet of the membrane, would not.

Genetic analysis of the phospholipase genes has revealed that the *plc*S gene is part of the three-gene *plc*SR operon, which includes *plc*R1 and *plc*R2, in-phase overlapping genes of unknown function.[125–127] These genes may play some role in activating the PLC-H protein, but this has not been substantiated.[125] Recently the *plc*S gene has been mapped to the 67-min position on the PAO chromosome.[128] Preliminary work indicates that the *plc*N structural gene resides on the opposite side of the *Pseudomonas* chromosome, *i.e.* at approximately 34 min.[125]

The role of the phospholipases in the virulence of *Pseudomonas* has yet to be defined. Initial studies indicated that purified PLC-H caused numerous pathologic consequences, including death, when injected into mice[129] and can cause the aggregation of human platelets.[130] Another study has shown that purified PLC-H induces a series of inflammatory responses in mice.[131] An earlier work using PLC-containing culture supernatants from *Pseudomonas* strains isolated from infected patients provided evidence that PLC caused the release of inflammatory mediators from rat peritoneal mast cells and human granulocytes.[132] Additional evidence in support of the importance of these factors in pathogenicity comes from an analysis of mutant strains in which the *plc*SR operon genes have been insertionally inactivated or deleted.[123] These mutant strains were tested in the BMM to determine the effect of the loss of the hemolytic phospholipase (PLC-H) or the *plc*R gene products on the virulence of the organism. When grown under phosphate-limiting conditions, the mutant strains exhibited a 200 to 10,000-fold reduction in virulence, in comparison with the PAO1 wild-type strain; however, under high phosphate conditions, only a modest difference (10-fold) was seen, perhaps because phosphate regulates the production of PLC-H. Of potential significance in these studies is the observation that the *plc*R mutant strain is more hemolytic, but less virulent than the wild-type PAO1 strain, which implies that the *plc*R gene products may have some role in pathogenesis. However, at the present time the role of the *plc*R genes remains unresolved.

6. IN CONCLUSION

During an infection *P. aeruginosa* secretes a complex assortment of virulence factors into the surrounding environment in the host organism. For this reason, as well as its metabolic diversity and ability to rapidly acquire antibiotic resistance, *Pseudomonas* infections represent a serious and unwelcome situation to the clinician. Because of its opportunistic nature and omnipresence in the environment, *Pseudomonas* will continue to remain a clinical threat to certain populations until means of preventing these infections are developed. Due to the varied nature and pathology associated with *Pseudomonas* infections, an effective approach appears to be the targeting of selected susceptible populations, *e.g.* CF patients, for vaccine development; indeed, this strategy is being employed. It is critically important to gain a detailed understanding of the mechanisms that cause the pathologic consequences associated with infections caused by *P. aeruginosa*. In recent years substantial progress has been made in understanding the nature of several of the secreted products of this organism. This information is critical to the development of therapeutic intervention to counter these virulence factors.

REFERENCES

1. Bennett, J. V., 1974, Nosocomial infections due to *Pseudomonas*, *J. Infect. Dis.* **130:**S4–7.
2. Flick, M. R., and Cluff, L. E., 1976, *Pseudomonas* bacteremia: Review of 108 cases, *Am. J. Med.* **60:**501–508.
3. Bodey, G. P., Bolivar, R., Fainstein, V., and Jadeja, L., 1983, Infections caused by *Pseudomonas aeruginosa*, *Rev. Infect. Dis.* **5:**279–313.
4. Baltch, A. L., Hammer, M., Smith, R. P., and Sutphen, N., 1979, *Pseudomonas aeruginosa* bacteremia: Susceptibility of 100 blood culture isolates to seven antimicrobial agents and its clinical significance, *J. Lab. Clin. Med.* **94:**201–214.
5. McManus, A. T., Mason, A. D. J., McManus, W. F., and Pruitt, B. A. J., 1985, Twenty-five year review of *Pseudomonas aeruginosa* bacteremia in a burn center, *Eur. J. Clin. Microbiol.* **4:** 219–223.
6. Stieritz, D. D., and Holder, I. A., 1975, Experimental studies of the pathogenesis of infections due to *Pseudomonas aeruginosa*: Description of a burned mouse model, *J. Infect. Dis.* **131:**688–691.
7. Holder, I. A., 1991, *P. aeruginosa* burn infections: Pathogenesis and treatment, in: *Microbial Pathogenesis and Immunity*, this volume (H. Freidman, M. Bendinelli and M. Campa, eds.), Plenum Publishing Corp., New York.
8. Pennington, J. E., 1979, Efficacy of lipopolysaccharide *Pseudomonas* vaccine for pulmonary infection, *J. Infect. Dis.* **139:**73–80.
9. Pennington, J. E., and Miller, J. J., 1979, Evaluation of a new polyvalent *Pseudomonas* vaccine in respiratory infections, *Infect. Immun.* **25:**1029–1034.
10. Cash, H. A., Woods, D. E., McCullough, B., Johanson, W. G., and Bass, J. A., 1979, A rat model of chronic respiratory infection with *Pseudomonas aeruginosa*, *Am. Rev. Respir. Dis.* **119:**453–459.
11. Woods, D. E., Cryz, S. J., Friedman, R. L., and Iglewski, B. H., 1982, Contribution of toxin A and elastase to virulence of *Pseudomonas aeruginosa* in chronic lung infections of rats, *Infect. Immun.* **36:**1223–1228.
12. Ziegler, E. J., and Douglas, H., 1979, *Pseudomonas aeruginosa* vasculitis and bacteremia following conjunctivitis: A simple model of fatal *Pseudomonas* infection in neutropenia, *J. Infect. Dis.* **139:**288–296.
13. Cryz, S. J. J., Furer, E., and Germanier, R., 1983, Simple model for the study of *Pseudomonas aeruginosa* infections in leukopenic mice, *Infect. Immun.* **39:**1067–1071.
14. Ohman, D. E., Burns, R. P., and Iglewski, B. H., 1980, Corneal infections in mice with toxin A and elastase mutants of *Pseudomonas aeruginosa*, *J. Infect. Dis.* **142:**547–555.
15. Liu, P. V., Abe, Y., and Bates, J. L., 1961, The roles of various fractions of *Pseudomonas aeruginosa* in its pathogenesis, *J. Infect. Dis.* **108:**218–228.
16. Allured, V. S., Collier, R. J., Carroll, S. F., and McKay, D. B., 1986, Structure of exotoxin A of *Pseudomonas aeruginosa* at 3.0A resolution, *Proc. Natl. Acad. Sci. USA* **83:**1320–1324.
17. FitzGerald, D. J, Willingham, M. C., and Pastan, I., 1988, *Pseudomonas* exotoxin—

Immunotoxins, in: *Immunotoxins*, (A. E. Frankel, ed.), Kluwer Academic Publishers, pp. 161–173.
18. Pastan, I., and FitzGerald, D., 1989, *Pseudomonas* exotoxin: Chimeric toxins, *J. Biol. Chem.* **264:**15157–15160.
19. Pollack, M., 1983, The role of exotoxin A in *Pseudomonas* disease and immunity, *Rev. Infect. Dis.* **5:**s979–s984.
20. Pollack, M., Taylor, N. S., and Callahan, L. T. III, 1977, Exotoxin production by clinical isolates of *Pseudomonas aeruginosa*, *Infect. Immun.* **15:**776–780.
21. Bjorn, M. J., Vasil, M. L., Sadoff, J. C., and Iglewski, B. H., 1977, Incidence of exotoxin production by *Pseudomonas* species, *Infect. Immun.* **16:**362–366.
22. Gill, D. M., 1982, Bacterial toxins: A table of lethal amounts, *Microbiol. Rev.* **46:**86–94.
23. Taylor, N. S., and Pollack, M., 1978, Purification of *Pseudomonas aeruginosa* exotoxin by affinity chromatography, *Infect. Immun.* **19:**66–70.
24. Leppla, S., 1976, Large scale purification and characterization of the exotoxin of *Pseudomonas aeruginosa*, *Infect. Immun.* **14:**1077–1086.
25. Pavlovskis, O. R., Callahan, L. T., III, and Pollack, M., 1975, *Pseudomonas aeruginosa* exotoxin, in: *Microbiology—1975*, (D. Schlessinger, ed.), Am. Soc. Microbiol., Washington, D. C., pp. 252–256.
26. Atik, M., Liu, P. V., Hanson, B. A., Amini, S., and Rosenberg, C. F., 1968, *Pseudomonas* exotoxin shock, *J.A.M.A.* **205:**134–140.
27. Pavlovskis, O. R., Iglewski, B. H., and Pollack, M., 1978, Mechanism of action of *Pseudomonas aeruginosa* exotoxin A in experimental mouse infections: Adenosine diphosphate ribosylation of elongation factor 2, *Infect. Immun.* **19:**29–33.
28. Saelinger, C. B., Snell, K., and Holder, I. A., 1977, Experimental studies in the pathogenesis of infections due to *Pseudomonas aeruginosa* equal direct evidence for toxin production during *Pseudomonas* infection of burned skin tissues, *J. Infect. Dis.* **136:**555–561.
29. Pavlovskis, O. R., and Gordon, F. B., 1972, *Pseudomonas aeruginosa* exotoxin: Effect on cell cultures, *J. Infect. Dis.* **125:**631–636.
30. Pollack, M. S., and Anderson, S. E. J., 1978, Toxicity of *Pseudomonas aeruginosa* exotoxin A for human macrophages, *Infect. Immun.* **19:**1092–1096.
31. Middlebrook, J. L., and Dorland, R. B., 1977, Response of cultured mammalian cells to the exotoxins of *Pseudomonas aeruginosa* and *Corynebacterium diphtheria*: differential cytotoxicity, *Can. J. Microbiol.* **23:**183–189.
32. Yamaizumi, M., Mekada, E., Uchida, T., and Okada, Y., 1978, One molecule of diphtheria toxin fragment A introduced into a cell can kill the cell, *Cell* **15:**245–250.
33. Iglewski, B. H., Liu, P. V., and Kabat, D., 1977, Mechanism of action of *Pseudomonas aeruginosa* exotoxin A: Adenosine diphosphate-ribosylation of mammalian elongation factor 2 in vitro and in vivo, *Infect. Immun.* **15:**138–144.
34. Brandhuber, B. J., Allured, V. S., Falbel, T. G., and McKay, D. B., 1988, Mapping the enzymatic active site of *Pseudomonas aeruginosa* exotoxin A, **3:**146–154.
35. Hwang, J., Fitzgerald, D. J., Adhya, S., and Pastan, I., 1987, Functional domains of *Pseudomonas aeruginosa* identified by deletion analysis of the gene expressed in E. coli, *Cell* **48:**129–136.
36. Carroll, S. F., and Collier, R. J., 1987, Active site of *Pseudomonas aeruginosa* exotoxin A: Glutamic Acid 553 is photolabeled by NAD and shows functional homology with glutamic Acid 148 of diphtheria toxin, *J. Biol. Chem.* **262:**8707–8711.
37. Galloway, D. R., Hedstrom, R. C., McGowan, J. L., Kessler, S. P., and Wozniak, D. J., 1989, Biochemical analysis of CRM 66: A nonfunctional *Pseudomonas aeruginosa* exotoxin A, *J. Biol. Chem.* **264:**14869–14873.
38. Wozniak, D. J., Hsu, L, and Galloway, D. R., 1988, His-426 of the *Pseudomonas aeruginosa* exotoxin A is required for ADP-ribosylation of elongation factor II, *Proc. Natl. Acad. Sci. USA* **85:**8880–8885.

39. McGowan, J. L., Kessler, S. P., Anderson, D. C., and Galloway, D. R., 1991, Immunochemical analysis of *Pseudomonas aeruginosa* exotoxin A: Analysis of the His 426 determinant, *J. Biol. Chem.*, in press.
40. Sadoff, J. C., Buck, G. A., Iglewski, B. H., Bjorn, M. J., and Groman, N. B., 1982, Immunological cross-reactivity in the absence of DNA homology between Pseudomonas toxin A and diphtheria toxin, *Infect. Immun.* **37**:250–254.
41. McGowan, J. L., Anderson, D. C., and Galloway, D. R., 1990, Structural basis for immunological cross-reactivity in ADP-ribosylating toxins, *ASM Ann. Meeting Abstr.* 1990:B-183, p. 57.
42. Carroll, S. F., and Collier, R. J., 1988, Amino acid sequence homology between the enzymic domains of diphtheria toxin and *Pseudomonas aeruginosa* exotoxin A, *Mol. Microbiol.* **2**:293–296.
43. FitzGerald, D., Morris, R. E., and Saelinger, C. B., 1980, Receptor-mediated internalization of *Pseudomonas* toxin by mouse fibroblasts, *Cell* **21**:867–873.
44. Ogata, M., Chaudhary, V. K., Pastan, I., and Fitzgerald, D. J., 1990, Processing of *Pseudomonas* exotoxin by a cellular protease results in the generation of a 37,000-Da toxin fragment that is translocated to the cytosol, *J. Biol. Chem.* **265**:20678–20685.
45. Leppla, S. H., Martin, O. C., and Muehl, L. A., 1978, Exotoxin A of *Pseudomonas aeruginosa*: A proenzyme having an unusual mode of activation, *Biochem. Biophys. Res. Commun.* **81**: 532–538.
46. Lory, S., and Collier, R. J., 1980, Expression of enzymic activity by exotoxin A from *Pseudomonas aeruginosa*, *Infect. Immun.* **28**:494–501.
47. Chung, D., and Collier, R. J., 1977, Enzymatically active peptide from the adenosine diphosphate-ribosylating toxin of *Pseudomonas aeruginosa*, *Infect. Immun.* **16**:832–841.
48. Vasil, M. L., Kabat, D., and Iglewski, B. H., 1977, Structure-activity relationships of an exotoxin of *Pseudomonas aeruginosa*, *Infect. Immun.* **16**:353–361.
49. Gray, G. L., Smith, D. H., Baldridge, J. S., Harkins, R. N., Vasil, M. L., Chen, E. Y., and Heyneker, H. L., 1984, Cloning, nucleotide sequence and expression in *Escherichia coli* of the exotoxin A structural gene of *Pseudomonas aeruginosa*, *Proc. Natl. Acad. Sci. USA* **81**: 2645–2649.
50. Pollack, M., 1980, *Pseudomonas aeruginosa* Exotoxin A, *N. Engl. J. Med.* **302**:1360–1361.
51. Liu, P. V., 1966, The roles of various fractions of *Pseudomonas aeruginosa* on its pathogenesis. II. Effects of lecithinase and protease, *J. Infect. Dis.* **116**:112–116.
52. Pavlovskis, O. R., Pollack, M., Callahan, L. T. III, and Iglewski, B. H., 1977, Passive protection by antitoxin in experimental *Pseudomonas aeruginosa* burn infections, *Infect. Immun.* **18**:596–602.
53. Pollack, M. S., and Young, L. S., 1979, Protective activity of antibodies to exotoxin A and lipopolysaccharide at the onset of *Pseudomonas aeruginosa* septicemia in man, *J. Clin. Invest.* **63**:276–286.
54. Cross, A. S., Sadoff, J. C., Iglewski, B. H., and Sokol, P. A., 1980, Evidence for the role of toxin A in the pathogenesis of infection with *Pseudomonas aeruginosa* in humans, *J. Infect. Dis.* **142**:538–546.
55. Klinger, J. D., Straus, D. C., Hilton, C. B., and Bass, J. A., 1978, Antibodies to proteases and exotoxin A of *Pseudomonas aeruginosa* in patients with cystic fibrosis: Demonstration by radioimmunoassay, *J. Infect. Dis.* **138**:49–58.
56. Jagger, K. S., Robinson, D. L., Franz, M. N., and Warren, R. L., 1982, Detection by enzyme-linked immunosorbent assays of antibody specific for *Pseudomonas* proteases and exotoxin A in sera from cystic fibrosis patients, *J. Clin. Microbiol.* **15**:1054–1058.
57. Pollack, M. S., Callahan, L. T. I., and Taylor, N. S., 1976, Neutralizing antibody to *Pseudomonas aeruginosa* exotoxin in human sera: Evidence for in vivo toxin production during infections, *Infect. Immun.* **14**:942–947.
58. Pavlovskis, O. R., and Shackelford, A. H., 1974, *Pseudomonas aeruginosa* exotoxin in mice: Localization and effect on protein synthesis, *Infect. Immun.* **9**:540–546.

59. Iglewski, B. H., and Kabat, D., 1975, NAD-Dependent inhibition of protein synthesis by *Pseudomonas aeruginosa* toxin, *Proc. Natl. Acad. Sci. USA* **72**:2284–2288.
60. Woods, D. E., and Iglewski, B. H., 1983, Toxins of *Pseudomonas aeruginosa*: New perspectives, *Rev. Infect. Dis.* **5**:S715–S722.
61. Blackwood, L. L., Stone, R. M., Iglewski, B. H., and Pennington, J. E., 1983, Evaluation of *Pseudomonas aeruginosa* exotoxin A and elastase as virulence factors in acute lung infection, *Infect. Immun.* **39**:198–201.
62. Snell, K., Holder, I. A., Leppla, S. A., and Saelinger, C. B., 1978, Role of exotoxin and protease as possible virulence factors in experimental infections with *Pseudomonas aeruginosa*, *Infect. Immun.* **19**:839–845.
63. Coburn, J., Dillon, S. T., Iglewski, B. H., and Gill, D. M., 1989, Exoenzyme S of *Pseudomonas aeruginosa* ADP-ribosylates the intermediate filament protein vimentin, *Infect. Immun.* **57**:996–998.
64. Coburn, J., Wyatt, R. T., Iglewski, B. H., and Gill, D. M., 1989, Several GTP-binding proteins, including p21 c-H-ras, are preferred substrates of *Pseudomonas aeruginosa* exoenzyme S, *J. Biol. Chem.* **264**:9004–9008.
65. Nicas, T. I., and Iglewski, B. H., 1985, Contribution of exoenzyme S to the virulence of *Pseudomonas aeruginosa*, *Antibiot. Chemother.* **36**:40–48.
66. Woods, D. E., and Que, J. U., 1987, Purification of *Pseudomonas aeruginosa* exoenzyme S, *Infect. Immun.* **55**:579–586.
67. Nicas, T. I., Frank, D. W., Stenzl, P., Lile, J. D., and Iglewski, B. H., 1985, Role of exoenzyme S in chronic *Pseudomonas aeruginosa* lung infections, *Eur. J. Clin. Microbiol.* **4**:175–179.
68. Woods, D. E., and Sokol, P. A., 1985, Use of transposon mutants to assess the role of exoenzyme S in chronic pulmonary disease due to *Pseudomonas aeruginosa*, *Eur. J. Clin. Microbiol.* **4**:163–169.
69. Nicas, T. I., and Iglewski, B. H., 1984, Isolation and characterization of a transposon induced mutant of *Pseudomonas aeruginosa* deficient in exoenzyme S, *Infect. Immun.* **45**:470–474.
70. Iglewski, B. H., Sadoff, J., Bjorn, M. J., and Maxwell, E. S., 1978, *Pseudomonas aeruginosa* exoenzyme S: An adenosine diphosphate ribosyltransferase distinct from toxin A, *Proc. Natl. Acad. Sci. USA* **75**:3211–3215.
71. Hedstrom, R. C., Funk, C. R., Kaper, J. B., Pavlovskis, O. R., and Galloway, D. R., 1986, Cloning of a gene involved in regulation of exotoxin A expression in *Pseudomonas aeruginosa*, *Infect. Immun.* **51**:37–42.
72. Bjorn, M. J., Pavlovskis, O. R., Thompson, M. R., and Iglewski, B. H., 1979, Production of exoenzyme S during *Pseudomonas aeruginosa* infections of burned mice, *Infect. Immun.* **24**:837–842.
73. Woods, D. E., Hwang, W. W., Shahrabadi, M. S., and Al, E., 1988, Alteration of pulmonary structure by *Pseudomonas aeruginosa* exoenzyme S. *J. Med. Microbiol.* **26**:133–141.
74. Simpson, D. A., and Woods, D. E., 1990, Binding of *Pseudomonas aeruginosa* exoenzyme S to eucaryotic cells, *ASM Ann. Meeting Abst.* B-180, p. 56.
75. Baker, N., Mino, V., Deal, C., Shahrabadi, M. S., Simpson, D. A., and Woods, D. E., 1991, *Pseudomonas aeruginosa* exoenzyme S is an adhesin, *Infect. Immun.* **59**:2859–2863.
76. Jensen, S. E., Phillipe, L., Teng Tseng, J., Stemke, G. W., and Campbell, J. N., 1980, Purification and characterization of exocellular proteases produced by a clinical isolate and a laboratory strain of *Pseudomonas aeruginosa*, *Can. J. Microbiol.* **26**:77–86.
77. Morihara, K. 1964, Production of elastase and proteinase by *Pseudomonas aeruginosa*, *J. Bacteriol.* **88**:745–757.
78. Morihara, K., Tsuzuki, T., Oka, J., Inoue, H., and Ebta, M., 1965, *Pseudomonas aeruginosa* elastase. Isolation, crystallization and preliminary characterization, *J. Biol. Chem.* **240**:3295–3304.

79. Thayer, M. M., Flaherty, K. M., and McKay, D. B., 1991, Three-dimensional structure of the elastase of *Pseudomonas aeruginosa* at 1.5 Angstrom resolution, *J. Biol. Chem.*, in press.
80. Bever, R. A., and Iglewski, B. H., 1988, Molecular characterization and nucleotide sequence of the *Pseudomonas aeruginosa* elastase structural gene, *J. Bacteriol.* **170**:4309–4314.
81. Fukushima, J., Yamamoto, S., Morihara, K., Atsumi, Y., Takeuchi, H., Kawamoto, S., and Okuda, K., 1989, Structural gene and complete amino acid sequence of *Pseudomonas aeruginosa* IFO 3455 elastase, *J. Bacteriol.* **171**:1698–1704.
82. Kessler, E., and Safrin, M., 1988, Partial purification and characterization of an inactive precursor of *Pseudomonas aeruginosa* elastase, *J. Bacteriol.* **170**:1215–1219.
83. Kessler, E., and Safrin, M., 1988, Synthesis, processing, and transport of *Pseudomonas aeruginosa* elastase, *J. Bacteriol.* **170**:5241–5247.
84. Goldberg, J. B., and Ohman, D. E., 1987, Activation of an elastase precursor by the lasA gene product of *Pseudomonas aeruginosa*, *J. Bacteriol.* **169**:4532–4539.
85. Schad, P. A., and Iglewski, B. H., 1988, Nucleotide sequence and expression in *Escherichia coli* of the *Pseudomonas aeruginosa* lasA gene, *J. Bacteriol.* **170**:2784–2789.
86. Ohman, D. E., Cryz, S. J., and Iglewski, B. H., 1980, Isolation and characterization of a *Pseudomonas aeruginosa* PAO mutant that produces altered elastase, *J. Bacteriol.* **142**:832–842.
87. Schad, P. A., Bever, R. A., Nicas, T. I., Leduc, F., Homme, L. F., and Iglewski, B. H., 1987, Cloning and characterization of elastase genes from *Pseudomonas aeruginosa*, *J. Bacteriol.* **169**:2691–2696.
88. Goldberg, J. B., and Ohman, D. E., 1987, Cloning and transcriptional regulation of the elastase lasA gene in mucoid and nonmucoid *Pseudomonas aeruginosa*, *J. Bacteriol.* **169**:1349–1351.
89. Peters, J. E., and Galloway, D. R., 1990, Purification and characterization of an active fragment of the LasA protein from *Pseudomonas aeruginosa*: Enhancement of elastase activity, *J. Bacteriol.* **172**:2236–2240.
90. Darzins, A., Peters, J. E., and Galloway, D. R., 1990, Revised nucleotide sequence of the lasA gene from *Pseudomonas aeruginosa* PAO1, *Nucleic Acids Res.* **18**:6444.
91. Wolz, C. Hellstern, E., Haug, M., Galloway, D. R., Vasil, M. L., and Doring, G., 1991, *Pseudomonas aeruginosa* lasB mutant constructed by insertional mutagenesis reveals elastolytic activity due to alkaline proteinase and LasA fragment, submitted.
92. Wretlind, B., and Pavlovskis, O. R., 1983, *Pseudomonas aeruginosa* elastase and its role in *Pseudomonas* infections, *Rev. Infect. Dis.* **5**:998–1004.
93. Nicas, T., and Iglewski, B. H., 1986, Production of elastase and other exoproducts by environmental isolates of *Pseudomonas aeruginosa*, *J. Clin. Microbiol.* **23**:967–969.
94. Wretlind, B., Heden, L., Sjoberg, L., and Wadstrom, T., 1973, Production of enzymes and toxins by hospital strains of *Pseudomonas aeruginosa* in relation to serotype and phage typing pattern, *J. Med. Microbiol.* **6**:91–100.
95. Wretlind, B., and Wadstrom, T., 1977, Purification and properties of a protease with elastase activity from *Pseudomonas aeruginosa*, *J. Gen. Microbiol.* **103**:319–327.
96. Meinke, G., Barum, J., Rosenberg, B., and Berk, R., 1970, In vivo studies with partially purified protease (elastase) from *Pseudomonas aeruginosa*, *Infect. Immun.* **2**:583–589.
97. Kawaharajo, K., Homma, J. Y., Aoyama, Y., and Morihara, K., 1975, In vivo studies on protease and elastase from *Pseudomonas aeruginosa*, *Jpn. J. Exp. Med.* **45**:89–100.
98. Schultz, D. R., and Miller, K. D., 1974, Elastase of *Pseudomonas aeruginosa*: Inactivation of complement components and complement-derived chemotactic and phagocytic factors, *Infect. Immun.* **10**:128–135.
99. Heck, L. W., Alarcon, P. G., Kulhavy, R. M., Morihara, K., Russell, M. W., and Mestecky, J. F., 1990, Degradation of IgA proteins by *Pseudomonas aeruginosa* elastase, *J. Immunol.* **144**:2253–2257.

100. Fick, R. B. J., Baltimore, R. S., Squier, S. V., and Reynolds, H. Y., 1985, IgG proteolytic activity of *Pseudomonas aeruginosa* in cystic fibrosis, *J. Infect. Dis.* **151**:589–598.
101. Doring, G., Obernesser, J., and Botzenhart, K., 1981, Extracellular toxins of *P. aeruginosa* II. Effect of two proteases on human immunoglobulins IgG, IgA and secretory IgA, *Zentralb. Bakteriol. Mikrobiol. Hyg.* I Abt. Orig. A **249**:89–98.
102. Heck, L. D., Morihara, K., McRae, W. B., and Miller, E. J., 1986, Specific cleavage of human type III and IV collagens by *Pseudomonas aeruginosa* elastase, *Infect. Immun.* **51**:115–118.
103. Morihara, K., Tsuzuki, H., and Oda, K., 1979, Protease and elastase of *Pseudomonas aeruginosa*: Inactivation of human plasma alpha-1-proteinase inhibitor, *Infect. Immun.* **24**: 188–193.
104. Horvat, R. T., Clabaugh, M., Duval-Jobe, C., and Parmely, M. J., 1989, Inactivation of human gamma interferon by *Pseudomonas aeruginosa* proteases: Elastase augments the effects of alkaline protease despite the presence of a2-macroglobulin, *Infect. Immun.* **57**: 1668–1674.
105. Gray, L. D., and Kreger, A., 1975, Rabbit corneal damage produced by *Pseudomonas aeruginosa* infection, *Infect. Immun.* **12**:419–432.
106. Gray, L. D., and Kreger, A., 1979, Microscopic characterization of rabbit lung damage produced by *Pseudomonas aeruginosa* proteases, *Infect. Immun.* **23**:150–159.
107. Azghani, A. O., Connelly, J. C., Peterson, B. T., Gray, L. D., Collins, M. L., and Johnson, A. R., 1990, Effects of *Pseudomonas aeruginosa* elastase on alveolar epithelial permeability in guinea pigs, *Infect. Immun.* **58**:433–438.
108. Pavlovskis, O. R., and Wretlind, B., 1979, Assessment of protease (elastase) as a possible virulence factor in experimental mouse burn infection, *Infect. Immun.* **24**:181–187.
109. Holder, I. A., and Haidaris, C. G., 1979, Experimental studies of the pathogenesis of infections due to *Pseudomonas aeruginosa*: Extracellular protease and elastase as *in vivo* virulence factors, *Can. J. Microbiol.* **25**:593–599.
110. Cicmanec, J. F., and Holder, I. A., 1979, Growth of *Pseudomonas aeruginosa* in normal and burned skin extract: role of extracellular proteases, *Infect. Immun.* **25**:477–483.
111. Bruce, M. C., Poncz, L., Klinger, J. D., Stern, R. C., and Tomashefski, J. F., Jr., 1985, Biochemical and pathological evidence for proteolytic destruction of lung connective tissue in cystic fibrosis, *Am. Rev. Respir. Dis.* **132**:529–535.
112. Baker, N., 1982, Role of exotoxin A and proteases of *Pseudomonas aeruginosa* in respiratory tract infections, *Can. J. Microbiol.* **28**:248–255.
113. Homma, J. Y., Tomiyama, T., Sano, H., Hirao, Y., and Saku, K., 1975, Passive hemagglutinin reaction test using formalinized sheep erythrocytes treated with tannic acid and coated with protease or elastase of *P. aeruginosa*, *Jpn. J. Exp. Med.* **45**:361–365.
114. Liu, P. V., 1979, Toxins of *Pseudomonas aeruginosa* in: *Pseudomonas aeruginosa*—Clinical manifestations of infection and current therapy (R. G. Doggett, ed.), Academic Press, New York, pp. 63–88.
115. Kurioka, S., and Liu, P. V., 1967, Effect of the hemolysin of *Pseudomonas aeruginosa* on phosphatides and on phospholipase C activity, *J. Bacteriol.* **93**:670–674.
116. Berka, R. M., and Vasil, M., 1982, Phospholipase C (heat-labile hemolysin) of *Pseudomonas aeruginosa*: Purification and preliminary characterization, *J. Bacteriol.* **152**:239–245.
117. Besterman, J. M., Duronio, V., and Cuatrecasas, P., 1986, Rapid formation of diacylglycerol from phosphatidylcholine: a pathway for generation of a second messenger, *Proc. Natl. Acad. Sci. USA* **83**:6785–6789.
118. Coleman, K., Dougan, G., and Arbuthnott, 1983, Cloning and expression in *Escherichia coli* K-12 of the chromosomal hemolysin (phospholipase C) determinant of *Pseudomonas aeruginosa*, *J. Bacteriol.* **153**:909–915.
119. Ding, J., Lory, S., and Tai, P. C., 1985, Orientation and expression of the cloned hemolysin gene of *Pseudomonas aeruginosa*, *Gene* **33**:313–321.

120. Lory, S., and Tai, P. C., 1983, Characterization of the phospholipase C gene of *Pseudomonas aeruginosa* cloned in *Escherichia coli*, *Gene* **32**:95–101.
121. Vasil, M. L., Berka, R. M., Gray, G. L., and Nakai, H., 1982, Cloning of a phosphate-regulated hemolysin gene (phospholipase C), *J. Bacteriol.* **152**:431–440.
122. Ostroff, R. M., and Vasil, M. L., 1987, Identification of a new phospholipase C activity by analysis of an insertional mutation in the hemolytic phospholipase C structural gene of *Pseudomonas*, *J. Bacteriol.* **169**:4597–4601.
123. Ostroff, R. M., Wretlind, B., and Vasil, M. L., 1989, Mutations in the hemolytic-phospholipase C operon result in decreased virulence of *Pseudomonas aeruginosa* PAO1 grown under phosphate-limiting conditions, *Infect. Immun.* **57**:1369–1373.
124. Vasil, M. L., 1989, Molecular Biology of exotoxin A and phospholipase C of *Pseudomonas aeruginosa*, in: *Pseudomonas: Biotransformations, Pathogenesis, and Evolving Biotechnology*, (S. Silver, A. M. Chakrabarty, B. H. Iglewski and S. Kaplan, eds.), Am. Soc. Microbiol., Washington, D. C., pp. 3–14.
125. Ostroff, R. M., Vasil, A. I., and Vasil, M., 1990, Molecular comparison of a nonhemolytic and a hemolytic phospholipase C from *Pseudomonas aeruginosa*, *J. Bacteriol.* **172**:5915–5923.
126. Pritchard, A. E., and Vasil, M. L., 1986, Nucleotide sequence and expression of a phosphate-regulated gene encoding a secreted hemolysin of *Pseudomonas aeruginosa*, *J. Bacteriol.* **167**:291–298.
127. Shen, B., Tai, P. C., Pritchard, A. E., and Vasil, M. L., 1987, Nucleotide sequences and expression in *Escherichia coli* of the in-phase overlapping *Pseudomonas aeruginosa* plcR genes, *J. Bacteriol.* **169**:4602–4607.
128. Lindgren, V., Ostroff, R. M., Vasil, M. L., and Wretlind, B., 1990, Genetic mapping of the structural gene for phospholipase C of *Pseudomonas aeruginosa* PAO, *J. Bacteriol.* **172**:1155–1156.
129. Berk, R. S., Brown, D., Coutinho, I., and Meyers, D., 1987, *In vivo* studies with two phospholipase C fractions from *Pseudomonas aeruginosa*, *Infect. Immun.* **55**:1728–1730.
130. Coutinho, I. R., Berk, R. S., and Mammen, E., 1988, Platelet aggregation by a phospholipase C from *Pseudomonas aeruginosa*, *Thromb. Res.* **51**:495–505.
131. Meyers, D. J., and Berk, R. S., 1990, Characterization of phospholipase C from *Pseudomonas aeruginosa* as a potent inflammatory agent, *Infect. Immun.* **58**:659–666.
132. Bergmann, U., Scheffer, J., Koller, M., Schonfeld, W., Erbs, G., Muller, F. E., and Konig, W., 1989, Induction of inflammatory mediators (histamine and leukotrienes) from rat peritoneal mast cells and human granulaocytes by *Pseudomonas aeruginosa* strains from burn patients, *Infect. Immun.* **57**:2187–2195.

7

The Role of Proteases in the Pathogenesis of *Pseudomonas aeruginosa* Infections

ROBERT STEADMAN, LOUIS W. HECK, and DALE R. ABRAHAMSON

1. INTRODUCTION

Pseudomonas aeruginosa is the most common gram-negative organism causing nosocomial infections and is a major pathogen in immuno- and myelosuppressed patients. Unlike many other gram-negative organisms, *P. aeruginosa* is non-fermentative and usually aerobic but will grow under anaerobic conditions in the presence of a suitable nitrogen source. The ability to adapt to varying oxygen concentrations is undoubtedly important in enabling *P. aeruginosa* to survive in soil, water, wounds and devitalized tissues.[1] The organism also has the ability to elaborate a large number of secretory products and proteins including extracellular proteases.[2,3] The specific functions or adaptive advantages gained by *P. aeruginosa* in the natural environment through the secretion of these proteases are not clear, but they are probably involved in nutrient scavenging, which provides the organism with

---

ROBERT STEADMAN • Institute of Nephrology, Cardiff Royal Infirmary, Cardiff, Wales CF2 1SZ   LOUIS W. HECK • Department of Medicine, Veterans Administration Medical Center, University of Alabama at Birmingham, UAB Station, Birmingham, Alabama 35294. DALE R. ABRAHAMSON • Department of Cell Biology, University of Alabama at Birmingham, UAB Station, Birmingham, Alabama 35294.

Pseudomonas aeruginosa as an Opportunistic Pathogen, edited by Mario Campa *et al.* Plenum Press, New York, 1993.

nitrogen-rich digestion products to allow growth. Two major potent proteases have been isolated, characterized and extensively studied: *Pseudomonas* elastase (PE) and an alkaline protease (PAP). *Pseudomonas* isolated from a variety of environmental sources and from the tissues of infected patients secrete these proteases,[4] which are probably instrumental in initiating and controlling the tissue invasion and necrosis characteristic of *Pseudomonas* infections.[5,6]

2. THE CONTROL OF PROTEASE SECRETION

The synthesis and extracellular release of PE and PAP are complex processes that proceed through two independent secretory mechanisms. PAP secretion seems to be similar to the secretion pathway in *Escherichia coli* for α-hemolysin.[7] The synthesis of PAP is initiated in late exponential or early stationary phase. PAP contains neither an attached signal sequence[8] nor does it accumulate intracellularly.[9] PAP is continuously secreted as a 48-kD protein to the extracellular medium where it has a pH optimum for activity of 8 to 9. PE, in contrast, is made as a 54-kD pre-pro enzyme.[10,11] A short signal sequence is removed during passage across the bacterial inner membrane after which a 14.5-kD pro-peptide is dissociated from the remaining protein, either in the periplasm or during secretion. The final zinc-metalloprotease is 39.5 kD and is also secreted during late exponential or stationary phase. Table I gives some of the biochemical characteristics of the two proteases. PE and PAP are active against several denatured protein substrates, such as casein, hemoglobin, and fibrin, and substrate-specificity studies have shown that PE has approximately five times greater specific proteolytic activity against casein on a molar basis than either trypsin or chymotrypsin. The specific caseinolytic activity of PAP, however, is approximately half that of trypsin.[6] Both PE and PAP are inhibited by metal chelators such as 1,10-phenanthroline, whereas other protease inhibitors, such as the serine protease inhibitor diisopropylphosphofluoridate have no effect on either PE or PAP. Whereas PAP has a relatively broad specificity in the sites at which it will

TABLE I
**Biochemical Characteristics of *P. aeruginosa*
Elastase and Alkaline Protease**[a]

	Elastase	Alkaline Protease
Molecular weight (kD)	39.5	48.4
Isoelectric point (pH)	5.9	4.1
Optimum pH for caseinolysis	7–8	8–9
Stable pH range	6–10	5–9

[a]From Morihara and Homma (6).

cleave, similar to that of proteases isolated from *Proteus* and *Serratia* species, PE has a comparatively restricted requirement for large or hydrophobic residues at the cleavage site.[6] In this respect it is typical of and functionally similar to several other bacterial neutral metalloproteases including that of *Legionella pneumophila*.[12] The products of at least four genes cooperate in the PE secretory pathway and are also involved in the trafficking and processing of many of the other secreted products of *P. aeruginosa* such as phospholipase C (PLC), exotoxin A (ETA), a lipase and an alkaline phosphatase.[8] In addition, there is recent evidence that a gene product of the accessory pilus biogenesis protein gene *pil* D is also involved in the export of the secreted *Pseudomonas* proteins.[13] Thus, although both PAP and PE are secreted at the same point in the *Pseudomonas* growth cycle, the mechanism of the secretion of each protease is independent. As with other gram-negative opportunistic pathogens such as *E. coli*,[14] *P. aeruginosa* elaborates an iron-sequestering mechanism[15] and the production of PE, PAP and other extracellular products is independently regulated by iron.[16] Little is known, however, about other environmental factors influencing the secretion of extracellular products by *Pseudomonas* or about the control mechanisms of protease synthesis or release.

3. PROTEASE INVOLVEMENT IN PATHOGENICITY

Whereas there is no clearly defined role for proteases in the growth of *Pseudomonas* in the natural environment, there is a wealth of direct and indirect evidence for their role in tissue invasiveness, injury, and necrosis in the host. Protease synthesis is associated with organisms isolated from acute lung infections.[17] Similarly, corneal infections,[18,19] and experimental alveolar necrosis and hemorrhage,[20] which closely resemble the pathology observed in patients with *P. aeruginosa* pneumonia, are also associated with protease production. In addition, purified proteases injected intradermally have hemorrhagic and necrotic effects in skin.[21-23] PE is probably responsible for the dissolution of the elastic lamina of blood vessels in the hemorrhagic vascular lesions associated with *Pseudomonas* septicemia.[24]

Two observations in particular indicate that proteases are released extracellularly *in vivo*. First, the proteases have been detected in the sputum of cystic fibrosis (CF) patients, many of whom suffer from chronic *Pseudomonas* infections of the respiratory tract.[25] Second, antibodies to the proteases are often detected in patients colonized by *Pseudomonas*.[26] The proteases themselves are not cytotoxic,[27] but degrade many extracellular matrix components that are constituents of connective tissues, including elastin, collagen types III and IV, and laminin.[24,28,29]

A polysaccharide matrix or glycocalyx is secreted by *P. aeruginosa* as an aid to colonization.[30,31] This glycocalyx is believed to provide a protected microenvironment, inside which the invading organism forms microcolonies and grows. Recent evidence has shown that the glycoprotein component of this matrix traps secreted proteases and contains metalloprotease activity.[32] These metalloproteases degrade collagenous and non-collagenous components of intact basement membranes to oligopeptides and other low molecular weight products. The extracellular release of proteases thus contributes to the virulence of the invading organism. The mechanisms controlling invasiveness and virulence within the host, however, are multifactorial. Thus, while the bacterial cell secretes a protective glycocalyx,[30,31] it is also releasing proteases breaking down basement membranes and tissues and secreting a variety of other products to impair host defenses. The proteases have been associated with subsequent bacterial dissemination,[33] but when infused alone have a low systemic toxicity,[34] probably due to large intravascular concentrations of α_2-macroglobulin and α_1-proteinase inhibitor.

4. TISSUE DAMAGE INDUCED BY PROTEASES

An example of the combined effects of glycocalyx and proteases is seen in *Pseudomonas* respiratory tract infections. The bacterial polysaccharide glycocalyx protects the bacterium against phagocytic cells and other host defenses,[35,36] while the principal target of the *Pseudomonas* proteases is the ciliary lining of the tract. Experiments *in vitro* have shown that dismembranated cilia, which retain ATP-dependent motility, show impaired motility after degradation by PE and PAP.[37] Each cilium was dissociated into isolated groups of one or two microtubules. In addition, a few individual proteins such as dynein were also cleaved. Approximately 90% of the structural proteins of the cilia, however, when analyzed by polyacrylamide gradient gel electrophoresis, were relatively resistant to proteolytic attack. Thus during the initial stages of airway colonization, it is possible that the proteases cause localized ciliary dysfunction. This would aid colonization of the respiratory epithelium, leading to enhanced tissue destruction as observed in several model systems.[20,38]

Because *Pseudomonas* proteases are able to degrade connective tissue constituents[24] and intact basement membranes,[32] a great deal of attention has been paid to the specific cleavage and degradation products of connective tissues. For example, Heck *et al.*[28] have investigated the effect of PE and PAP on the major fibrillar, components of connective tissue, interstitial and basement membrane collagens, types I, II, III, IV, and V. PE converted crosslinked type I collagen β-chains to monomeric α chains. The degradation of the type I collagen helical structure by both PE and PAP, however, was slow. Both type II and type V collagens were completely resistant to cleavage by either enzyme (Fig. 1). There was extensive degradation, however, of soluble native type III and type IV collagens by PE to specific, defined fragments

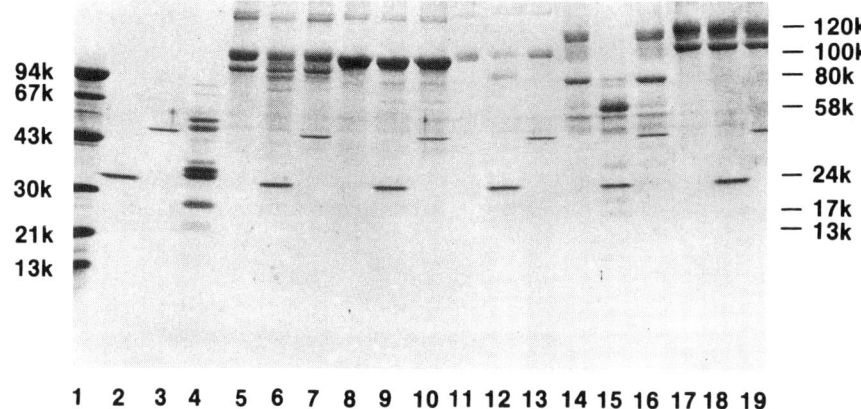

FIGURE 1. Coomassie blue staining pattern of SDS polyacrylamide gradient gel electrophoresis run under reducing conditions after incubating PE and PAP with types I, II, III, IV, and V collagens. In lanes 1 and 4 are the respective globular protein and collagen peptide mol. wt. standards. In lanes 2 and 3 are 1 μg each of PE and PAP, respectively. In lanes 5, 8, 11, 14, and 17 are 10 μg each of type I, II, III, IV, and V collagens incubated without enzyme. In lanes 6, 9, 12, 15, and 18 are 10 μg each of type I, II, III, IV, and V collagens incubated with 1 μg of PE. In lanes 7, 10, 13, 16, and 19 are 10 μg each of type I, II, III, IV, and V collagens incubated with 1 μg of PAP. All incubations were for 16 hr at 25°C. (Reproduced from ref. 28, with permission.)

(Fig. 2). Type III collagen is abundant in the interstitium of blood vessel walls, dermis, and lungs. In contrast, type IV collagen is primarily localized to basement membranes and is thus a major component of all vascular tissues.

Many of the pathological changes associated with *Pseudomonas*-induced tissue destruction may thus be attributed to an effect on the integrity of the collagen component of the tissue. The use of polyacrylamide gradient gel electrophoresis to identify proteolytic degradation products allowed Heck et al.[28] a direct method to characterize proteolytic activity. Their finding of limited type I collagen cleavage and the breaking of cross-links supports earlier findings,[39] showing conversion of cross-linked regions to form monomeric α chains with only limited α chain degradation. The cleavage products of types III and IV collagen generated by PE closely resemble those generated by human neutrophil elastase[40,41] and are distinctly different from those formed by other elastase types that are relatively inactive against these forms of collagen.[28]

In other experiments, the effects of PE and PAP on laminin were studied.[29] Laminin is the major non-collagenous component of all basement membranes[42] and promotes the adhesion of a variety of cell types to basal lamina.[43] Laminin also functions as a specific binding protein for a variety of other basement membrane constituents such as type IV collagen[44] and heparan sulfate proteoglycans.[45] Laminin, therefore, plays a central role in

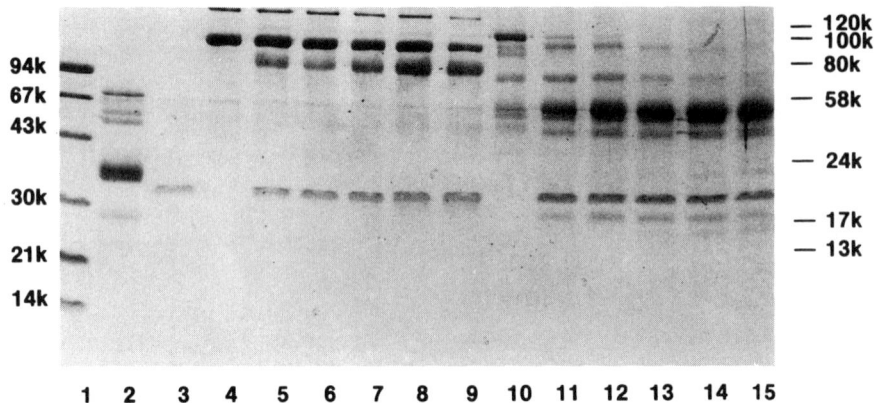

FIGURE 2. Coomassie blue staining pattern of SDS polyacrylamide gradient gel electrophoresis run under reducing conditions after incubating PE with type III and IV collagens for various times. In lanes 1 and 2, respectively, are the globular protein and collagen peptide mol. wt. standards. In lane 3 is 1 μg of PE. In lanes 4 and 10 are 10 μg each of type III and IV collagens incubated without enzyme. In lanes 5 through 9 is 10 μg of type III collagen incubated with 1 μg of PE for 1, 2, 4, 8, and 16 hr, respectively. In lanes 11 through 15 is 10 μg of type IV collagen incubated with 1 μg of PE for 1, 2, 4, 8, and 16 hr, respectively. All incubations were at 25°C. (Reproduced from ref. 28, with permission.)

maintaining the integrity of basement membranes. PE extensively degraded the laminin A and B chains when incubated with soluble purified laminin[29] (Fig. 3). In separate experiments, the A chains were also cleaved by PAP. The laminin B chains, however, were relatively resistant to PAP degradation; a large disulfide-rich region is responsible for this resistance to PAP proteolysis. At extended times of incubation with higher concentrations of PAP, however, B chain degradation did occur (Fig. 4). Whereas this degradation was slow, there is clearly an interesting difference between the susceptibility of collagens and laminin to PAP proteolysis, because laminin is cleaved by PAP more readily than the collagens. In the same study, cryostat sections of rat kidneys were incubated with PE and PAP. Immunoreactive laminin epitopes were proteolytically degraded and lost from the intact basement membrane after incubation with the proteases (Fig. 5). The results of these and other studies suggest that PE and PAP, when released, would cause extensive lesions in basement membranes. Histologic findings in other tissues infected with *P. aeruginosa*, or with tissues inoculated with *Pseudomonas* proteases, also indicate proteolytic damage to basement membranes.[46,47] The loss of integrity of basement membranes following *Pseudomonas* protease attack is likely to lead to the formation of necrotic lesions once the kinetics of degradation exceed those of re-synthesis of matrix constituents.

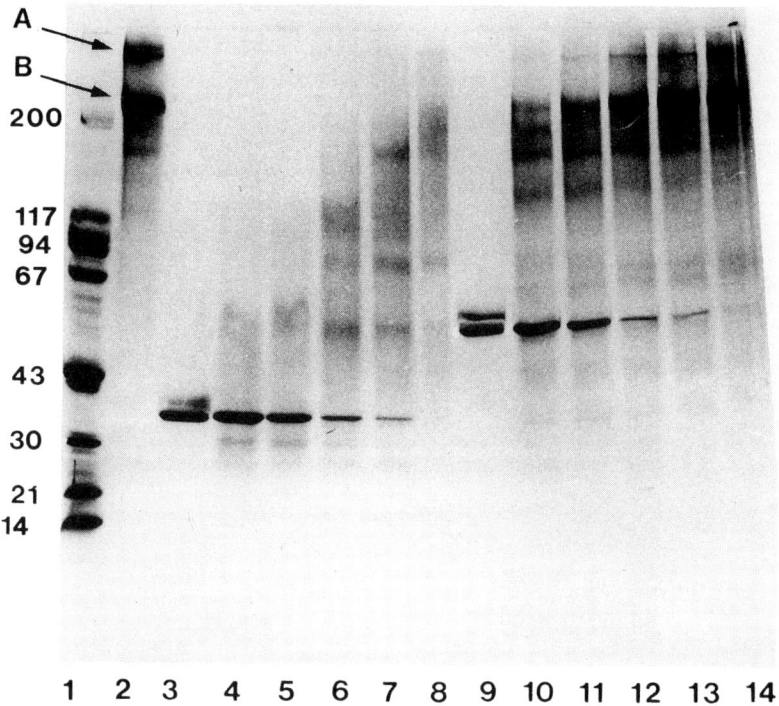

FIGURE 3. Coomassie blue staining of SDS-polyacrylamide gradient gel electrophoresis run under reducing conditions after incubating various amounts of PE or PAP with constant amounts of laminin at a fixed time and temperature. In lane 1 are the globular protein mol. wt. standards, and their approximate $M_r \times 1000$ are shown on the left. In lane 2 is 30 μg of mouse EHS tumor laminin, and its A and B chains are shown. In lanes 3 and 9 are 10 μg of PE and PAP, respectively. In lanes 4 through 8 are 30 μg of laminin incubated with 10, 5, 1, 0.5, and 0.1 μg of PE, respectively, In lanes 10 through 14 are 30 μg of laminin incubated with 10, 5, 1, 0.5, and 0.1 μg of PAP, respectively. All samples in lanes 2 through 14 were incubated for 30 min at 37°C. (Reproduced from ref. 29, with permission.)

5. EFFECTS OF PROTEASES ON THE IMMUNE SYSTEM

In addition to their damaging effects on intact basement membranes and on isolated basement membrane constituents, there is increasing evidence that both PE and PAP affect many of the functions of the immune system. For example, the proteases are reported to inhibit the chemotaxis, phagocytosis and oxidative metabolism of human neutrophils.[48–50] The mechanism of this inhibition involves proteolytic cleavage of cell surface receptors on neutrophils, and a similar proteolytic mechanism has been

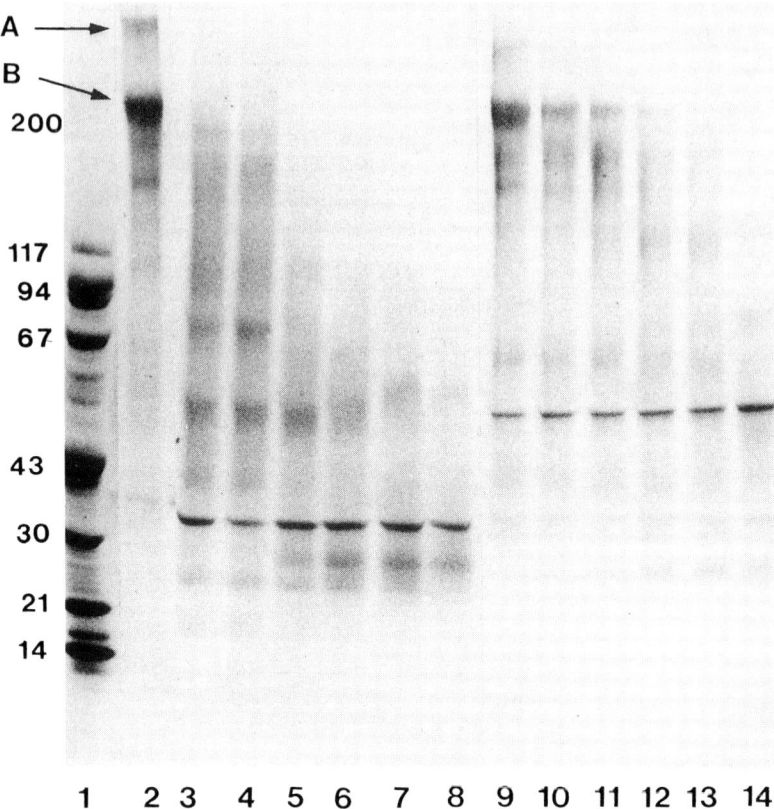

FIGURE 4. Coomassie blue staining of SDS-polyacrylamide gradient gel electrophoresis run under reducing conditions after incubating constant amounts of mouse laminin with PE or PAP for variable times at 37°C. In lane 1 are the globular protein mol. wt. standards. In lane 2 is 30 μg of laminin. In lanes 3 through 8 are 30 μg of laminin incubated with 1 μg of PE for 5, 15, 60, 120, and 240 min, respectively. In lanes 9 through 14 are 30 μg of laminin incubated with 1 μg of PAP for 5, 15, 60, 120, and 240 min, respectively. (Reproduced from ref. 29, with permission.)

described for the inhibition of natural killer (NK) cell activity by *Pseudomonas* proteases.[51] The proteases affected the binding of NK cells to target cells and the binding of a specific monoclonal antibody to the Fc receptor (CD 16). This effect was attributed to the proteolytic activity of the proteases on NK cell receptors although no specific cleavage was demonstrated. The proteases are selective in the cell surface markers that they will attack and do not prevent monoclonal antibody binding to HLA-ABC, HLA-DR, HLA-DQ, HLA-DP/DR, β_2-microglobulin or to several lymphocyte markers. They do, however, affect binding to the CD-4 surface marker of T helper cells.[52] The effect on

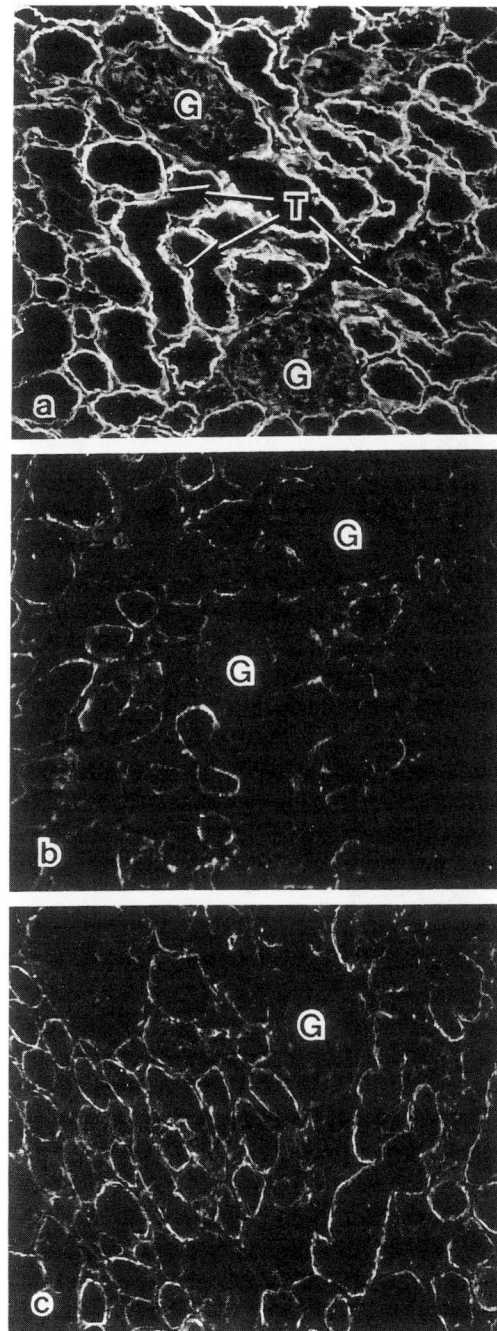

FIGURE 5. Immunofluorescent photomicrographs of cryostat sections of unfixed rat kidney. Sections were treated for 2 min with buffer (a), PE (b), or PAP (c). Sections were then sequentially labeled with affinity-purified sheep anti-laminin IgG and fluorescein anti-sheep IgG. In sections treated with buffer only (a), there was intense fluorescence from basement membranes of glomeruli (G) and tubules (T). After treatment with PE (b) or PAP (c), there was a marked reduction in binding of anti-laminin IgG. Magnification ×200. (Reproduced from ref. 29, with permission.)

binding is relatively specific and is not mimicked by porcine elastase. The decreased binding is dependent on proteolytic activity, however, and is inhibited by metalloprotease inhibitors, such as EDTA and 1, 10-phenanthroline. Thus, while many cell surface receptors are resistant to protease attack, there are several receptor molecules on distinct cell types that are sensitive to the *Pseudomonas* proteases. Studies *in vitro* have shown that serum will slow but not abolish the rate of this proteolytic inactivation of receptor functions.[50] Therefore, the proteolytic activity released by *Pseudomonas in vivo* would still function despite the presence of serum-derived protease inhibitors.

Besides this direct effect on immune cell function, several lines of evidence indicate that PE and PAP can also affect the mediators of inflammatory responses such as cytokines and immunoglobulins.[53,54] Furthermore, *P. aeruginosa* inoculation into mice suppresses immunity and delayed hypersensitivity reactions to an unrelated pathogen such as *Listeria monocytogenes*.[55,56] Thus, *Pseudomonas* or its secreted products also indirectly impair cellular immune functions. Using T-cell clones, Horvat and Parmely[57] demonstrated that a heat- and trypsin-sensitive protease was active in *Pseudomonas* bacterial filtrates that inhibited interferon gamma (IFN-γ) production from the T cells. This inhibition was due to proteolytic attack on IFNγ by PAP and there was altered migration of IFN-γ on gel electrophoresis following PAP treatment. In a later study,[57] the effect of PE to degrade IFN-γ was demonstrated. Interestingly, the effect of PE but not that of PAP was reduced in the presence of serum. This inhibition was attributed to the serum protease inhibitor, α_2 macroglobulin (α_2M). There was synergy, however, between PE and PAP to enhance IFN-γ degradation. This synergy occurred even in the presence of serum and α_2M. Since PE and PEP did not show a similar synergistic effect on IFN-α, IFN-β, or casein, and since PAP did not inactivate α_2M, the possibility exists that PAP partly modifies IFN-γ, making it accessible to the PE-active site inside the PE/α_2m complex.[58]

IFN-γ is a T-cell product that has a central role in controlling a variety of immune cell functions, including the initiation of transcription of a variety of mediators and cytokines.[59] IFN-γ also controls the expression of type II major histocompatibility complex molecules[60,61] and Fc receptors on immune cells.[61] Other cytokines such as interleukin 1 (IL-1) α and IL-1 β are resistant to the *Pseudomonas* proteases.[53] Tumor necrosis factor-α and IL-2, however, are proteolytically inactivated by PE and PAP.[53,63] These results demonstrate a range of possible substrates for the proteases among the proteins and peptides involved in controlling the immune response. Combined with earlier data demonstrating inactivation of components of the complement cascade[64] and of immunoglobulin G,[65] the importance of the proteases for the maintenance of *Pseudomonas* infection becomes clearer. In addition, PE proteolytically degrades IgA that constitutes one of the major lines of defense at mucosal surfaces.[54] The specific sites of PE cleavage on the IgA molecule, however, are uncertain.[54] Nevertheless the results demonstrate a specific mechanism whereby *Pseudomonas* evades a major mechanism of host defense.

This evasion and the continued erosion of cell and humoral-mediated immunity assists not only in the colonization of tissues but also in the persistence of infection. Combined with the ability to degrade and erode tissues and basement membranes, the *Pseudomonas* proteases provide an extremely potent virulence-associated mechanism.

6. INHIBITION OF PROTEASES

The major serum inhibitor of proteases, α_2M, is inhibitory to PE but not to PAP and not to the combined effects of PE and PAP.[58] Similarly, whereas PAP is inhibited by serum α_1-proteinase inhibitor (α_1-PI), PE is unaffected by α_1-PI and the inhibitor itself is a proteolytic substrate for PE.[66] Further detailed studies have been carried out to evaluate other serum-derived protease inhibitors. For example, connective tissues contain amyloid P as a component of elastic fibers. Amyloid P is a potent inhibitor of PE[67] and is also found in high concentrations in serum. Unlike many of the other serum-derived proteinase inhibitors (such as α_1-PI), which are inactivated by reactive oxygen metabolites, amyloid P is resistant to the effects of inflammatory cell-derived oxidants,[67] and is therefore likely to be of great inhibitory importance at sites of *Pseudomonas* infection. The broad protease inhibitor aprotinin, which is found in many tissues including the lung and pancreas,[68] does not protect against protease damage to rabbit corneas[69] when *P. aeruginosa* is injected intrastromally.[70] Further, neither aprotinin[70] or other protease inhibitors[72] enhance the effectiveness of antibiotic therapy in this model.

A recent report has demonstrated that antibiotics may have an important role to play in controlling *Pseudomonas* protease damage *in vivo*.[72] Cultures of *Pseudomonas* decreased their release of secreted products (including the proteases) during culture in the presence of sub-inhibitory doses of ciprofloxacin, tobramycin and ceftazidime. In the same study rats were chronically infected by intra-tracheal inoculation with *P. aeruginosa*. While the lungs of those treated with low doses of antibiotics and those that were not treated had the same bacterial count, histological damage was significantly reduced in the antibiotic-treated group. These results confirm the importance of the secreted proteases in mediating tissue injury. They also demonstrate that the suppression of protease release reduces progressive tissue damage during chronic infections.

7. SUMMARY

As with a number of opportunistic bacterial pathogens, the virulence of *P. aeruginosa* is multifactorial and depends on both the adaptability of the bacteria and the susceptibility of the host. *Pseudomonas* infections of the uncompromised host are unusual. However in compromised individuals, such as burn victims, neutropenic or cystic fibrosis patients, *P. aeruginosa* is a major pathogen.

P. aeruginosa causes extensive tissue injury during infection. Tissue invasion is associated with necrosis, microabscess formation, vascular lesions, and hemorrhage. Both this tissue damage, with extensive degradation of basement membrane constituents, and modifications of the cellular and humoral immune responses, result from the activity of proteases synthesized and secreted by the organism. While the secretion of proteases is only one of several virulence-associated traits contributing to the success of the organism, extracellular proteolysis is obviously instrumental in promoting and maintaining the infection. The secreted proteases of *P. aeruginosa* are thus an essential part of the virulence mechanisms developed by the organism.

REFERENCES

1. Rhame, F. S., 1980, The ecology and epidemiology of *Pseudomonas aeruginosa*, In: *Pseudomonas aeruginosa: The Organism, Diseases it Causes and their Treatment* (L. D. Sabath, ed.), Hans Huber Publishers, Bern, Switzerland, pp. 31–51.
2. Liu, P. V., 1974, Extracellular toxins of *Pseudomonas aeruginosa*, *J. Infect. Dis.* **130**:S94–S99.
3. Nicas, T. I., and Iglewski, B. H., 1985, The contribution of exoproducts to virulence of *Pseudomonas aeruginosa, Can. J. Microbiol.* **31**:387–392.
4. Nicas, T. I., and Iglewski, B. H., 1986, Production of elastase and other exoproducts by environmental isolates of *Pseudomonas aeruginosa, J. Clin. Microbiol.* **23**:967–969.
5. Homma, J. Y., Marsuura, M., Shibata, M., Kazuyama, Y., Uamamoto, M., Kubota, Y., Hirayama, T., and Kato, I., 1984, Production of leucocidin by clinical isolates of *Pseudomonas aeruginosa* and antileucocidin antibody from sera of patients with diffuse panbronchitis, *J. Clin. Microbiol.* **20**:855–859.
6. Morihara, K., and Homma, J. Y., 1985, *Pseudomonas* proteases, in *Bacterial Enzymes and Virulence* (I. Holder, ed.), CRC Press, Inc., Boca Raton, FL, pp. 41–75.
7. Gray, L., Kenny, B., Mackman, N., Haigh, R., and Holland, I. B., 1989, A novel C-terminal signal sequence targets *Escherichia coli* haemolysin directly to the medium, *J. Cell Sci. Suppl.* **11**:45–57.
8. Lazdunski, A., Guzzo, J., Filloux, A., Bally, M., and Murgier, M., 1990, Secretion of extracellular proteins by *Pseudomonas aeruginosa. Biochimie* **72**:147–156.
9. Guzzo, J., Murgier, M., Filloux, A., and Lazdunski, A., 1990, Cloning of the *Pseudomonas aeruginosa* alkaline protease gene and secretion of the protease into the medium by *Escherichia coli, J. Bacteriol.* **172**:942–948.
10. Kessler, G., and Saffrin, M., 1988, Synthesis, processing, and transport of *Pseudomonas aeruginosa* elastase, *J. Bacteriol.* **170**:5241–5247.
11. Berer, R. A., and Iglewski, B. H., 1988, Molecular characterization and nucleotide sequence of the *Pseudomonas aeruginosa* elastase structural gene, *J. Bacteriol.* **170**:4309–4314.
12. Black, W. J., Quinn, F. D., and Tompkins, L. S., 1990, *Legionella pneumophila* zinc metalloprotease is structurally and functionally homologous to *Pseudomonas aeruginosa* elastase, *J. Bacteriol.* **172**:2608–2613.
13. Strom, S. M., Nunn, D., and Lory, S., 1991, Multiple roles of the pilus biogenesis protein PilD: Involvement of PilD in excretion of enzymes from *Pseudomonas aeruginosa, J. Bacteriol.* **173**: 1175–1180.

14. Bullen, J. J., 1985, Iron and infection, *Eur. J. Clin. Microbiol.* **4:**537–539.
15. Cox, C. D., 1985, Iron transport and serum resistance in *Pseudomonas aeruginosa*, *Antibiot. Chemother.* **36:**1–12.
16. Bjorn, M. J., Sokol, P. A., and Iglewski, B. H., 1979, Influence of iron on yields of extracellular product in *Pseudomonas aeruginosa* cultures, *J. Bacteriol.* **138:**193–200.
17. Woods, D. E., Schaffer, M. S., Rabin, H. R., Campbell, G. D., and Sokol, P. A., 1986, Phenotypic comparison of *Pseudomonas aeruginosa* strains isolated from a variety of clinical sites, *J. Clin. Microbiol.* **24:**260–264.
18. Gray, L. D., and Kreger, A. S., 1975, Rabbit corneal damage produced by *Pseudomonas aeruginosa* infection, *Infect. Immun.* **12:**419–432.
19. Kreger, A. S., and Gray, L. D., 1978, Purification of *Pseudomonas aeruginosa* proteases and microscopic characterization of pseudomonal protease-induced rabbit corneal damage, *Infect. Immun.* **19:**630–648.
20. Gray, L. D., and Kreger, A. S., 1979, Microscopic characterization of rabbit lung damage produced by *Pseudomonas aeruginosa* proteases, *Infect. Immun.* **23:**150–159.
21. Liu, P. V., 1966, The roles of various fractions of *Pseudomonas aeruginosa* in its pathogenesis. II. Effects of lecithinase and protease, *J. Infect. Dis.* **116:**112–116.
22. Kreger, A. S., and Griffin, O. K., 1974, Physicochemical fractionation of extracellular cornea-damaging proteases of *Pseudomonas aeruginosa*, *Infect. Immun.* **9:**828–834.
23. Kawaharajo, K., Homma, J. Y., Aoyama, Y., and Morihara, K., 1975, In vivo studies on protease and elastase from *Pseudomonas aeruginosa*, *Jpn. J. Exp. Med.* **45:**89–100.
24. Mull, J. D., and Callahan, W. S., 1965, The role of the elastase of *Pseudomonas aeruginosa* in experimental infection, *Exp. Mol. Pathol.* **4:**567–575.
25. Döring, G., Obernesser, H. J., Botzenhart, K., Flehming, B., Holly, N., and Hofmann, A., 1983, Proteases of *Pseudomonas aeruginosa* in patients with cystic fibrosis, *J. Infect. Dis.* **147:**744–750.
26. Klinger, J. D., Straus, D. C., Hilton, C. B., and Bass, J. A., 1978, Antibodies to proteases and exotoxin A of *Pseudomonas aeruginosa* in patients with cystic fibrosis: Demonstration by radioimmunoassay, *J. Infect. Dis.* **138:**49–58.
27. Wretlind, B., and Pavlovskis, O. R., 1981, The role of proteases and exotoxin A in the pathogenicity of *Pseudomonas aeruginosa* infections, *Scand. J. Infect. Dis.* **29:**13–19.
28. Heck, L. W., Morihara, K., McRae, W. B., and Miller, E. J., 1986, Specific cleavage of human type III and IV collagens by *Pseudomonas aeruginosa* elastase, *Infect. Immun.* **51:**115–118.
29. Heck, L. W., Morihara, K., and Abrahamson, D. R., 1986, Degradation of soluble laminin and depletion of tissue-associated basement membrane laminin by *Pseudomonas aeruginosa* elastase and alkaline protease, *Infect. Immun.* **54:**149–153.
30. Costerton, J. W., Brown, M. R. W., and Sturgess, J. M., 1979, The cell envelope: Its role in infection, in: *Pseudomonas aeruginosa: Clinical Manifestations of Infection and Current Therapy*, (R. G. Doggett, ed.), Academic Press, New York, pp. 41–62.
31. Lam, J., Chan, R., Lam, K., and Costerton, J. W., 1980, Production of mucoid microcolonies by *Pseudomonas aeruginosa* within infected lungs in cystic fibrosis, *Infect. Immun.* **28:**546–556.
32. Anastassiou, E. D., Karakiulakis, G., Missirhs, E., Maragoudakis, M. E., and Dimitracopoulos, G., 1989, Comparative evaluation of mitogenicity and basement-membrane-degrading activity of *Pseudomonas aeruginosa* slime glycolipoprotein and alginate, *J. Clin. Microbiol.* **27:**490–494.
33. Janda, J. M., and Bottone, E. J., 1981, *Pseudomonas aeruginosa* enzyme profiling: Predictor of potential invasiveness and use as an epidemiological tool, *J. Clin. Microbiol.* **14:**55–60.
34. Wretlind, B., and Pavlovskis, O. R., 1981, The role of proteases and exotoxin A in the pathogenicity of *Pseudomonas aeruginosa* infections, *Scand. J. Infect. Dis.* **29:**13–19.
35. Schwartzmann, S., and Boring, J. R., III, 1971, Antiphagocytic effect of slime from a mucoid strain of *Pseudomonas aeruginosa*, *Infect. Immun.* **3:**762–767.
36. Baltimore, R. S., and Mitchell, M., 1980, Immunologic investigation of mucoid strains of

Pseudomonas aeruginosa: Comparison of susceptibility of opsonic antibody in mucoid and nonmucoid strains, *J. Infect. Dis.* **141:**238–247.
37. Hinglay, S. T., Hastie, A. T., Kueppers, F., and Higgins, M. L., 1986, Disruption of respiratory cilia by proteases including those of *Pseudomonas aeruginosa*, *Infect. Immun.* **54:**379–385.
38. Woods, D. E., Cryz, S. J., Friedman, R. L., and Iglewski, B. H., 1982, Contribution of toxin A and elastase to virulence of *Pseudomonas aeruginosa* in chronic lung infections of rats, *Infect. Immun.* **36:**1223–1228.
39. Kessler, E., Kennah, H. E., and Brown, S. I., 1977, *Pseudomonas* proteases. Purification, partial characterization and its effect on collagen, proteoglycan and rabbit corneas, *Invest. Ophthalmol. Visual Sci.* **16:**488–497.
40. Gadeck, J. E., Fells, G. A., Wright, D. G., and Crystal, R., 1980, Human neutrophil elastase functions as a type III collagen "collagenase," *Biochem. Biophys. Res. Commun.* **95:**1815–1822.
41. Mainardi, C. L., Dixit, S., and Kang, A. H., 1980, Degradation of type IV (basement membrane) collagen by a proteinase isolated from human polymorphonuclear leukocyte granules, *J. Biol. Chem.* **255:**5435–5441.
42. Timpl, R., Ronde, H., Robey, P. G., Rennard, S. I., Foidart, J.-M., and Martin, G. R., 1979, Laminin—a glycoprotein from basement membranes, *J. Biol. Chem.* **254:**9933–9937.
43. Kleinmann, H. R., McCarrey, M. L., Hassell, J. R., Martin, G. R., Van Evercooren, A. B., and Dubois-Dakq, M., 1984, Role of laminin in basement membrane and in growth, adhesion and differentiation of cells, in: *Role of Extracellular Matrix in Development* (R. T. Trelstad, ed.), Alan R. Liss Inc., New York, pp. 123–143.
44. Terranova, V. P., Rohrbach, D. H., and Martin, G. R., 1980, Role of laminin in the attachment of PAM 212 (epithelial) cells to basement membrane collagen, *Cell* **22:**719–726.
45. Woodley, G. T., Rao, C. N., Hassell, J. R., Liotta, L. A., Martin, G. R., and Kleinmann, H. K., 1983, Interaction of basement membrane components, *Biochem. Biophys. Acta* **761:**278–283.
46. Blackwood, L. L., Stone, R. M., Iglewski, B. H., and Pennington, J. E., 1983, Evaluation of *Pseudomonas aeruginosa* exotoxin A and elastase as virulence factors in acute lung infection, *Infect. Immun.* **39:**198–201.
47. Döring, G., Dalhoff, A., Vogel, O., Brunner, H., Dröge, U., and Botzenhart, K., 1984, *In vivo* activity of proteases in *Pseudomonas aeruginosa* in a rat model, *J. Infect. Dis.* **149:**532–537.
48. Kharazmi, A., Döring, G., Høiby, N., and Valenius, N. H., 1984, Interaction of *Pseudomonas aeruginosa* alkaline protease and elastase with human polymorphonuclear leukocytes *in vitro*, *Infect. Immun.* **43:**161–165.
49. Kharazmi, A., Høiby, N., Döring, G., and Valerius, N. H., 1984, *Pseudomonas aeruginosa* exoproteases inhibit human neutrophil chemiluminescence, *Infect. Immun.* **44:**587–591.
50. Kharazmi, A., Eriksen, H.O., Döring, G., Goldstein, W., and Høiby, N., 1986, Effect of *Pseudomonas aeruginosa* proteases on human leukocyte phagocytosis and bactericidal activity, *Acta Pathol. Microbiol. Immunol. Scand. Sect. C* **94:**175–179.
51. Pedersen, B. K., and Kharazmi, A., 1987, Inhibition of human natural killer cell activity by *Pseudomonas aeruginosa* alkaline protease and elastase, *Infect. Immun.* **55:**986–989.
52. Pedersen, B. K., Kharazmi, A., Theanoler, T. G., Ødum, N., Andersen, V., and Bendtzen, K., 1987, Selective modulation of the CD4 molecular complex by *Pseudomonas aeruginosa* alkaline protease and elastase, *Scand. J. Immunol.* **26:**91–94.
53. Parmely, M., Gale, A., Clabaugh, M., Horvat, R., and Zhou, W.-W., 1990, Proteolytic inactivation of cytokines by *Pseudomonas aeruginosa*, *Infect. Immun.* **58:**3009–3014.
54. Heck, L. W., Alarcon, P. G., Kukhavy, R. M., Morihara, K., Russell, M. W., and Mestecky, J. F., 1990, Degradation of IgA proteins by *Pseudomonas aeruginosa* elastase, *J. Immunol.* **144:**2253–2257.
55. Blackwood, L. L., Lin, T., and Rowe, J. I., 1987, Suppression of the delayed-type hypersensitivity and cell-mediated immune responses to Listeria monocytogenes induced by *Pseudomonas aeruginosa*, *Infect. Immun.* **55:**639–644.

56. Petit, J.-C., Richard, G., Albert, B., and Daquet, G.-L., 1982, Depression by *Pseudomonas aeruginosa* of two T-cell mediated responses, anti-Listeria immunity and delayed-type hypersensitivity to sheep erythrocytes, *Infect. Immun.* **35**:900–908.
57. Horvat, R. T., and Parmely, M. J., 1988, *Pseudomonas aeruginosa* alkaline protease degrades human gamma interferon and inhibits its bioactivity, *Infect. Immun.* **56**:2925–2932.
58. Horvat, R. T., Clabaugh, M., Duval-Jobe, C., and Parmely, M. J., 1989, Inactivation of human gamma interferon by *Pseudomonas aeruginosa* proteases: Elastase augments the effects of alkaline protease despite the presence of α_2-macroglobulin, *Infect. Immun.* **57**:1668–1674.
59. Colbert, M. A, Belin, D., Vassalli, J.-D., de Kossodo, S., and Vassalli, P., 1986, Interferon enhances macrophage transcription of the tumor necrosis factor/cachectin, interleukin 1, and urokinase genes, which are controlled by short-lived repressors, *J. Exp. Med.* **164**:2113–2118.
60. Pober, J. S., Gimbrone, M. A., Cotran, R. S., Reiss, C. S., Burakoff, S. J., Fiers, W., and Aults, K. A., 1983, Ia expression by vascular endothelium is inducible by activated T cells and by human γ-interferon, *J. Exp. Med.* **157**:1339–1353.
61. Wong, G. H. W., Clark-Lewis, I., McKimm-Breschkin, J. L., Harris, A. W., and Schrader, J. W., 1983, Interferon-γ induces enhanced expression of Ia and H-2 antigens on B lymphoid, macrophage, and myeloid cell lines, *J. Immunol.* **131**:788–793.
62. Guyre, P. M., Morganelli, P. M., and Miller, R., 1983, Recombinant immune interferon increases immunoglobulin G Fc receptors on cultured human mononuclear phagocytes, *J. Clin. Invest.* **72**:393–397.
63. Theander, T. G., Kharazmi, A., Pedersen, B. K., Christensen, L. D., Tvede, N., Poulsen, L. K., Ødum, N., Svenson, M., and Bendtzen, K., 1988, Inhibition of human lymphocyte proliferation and cleavage of interleukin-2 by *Pseudomonas aeruginosa* proteases, *Infect. Immun.* **56**:1673–1677.
64. Schultz, D. R., and Miller, K. D., 1974, Elastase of *Pseudomonas aeruginosa*: inactivation of complement components and complement derived chemotactic and phagocytic factors, *Infect. Immun.* **10**:128–135.
65. Holder, I. A., and Wheeler, R., 1984, Experimental studies of the pathogenesis of infections owing to *Pseudomonas aeruginosa* elastase, an IgG protease, *Can J. Microbiol.* **30**:1118–1124.
66. Morihara, K., Tsuzuki, H., and Oda, K., 1979, Protease and elastase of *Pseudomonas aeruginosa*: Inactivation of human plasma α_1-proteinase inhibitor, *Infect. Immun.* **24**: 188–193.
67. Vachino, G., Heck, L. W., Gelfand, J. A., Kaplan, M. M., Burke, J. F., Berninger, R. W., and McAdam, K. P. W. J., 1988, Inhibition of human neutrophil and *Pseudomonas* elastases by the amyloid P component: A constituent of elastic fibers and amyloid deposits, *J. Leuk. Biol.* **44**: 529–534.
68. Fritz, H., and Wunderer, G., 1983, Biochemistry and applications of aprotinin, the kallikrein inhibitor from bovine organs, *Arzneim Forsch.* **33**:479–494.
69. Twining, S. S., Davis, S. D., and Hyndink, R. A., 1986, Relationship between proteases and descemetocele formation in experimental *Pseudomonas* keratitis, *Curr. Eye Res.* **5**:503–510.
70. Stuart, J. C., Turgeon, P. T., and Kowalski, R. P., 1991, Aprotinin treatment of Pseudomonal corneal infection, *Cornea* **10**:63–66.
71. Bohigian, G., Valenton, M., Okamoto, M., and Carraway, B. L., 1976, Collagenase inhibitors in *Pseudomonas* keratitis, *Arch. Ophthalmol.* **91**:52–56.
72. Grimwood, K., To, M., Rabin, H. R., and Woods, D. E., 1989, Inhibition of *Pseudomonas aeruginosa* exoenzyme expression by subinhibitory antibiotic concentrations, *Antimicrob. Ag. Chemother.* **33**:41–47.

8

Genetic Regulation and Expression of Elastase in *Pseudomonas aeruginosa*

JANEL HECTOR, ALI AZGHANI, and ALICE JOHNSON

1. INTRODUCTION

Pseudomonas aeruginosa, a gram-negative organism, is a frequent cause of lung infections in cystic fibrosis (CF) or in debilitated and immunosuppressed individuals. Elastase secreted by *P. aeruginosa* not only promotes entry of the bacteria through the respiratory tract but also contributes to the pulmonary damage during infection. Chronic *Pseudomonas* infections are commonly difficult to resolve even with antibiotic therapy. Therefore, the genetic regulation of virulence factors, such as elastase, is of primary concern.

P. aeruginosa can survive in almost any environment.[1] It can endure higher temperatures than enteric organisms and can use more than 50 simple organic compounds for growth. *Pseudomonas* can grow in distilled water, disinfectant solutions, and hospital scrub sinks as well as in soil. This hardy organism thrives on amino acids and small peptides from human respiratory tract secretions.[2]

Compared with other gram-negative organisms, *P. aeruginosa* is atypical because it secretes a large number of proteins during growth. In most other

---

JANEL HECTOR, ALI AZGHANI, and ALICE JOHNSON • Department of Biochemistry, University of Texas Health Science Center at Tyler, Tyler, Texas 75710.

Pseudomonas aeruginosa as an Opportunistic Pathogen, edited by Mario Campa *et al.* Plenum Press, New York, 1993.

gram-negative bacteria, such as *E. coli*, a selectively permeable outer membrane retains secreted proteins within the periplasm.[3]

1.1. *Pseudomonas* Elastase

Elastolytic activity accounts for 88% of *P. aeruginosa* proteolytic activity.[4] The bacterial elastase is a zinc-requiring metalloprotease; its active site is blocked by zinc ligands.[4] It is both proteolytic and elastolytic, and digests many different human structural and functional proteins: collagen types III and IV,[5] fibronectin,[6] lung elastin,[7] laminin A and B chains,[8] immunoglobulins A[9,10] and G,[11,12] gamma interferon,[13] gastric mucin,[14] complement components, fibrin, and transferrin.[15] By degradation of potentially protective proteins, such as α-1 proteinase inhibitor[16–19] it can further enhance tissue injury and infection.

1.2. Chemistry

Morihara *et al.*[20] were the first investigators to isolate and crystallize *P. aeruginosa* elastase. Further studies by Morihara and his colleagues defined this enzyme as a protein with an isoelectric point of 5.9. They determined that the optimum pH for elastin hydrolysis was between 7 and 8, but the enzyme was stable over a pH range of 6 to 10.[4]

The activity of *P. aeruginosa* elastase can be measured with various synthetic peptide substrates, including Ala-Gly-Leu-Ala, Phe-Gly-Leu-Ala, or Ala-Leu-Ala.[4] Elastolytic activity is inhibited by metal chelators such as EDTA and o-phenanthroline,[21] zinc ligands such as phosphoramidon,[4] and functional groups including hydroxamic acid,[4,22] N-hydroxypeptide,[4] thiol,[4] and 3-(2-furyl)acrylolyl-glycyl-L-phenylalanyl-L-phenylalanine.[23] However, elastase is not blocked by chloro-4-(1-hydroxyoctadecyl)benzoic acid, an inhibitor of neutrophil elastase.[24]

P. aeruginosa elastase is similar to metalloproteases from other organisms. The zinc metalloprotease from *Legionella pneumophilia* appears structurally and functionally homologous to *P. aeruginosa* elastase.[25] Thermolysin from *Bacillus thermoproteolyticus* is similar but not identical. Homology studies comparing elastase with thermolysin indicate an overall amino acid homology of 49%. Although the amino and carboxy termini of elastase and thermolysin are different, the central portions of the two proteins are 67% homologous.[26] X-ray diffraction studies of thermolysin predict that *P. aeruginosa* elastase will have three zinc ligands: His 140, His 144 and Glu 164. His 223 is believed to be part of the active site, but full elastase activity may require Glu 141 and Asp 221.[15,26]

Physical characteristics of elastase produced by mucoid and nonmucoid strains appear identical. Hastie *et al.*[27] determined that elastase from both mucoid and nonmucoid strains have a pI of approximately 6.3. Analysis of elastase by polyacrylamide gel electrophoresis (PAGE) showed that the purified enzyme does not migrate in low-pH gels. In high-pH gels elastase from mucoid and nonmucoid *P. aeruginosa* strains migrated at the same rate and hydrolyzed elastin in gels impregnated with the substrate.

When rates of migration of mature elastase were compared with protein standards in PAGE gels elastase had a molecular weight of approximately 39,000.[4,27] When the nucleotide sequence of the elastase gene was determined, however, the molecular weight was determined more accurately at 32,926.[26,28] *P. aeruginosa* elastase is initially synthesized as a larger, nonelastolytic protein (pre-proelastase) with a molecular weight of approximately 53.6 kDa.[26,28] Processing occurs prior to secretion, and two proenzyme forms have been identified.[29,30] One modifying enzyme (gene *las*A) has been identified in *P. aeruginosa*.[31]

1.3. Biological Effects

The pathogenic role of *Pseudomonas* elastase is still poorly understood. *In vivo* studies using bacterial mutants deficient in elastase secretion indicate that this enzyme plays a major role in lung infections.[32,33] Elastase damages most tissues on contact. Many investigators found destructive changes after exposure to either the intact bacteria or isolated elastase. Electron micrographs published by Baker[34] show extensive damage to hamster tracheal epithelium by *Pseudomonas* organisms. Kawaharajo *et al.*[35] showed that the isolated elastase injected intravenously into mice caused hemorrhage in lungs, renal medulla, cerebral ventricles, and stomach. Intraperitoneal injections caused similar lesions in the lung, diaphragm, peritoneum, and the serosa of the gastrointestinal tract. Intrapleural injections primarily damaged lung and diaphragm.

Because of its ability to degrade a large number of different proteins, *P. aeruginosa* elastase can affect various functions in the lung. It can cause direct structural damage by degradation of elastin[7] and other extracellular matrix components,[36] but it also disrupts cilial function,[37] with potentially serious consequences. By initiation of the human Hageman factor cascade *P. aeruginosa* elastase enhances inflammation,[22,38] but it also may blunt immune defense mechanisms by inhibiting the activity of natural killer (NK) cells.[39] Elastase damage to host tissue is probably confined to the early stages of infection because the host immune response and subsequent accumulation of antibodies against bacterial elastase will limit its actions.[4,19]

Experiments from our laboratory showed that deposition by aerosol of low concentrations (0.1-5 μg/ml) of *P. aeruginosa* elastase into guinea pig lungs increased the permeability of pulmonary epithelium to labeled albumin, without disruption of either epithelial or subepithelial morphology.[40] Fig. 1 shows that elastase probably damages the epithelial intercellular tight junctions. When we injected an electron-dense horseradish peroxidase tracer

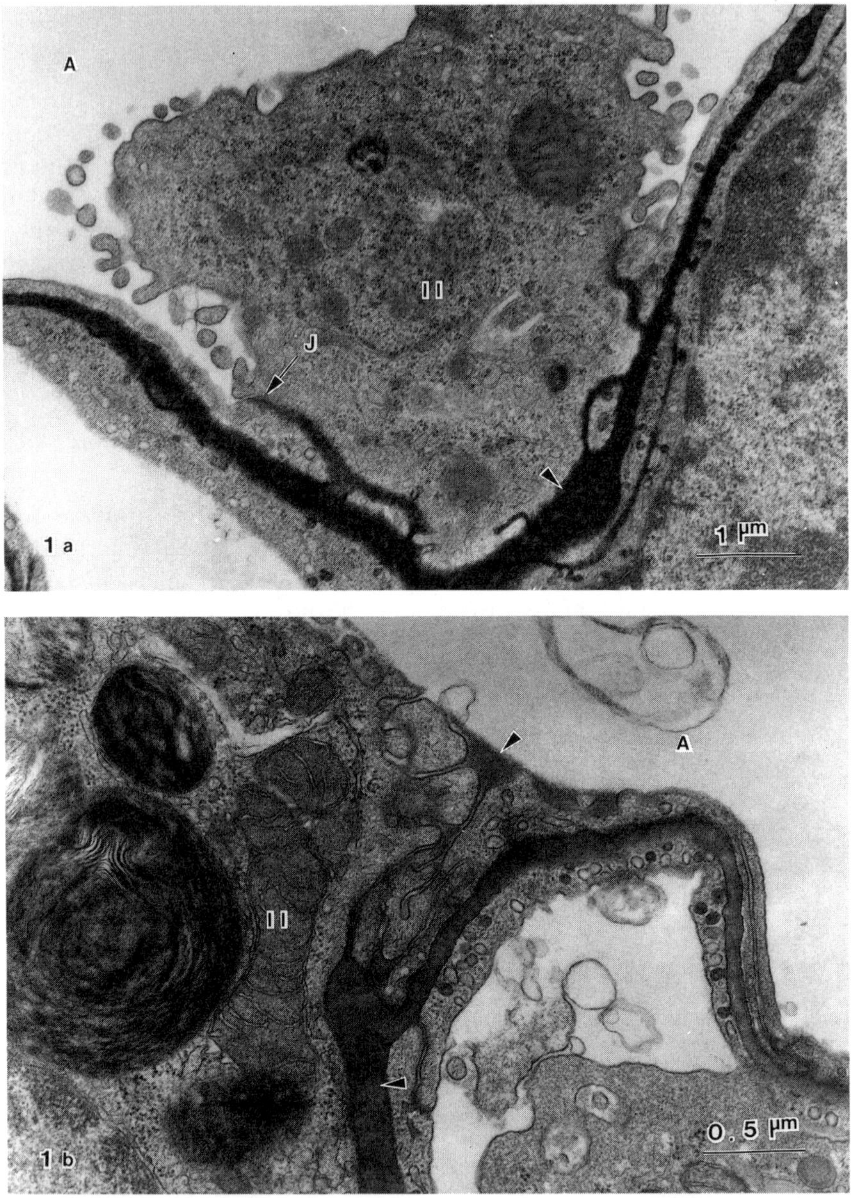

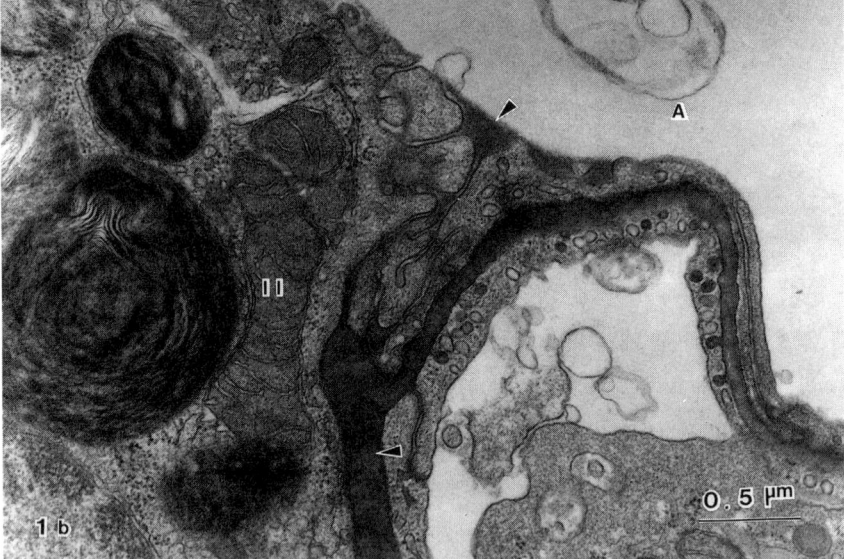

FIGURE 1. Horseradish peroxidase (HPR) tracer studies in lungs of control and *Pseudomonas* elastase (n = 5) treated guinea pigs. Animals received 300 mg HRP in 3 ml saline intravascularly prior to the end of a 3 hr-study. (a) HRP is in the intercellular space (arrow) but stops at the tight junction (J) level of a type-II pneumocyte (II). (b) HRP is shown in the intercellular space (arrow head) and on the alveolar (A) surfaces of type-II cells (II) of an elastase-treated animal. Data from Azghani et al.[40]

intravenously after elastase exposure, the tracer penetrated the intercellular junctions and appeared on the epithelial surface. This experimental work indicates that even low concentrations of P. aeruginosa elastase can cause subtle damage and may facilitate penetration of bacterial toxins or bacteria into the lungs.

1.4. Bacterial Adherence

Adhesion of pathogens to host cells is thought to be the initial step in bacterial colonization of the tissue and onset of infection.[41-43] Colonization of P. aeruginosa in the respiratory tract requires bacterial adherence to epithelial cells. Mechanisms such as pili[36,44] and alginate,[13,14] an acetylated exopolysaccharide,[2] enable the bacteria to adhere to respiratory epithelium. In a study of patients in an intensive care unit, Todd and associates noted more colonization with P. aeruginosa in individuals with pneumonitis than in those with nonpulmonary diseases, but bacterial adherence did not correlate with intubation.[45] The tenacious adherence of this organism to pulmonary epithelium affords secreted elastase almost immediate access to the parenchymal tissues of the lung.

Early studies *in vitro* indicated that cell surface fibronectin protected against adherence of gram-negative bacteria to epithelial cells. Woods *et al.*[33,46] showed that removal of fibronectin from the epithelial surfaces promoted adherence of P. aeruginosa. Work in our laboratory showed that P. aeruginosa elastase can degrade purified fibronectin, and also fibronectin and fibronectin receptors on the surface of human lung fibroblasts. We also found that elastase treatment of fibroblasts enhanced adherence of bacteria in comparison with control (untreated) cells.[6,47]

Elastase production appears to correlate with bacterial virulence, and it has a direct effect on the clinical status of infected patients.[48] Elastase-producing strains of *Pseudomonas* are more difficult to clear from the lungs of experimental animals than are non-elastase-producing strains.[32] Further, rats with lungs already damaged by neutrophil elastase were unable to clear challenging P. aeruginosa colonies.[49]

2. ENVIRONMENTAL EFFECTS ON ELASTASE PRODUCTION

Elastase produced by P. aeruginosa contributes to a variety of infections. Factors that control the amount and activity of this enzyme *in vivo* are still unknown. Elastase production is independent of serotype,[50,51] but it might be influenced by factors within the immediate environment of infection. We related elastase production to environmental conditions, hoping to gain clues to the regulation of this enzyme.

2.1. Source

A large proportion *Pseudomonas* isolates from CF patients produce elastase.[27] Comparison of *P. aeruginosa* strains from burn wounds, skin wounds, urine, CF sputum, acute pneumonia sputum, and blood indicated that elastase production is highest in isolates from acute lung infections, intermediate in isolates from burns, wounds and urine, and lowest in isolates from CF sputum and blood.[48] Another study detected elastase production in *P. aeruginosa* isolates from sputum, throat swabs, pus, blood and urine, but not in isolates from ear discharges.[51] Elastase production by environmental isolates is similar to that of clinical samples.[52] Comparison of *Pseudomonas* isolates from different sources has revealed no obvious mechanisms that regulate elastase activity.

2.2. Antibiotics

Antibiotics that inhibit growth of the bacteria *in vivo* might be expected to alter their characteristics. Ciprofloxacin and tobramycin can reduce elastase activity *in vitro* and in experimental animals (rat), and pretreatment with these agents results in decreased elastase activity as well as decreased lung damage.[53] No antibiotic, however, is known to suppress elastase synthesis or secretion.

2.3. Culture Conditions

Because the synthesis of some bacterial enzymes is regulated by substrate/inhibitor feedback systems, the next step in the study of the regulation of elastase was to try to correlate the presence or absence of various substrates or phenotypic characteristics of different strains with the production of elastolytic activity. The studies of Jensen and colleagues defined the effects of media composition.[21]

2.4. Media Composition

The composition of growth media can influence elastase production by *P. aeruginosa*. Eight strains from both clinical and environmental sources were grown on various combinations of nutrients.[21] Elastase production, based on elastase activity in azocasein-impregnated gels, was measured from the media supernatants. Glucose was the best carbon source, and elastase production increased as the glucose concentration increased up to 0.07M. Activity then declined at higher glucose concentrations. Ammonia inhibited elastase production, while glutamate or Gln, if these were the sole sources of nitrogen, promoted elastase production. Elastase production further increased with the addition of Val and Phe, although these amino acids alone were insufficient as nitrogen sources. Zinc and iron were both necessary for maximum elastase production. Because elastase is a zinc metalloprotease, zinc is necessary for elastolytic activity, but the reason for the iron requirement is obscure. Calcium and magnesium added to prevent clumping of cells did not affect elastase production. Maximum production of elastase occurred in media containing sodium glutamate, Val, Phe, glucose, NaCl, K_2HPO_4, $MgSO_4$, $CaCl_2$, $FeSO_4$, and $ZnSO_4$. Protein was not required to induce elastase synthesis, nor was production repressed by the presence of free amino acids. Because glucose increased elastase production, elastase production was not controlled by catabolite repression. Although levels of elastase production could be influenced, no on/off regulatory mechanism was found.[21]

2.5. Duration of Culture

The amount of elastase produced also depends upon the age of the bacteria in culture. Of 132 fresh *P. aeruginosa* strains collected from CF patients, 86% had elastase activity. After 6 months' growth in nutrient agar, 20% of these active strains lost elastase activity. After 3 years, only 35% of the 20 strains that were previously positive still made elastase. Because genes that produce proteins unessential for survival of the bacteria are likely shut off, the loss of elastase activity is not surprising. Elastase activity was restored when the elastase-negative strains were grown in trypticase soy broth or bouillon. The form of culture, whether solid, static fluid or shaking fluid, did not influence recovery.[4]

The time course of enzyme release by elastase-producing strains also indicated a definite pattern. Elastase in the culture supernatant increased to a maximum 24–48 hr after inoculation, then dropped off at 83–85 hr,[27] indicating that fresh culture media stimulated elastase production. Both mucoid and nonmucoid strains secreted elastase, and the amounts of elastase detected were not significantly different between mucoid and nonmucoid strains.

This finding was contradicted by another report. Ohman and Chakrabarty[2] tested seven alginate-producing strains cultured from individuals with CF, and their respective alginate negative mutants. Four of the seven positive/negative pairs produced no detectable elastase. Of the remaining three pairs, the mucoid strains produced less elastase than their nonmucoid variants. Also, when grown in medium containing sputum from the patients, two alginate-positive strains produced less elastase than the respective alginate-negative mutants. These investigators concluded that the alginate formed a barrier around the cell that interfered with production and/or secretion of elastase. In a later study, Flynn and Ohman[54] cloned the alginate gene and found that mucoid production or nonproduction reflect two different phenotypes, and conversion from one to the other can occur spontaneously.

Data from our own laboratory indicate no consistent relationship between the amount of elastase produced in culture and the mucoid phenotype of the *P. aeruginosa* strain. All strains of *P. aeruginosa* isolated from our group of CF patients produced elastase when grown in complex media (unpublished data). The use of rhodamine-conjugated elastin in culture overlays enabled us to detect elastase activity in all cystic fibrosis isolates, while Ohman and Chakrabarty detected elastase in only three of their seven mucoid/nonmucoid paired isolates. Thus, the variation in results from one laboratory to another is probably due to differences in culture techniques or in the sensitivity of elastase assays.

When we cultured mucoid/nonmucoid paired strains from CF patients, and analyzed their DNA by pulsed-field gel electrophoresis (PFGE), we found identical restriction fragment patterns in mucoid and nonmucoid strains taken from the same patient, indicating that these strains were phenotypic variants of one strain. There was no significant difference in elastase activity of the paired mucoid/nonmucoid strains. Further, when strains taken from various unrelated patients were analyzed, restriction fragment patterns were distinctly different. Elastase production did vary between strains. Fig. 2 shows the PFGE DNA restriction patterns obtained with bacteria cultured from several different CF individuals. Grothues *et al.*[55] also observed different restriction band patterns when isolates from a CF population were compared using field inversion gel electrophoresis.

Because the PFGE patterns revealed no obvious differences in DNA fragments from isolates from the same patient, we conclude that mucoid and nonmucoid colonies are variants of the same strain and differ only in their regulation of the alginate gene. Further, elastase production appears to be independent of alginate production.

3. MOLECULAR BIOLOGY STUDIES

The study of any regulatory system depends on the discovery of mutations that affect that system. Naturally occurring strains of *P. aeruginosa* have been reported that produce little or no elastase.[52,56] However, mutations affecting elastase secretion were difficult to obtain, and most mutations affected the secretion of a number of extracellular proteins in addition to elastase.[57,58] Recently, however, several mutants have been discovered and analyzed, first with complement studies, and then by molecular biology techniques.

3.1. Elastase-Deficient Mutants

The first mutant to affect elastase production specifically was obtained after treating PAO1 wild-type cells with the mutagen n-methyl-n'-nitroso-

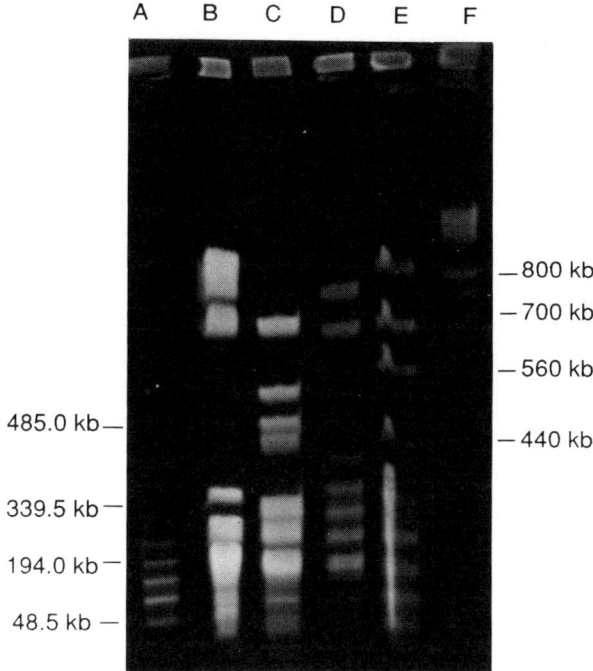

FIGURE 2. Pulsed-field gel electrophoresis of *Pseudomonas aeruginosa* strains from CF patients. Lane A: lambda concatemer (48.5 kilobase) standard, lane B–E: *P. aeruginosa* isolates from four different CF patients, lane F: *Saccharomyces cerevisiae* chromosomal DNA standard.

guanidine.[59] The resulting strain, designated PAO-E64, had normal proteolytic activity but no elastolytic activity above 32°C.[60] This mutation was named *las*A1.[59] Although elastolytic activity disappeared at temperatures above 32°C, an antibody to elastase detected the antigen at levels equal to those produced by the parent strain. All other exoproducts were secreted normally.[59] This mutant was less virulent than its parent strain when tested in animal models, including chronic lung infection in rats, acute lung infection in guinea pigs, and burned mice. However, when the *las*A1 mutant was introduced into a mouse model for corneal infections, this differential disappears, probably because there is no elastin in the mouse cornea.[46]

This mutant might explain another observation. Morihara and Homma[4] noted that elastolytic activity of some cultures of *Pseudomonas* decreased in the presence of MgCl concentrations greater than 0.1M, but proteolytic activity was unaffected. Although these workers did not evaluate temperature sensitivity of the enzyme, the pattern of decreased elastolytic activity with normal proteolytic activity fits the *las*A1 pattern.

Other *las*A mutants have normal proteolytic activity but little elastolytic activity.[60] These mutants have defective processing of proelastase to elastase. The lasA2 mutant was derived from an engineered plasmid containing the lasA gene, and it contains an insertion of the transposon (Tn10)-kan within the lasA coding sequence. This mutant does not complement the lasA1 mutation.[60] The lasA3 mutant was developed from the lasA2 plasmid, which had lost about 3.3 kilobase of DNA (2.1 kilobase of the P. aeruginosa lasA gene and 1.3 kilobase of the transposon DNA) and thus had lost most of the lasA coding sequence.[61] Both mutants produce a protein that reacts with anti-elastase antibodies just as the wild-type elastase does, indicating that none of the major antigenic sites of wild-type elastase are lost.[60]

Other mutants that make no elastase at all are defined as elastase null mutants, and have no elastase antigenic or elastolytic activity. One null mutant, strain PAO-E105, is a Tn501 mutation of wild-type PAO1.[31]

3.2. Elastase Genes

Complementation and molecular biology techniques helped to determine which genes are required for production of mature elastase. When a gene bank was constructed from wild-type PAO1, then used to complement the lasA1 and elastase-null mutants, two separate genes were identified.[31] The first gene (lasA) complemented the lasA1 mutant, and the combination resulted in normal elastase production. However, lasA did not complement the PAO-E105 null mutant, and it did not produce elastase when inserted in E. coli. Oligonucleotide probes constructed to complement the elastase gene did not hybridize with this gene.[31] When the lasA gene was expressed in E. coli, it encoded a protein of 31,000 mol wt. This lasA protein could activate the proteolytic but not elastolytic lasA elastase antigen, and the resulting protein was identical to mature elastase.[61] The lasA gene, therefore, is not the structural elastase gene, but is a modifier gene essential for modification of proelastase to mature elastase. The active regions of the lasA protein are currently being defined.[62]

The second gene (lasB) is the structural elastase gene.[31] This gene complements the null PAO-E105 mutant but not the lasA1 mutant strain, PAO-E64. The gene hybridized with oligonucleotide probes constructed to complement the elastase gene, and when expressed in E. coli, it produced an elastase that reacted with anti-elastase.[31,63] Because E. coli produced functional elastase, the P. aeruginosa promoter and translation initiation sites were functional within E. coli.[26]

The nucleotide sequence of the elastase structural gene lasB) contains a 1491-base-pair reading frame (G+C 64.3%) that codes for 498 amino acids. This product has a molecular weight of 53,600, which corresponds to that estimated for pre-proelastase.[26,28] The reading frame includes a signal sequence followed by a "pro" sequence (197 amino acids), a short pro fragment, and the sequence for the mature elastase protein (301 amino acids, 32,926 mol. wt.).[26,28] This relationship is depicted in Fig. 3. It is clear that both *las*A and *las*B genes are necessary to produce the fully mature elastolytic enzyme. *Las*B is a structural gene that encodes the amino acid sequence of elastase, and *las*A encodes a completely separate enzyme that acts as a modifier. This modifying enzyme cleaves proelastase (proenzyme II), which is proteolytic but not elastolytic, to produce a smaller, mature proteolytic elastolytic enzyme. The *las*A gene has been sequenced[64] and mapped to the *P. aeruginosa* chromosomal DNA at 51' (on a 75' map),[59] and at 75' on a 95' map.[65] A physical map of the *P. aeruginosa* genome is also available.[66]

3.3. Processing of Elastase

Three systems have been used to study *P. aeruginosa* elastase production: a cell-free transcription–translation system, intact *E. coli*, and intact *P. aeruginosa*. Host regulation–modification systems in *E. coli* and *P. aeruginosa* organisms may alter the product, whereas the cell-free system produces the proenzyme without post-translational modifications.

Bever and Iglewski[26] used an *E. coli* cell-free transcription–translation system to synthesize elastase from a 3.0 kilobase EcoRI-KpnI DNA fragment from *P. aeruginosa* that contained the *las*B gene. They found that the *las*B gene produced two products of 54,000 and 50,000 mol. wt., determined by PAGE. Both of these proteins reacted with anti-elastase. The authors concluded that the 54-kDa protein was preproelastase, since it matched the predicted 53,600 mol. wt. *las*B gene product from the nucleotide sequence of the *las*B gene.[26,28] The 50,000 mol. wt. protein appears to be a proenzyme form (proelastase I) that in the cell is located in the periplasm, but it has a short half-life.[29,30] Because no initiation site was found in the *las*B gene to account for the presence of a 50,000-mol. wt. protein, Bever and Iglewski[26] concluded that the 54,000-mol. wt. protein is modified within the cell, and that this modification is required for the 50,000-mol. wt. proelastase I to cross

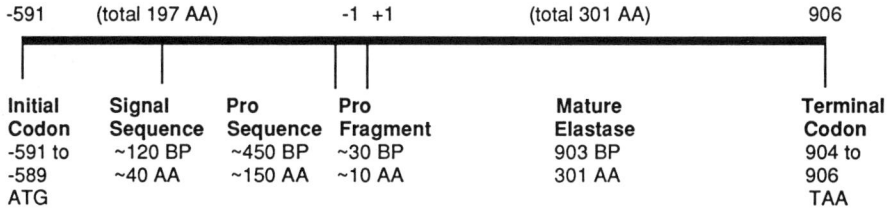

FIGURE 3. Structure of the *Pseudomonas aeruginosa* elastase structural gene. Three preliminary sequences, including the signal sequence, pro sequence and pro fragment, total 591 nucleotides (197 amino acids). The mature elastase protein is coded for by 903 nucleotides (301 amino acids). Taken from DNA sequences with initiator, proenzyme and signal sequences proposed by Bever and Iglewski,[26] Kessler and Safrin,[29,30] and Fukushima et al.[28]

the inner cytoplasmic membrane. The cell-free system transcribes and translates the gene, but the protein is not modified without the *las*A enzyme.

Bever and Iglewski[26] and Fukushima et al.[28] have used *E. coli* to express the elastase gene that was inserted by a plasmid vector. When translated in *E. coli*, the *las*B gene produced a 33,000-mol. wt. protein that reacted with anti-elastase. This protein was proteolytic as well as elastolytic; it was found in the cell membrane fraction and in the supernatant of sonicated bacteria but was not released into the culture supernatant.[26,28,63] It is interesting to note that the elastase gene, when inserted in *E. coli*, is modified to a molecular weight of 33,000 as in *P. aeruginosa*; thus *E. coli* must contain a modifier enzyme that cleaves the elastase precursor in the same way as the *las*A enzyme. However, *E. coli* appears to lack the secretory mechanism present in *P. aeruginosa*, because elastase accumulates within *E. coli* cells.[60] Also, elastase produced by *P. aeruginosa* is not elastolytic until released into the supernatant, but in *E. coli* the intracellular elastase is elastolytic.[67,68]

Goldberg and Ohman[61] expressed the modifying gene *las*A in *E. coli* and found a protein product of 31 kDa. This *las*A protein activated proelastase produced by *las*A mutants to a protein with elastolytic activity, and a molecular weight of 37,000 (PAGE), which corresponds to the 33,000-mol. wt. protein found by Fukushima and co-workers using sequence data,[26,28] and was identical to purified elastase. The *las*A protein did not react with anti-elastase, and was not elastolytic. They concluded that the *las*A protein activated the elastolytic function of elastase and broadened the specificity of elastase, because the pre-proelastase is proteolytic, and mature elastase is both proteolytic and elastolytic. It is unusual, however, for an enzyme to undergo a broadening of substrate-specificity during processing.[15]

Goldberg and Ohman[61] also studied a nonmucoid strain of *P. aeruginosa*, in which the *las*B gene product *is* elastolytic. It reacts with anti-elastase, and it is released into the supernatant in high levels. SDS-PAGE was used to estimate molecular weights. From this method they identified low levels of a 37-kDa mature elastase that corresponds to the 33-kDa sequenced protein in the periplasmic fraction. They also found a 47-kDa proelastase I (proteolytic but not elastolytic) in the membrane-associated protein-enriched fraction and also, at low levels, in the soluble fraction. SDS-PAGE was used to estimate molecular weights. In a *las*A mutant, they found a 47-kDa membrane-associated protein that accumulated in large amounts in the soluble fraction of the cell. These 47-kDa proteins appear to correspond to proelastase I (50 kDa). They also found a 37-kDa protein in *las*A mutants that was proteolytic but not elastolytic, and which appears to be proelastase II. *Las*A mutants and elastase-producing strains had similar amounts of elastase antigen; however, the final product of the *las*A mutant was proelastase II (molecular weight similar to that of mature elastase), whereas mature elastase was the final product of the elastolytic nonmucoid strain.

3.4. Secretion

Kessler and Safrin[29,30] performed pulse-labeling experiments using [^{35}S]-methionine in *P. aeruginosa* and provided substantial evidence that elastase exists in four forms. A pre-proelastase of 60 kDa (SDS-PAGE), corresponding to the 53.6-kDa protein,[26,28] was found in the membrane fraction. This pre-proelastase was not detected after 15-sec pulses, unless inhibitors were used, and thus is processed rapidly. During processing for transport, a proelastase (I) of 56,000 mol. wt. (SDS-PAGE), corresponding to the 50-kDa protein,[26] is seen in the periplasm; it is also short-lived. A second proelastase (II) of 36 kDa (slightly larger than mature elastase at 32.9 kDa)[28] is also found in the periplasm, probably as a complex with the 20-kDa fragment released from the first proelastase. Secretion of the mature elastase 35 kDa (corresponding to 32.9 kDa) requires dissociation of the 20-kDa fragment[30] and probably proteolytic removal of a small peptide of 500–1000 mol. wt.[29] Kessler and Safrin[30] also identified several inhibitors of the elastase cleavage sequence. The formation of proelastase I from pre-proelastase was inhibited by ethanol (with or without EDTA), dinitrophenol with EDTA, or carbonyl cyanide m-chlorophenyl hydrazone with EDTA. The conversion of proelastase I to proelastase II was inhibited by EDTA, but not by EGTA [ethylene glycol-bis(β-aminoethyl ether)-N,N,N',N'-tetraacetic acid]. Also, trypsin converted proelastase II to mature elastase.[29]

A change in hydrophobicity, perhaps due to a change in conformation, may also be required for secretion of elastase.[68] Activation by *las*A allows elastase to exist within the bacterial cell as the proenzyme form proelastase II. The enzyme becomes toxic only when altered by the *las*A protein and released into the environment.[28] The *las*A protein is also assumed to play some undefined role in the secretion of mature elastase, because *las*A mutants accumulate proelastase II within the cell.[26] According to evidence presented by Kessler and Safrin,[29] the activation of proelastase II is due to proteolytic removal of a small fragment of approximately 10 amino acids. This uncleaved pro fragment appears to render the elastase elastolytically inactive within the host.

In conclusion, the cell-free transcription–translation system, along with *E. coli* and *P. aeruginosa* studies and sequencing of the *las*B gene, indicate four forms of elastase (see Fig. 3 and 4). Elastase is first translated in a pre-proenzyme form of 53.6 kDa composed of 1491 nucleotide base pairs and 498 amino acids. Pre-proelastase, located in the membrane fraction, is proteolytic but not elastolytic, has a short half-life, and reacts with antielastase antibodies. A small signal sequence (about 4 kDa) is cleaved off and the enzyme, now designated proelastase I, crosses the inner cytoplasmic membrane into the periplasm. Proelastase I (50 kDa) reacts with anti-elastase and with antibody to the 20-kDa protein, and it also has a short half-life.

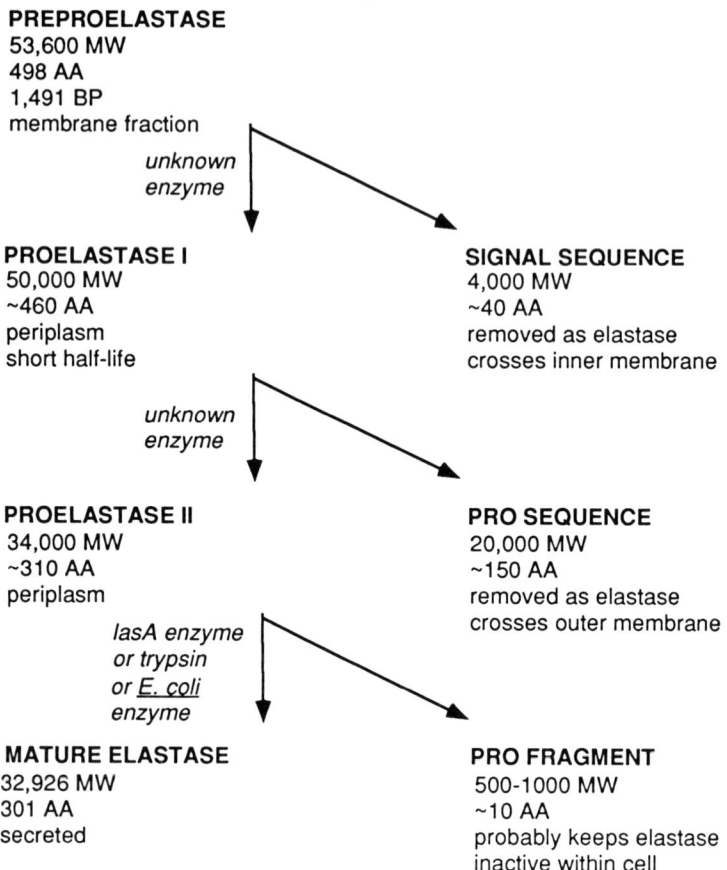

FIGURE 4. Specific cleavage of elastase-precursor protein generates mature elastase. Elastase is found in four forms in *Pseudomonas aeruginosa*, and three different "pro" sequences are removed during processing. MW = molecular weight, AA = amino acid, BP = nucleotide base pair. This cleavage pattern is derived from patterns proposed by Bever and Iglewski,[26] Kessler and Safrin,[29,30] and Fukushima et al.[28]

Proelastase I is cleaved into proelastase II (34 kDa) and a pro sequence (20 kDa). The pro sequence is neither proteolytic nor elastolytic, and it dissociates from proelastase II as it crosses the outer membrane. Proelastase II is proteolytic but not elastolytic, reacts with anti-elastase, is slightly larger than mature elastase, and accumulates in the periplasm. The final step of elastase processing is the removal of a small pro fragment by the *las*A enzyme, which appears to render elastase inactive within the cell. Mature elastase, both proteolytic and elastolytic, is then secreted into the medium.

4. CONCLUSIONS

P. aeruginosa is a remarkably adaptable organism. Not only can it adapt to limited growth conditions, it also adapts to secretion of one of its major virulence factors, elastase. Elastase production begins with the synthesis of an elastolytically inactive pre-proenzyme. As this molecule crosses the cytoplasmic membrane it is cleaved to an antigenically reactive enzyme, proelastase I, and a small signal sequence. Proelastase I is composed of two protein units, a 34-kDa proelastase II and a 20-kDa pro sequence, that associate noncovalently within the periplasm. The larger unit crosses the outer membrane where it is activated by the *las*A enzyme, and only then does the enzyme become fully elastolytic and capable of damaging tissues.

We have achieved a preliminary understanding of elastase regulation. First, elastase production can be influenced only slightly by media conditions or antibiotics. Second, elastase production is independent of alginate production, as shown using PFGE to identify DNA identical alginate positive/negative pairs. Third, the major steps of elastase synthesis, including precursors and one enzyme (*las*A) have been identified. And finally, the elastase gene has been sequenced. *P. aeruginosa* is a tenacious organism and difficult to eradicate from infected patients. However, our increased understanding of the regulation of elastase, one of the major toxins of this organism, may provide the means for controlling elastase toxicity in *P. aeruginosa* infections.

REFERENCES

1. Vasil, M. L., 1986, *Pseudomonas aeruginosa*: Biology, mechanisms of virulence, epidemiology, *J. Pediatr.* **108**:800–805.
2. Ohman, D. E., and Chakrabarty, A. M., 1982, Utilization of human respiratory secretions by mucoid *Pseudomonas aeruginosa* of cystic fibrosis origin, *Infect. Immun.* **37**:662–669.
3. Nielsen, J. B. K., Mezes, P. S. F., and Lampen, J. O., 1983, Secretion by *Pseudomonas aeruginosa*: Fate of a cloned gram-positive lipoprotein deletion mutant, *J. Bacteriol.* **156**:559–566.
4. Morihara, K., and Homma, J. Y., 1985, *Pseudomonas* proteases, in: *Bacterial Enzymes and Virulence*, (J. A. Holder, ed.), CRC Press Inc., Boca Raton, Florida, pp.
5. Heck, L. W., Morihara, K., McRae, W. B., and Miller, E. J., 1986, Specific cleavage of human type III and IV collagens by *Pseudomonas aeruginosa* elastase, *Infect. Immun.* **51**:115–118.
6. Asghani, A. O., and Johnson, A. R., 1990, Elastase from *Pseudomonas aeruginosa* alters fibronectin and fibronectin receptors of cultured human lung fibroblasts, *Am. Soc. Microbiol. Annu. Meet.* abstract B175.
7. Hamdaoui, A., Wund-Bisseret, F., and Bieth, J. G., 1987, Fast solubilization of human lung elastin by *Pseudomonas aeruginosa* elastase, *Am. Rev. Respir. Dis.* **135**:860–863.
8. Heck, L. W., Morihara, K., and Abrahamson, D. R., 1986, Degradation of soluble laminin and depletion of tissue-associated basement membrane laminin by *Pseudomonas aeruginosa* elastase and alkaline protease, *Infect. Immun.* **54**:149–153.
9. Niederman, M. S., Merrill, W. W., Polomski, L. M., Reynolds, H. Y., and Gee, J. B., 1986,

Influence of sputum IgA and elastase on tracheal cell bacterial adherence, *Am. Rev. Respir. Dis.* **133:**255–260.
10. Heck, L. W., Alarcon, P. G., Kulhavy, R. M., Morihara, K., Russell, M. W., and Mestecky, J. F., 1990, Degradation of IgA proteins by *Pseudomonas aeruginosa* elastase, *J. Immunol.* **144:** 2253–2257.
11. Holder, I. A., and Wheeler, R., 1984, Experimental studies of the pathogenesis of infections due to *Pseudomonas aeruginosa*. Elastase: A IgG protease, *Can. J. Microbiol.* **30:**1118–1124.
12. Bainbridge, T., and Fick, R. B., Jr., 1989, Functional importance of cystic fibrosis immunoglobulin G fragments generated by *Pseudomonas aeruginosa* elastase, *J. Lab. Clin. Med.* **114:** 728–733.
13. Horvat, R. T., Clabaugh, M., Duval-Jobe, C., and Parmely, M. J., 1989, Inactivation of human gamma interferon by *Pseudomonas aeruginosa* proteases: Elastase augments the effects of alkaline protease despite the presence of alpha 2-macroglobulin, *Infect. Immun.* **57:**1668–1674.
14. Poncz, L., Jentoft, N., Ho, M. C. D., and Dearborn D. G., 1988, Kinetics of proteolysis of hog gastric mucin by human neutrophil elastase and by *Pseudomonas aeruginosa* elastase, *Infect. Immun.* **56:**703–704.
15. Iglewski, B., 1989, Probing *Pseudomonas aeruginosa*, an opportunistic pathogen, *ASM News* **55:**303–307.
16. Goldstein, W., and Doring, G., 1986, Lysosomal enzymes from polymorphonuclear leukocytes and proteinase inhibitors in patients with cystic fibrosis. *Am. Rev. Respir. Dis.* **134:** 49–56.
17. Morihara, K., Tsuzuki, H., and Oda, K., 1979, Protease and elastase of *Pseudomonas aeruginosa*: Inactivation of human plasma α_1-proteinase inhibitor, *Infect. Immun.* **24:**188–193.
18. Perlmutter, D. H., and Punsal, P. I., 1988, Distinct and additive effects of elastase and endotoxin on expression of α_1-proteinase inhibitor in mononuclear phagocytes, *J. Biol. Chem.* **263:**16499–16503.
19. Doring, G., Goldstein, W., Roll, A., Schiotz, P. O., Hoiby, N., and Botzenhart, K., 1985, Role of *Pseudomonas aeruginosa* exoenzymes in lung infections of patients with cystic fibrosis, *Infect. Immun.* **49:**557–562.
20. Morihara, K., Tsuzuki, H., Oka, T., Inoue, H., and Ebata, M., 1965, *Pseudomonas aeruginosa* elastase isolation, crystallization, and preliminary characterization, *J. Biol. Chem.* **240:**3295–3304.
21. Jensen, S. E., Fecycz, I. T., and Campbell, J. N., 1980, Nutritional factors controlling exocellular protease production by *Pseudomonas aeruginosa*, *J. Bacteriol.* **144:**844–847.
22. Yamamoto, T., Shibuya, Y., Nishino, N., Okabe, H., and Kambara, T., 1990, Activation of human Hageman factor by *Pseudomonas aeruginosa* elastase in the presence or absence of negatively charged substance in vitro, *Biochem. Biophys. Acta.* **1038:**231–239.
23. Poncz, L., 1988, Substrate inhibition of *Pseudomonas aeruginosa* elastase by 3-(2-furyl)-acryloyl-glycyl-L-phenylalanyl-L-phenylalanine, *Arch. Biochem. Biophys.* **266:**508–515.
24. Nakao, A., Partis, R. A., Jung, G. P., and Mueller, R. A., 1987, SC-39026, a specific human neutrophil elastase inhibitor. *Biochem. Biophys. Res. Commun.* **147:**666–674.
25. Black, W. J., Quinn, F. D., and Tompkins, L. S., 1990, *Legionella pneumophila* zinc metalloprotease is structurally and functionally homologous to *Pseudomonas aeruginosa* elastase, *J. Bacteriol.* **172:**2608–2613.
26. Bever, R. A., and Iglewski, B. H., 1988, Molecular characterization and nucleotide sequence of the *Pseudomonas aeruginosa* elastase structural gene, *J. Bacteriol.* **170:**4309–4314.
27. Hastie, A. T., Hingley, S. T., Kueppers, F., Higgins, M. L., Tannenbaum, C. S., and Weinbaum, G., 1983, Protease production by *Pseudomonas aeruginosa* isolates from patients with cystic fibrosis, *Infect. Immun.* **40:**506–513.
28. Fukushima, J., Yamamoto, S., Morihara, K., Atsumi, Y., Takeuchi, H., Kawamoto, S., and Okuda, K., 1989, Structural gene and complete amino acid sequence of *Pseudomonas aeruginosa* IFO 3455 elastase, *J. Bacteriol.* **171:**1698–1704.

29. Kessler, E., and Safrin, M., 1988, Partial purification and characterization of an inactive precursor of *Pseudomonas aeruginosa* elastase, *J. Bacteriol.* **170:**1215–1219.
30. Kessler, E., and Safrin, M., 1988, Synthesis, processing, and transport of *Pseudomonas aeruginosa* elastase, *J. Bacteriol.* **170:**5241–5247.
31. Schad, P. A., Bever, R. A., Nicas, T. I., Leduc, F., Hanne, L. F., and Iglewski, B. H., 1987, Cloning and characterization of elastase genes from *Pseudomonas aeruginosa*, *J. Bacteriol.* **169:** 2691–2696.
32. Blackwood, L. L., Stone, R. M., Iglewski, B. H., and Pennington, J. E., 1983, Evaluation of *Pseudomonas aeruginosa* exotoxin A and elastase as virulence factors in acute lung infection, *Infect. Immun.* **39:**198–201.
33. Woods, D. E., Cryz, S. J., Friedman, R. L., and Iglewski, B. H., 1982, Contribution of toxin A and elastase to virulence of *Pseudomonas aeruginosa* in chronic lung infections of rats, *Infect. Immun.* **36:**1223–1228.
34. Baker, N. R., 1982, Role of exotoxin A and proteases of *Pseudomonas aeruginosa* in respiratory tract infections, *Can. J. Microbiol.* **28:**248–255.
35. Kawaharajo, J., Homma, Y., Aoyama, Y., and Morihara, K., 1975, In vivo studies on protease and elastase from *Pseudomonas aeruginosa*, *J. Exp. Med.* **45:**89–100.
36. Roberts, D. D., 1990, Interactions of respiratory pathogens with host cell surface and extracellular matrix components, *Am. J. Respir. Cell Mol. Biol.* **3:**181–186.
37. Hingley, S. T., Hastie, A. T., Kueppers, F., and Higgins, M. L., 1986, Disruption of respiratory cilia by proteases including those of *Pseudomonas aeruginosa*, *Infect. Immun.* **54:** 379–385.
38. Holder, I. A., and Neely, A. N., 1989, *Pseudomonas* elastase acts as a virulence factor in burned hosts by Hageman factor-dependent activation of the host kinin cascade, *Infect. Immun.* **57:**3345–3348.
39. Pedersen, B. K., and Kharazmi, A., 1987, Inhibition of human natural killer cell activity by *Pseudomonas aeruginosa* alkaline protease and elastase, *Infect. Immun.* **55:**986–989.
40. Azghani, A. O., Connelly, J. C., Peterson, B. T., Gray, L. D., Collins, M. L., and Johnson, A. R., 1990, Effects of *Pseudomonas aeruginosa* elastase on alveolar epithelial permeability in guinea pigs, *Infect. Immun.* **58:**433–438.
41. Johanson, W. G., Jr., Woods, D. E., and Chaudhuri, T., 1979, Association of respiratory tract colonization with adherence of gram-negative bacilli to epithelial cells, *J. Infect. Dis.* **139:** 667–673.
42. Beachey, E. H., 1981, Bacterial adherence: Adhesin receptor interactions mediating the attachment of bacteria to mucosal surfaces, *J. Infect. Dis.* **143:**325–345.
43. Fowler, J. E., Jr., and Stamey, T. A., 1977, Studies on introital colonization in women with recurrent urinary tract infections. VII. The role of bacterial adherence, *J. Urol.* **117:**472–476.
44. Doig, P. Todd, T., Sastry, P. A., Lee, K. K., Hodges, R. S., Paranchych, W., and Irvin, R. T., 1988, Role of pili in adhesion of *Pseudomonas aeruginosa* to human respiratory epithelial cells, *Infect. Immun.* **56:**1641–1646.
45. Todd, T. R. J., Franklin, A., Mankinen-Irvin, P., Gurman, G., and Irvin, R. T., 1989, Augmented bacterial adherence to tracheal epithelial cells is associated with gram-negative pneumonia in an intensive care unit population, *Am. Rev. Respir. Dis.* **140:**1585–1589.
46. Woods, D. E., and Iglewski, B. H., 1983, Toxins of *Pseudomonas aeruginosa*: New perspectives, *Rev. Infect. Dis.* **5:**S715–S722.
47. Azghani, A. O., Kondepudi, A. Y., and Johnson, A. R., 1991, Adherence of *Pseudomonas aeruginosa* fibroblasts: Role of *Pseudomonas* elastase and cell surface fibronectin, *Amer. Soc. Microbiol. Annu. Meet.* abstract B132.
48. Woods, D. E., Schaffer, M. S., Rabin, H. R., Campbell, G. D., and Sokol, P. A., 1986, Phenotypic comparison of *Pseudomonas aeruginosa* strains isolated from a variety of clinical sites, *J. Clin. Microbiol.* **24:**260–264.
49. Doring, G., and Dauner, H. M., 1988, Clearance of *Pseudomonas aeruginosa* in different rat lung models, *Am. Rev. Respir. Dis.* **138:**1249–1253.

50. Elsheikh, L. E., Bergman, R., Cryz, S. J., and Wretlind, B., 1986, A comparison of different methods for determining elastase activity of *Pseudomonas aeruginosa* strains from mink, *Acta Pathol. Microbiol. Immunol. Scand.* **94**:135–138.
51. Iida, T., Katoh, M., Tsukiyama, F., Nakamura, K., Watanabe, T., Ikeda, M., Muroki, K., Fujiue, Y., and Kuwabara, M., 1982, Protease and elastase production in relation to serotype of *Pseudomonas aeruginosa*, *Hiroshima J. Med. Sci.* **31**:181–185.
52. Nicas, T. I., and Iglewski, B. H., 1986, Production of elastase and other exoproducts by environmental isolates of *Pseudomonas aeruginosa*, *J. Clin. Microbiol.* **23**:967–969.
53. Grimwood, K., To, M., Rabin, H. R., and Woods, D. E., 1989, Inhibition of *Pseudomonas aeruginosa* exoenzyme expression by subinhibitory antibiotic concentrations, *Antimicrob. Agents Chemother.* **33**:41–47.
54. Flynn, J. L., and Ohman, D. E., 1988, Cloning of genes from mucoid *Pseudomonas aeruginosa* which control spontaneous conversion to the alginate production phenotype, *J. Bacteriol.* **170**:1452–1460.
55. Grothues, D., Koopmann, U., von der Hardt, H., and Tummler, B., 1988, Genome fingerprinting of *Pseudomonas aeruginosa* indicates colonization of cystic fibrosis siblings with closely related strains, *J. Clin. Microbiol.* **26**:1973–1977.
56. Janda, J. M., Atang-Nomo, S., Bottone, E. J., and Desmond, E. P., 1980, Correlation of proteolytic activity of *Pseudomonas aeruginosa* with site of isolation, *J. Clin. Microbiol.* **12**:626–628.
57. Wretlind, B., and Pavlovskis, O. R., 1984, Genetic mapping and characterization of *Pseudomonas aeruginosa* mutants defective in the formation of extracellular proteins, *J. Bacteriol.* **158**:801–808.
58. Wretlind, B., Sjoberg, L., and Wadstrom, T., 1977, Protease-deficient mutants of *Pseudomonas aeruginosa*: Pleiotropic changes in activity of other extracellular enzymes, *J. Gen. Microbiol.* **103**:329–336.
59. Ohman, D. E., Cryz, S. J., and Iglewski, B. H., 1980, Isolation and characterization of a *Pseudomonas aeruginosa* PAO mutant that produces altered elastase, *J. Bacteriol.* **142**:836–842.
60. Goldberg, J. B., and Ohman, D. E., 1987, Activation of an elastase precursor by the *las*A gene product of *Pseudomonas aeruginosa*, *J. Bacteriol.* **169**:4532–4539.
61. Goldberg, J. B., and Ohman, D. E., 1987, Cloning and transcriptional regulation of the elastase *las*A gene in mucoid and nonmucoid *Pseudomonas aeruginosa*, *J. Bacteriol.* **169**:1349–1351.
62. Peters, J. E., and Galloway, D. R., 1990, Purification and characterization of an active fragment of the LasA protein from *Pseudomonas aeruginosa*: Enhancement of elastase activity, *J. Bacteriol.* **172**:2236–2240.
63. Yamamoto, S., Fukushima, J., Atsumi, Y., Takeuchi, H., Kawamoto, S., Okuda, K., and Morihara, K., 1988, Cloning and characterization of elastase structural gene from *Pseudomonas aeruginosa* IFO 3455, *Biochem. Biophys. Res. Commun.* **152**:1117–1122.
64. Schad, P. A., and Iglewski, B. H., 1988, Nucleotide sequence and expression in *Escherichia coli* of the *Pseudomonas aeruginosa las*A gene, *J. Bacteriol.* **170**:2784–2789.
65. Howe, T. R., Wretlind, B., and Iglewski, B. H., 1983, Comparison of two methods of genetic exchange in determination of the genetic locus of the structural gene for *Pseudomonas aeruginosa* elastase, *J. Bacteriol.* **156**:58–61.
66. Romling, U., Grothues, D., Bautsch, W., and Tummler, B., 1989, A physical genome map of *Pseudomonas aeruginosa* PAO, *EMBO J.* **8**:4081–4089.
67. Fecycz, I. T., and Campbell, J. N., 1985, Mechanisms of activation and secretion of a cell associated precursor of an exocellular protease of *Pseudomonas aeruginosa* 34362A, *Eur. J. Biochem.* **146**:35–42.
68. Jensen, S. E., Fecycz, I. T., Stemke, G. W., and Campbell, J. N., 1980, Demonstration of a cell associated, inactive precursor of an exocellular protease produced by *Pseudomonas aeruginosa*, *Can. J. Microbiol.* **26**:77–86.

9

Pseudomonas aeruginosa–Phagocytic Cell Interactions

DAVID P. SPEERT

1. INTRODUCTION

Phagocytic cells are critically important in defending against infection by extracellular pathogens. Their role in protecting against infections with *Pseudomonas aeruginosa* is demonstrated dramatically in patients whose neutrophil-mediated functions are compromised (by neutropenia, after thermal burns, and by congenital phagocytic dysfunction).[1] The interplay between *P. aeruginosa* and phagocytic cells is dynamic, and its outcome is determined by both bacterial and host-determined factors. Although neutrophils and macrophages are armed with an array of antibacterial products, *P. aeruginosa* can counter with an awesome array of cell-associated and secreted products capable of abrogating normal host defenses. The armed struggle that ensues when host meets pathogen may be waged with such intensity that host tissues are laid waste by the combined effects of toxins derived from both bacteria and phagocytic cells. This chapter provides an overview of the nature of this dynamic interaction.

DAVID P. SPEERT • Departments of Pediatrics and Microbiology and the Canadian Bacterial Diseases Network, University of British Columbia, and Division of Infectious and Immunological Diseases, British Columbia's Children's Hospital, Research Centre, Vancouver, British Columbia, Canada V5Z 4H4.

Pseudomonas aeruginosa as an Opportunistic Pathogen, edited by Mario Campa *et al.* Plenum Press, New York, 1993.

2. MECHANISMS OF PHAGOCYTOSIS

2.1. Professional Phagocytic Cells: In Defense against Infection

Although a wide range of cells have some phagocytic capacity, those that are well-suited to the task are referred to as professional phagocytes. These cells include both mononuclear phagocytes (monocytes and macrophages) and polymorphonuclear leucocytes (neutrophils or PMN).

2.1.1. Mononuclear Phagocytes

The mononuclear phagocytic system consists of both circulating monocytes and fixed or adherent macrophages. Macrophages appear to be derived from monocytes and their phenotypic characteristics may be determined in part by the local conditions in the tissues where they come to reside.[2] Macrophages are found fixed in tissues (such as the Kupffer cells of the liver) and loosely attached to surfaces (such as in the pulmonary alveoli). They are widely distributed throughout the body, and in the mouse are found in highest concentration in the liver, large and small bowel, bone marrow, spleen, lymph nodes, and kidneys.[3] These fixed-tissue macrophages may function to clear the blood of circulating bacteria.[4] Pulmonary alveolar macrophages appear to serve as the first line of defense against inhaled microorganisms[5] and as such may have to perform their phagocytic role unaided by opsonizing antibody and complement. These cells appear to be of critical importance in defense of the lung against infection by *P. aeruginosa*.

2.1.2. Polymorphonuclear Leukocytes

Neutrophils are the principal phagocytic cell in the circulation and are critical in defense against invasive bacterial pathogens. They serve as the antibacterial "foot soldiers" and are recruited to sites of extravascular infection when the first line of defense (the mononuclear phagocytes) are overwhelmed. *P. aeruginosa* is killed more efficiently by human neutrophils than by peripheral monocytes; this difference may be due to more efficient bacterial phagocytosis by PMN.[6,7] PMN also appear to play a critically important role in clearance of *P. aeruginosa* from the lungs of experimentally infected animals.[8] The central role of neutrophils in defense against *Pseudomonas* infections is illustrated in patients who lack this line of defense, as a result of malignancy, ablative chemotherapy, or congenital deficiency.

2.2. The Process of Phagocytosis

Phagocytosis is a dynamic process whereby a foreign particle is bound by specific phagocytic receptors, ingested with the aid of contiguous receptors and killed by oxidative and/or nonoxidative mechanisms.[9,10] Recent studies have suggested that the fate of an ingested particle is determined, in part, by the receptor mediating its phagocytosis. For instance, ligation of receptors that recognize the Fc portion of IgG triggers a respiratory burst with generation of reactive oxygen radicals. On the other hand, particles that are coated with the iC3b complement breakdown product bind to macrophage complement receptor 3, but are neither internalized nor do they trigger a respiratory burst unless the macrophage is activated.[11,12]

For ingestion to occur, a particle must be covered circumferentially with phagocytosis-promoting ligands. This observation has given rise to the "zipper hypothesis" of phagocytosis, which describes a process of sequential ligation of phagocytic receptors, leading to envelopment of the particle within a membrane-bound phagosome.[13,14] If the phagocytosis-promoting ligand is present on only one pole of the particle, binding without ingestion will occur.

The various receptors that may play a role in the phagocytosis of *P. aeruginosa* and the complementary ligands they recognize are listed in Table I. Details on the different phagocytic receptors and other aspects of the phagocytic process can be found in a recent review.[10]

2.3. Opsonic and Nonopsonic Phagocytosis

Phagocytosis of bacteria is greatly enhanced in the presence of specific serum opsonins. The process of opsonic phagocytosis enables a wide array of foreign particles to be ingested by a limited number of macrophage and neutrophil phagocytic receptors. In addition to the "conventional" opsonins (immunoglobulin and complement), other serum proteins and glycoproteins may bind directly to certain gram-negative bacteria and enhance their phagocytosis. Opsonins that may enhance the phagocytosis of *P. aeruginosa* are discussed in section 3.1.

TABLE I
Human Phagocytic Receptors

Receptor	Ligand
Fc-gamma receptors	IgG1–4
Fc-alpha receptor	IgA
Complement receptor 1	C3b
Complement receptor 3	iC3b
C1q receptor	Mannose-binding protein
	Lung surfactant protein A
CD14	LPS-binding protein
Mannosyl/fucosyl receptor	Mannose residues
Adhesion-promoting receptors (CD18)	Bacterial LPS

A great number of bacterial species, parasites and fungi are also ingested by neutrophils and/or macrophages in the absence of opsonins. This process of nonopsonic phagocytosis may be of critical importance in antibacterial defense of the nonimmune host at sites such as the endobronchial space which normally has low levels of opsonizing antibody and complement. Macrophages appear to be well-suited for opsonin-independent phagocytosis, and receptors mediating these processes have been characterized recently.[15,16]

3. PHAGOCYTOSIS OF *PSEUDOMONAS AERUGINOSA*

3.1. Opsonic Phagocytosis

Serum opsonins play a central role in enhancing both phagocytosis and killing of pyogenic extracellular bacterial pathogens.[9,17] Some of the most efficient and virulent pathogens are those that resist phagocytosis except in the presence of specific opsonizing antibody. Phagocytosis of *P. aeruginosa* is enhanced substantially in the presence of serum factors, including IgG, complement, and fibronectin.

3.1.1. Complement

The importance of complement in phagocytosis of *P. aeruginosa* has been demonstrated clearly *in vitro* and *in vivo*. Phagocytosis by human neutrophils is enhanced markedly by the first four components of complement.[18] Opsonic forms of complement component C3 are deposited on the bacterial surface via the classical or alternative pathway of activation.[19,20] Complement is particularly important in enhancing phagocytosis of *P. aeruginosa* in the absence of specific opsonizing antibody.[21,22]

Complement also plays an important role in aiding clearance of *P. aeruginosa* from the lung, functioning as both opsonin and chemotaxin. This role of complement has been demonstrated clearly in animals that are either congenitally complement-deficient or depleted of complement by treatment with cobra venom factor.[23–26]

Complement also contributes to defense against *P. aeruginosa* infection by directly mediating bacterial lysis. Most strains of *Pseudomonas* from patients with invasive infection and bacteremia are resistant to the bactericidal effect of serum complement. However, strains from patients with cystic fibrosis (CF) are serum-sensitive by virtue of their rough lipopolysaccharide (LPS).[27] These LPS-rough strains may be killed by human serum via activation of the alternative pathway of complement in an antibody-independent fashion.[28] Both serum-sensitive and serum-resistant strains of *P. aeruginosa* are able to activate complement and consume components, including C9;

however, sensitivity to serum appears to depend upon the capacity for complement to be deposited into the bacterial membrane in a stable position.[29]

3.1.2. Immunoglobulin

Phagocytosis of *P. aeruginosa* by both neutrophils and macrophages is enhanced substantially in the presence of specific opsonizing antibody.[18,30–34] Mucoid strains from patients with CF require higher titers of specific antibody for neutrophil-mediated killing than do isogeneic nonmucoid variants. All immunoglobulin isotypes appear to have opsonic capacity, but IgG is the most effective. IgM is opsonic by enhancing deposition of complement components; phagocytic receptors for this immunoglobulin isotype have not been demonstrated. Both IgG and IgA are found in immune bronchial secretions, but IgG is far more efficient as an opsonin for phagocytosis by macrophages.[32–34] Although both complement and immunoglobulins each can opsonize many strains of *P. aeruginosa* independently, they function optimally in concert with one another.[21]

3.1.3. Fibronectin

Phagocytosis of *P. aeruginosa* may also be influenced by the presence of fibronectin. This glycoprotein has been shown to enhance macrophage phagocytosis of *Pseudomonas*[35] by direct action on the macrophage, rather than as a conventional opsonin[36] in a manner analogous to that seen with complement receptors. In the presence of fibronectin, macrophage complement receptors are able to ingest complement-coated particles; in its absence, the particles are simply bound to the phagocytic membrane.[12] The presence of fibronectin does not influence neutrophil phagocytosis of *P. aeruginosa*.[37]

3.2. Nonopsonic Phagocytosis

Macrophages appear well-equipped to phagocytose certain strains of *P. aeruginosa* in the absence of serum. Normal bronchopulmonary secretions lack the rich panoply of opsonins available in the blood. Therefore, the phenomenon of nonopsonic phagocytosis may be an important aspect of host defense of the lung early in the course of respiratory tract contamination/infection, prior to the evolution of the inflammatory response and before the influx of neutrophils and serum proteins. The pulmonary alveolar macrophage must be able to dispatch invading pathogens unaided by serum levels of complement, immunoglobulin, and other less well-defined circulating opsonins. Furthermore, many strains of *P. aeruginosa* from patients with CF are susceptible to the bactericidal effect of serum.[27] Opsonin-dependent phagocytosis of these strains is difficult to evaluate, because the concentrations of fresh serum necessary for opsonization are also bactericidal. The process of nonopsonic phagocytosis is complex, and is influenced by a wide array of bacterial and phagocytic physical and chemical properties.

3.2.1. Bacterial Factors

Only certain strains of *P. aeruginosa* are susceptible to nonopsonic phagocytosis, a phenomenon depending in part upon bacterial surface characteristics.[38,39] Susceptibility of different strains to nonopsonic phagocytosis is correlated with their partitioning characteristics in a two-phase system of dextran and polyethylene glycol (PEG); those strains that segregate preferentially to the PEG phase are phagocytosed with greatest avidity by both neutrophils and macrophages.[40,41] The partitioning characteristics of these strains appear to be determined in part by their degree of piliation.[40] Furthermore, piliated phagocytosis-susceptible strains become resistant to ingestion by neutrophils and macrophages if they are rendered pili-deficient with heat, UV irradiation, or by growth in shaken broth.[40]

3.2.2. Phagocytic receptors

Receptors mediating opsonin-independent phagocytosis of *P. aeruginosa* have been characterized functionally using human monocyte-derived macrophages.[16] These receptors have most of the characteristics of the mannosyl/fucosyl receptor, but their function is blocked most effectively by antibodies directed at the common β chain of the integrin family of macrophage adhesion-promoting receptors (LFA-1, Mac1, p150,95). The specific biochemical identity of this nonopsonic receptor is under investigation.

4. PHAGOCYTIC KILLING OF *PSEUDOMONAS AERUGINOSA*

4.1. Bactericidal Mechanisms of Phagocytic Cells

Phagocytes are capable of killing ingested bacteria by both oxidative and nonoxidative mechanisms. Neutrophil bactericidal capacity exceeds that of the unactivated macrophage, a fact that derives in part from the superior capacity of the former to generate reactive oxygen radicals. Most of current knowledge about phagocytic bactericidal function is derived from studies with neutrophils. Nonetheless, with a few exceptions, observations from PMN can be extrapolated to macrophages.

4.1.1. Oxidative Microbicidal Mechanisms

Upon stimulation by either soluble or particulate factors, phagocytic cells produce an array of reactive oxygen radicals with the capacity to kill ingested microbes.[42,43] Oxygen is consumed in a reaction involving the one electron reduction of oxygen to superoxide anion. Superoxide is further reduced by both myeloperoxidase-dependent and -independent mechanisms to generate oxidative radicals (hydrogen peroxide, hydroxyl radical, singlet oxygen, and hypochlorite anion) with potent antibacterial activity. The role of these reactive oxygen radicals in killing specific species of bacteria can be deduced from studies performed under anaerobic conditions[44] and with phagocytes from patients with chronic granulomatous disease, whose cells lack the ability to generate reactive oxygen radicals.[43]

4.1.2. Nonoxidative Microbicidal Mechanisms

Neutrophils and macrophages are well-equipped to kill ingested microbes via mechanisms independent of oxidative metabolism. Several different proteins with antimicrobial activity are packaged within phagocytic lysosomes and are delivered to the site of ingested bacteria upon phagosome–lysosome fusion. These natural phagocyte-derived antibiotics (including defensins, cathepsin G, bactericidal permeability-inducing protein, myeloperoxidase, lysozyme, and lactoferrin) are discussed in detail in recent review articles.[42,45–47]

4.2. Mechanism of *Pseudomonas aeruginosa* Killing

Data on the killing of *P. aeruginosa* are derived predominantly from studies with human neutrophils. Nonoxidative mechanisms appear to play an important role in the bactericidal process. This conclusion is based upon the following evidence: (1) *P. aeruginosa* is killed by purified bactericidal proteins from neutrophils;[48] (2) macrophage cationic proteins increase the permeability of the *P. aeruginosa* outer membrane;[49] (3) neutrophils are able to kill *P. aeruginosa* under anaerobic conditions after nitrogen washout;[44] and (4) *P. aeruginosa* rarely causes infections in patients with chronic granulomatous disease, although *Pseudomonas cepacia* is emerging as an important pathogen.[50] These studies establish a role for nonoxidative mechanisms in killing *P. aeruginosa* but do not demonstrate whether or not oxidative radicals are bactericidal. Further studies using cell-free or whole-cell bactericidal assays will be necessary to establish whether reactive oxygen radicals are potentially bactericidal for *P. aeruginosa*.

5. *PSEUDOMONAS AERUGINOSA* PRODUCTS WITH EFFECTS ON PHAGOCYTOSIS

P. aeruginosa is an opportunistic pathogen that rarely causes invasive infections, except in patients with defects in local or systemic immunity.

Immune functioning is further compromised by direct action of *Pseudomonas* and its products on phagocytic cells and other accessory elements in the phagocytic process. It is therefore difficult to draw conclusions about the specific role of bacterial or host factors in the profound pathology typical of acute and chronic *Pseudomonas* infections. Most conclusions regarding the effects of *P. aeruginosa* and its products on the phagocytic process are deduced therefore from *in vitro* studies (summarized in Table II).

5.1. Cytotoxins

Direct toxic effects of *P. aeruginosa* products on phagocytic cells have been described by several different groups of investigators and the toxins are termed variously leukocidin, cytotoxin, and neutrophil inhibitor. A leukocidin, purified from *P. aeruginosa* by autolysis, is a 27-kD protein with broad reactivity against leukocytes of different animal species.[51] It is lethal for mice when 1 μg is given intravenously. The toxin creates structural changes in neutrophils, characterized by rounding up with extrusion of protoplasmic blebs. Leukocytes intoxicated by this or related cytotoxins lose their mo-

TABLE II
Pseudomonas aeruginosa Products with Effects of Phagocytes and/or Phagocytosis

Pseudomonas product	Effect	Reference
Leukocidin	↓ motility	52
	↓ bactericidal effect	53
	↓ phagocytosis	54
Neutrophil inhibitor	↓ chemotaxis	50, 57
	↓ phagocytosis	50, 57
	↓ bactericidal effect	50, 57
Elastase	↓ chemotaxis	59
	↓ oxidative burst	59, 69
	Degradation complement	61
	Cleavage of IgG	62
	Cleavage of IgA	64
Exotoxin A	↓ macrophage phagocytosis	68
	Neutriphil cytotoxicity	69
Mucoid exopolysaccharide	↓ opsonic phagocytosis	20, 75
	↓ nonopsonic phagocytosis	38, 41, 76
	↓ chemotaxis	80
	Quenches reactive oxygen radicals	81, 82
Slime glycolipoprotein	Leukopenia	84
	↓ motility	86
	↓ phagocytosis	86
	Activates complement	87
Pyocyanine	↑ or ↓ superoxide anion production	90

tility,[52] develop impaired bactericidal capacity,[53] and lose their ability to phagocytose opsonized particles.[54] At higher concentrations, it lyses PMN.[53] The cytotoxin is located in the bacterial periplasmic space[54] and binds to neutrophils via an integral protein of the plasma membrane.[55] The binding site on rabbit PMN is a protein of 50 kD.[56]

Another substance, called neutrophil inhibitor, is a 65-kD protein that interferes with various neutrophil functions. It is purified from the supernatant of a strain of *P. aeruginosa*.[57] This toxin is distinct from elastase and protease and interferes with neutrophil chemotaxis and phagocytosis of latex. The inhibitor also interferes with the capacity of neutrophil extracts to kill *Escherichia coli*, but it does not inhibit release of lysosomal enzymes.[58]

5.2. Elastase

Both phagocytic cells and opsonins are affected adversely by the elastase elaborated by *P. aeruginosa*. Direct effects on phagocytic cell functioning include inhibition of neutrophil chemotaxis, superoxide production,[59] and myeloperoxidase-mediated chemiluminescence.[60] Opsonic phagocytosis is further impaired by elastase via enzymatic digestion of both complement and immunoglobulin. The enzyme can degrade cell-bound C1 and C3 as well as fluid-phase C5, C8, and C9.[61] When opsonized *P. aeruginosa* is exposed to elastase, phagocytosis is impaired, presumably by degradation of opsonic forms of C3.[61] Proteolytic activity capable of digesting opsonic IgG is found in the bronchial secretions of patients with CF. This may be due to the effects of neutrophil- and/or *P. aeruginosa*-derived enzymes. An elastase extracted from *P. aeruginosa* is capable of cleaving IgG subclasses 1 and 3, whereas subclasses 2 and 4 are relatively resistant.[62] Immunoglobulins with high titers against *P. aeruginosa* can be cleaved into Fcγ and $F(ab')_2$ fragments by *Pseudomonas*. These fragments inhibit phagocytosis of *P. aeruginosa*, and are actually *less* effective than normal saline in promoting phagocytosis by human neutrophils.[63] *P. aeruginosa* elastase is also capable of cleaving human IgA of subclasses 1 and 2, thereby rendering this aspect of host defense at mucosal surfaces ineffective.[64]

5.3. Exotoxin A

Exotoxin A (ETA) is an important virulence factor, considered by some authors to be the most toxic extracellular product of *P. aeruginosa*.[65] It exerts its toxic effects by inhibiting NAD-dependent protein synthesis.[66] Patients with cancer who have antibodies to ETA are relatively protected against fatal *Pseudomonas* infections.[67] This toxin compromises macrophage function; at concentrations as low as 10 ng/ml, phagocytosis is impaired.[68] It also has adverse effects on human neutrophils.[69] Although neutrophil phagocytic function is not impaired by ETA, ultrastructural changes are seen.

5.4. Mucoid Exopolysaccharide

Strains of *P. aeruginosa* isolated from patients with CF have a peculiar mucoid colonial morphology. This morphotype is due to the exuberant production of a mucoid exopolysaccharide (MEP), composed of mannuronic and guluronic acids with associated O-acetylation.[70] Production of MEP by these strains of *P. aeruginosa* likely provides the bacteria with some survival advantage within the CF lung.[71] These strains produce MEP *in vivo*, as evidenced by the presence of antibody in colonized CF patients[39,72,73] and as demonstrated by immunofluorescence studies of infected CF lungs from autopsy specimens.[74] MEP interferes with a number of phagocytic cell functions. Mucoid strains of *P. aeruginosa* are relatively resistant to both opsonic[30] and nonopsonic[38,41] phagocytosis. Purified MEP is antiphagocytic; it interferes with ingestion by rabbit and human neutrophils[75,76] and murine and rat macrophages.[77-79] MEP further impairs phagocytic cell function by interfering with chemotaxis[80] and by quenching reactive oxygen radicals with potential bactericidal activity.[81,82] This latter effect might not influence the survival of *P. aeruginosa*, which appears to be killed primarily by nonoxidative means.

5.5. Slime Glycolipoprotein

An extracellular slime glycolipoprotein can be extracted from non-mucoid strains of *P. aeruginosa*.[83] This material is distinct from lipopolysaccharide and is composed of polysaccharides, lipids and proteins. The extracted material exhibits many of the biological activities of intact *P. aeruginosa* when injected intraperitoneally into mice,[84] notably leukopenia and death. These toxic manifestations can be blocked by active or passive immunization. Substantial *in vitro* work has been done to provide explanations for these *in vivo* effects. The glycolipoprotein has been modified by chemical and enzymatic treatment to determine which component(s) determine its biological activities.[85] Removal of proteins does not alter the biological activities, but treatment with acetic acid to remove lipid, but not protein or carbohydrate, abrogates its capacity to produce leukopenia and death in mice.

Slime glycolipoprotein exerts adverse effects upon phagocyte–bacterial interactions in addition to the simple induction of leukopenia. It interferes with a variety of human neutrophil functions, including motility (both random and directed) and ingestion of *Saccharomyces cerevisiae*.[86] Interference with nitroblue tetrazolium dye reduction (a measure of the metabolic burst accompanying phagocytosis) is probably due to a decrease in the number of particles ingested rather than to a direct influence on oxidative metabolism.

This material also has effects upon opsonin-dependent phagocytosis. It activates complement via the alternative pathway.[87] This could enhance or interfere with phagocytosis, depending upon whether or not the slime is associated with the bacterial surface. If complement is activated at a distance from the bacterial surface, opsonically-active components of C3 would not be able to cross-ligate the bacteria to phagocytic membrane receptors. However, if the slime is surface-associated, it would serve as the site for deposition of opsonically active complement. Glycolipoprotein is able to stimulate the production of opsonically active antibody, which enhances macrophage phagocytosis of *P. aeruginosa*.[88] Phagocytosis is enhanced by this antiserum independent of the presence of complement.

5.6. Pyocyanine

Among the phenazine pigments produced by *P. aeruginosa*, pyocyanine exerts broad toxic effects on cells of the human immune system. Its inhibitory effects on lymphocyte blastogenesis have been well-described by Sorensen and coworkers.[89] In addition, it influences superoxide anion production by neutrophils.[90] The effect is dose-dependent, with inhibition at 50 μM concentration and enhancement at 1 μM. Because *P. aeruginosa* appears to be killed by nonoxidative means and reactive oxygen radicals can damage infected tissues, inhibition of superoxide production may be beneficial to the host. The enhanced superoxide production at low concentrations of phenazine pigment may, conversely, augment tissue destruction.

6. DISEASE STATES IN WHICH PHAGOCYTIC DYSFUNCTION MAY PREDISPOSE TO INFECTIONS WITH *PSEUDOMONAS AERUGINOSA*

6.1. Neutropenia

Neutrophils play a central role in host defense against invasive bacterial infection.[91,92] Nowhere is this fact more obvious than in patients who are neutropenic, particularly secondary to hematological malignancy or chemotherapy. It has been predicted that 138,000 cases of bacteremia due to Enterobacteriaciae and Pseudomonadaceae occur annually in the United States and that approximately 10% are due to *P. aeruginosa*.[72] These cases are predominantly nosocomial and associated with neutropenia. The mortality rate from these infections is higher than for other gram-negative infections (40–50%) and often unresponsive to early aggressive antimicrobial therapy.[72,93] Patients with leukemia constitute the largest group at risk for *P. aeruginosa* bacteremia.[94] This is probably due to the large numbers at risk, the frequency with which they are neutropenic, and their low levels of serum opsonic activity.[95]

6.2. Thermal Burns

Bacteremia and sepsis from *P. aeruginosa* are common among patients who have suffered extensive thermal injuries. In a large study over a 25-year period, approximately 10% of nearly 6,000 patients developed *P. aeruginosa* bacteremia; among those the mortality due to the infection was 28%.[96] This problem has increased in scope with the advent of improved methods for dealing with severely burned patients and the development of improved expanded-spectrum antibiotics. Various aspects of neutrophil function are deranged in patients with severe thermal burns; the best-documented abnormality is decreased neutrophil chemotaxis from these patients.[97,98] In a rat burn infection model, intraperitoneal inflammation after injection with heat-killed *P. aeruginosa* was diminished, as was the number of marginating neutrophils and adherence of neutrophils to nylon wool.[99] Serum from burned rats impaired the adherence and chemotaxis of neutrophils from normal unburned rats.

6.3. Cystic Fibrosis

Patients with CF are at greatly enhanced risk of infection with *P. aeruginosa*. The infection is rarely invasive and is generally confined to the endobronchial spaces until late in the course of disease. This is in marked contrast with neutropenic and burned patients in whom invasive and bacteremic infections are the rule. A phagocytic cellular defect has been proposed to explain the peculiar predisposition of CF patients to infection with *P. aeruginosa*, but none has been demonstrated (reviewed in 71). Nonetheless, compromised *in vitro* phagocytosis due to alterations in receptor and opsonic function has been documented using CF leukocytes and serum. These observations are described briefly here.

6.3.1. Fragmented Immunoglobulins

Biggar *et al.*[100] demonstrated that serum from patients with CF inhibited macrophage phagocytosis of *P. aeruginosa*. An explanation for this phenomenon was provided by Fick and co-workers[101,102] who demonstrated that the specific anti-*Pseudomonas* immunoglobulin from serum and bronchial secretions of patients with CF is anti-phagocytic by virtue of fragmentation into Fab and Fc components. Although the Fab fragment can bind to the bacterial surface, it lacks the Fc domain for ligation of macrophage phagocytic receptors.

6.3.2. Nonopsonic Antibody

Most older patients with CF have high titers of antibody to the major *Pseudomonas* cellular and extracellular products (reviewed in 71). Nonetheless, these patients are unable to eradicate colonization/infection, suggesting that the humoral immunity is in some way dysfunctional. Pier et al.[73] demonstrated that older *noncolonized* CF patients have antibody to the MEP of mucoid *P. aeruginosa*, which is able to opsonize the bacteria for killing by normal neutrophils. Although older *colonized* patients also have high titers of opsonophagocytic killing antibody, it is directed at epitopes other than the MEP. These authors speculate that some patients remain uncolonized because their opsonic antibody repertoire is functional in enhancing clearance of *P. aeruginosa* from the respiratory tract.

These observations have been extended by Eichler et al..[103] They found that patients with CF who are colonized with *P. aeruginosa* have nonopsonic antibody directed against *Pseudomonas* lipopolysaccharide. When this antibody is removed from their serum by adsorption, the opsonic activity increases. These observations were explained on the basis of the immunoglobulin isotype composition of the CF serum; certain isotypes are more effective than others in opsonizing *P. aeruginosa* for phagocytosis by PMN.

6.3.3. Immunoglobulin Subclass Distribution

Other investigators have examined the IgG subclass distribution in CF serum to try to explain its anti-opsonic activity. Although these sera have high titers of antibody to *P. aeruginosa* lipopolysaccharide, with elevation of IgG2, levels of IgG1 are depressed.[104,105] This alteration from the norm in subclass distribution might provide a partial explanation for the opsonic incompetence of CF serum. Since pulmonary alveolar macrophages have Fcγ receptors for IgG1 and IgG3, opsonization with serum deficient in these subclasses could result in receptor–ligand mismatch and suboptimal phagocytosis. Furthermore, the high levels of IgG2 in CF serum promotes the formation of immune complexes, which are also antiphagocytic.[106]

6.3.4. Proteolytic Activity in Bronchial Secretions

Free granulocyte elastase is found in the bronchial secretions of CF patients who are infected with *P. aeruginosa*.[107,108] This protease has the ability to cleave a wide range of proteins, including C3,[109] thereby interfering with phagocytosis and clearance of *P. aeruginosa* from infected bronchial secretions of CF patients. The levels of granulocyte elastase are correlated with the severity of pulmonary pathology in CF, providing some evidence for its role in pathogenesis of respiratory disease.[107]

6.3.5. Phagocytic Receptor Expression

Complement receptors play an important role in the phagocytosis of opsonized *P. aeruginosa*. Peripheral blood PMN from patients with CF have normal expression and up-regulation of these complement receptors, but neutrophils from CF bronchial secretions have markedly depressed expression of complement receptor 1 (that recognizes C3b).[110] These observations have been explained by *in vitro* studies demonstrating that complement receptor 1 but not 3 is cleaved from normal PMN by PMN elastase. Furthermore, complement component iC3b (recognized by complement receptor 3) is cleaved from opsonized *P. aeruginosa* by either *Pseudomonas* or PMN elastase.[111] Cleavage of both receptor (complement receptor 1) and ligand (iC3b) by bacterial and host elastases establishes a receptor–ligand mismatch and interferes with phagocytosis, superoxide production, and bactericidal activity of the neutrophils. This provides another possible explanation for the persistence of *P. aeruginosa* in the CF lung and the inability of normal host defenses to dispense with this intransigent parasite.

REFERENCES

1. Bodey, G. P., Bolivar, R., Fainstein, V., and Jadeja, L., 1983, Infections caused by *Pseudomonas aeruginosa*, *Rev. Infect. Dis.* **5:**279–313.
2. Gordon, S., Perry, V. H., Rabinowitz, S., Chung, L., and Rosen, H., 1988, Plasma membrane receptors of the mononuclear phagocyte system, *J. Cell Sci. Suppl.* **39:**31–36.
3. Lee, S.-H., Starkey, P. M., and Gordon, S., 1985, Quantitative analysis of total macrophage content in adult mouse tissues: Immunochemical studies with monoclonal antibody F4/80, *J. Exp. Med.* **161:**475–489.
4. Frank, M. M., 1989, The role of macrophages in blood stream clearance, in: *Human Monocytes*, (M. Zembala, and G. L. Asherson, eds.), Academic Press, London, pp. 337–344.
5. Fels, A. O. S., and Cohn, Z. A., 1986, The alveolar macrophage, *J. Appl. Physiol.* **60:**353–369.
6. Peterson, P. K., Verhoef, J., Schmeling, D., and Quie, P. G., 1977, Kinetics of phagocytosis and bacterial killing by human polymorphonuclear leukocytes and monocytes, *J. Infect. Dis.* **136:**502–509.
7. Steigbigel, R. T., Lambert, L. H., Jr., and Remington, J. S., 1974, Phagocytic and bactericidal properties of normal human monocytes, *J. Clin. Invest.* **53:**131–142.
8. Rehm, S. R., Gross, G. N., and Pierce, A. K., 1980, Early bacterial clearance from murine lungs: Species-dependent phagocyte response, *J. Clin. Invest.* **66:**194–199.
9. Horwitz, M. A., 1982, Phagocytosis of microorganisms, *Rev. Infect. Dis.* **4:**104–123.
10. Silverstein, S. C., Greenberg, S., Di Virgilio, F., and Steinberg, T. H., 1989, Phagocytosis, in: *Fundamental Immunology* (W. E., Paul, ed.), Raven Press, New York, pp. 703–720.
11. Bianco, C., Griffin, F. M., Jr., and Silverstein, S. C., 1975, Studies of the macrophage complement receptor: Alteration of receptor function upon macrophage activation, *J. Exp. Med.* **141:**1278–1290.
12. Wright, S. D., and Silverstein, S. C., 1982, Tumor-promoting phorbol esters stimulate C3b and C3b' receptor-mediated phagocytosis in cultured human monocytes, *J. Exp. Med.* **156:**1149–1164.
13. Griffin, F. M., Jr., Griffin, J. A., Leider, J. E., and Silverstein, S. C., 1975, Studies on the mechanism of phagocytosis. I. Requirements for circumferential attachment of particle-bound ligands to specific receptors on the macrophage plasma membrane, *J. Exp. Med.* **142:**1263–1282.
14. Griffin, F. M., Jr., Griffin, J. A., and Silverstein, S. C., 1976, Studies on the mechanism of

phagocytosis. II. The interaction of macrophages with anti-immunoglobulin IgG-coated bone marrow derived lymphocytes, *J. Exp. Med.* **144:**788–809.
15. Wright, S. D., and Jong, M. T. C., 1986, Adhesion-promoting receptors on human macrophages recognize *Escherichia coli* by binding to lipolysaccharide, *J. Exp. Med.* **164:**1876–1888.
16. Speert, D. P., Wright, S. D., Silverstein, S. C., and Mah, B., 1988, Functional characterization of human macrophage receptors for *in vitro* phagocytosis of unopsonized *Pseudomonas aeruginosa*, *J. Clin. Invest.* **82:**872–879.
17. Leijh, P. C. J., van den Barselaar, M. T., van Zwet, L., Daha, M. R., and van Furth, R., 1979, Requirement of extracellular complement and immunoglobulin for intracellular killing of microorganisms by human monocytes, *J. Clin. Invest.* **63:**772–784.
18. Young, L. S., and Armstrong, D., 1972, Human immunity to *Pseudomonas aeruginosa*: I. *In vitro* interaction of bacteria, polymorphonuclear leukocytes, and serum factors, *J. Infect. Dis.* **126:**257–276.
19. Bjornson, A. B., and Michael, J. G., 1974, Factors in human serum promoting phagocytosis of *Pseudomonas aeruginosa*. I. Interaction of opsonins with the bacterium, *J. Infect. Dis.* **130:**S119–S126.
20. Baltimore, R. S., and Shedd, D. G., 1983, The role of complement in the opsonization of mucoid and non-mucoid strains of *Pseudomonas aeruginosa*, *Pediatr. Res.* **17:**952–958.
21. Peterson, P. K., Kim, Y., Schmeling, D., Lindemann, M., Verhoef, J., and Quie, P. G., 1978, Complement-mediated phagocytosis of *Pseudomonas aeruginosa*, *J. Lab. Clin. Med.* **92:**883–894.
22. Murphey, S. A., Root, R. K., and Schreiber, A. D., 1979, The role of antibody and complement in phagocytosis by rabbit alveolar macrophages, *J. Infect. Dis.* **140:**896–903.
23. Cerquetti, M. C., Sordelli, D. O., Bellanti, J. A., and Hooke, A. M., 1986, Lung defenses against *Pseudomonas aeruginosa* in C5-deficient mice with different genetic backgrounds, *Infect. Immun.* **52:**853–857.
24. Gross, G. N., Rehm, S. R., and Pierce, A. K., 1978, The effect of complement depletion on lung clearance of bacteria, *J. Clin. Invest.* **62:**373–378.
25. Heidbrink. P. J., Toews, G. B., Gross, G. N., and Pierce, A. K., 1982, Mechanisms of complement-mediated clearance of bacteria from the murine lung, *Am. Rev. Respir. Dis.* **125:**517–520.
26. Larsen, G. L., Mitchell, B. C., Harper, T. B., and Henson, P. M., 1982, The pulmonary response of C5 sufficient and deficient mice to *Pseudomonas aeruginosa*, *Am. Rev. Respir. Dis.* **126:**306–311.
27. Hancock, R. E., Mutharia, L. M., Chan, L., Darveau, R. P., Speert, D. P., and Pier, G. B., 1983, *Pseudomonas aeruginosa* isolates from patients with cystic fibrosis: A class of serum-sensitive, nontypable strains deficient in lipopolysaccharide O side chains, *Infect. Immun.* **42:**3170–3177.
28. Pier, G. B., and Ames, P., 1984, Mediation of the killing of rough, mucoid isolates of *Pseudomonas aeruginosa* from patients with cystic fibrosis by the alternative pathway of complement, *J. Infect. Dis.* **150:**223–228.
29. Schiller, N. L., and Joiner, K. A., 1986, Interaction of complement with serum-sensitive and serum-resistant strains of *Pseudomonas aeruginosa*, *Infect. Immun.* **54:**689–694.
30. Baltimore, R. S., and Mitchell, M., 1980, Immunologic investigations of mucoid strains of *Pseudomonas aeruginosa*: Comparison of susceptibility to opsonic antibody in mucoid and nonmucoid strains, *J. Infect. Dis.* **141:**238–247.
31. Bjornson, A. B., and Michael, J. G., 1970, Biological activities of rabbit immunoglobulin M and immunoglobulin G antibodies to *Pseudomonas aeruginosa*, *Infect. Immun.* **2:**453–461.
32. Reynolds, H. Y., 1974, Pulmonary host defenses in rabbits after immunization with *Pseudomonas* antigens: The Interaction of bacteria, antibodies, macrophages, and lymphocytes, *J. Infect. Dis.* **130:**S134–S142.
33. Reynolds, H. Y., and Thompson, R. E., 1973, Pulmonary host defenses: II. Interaction of

Respiratory antibodies with *Pseudomonas aeruginosa* and alveolar macrophages, *J. Immunol.* **111**:369–380.
34. Reynolds, H. Y., Kazmierowski, J. A., and Newball, H. H., 1975, Specificity of opsonic antibodies to enhance phagocytosis of *Pseudomonas aeruginosa* by human alveolar macrophages, *J. Clin. Invest.* **56**:376–385.
35. Kluftinger, J. L., Kelly, N. M., Jost, B. H., and Hancock, R. E. W., 1989, Fibronectin as an enhancer of nonopsonic phagocytosis of *Pseudomonas aeruginosa* by macrophages, *Infect. Immun.* **57**:2782–2785.
36. Kluftinger, J. L., Kelly, N. M., and Hancock, R. E. W., 1989, Stimulation by fibronectin of macrophage-mediated phagocytosis of *Pseudomonas aeruginosa*, *Infect. Immun.* **57**:817–822.
37. Boulanger, M. J., Smith, R. P., Baltch, A. L., Blumenstock, F. A., and Saba, T. M., 1985, Human plasma fibronectin effect on serum-mediated uptake of *Pseudomonas aeruginosa* PA 1348A by human graulocytes, *Complement* **2**:230–234.
38. Krieg, D. P., Helmke, R. J., German, V. F., and Mangos, J. A., 1988, Resistance of mucoid *Pseudomonas aeruginosa* to nonopsonic phagocytosis by alveolar macrophages *in vitro*, *Infect. Immun.* **56**:3173–3179.
39. Speert, D. P., Eftekhar, F., and Puterman, M. L., 1984, Nonopsonic phagocytosis of strains of *Pseudomonas aeruginosa* from cystic fibrosis patients, *Infect. Immun.* **43**:1006–1011.
40. Speert, D. P., Loh, B. A., Cabral, D. A., and Salit, I. E., 1986, Nonopsonic phagocytosis of nonmucoid *Pseudomonas aeruginosa* by human neutrophils and monocyte-derived macrophages is correlated with bacterial piliation and hydrophobicity, *Infect. Immun.* **53**:207–212.
41. Cabral, D. A., Loh, B. A., and Speert, D. P., 1987, Mucoid *Pseudomonas aeruginosa* resists nonopsonic phagocytosis by human neutrophils and macrophages, *Pediatr. Res.* **22**:429–431.
42. Andrew, P. W., Jackett, P. S., and Lowrie, D. B., 1985, Killing and degradation of microorganisms by macrophages, in: *Mononuclear Phagocytes: Physiology and Pathology* (R. T. Dean, and W. Jessup, eds.), Elsevier, New York, pp. 311–325.
43. Curnutte, J. T., and Babior, B. M., 1987, Chronic granulomatous disease, *Adv. Hum. Genet.* **16**:229–295.
44. Mandell, G. L., 1974, Bactericidal activity of aerobic and anaerobic polymorphonuclear neutrophils, *Infect. Immun.* **9**:337–341.
45. Ganz, T. Selsted, M. E., and Lehrer, R. I., 1986, Antimicrobial activity of phagocyte granule proteins, *Semin. Resp. Infect.* **1**:107–117.
46. Spitznagel, J. K., and Shafer, W. M., 1985, Neutrophil killing of bacteria by oxygen-independent mechanisms: A historical summary, *Rev. Infect. Dis.* **7**:398–402.
47. Spitznagel, J. K., 1990, Antibiotic proteins of human neutrophils, *J. Clin. Invest.* **86**:1381–1386.
48. Hovde, C. J., and Gray, B. H., 1986, Physiological effects of a bactericidal protein from human polymorphonuclear leukocytes on *Pseudomonas aeruginosa*, *Infect. Immun.* **52**:90–95.
49. Sawyer, J. G., Martin, N. L., and Hancock, R. E. W., 1988, Interaction of macrophage cationic proteins with the outer membrane of *Pseudomonas aeruginosa*, *Infect. Immun.* **56**:693–698.
50. O'Neill, K. M., Herman, J. H., Modlin, J. F., Moxon, E. R., and Winkelstein, J. A., 1986, *Pseudomonas cepacia*: An emerging pathogen in chronic granulomatous disease, *J. Pediatr.* **108**:940–942.
51. Scharmann, W., 1976, Purification and characterization of leukocidin from *Pseudomonas aeruginosa*, *J. Gen. Microbiol.* **93**:292–302.
52. Scharmann, W., Jacob, F., and Postendörfer, J., 1976, Cytotoxic action of leucocidin from *Pseudomonas aeruginosa* on human polymorphonuclear leukocytes, *J. Gen. Microbiol.* **93**:303–308.
53. Baltch, A. L., Hammer, M. C., Smith, R. P., Obrig, T. G., Conroy, J. V., Bishop, M. B., Egy,

M. A., and Lutz, F., 1985, Effects of *Pseudomonas aeruginosa* cytotoxin on human serum and granulocytes and their microbicidal, phagocytic, and chemotactic functions, *Infect. Immun.* **48:**498–506.
54. Kluftinger, J. L., Lutz, F., and Hancock, R. E. W., 1989, *Pseudomonas aeruginosa* cytotoxin: Periplasmic localization and inhibition of macrophages, *Infect. Immun.* **57:**882–886.
55. Scharmann, W., 1976, Interaction of purified leucocidin from *Pseudomonas aeruginosa* with bovine polymorphonuclear leukocytes, *Infect. Immun.* **13:**1046–1053.
56. Hirayama, T. Noda, M., Matsuda, F., Nagamori, M., and Kato, I., 1984, Binding of Pseudomonal leukocidin to rabbit polymorphonuclear leukocytes, *Infect. Immun.* **46:**631–634.
57. Nonoyama, S., Kojo, H., Mine, Y., Nishida, M., Goto, S., and Kuwahara, S., 1979, Inhibitory effect of *Pseudomonas aeruginosa* on the phagocytic and killing activities of rabbit polymorphonuclear leukocytes: Purification and characterization of an inhibitor of polymorphonuclear leukocyte function, *Infect. Immun.* **24:**394–398.
58. Nonoyama, S., Kojo, H., Mine, Y., Nishida, M., Goto, S., and Kuwahara, S., 1979, Inhibitory effect of *Pseudomonas aeruginosa* on the phagocytic and killing activity of rabbit polymorphonuclear leukocytes: Mechanisms of action of a polymorphonuclear leukocyte inhibitor, *Infect. Immun.* **24:**399–403.
59. Kharazmi, A., Döring, G., Høiby, N., and Valerius, N. H., 1984, Interaction of *Pseudomonas aeruginosa* alkaline protease and elastase with human polymorphonuclear leukocytes *in vitro*, *Infect. Immun.* **43:**161–165.
60. Kharazmi, A., Høiby, N., Döring, G., and Valerius, N. H., 1984, *Pseudomonas aeruginosa* exoproteases inhibit human neutrophil chemiluminescence, *Infect. Immun.* **44:**587–591.
61. Schultz, D. R., and Miller, K. D., 1974, Elastase of *Pseudomonas aeruginosa*: Inactivation of complement components and complement-derived chemotactic and phagocytic factors, *Infect. Immun.* **10:**128–135.
62. Fick, R. B., Jr., Baltimore, R. S., Squier, S. U., and Reynolds, H. Y., 1985, IgG proteolytic activity of *Pseudomonas aeruginosa* in cystic fibrosis, *J. Infect. Dis.* **151:**589–598.
63. Bainbridge, T., and Fick, R. B., Jr., 1989, Functional importance of cystic fibrosis immunoglobulin G fragments generated by *Pseudomonas aeruginosa* elastase, *J. Lab. Clin. Med.* **114:** 728–733.
64. Heck, L. W., Alarcon, P. G., Kulhavy, R. M., Morihara, K., Russell, M. W., and Mestecky, J. F., 1990, Degradation of IgA proteins by *Pseudomonas aeruginosa* elastase, *J. Immunol.* **144:** 2253–2257.
65. Woods, D. E., and Iglewski, B. H., 1983, Toxins of *Pseudomonas aeruginosa*: New perspectives, *Rev. Infect. Dis.* **5:**S715–S722.
66. Iglewski, B. H., and Kabat, D., 1975, NAS-dependent inhibition of protein synthesis by *Pseudomonas aeruginosa* toxin, *Proc. Nat. Acad. Sci. USA* **72:**2284–2288.
67. Pollack, M., and Young, L. S., 1979, Protective activity of antibodies to exotoxin A and lipopolysaccharide at the onset of *Pseudomonas aeruginosa* septicemia in man, *J. Clin. Invest.* **63:**276–286.
68. Pollack, M., and Anderson, S. E., Jr., 1978, Toxicity of *Pseudomonas aeruginosa* exotoxin A for human macrophages, *Infect. Immun.* **19:**1092–1096.
69. Bishop, M. B., Baltch, A. L., Hill, L. A., Smith, R. P., Lutz, F., and Pollack, M., 1987, The effect of *Pseudomonas aeruginosa* cytotoxin and toxin A on human polymorphonuclear leukocytes, *J. Med Microbiol.* **24:**315–324.
70. Evans, L. R., and Linker, A., 1973, Production and characterization of the slime polysaccharide of *Pseudomonas aeruginosa*, *J. Bacteriol.* **116:**915–924.
71. Speert, D. P., 1985, Host defenses in patients with cystic fibrosis: Modulation by *Pseudomonas aeruginosa*, *Surv. Synth. Path. Res.* **4:**14–33.
72. Bryan, C. S., Reynolds, K. L., and Brenner, E. R., 1983, Analysis of 1,186 episodes of gram-negative bacteremia in non-university hospitals: The effects of antimicrobial therapy, *Rev. Infect. Dis.* **5:**629–638.

73. Pier, G. B., Saunders, J. M., Ames, P., Edwards, M. S., Auerbach, H., Goldfarb, J., Speert, D. P., and Hurwitch, S., 1987, Opsonophagocytic killing antibody to *Pseudomonas aeruginosa* mucoid exopolysaccharide in older noncolonized patients with cystic fibrosis, *N. Engl. J. Med.* **317:**793–798.
74. Speert, D. P., Dimmick, J. E., Pier, G. B., Saunders, J. M., Hancock, R. E. W., and Kelly, N., 1987, An immunohistological evaluation of *Pseudomonas aeruginosa* pulmonary infection in two patients with cystic fibrosis, *Pediatr. Res.* **22:**743–747.
75. Schwarzmann, S., and Boring, J. R., III, 1971, Antiphagocytic effect of slime from a mucoid strain of *Pseudomonas aeruginosa*, *Infect. Immun.* **3:**762–767.
76. Bayer, A. S., Speert, D. P., Park, S., Tu, J., Witt, M., Nast, C. C., and Norman, D. C., 1991, Functional role of mucoid exopolysaccharide (alginate) upon antibiotic-induced and polymorphonuclear leukocyte-mediated killing of *Pseudomonas aeruginosa*, *Infect. Immun.* **59:**302–308.
77. Oliver, A. M., and Weir, D. M., 1983, Inhibition of bacterial binding to mouse macrophages by *Pseudomonas* alginate, *Clin. Lab. Immunol.* **10:**221–224.
78. Oliver, A. M., and Weir, D. M., 1985, The effect of *Pseudomonas* alginate on rat alveolar macrophage phagocytosis and bacterial opsonization, *Clin. Exp. Immunol.* **59:**190–196.
79. Simpson, J. A., Smith, S. E., and Dean, R. T., 1988, Alginate inhibition of the uptake of *Pseudomonas aeruginosa* by macrophages, *J. Gen. Microbiol.* **134:**29–36.
80. Stiver, H. G., Zachidniak, K., and Speert, D. P., 1988, Inhibition of polymorphonuclear chemotaxis by the mucoid exopolysaccharide of *Pseudomonas aeruginosa*, *Clin. Invest. Med.* **11:**247–252.
81. Learn, D. B., Brestel, E. P., and Seetharama, S., 1987, Hypochlorite scavenging by *Pseudomonas aeruginosa* alginate, *Infect. Immun.* **55:**1813–1818.
82. Simpson, J. A., Smith, S. E., and Dean, R. T., 1989, Scavenging by alginate of free radicals released by macrophages, *Free Radic. Biol. Med.* **6:**347–353.
83. Bartell, P. F., Orr, T. E., and Chudio, B., 1970, Purification and chemical composition of the protective slime antigen of *Pseudomonas aeruginosa*, *Infect. Immun.* **2:**543–548.
84. Sensakovic, J. W., and Bartell, P. F., 1974, The slime of *Pseudomonas aeruginosa*: Biological characterization and possible role in experimental infection, *J. Infect. Dis.* **129:**101–109.
85. Sensakovic, J. W., and Bartell, P. F., 1975, Biological activity of fragments derived from the extracellular slime glycolipoprotein of *Pseudomonas aeruginosa*, *Infect. Immun.* **12:**808–812.
86. Laharrague, P. F., Corberand, J. X., Fillola, G., Gleizes, B. J., Fontanilles, A. M., and Gyrard, E., 1984, *In vitro* effect of the slime of *Pseudomonas aeruginosa* on the function of human polymorphonuclear neutrophils, *Infect. Immun.* **44:**760–762.
87. Lambris, J. Papamichail, M., Ioannidis, C., and Dimitracopoulos, G., 1982, Activation of the alternative pathway of human complement by the extracellular slime glycolipoprotein of *Pseudomonas aeruginosa*, *J. Infect. Dis.* **145:**78–82.
88. Bartell, P. F., and Krikszens, A., 1980, Influence of anti-slime glycolipoprotein serum on the interaction between *Pseudomonas aeruginosa* and macrophages, *Infect. Immun.* **27:**777–783.
89. Sorensen, R. U., Klinger, J. D., Cash, H. A., Chase, P. A., and Dearborn, D. G., 1983, *In vitro* inhibition of lymphocyte proliferation by *Pseudomonas aeruginosa* phenazine pigments, *Infect. Immun.* **41:**321–330.
90. Miller, K. M., Dearborn, D. G., and Sorensen, R. U., 1987, *In vitro* effect of synthetic pyocyanine on neutrophil superoxide production, *Infect. Immun.* **55:**559–563.
91. Malech, H. L., and Gallin, J. I., 1987, Neutrophils in human diseases, *N. Engl. J. Med.* **317:**687–694.
92. Lehrer, R. I., Ganz, T., Selsted, M. E., Babior, B. M., and Curnutte, J. T., 1988, Neutrophils and host defense, *Ann. Intern. Med.* **109:**127–142.
93. Bisbe, J. Gatell, J. M., Puig, J., Mallolas, J., Martinez, J. A., Jimenez de Anta, M. T., and Soriano, E., 1988, *Pseudomonas aeruginosa* bacteremia: Univariate and multivariate analysis of factors influencing the prognosis in 133 episodes, *Rev. Infect. Dis.* **10:**629–635.

94. Bodey, G. P., Jadeja, L., and Elting, L., 1985, *Pseudomonas* bacteremia, *Arch. Intern. Med.* **145:**1621–1629.
95. Wollman, M. R., Young, L. S., Armstrong, D., and Haghbin, M., 1975, Anti-*Pseudomonas* heat-stable opsonins in acute lymphoblastic leukemia of childhood, *J. Pediatr.* **86:**376–381.
96. McManus, A. T., Mason, A. D., Jr., McManus, W. F., and Pruitt, B. A., Jr., 1985, Twenty-five year review of *Pseudomonas aeruginosa* bacteremia in a burn center, *Eur. J. Clin. Microbiol.* **4:** 219–223.
97. Warden, G. D., Mason, A. D., Jr., and Pruitt, B. A., Jr., 1974, Evaluation of leukocyte chemotaxis *in vitro* in thermally injured patients, *J. Clin. Invest.* **54:**1001–1004.
98. Davis, J. M., Dineen, P., and Gallin, J. I., 1980, Neutrophil degranulation and abnormal chemotaxis after thermal injury, *J. Immunol.* **124:**1467–1471.
99. McManus, A. T., 1983, Examination of neutrophil function in a rat model of decreased host resistance following burn trauma, *Rev. Infect. Dis.* **5:**S898–S907.
100. Biggar, W. D., Holmes, B., and Good, R. A., 1971, Opsonic defect in patients with cystic fibrosis of the pancreas, *Proc. Nat. Acad. Sci. USA* **68:**1716–1719.
101. Fick, R. B., Jr., Naegel, G. P., Matthay, R. A., and Reynolds, H. Y., 1981, Cystic fibrosis *Pseudomonas* opsonins, *J. Clin. Invest.* **68:**899–914.
102. Fick, R. B., Jr., Naegel, G. P., Squier, S. U., Wood, R. E., Gee, J. B. L., and Reynolds, H. Y., 1984, Proteins of the cystic fibrosis respiratory tract: Fragmented immunoglobulin G opsonic antibody causing defective opsonophagocytosis, *J. Clin. Invest* **74:**236–248.
103. Eichler, I., Joris, L., Hsu, Y. P., Van Wye, J., Bram, R., and Moss, R., 1989, Nonopsonic antibodies in cystic fibrosis: *Pseudomonas aeruginosa* lipopolysaccharide-specific immunoglobulin G antibodies from infected patient sera inhibit neutrophil oxidative responses, *J. Clin. Invest.* **84:**1794–1804.
104. Fick, R. B., Jr., Olchowski, J., Squier, S. U., Merrill, W. W., and Reynolds, H. Y., 1986, Immunoglobulin-G subclasses in cystic fibrosis: IgG2 response to *Pseudomonas aeruginosa* lipopolysaccharide, *Am. Rev. Respir. Dis.* **133:**418–422.
105. Shryock, T. R., Mollé, J. S., Klinger, J. D., and Thomassen, M. J., 1986, Association with phagocytic inhibition of anti-*Pseudomonas aeruginosa* immunoglobulin G antibody subclass levels in serum from patients with cystic fibrosis, *J. Clin. Microbiol.* **23:**513–516.
106. Hornick, D. B., and Fick, R. B., Jr., 1990, The immunoglobulin G subclass composition of immune complexes in cystic fibrosis: Implications for the pathogenesis of the *Pseudomonas* lung lesion, *J. Clin. Invest.* **86:**1285–1292.
107. Suter, S. Schaad, U. B., Roux, L. Nydegger, U. E., and Waldvogel, F. A., 1984, Granulocyte neutral proteases and *Pseudomonas* elastase as possible causes of airway damage in patients with cystic fibrosis, *J. Infect. Dis.* **149:**523–531.
108. Suter, S. Schaad, U. B., Tegner, H., Ohlsson, K., Desgrandchamps, D., and Waldvogel, F. A., 1986, Levels of free granulocyte elastase in bronchial secretions from patients with cystic fibrosis: Effect of antimicrobial treatment against *Pseudomonas aeruginosa*, *J. Infect. Dis.* **153:** 902–909.
109. Suter, S., Nydegger, U. E., Roux, L., and Waldvogel, F.A, 1981, Cleavage of C3 by neutral proteases from granulocytes in pleural empyema, *J. Infect. Dis.* **144:**499–508.
110. Berger, M., Sorensen, R. U., Tosi, M. F., Dearborn, D. G., and Döring, G., 1989, Complement receptor expression on neutrophils at an inflammatory site, the *Pseudomonas*-infected lung in cystic fibrosis, *J. Clin. Invest.* **84:**1302–1313.
111. Tosi, M. F., Zakem, H., and Berger, M., 1990, Neutrophil elastase cleaves C3bi on opsonized *Pseudomonas* as well as CR1 on neutrophils to create a functionally important opsonin receptor mismatch, *J. Clin. Invest.* **86:**300–308.

10

Genetic Regulation of the Murine Corneal and Non-Corneal Response to *Pseudomonas aeruginosa*

RICHARD S. BERK

1. INTRODUCTION

During the past several years an active interest has developed in genetic regulation of host susceptibility and resistance to both infection and malignancy.[1] The potential role of genetic makeup of individuals as a major determinant of susceptibility to a variety of infectious agents receives strong support from epidemiologic data. Concomitantly, the widespread development of genetically defined strains of mutant, congenic, and recombinant inbred mice have made it possible for investigators to make new advances in this field. According to Skamene,[1] this allows for detailed mapping of the murine genome, resulting in the identification of the various chromosomal loci controlling resistance and susceptibility to a given infectious or oncogenic stimulus. This strategy has already resulted in the identification of several chromosomal loci involved in regulation of various traits. As Skamene points out, resistance genes to various infectious or malignant agents appear to map

---

RICHARD S. BERK • Department of Immunology and Microbiology, Wayne State University School of Medicine, Detroit, Michigan 48201.

Pseudomonas aeruginosa as an Opportunistic Pathogen, edited by Mario Campa *et al.* Plenum Press, New York, 1993.

to the same locus.[1] This suggests that there may be common mechanisms of host resistance to combat a variety of unrelated agents. Once these various genes have been identified, we can then begin to investigate the various cellular and molecular mechanisms that underlie the traits of resistance and susceptibility, thereby developing a better understanding of host defense mechanisms along with the potential for developing remedial measures.

Depending on the nature of the infectious agents, *i.e.*, extracellular or intracellular parasites, the major immune response can be categorized into: (1) phagocytosis and bactericidal activity by macrophages or neutrophils; (2) antigen processing and presentation; (3) cell-mediated immunity based on T-lymphocyte activity; and (4) the humoral response of B cells. Quantitative variation in one or more of these activities may determine the degree of susceptibility or resistance to an infectious agent. As a general rule, macrophage phagocytic activity plays a dominant role in chronic infections caused by intracellular bacteria, whereas a neutrophilic response appears to be of greater importance in extracellular, acute infections such as those caused by *Pseudomonas aeruginosa*. However, in acute infections, antibody production and function, rather than cellular immunity, are of major protective importance. As pointed out by Biozzi *et al.*,[2] T-cell-mediated immunity may also be involved in some bacterial infections through lymphokine-induced macrophage stimulation and/or local inflammation. One can postulate that in some cases, more than one of the resistance mechanisms may play an interdependent role in both innate and acquired resistance. This would depend on the nature of the immunogen(s), dosage, route of infection, and genetic makeup of the infected animal. In addition, nonspecific factors such as differences in inflammatory response and rate and degree of tissue repair of locally infected sites such as the cornea of resistant and susceptible animals may also participate in the overall response.

The clinical importance of genetic background as it relates to susceptibility to infection by *P. aeruginosa* is strikingly apparent in cystic fibrosis (CF) patients. CF is caused by an autosomal recessive gene and is characterized by congenital bronchiectasis with a generalized disorder of exocrine gland secretions, which results in the accumulation of abnormally viscid tracheobronchial secretions.[3-4] In these patients, progressive pulmonary infection is the major cause of morbidity and mortality. Although these respiratory infections may involve *Staphylococcus aureus* and other organisms, a chronic *P. aeruginosa* bronchiolitis and bronchitis ultimately can be found in almost all CF patients. At the present time, the underlying basis for this unique association between *P. aeruginosa* and CF patients is not known. Infection is limited to the lungs whereas the extrapulmonary tissues are resistant to *P. aeruginosa* infection. A number of researchers have investigated the basic abnormality that results in chronic pulmonary infection of CF patients.[5-8] Parameters such as defects in mucociliary clearance mechanisms and ability to synthesize immunoglobulins specific to *P. aeruginosa* have been examined, but without findings that would explain the inherent susceptibility to *P. aeruginosa* infection.

2. NON-OCULAR STUDIES

2.1. Systemic Infections—Genetic Studies

Pennington and Williams[9] published the first paper on the influence of genetic factors on susceptibility or natural resistance of experimental animals to *P. aeruginosa*. They pointed out that predisposition of certain patients to *P. aeruginosa* infection can be associated with various degrees of immunosuppression such as burns or acute respiratory failure. They also stated that certain patients are more prone than others to infection, even when similar environmental risk factors are present. However, other than the case of CF, genetic background has not been shown to play a major role for human infection caused by *P. aeruginosa*. Their initial genetic studies employed intraperitoneal infection of 16 inbred mouse strains with *P. aeruginosa* strain PA-103 and then compared their survival rates with Swiss–Webster mice.[9] The LD_{50} value for this outbred strain was 10^6 colony-forming units (CFU). The mouse strains tested were the following and they varied in H-2 haplotypes and genome: BALB/c, DBA/2J, B10.D2/nSn, B10.D2/oSn, C3H/HeJ, C3H/HeSn, C3h.SW/Sn, A/J, A/WySn, A.BY, C57BL/6J, C57BL/10nSn, B10/A/SgSn, B10.BR, B10.A(2R)/SgSn and B10/A(5R)/SgSn. These investigators found no significant differences among the survival rates of most of the mouse strains. However, they found a major difference in survival rates between mice of the C3H and those of A genome indicating the latter mice have less natural resistance to *Pseudomonas* infection. They also concluded that the enhanced resistance of C3H mice was independent of both the H-2 haplotype and the bactericidal activity of their respective sera. This differential susceptibility to infection was seen only when *P. aeruginosa* was the infecting agent, because no difference in susceptibility was observed when the two mouse strains were challenged with either *S. aureus* or *Escherichia coli*.

2.2. T-cell Immunity—Genetic Studies

One of the first examples of a genetic basis for the diverse responses of different mouse strains to an immunogen was described by Pier[10] in 1982. He found that after immunization of BALB/c and C3H/ANF mice with Fisher immunotype IT-1 polysaccharide, they differed in their ability to make antibody cross-reactive to the Fisher–Devlin *P. aeruginosa* immunotype 2 (IT-2) polysaccharide from culture supernatants. In addition, C3H mice were able to make antibody after immunization with low doses of antigen (1 μg), whereas BALB/c were not. Markham and Pier[11] then attempted to determine whether these differences were associated with either the mouse major histocompatibility (H-2) complex, with a single gene outside the H-2 locus or with sex-linked genes. They concluded that the dissimilar response of the BALB/c and C3H mice was inherited independently and was not sex-linked, H-2-linked or due to a single gene outside the H-2 complex. Thus, there were two distinct response patterns, which varied both by the limiting immunogen dose as well as by the specificity of the generated antibodies. It was thought the two mouse strains process the immunogen differently. BALB/c mice produced antibody that cross-reacted with IT-2 polysaccharide, but C3H did not, so they may be recognizing different determinants. It may be that the BALB/c mice respond to the immunogen with a heteroclitic response to IT-2. Therefore, anti–IT-2 polysaccharide antibody reacts with heterologous antigen, but does not react with the homologous IT-1 polysaccharide. Other studies[12] indicated that the BALB/c mice immunized with IT-1 polysaccharide developed protective T-cell immunity to bacterial challenge. This was determined by adoptive cell transfer of resistance to infection to naive or nonimmunized animals. Subsequently, it was demonstrated that splenic T cells obtained from immunized mice could kill the organism *in vitro*. After re-exposure to the immunogen, T cells from the immune mice produced a lymphokine that exhibited a broad range of bactericidal activity against both gram-positive and gram-negative bacteria.[13]

The phenotype of the murine T cell was of the Lyt-$1^-,2^+$ and reacted with monoclonal antibodies directed at the putative I-J^d antigen. In addition, macrophages were required only as a source of interleukin 1 (IL-1) and did not appear to function in antigen presentation or in phagocytosis.[14] However, the CB.20 mouse strain, which is congenic with BALB/c mice at the *Igh-1* locus, was unable to kill *P. aeruginosa in vitro*. This nonresponsiveness was attributed by Markham *et al.*[14] to the activity of suppressor cells.

Powderly *et al.*[15] attempted to determine the significance of T-lymphocyte-mediated immune response by use of a model of mouse granulocytopenia. They demonstrated protection by adoptive transfer of immune T cells even when granulocytes were absent in the recipient. However, no protection was detected when nonimmune T or B cells were used. In addition, T cells from CB.20 mice were also unable to adoptively transfer *in vivo* protection with the bactericidal, immune T cells. Additional studies indicated that IT-1 immune T cells were unable to confer protection against *P. aeruginosa* immunotype IT-3, but did protect against simultaneous challenge with both IT-1 and IT-3 by adoptive transfer. These results suggest that *in vivo* re-exposure to the homologous IT-1 immunogen resulted in a nonspecific protective response against IT-3.

Powderly *et al.* attributed the inability of cells from immunized CB.20 mice to kill *P. aeruginosa* to the inactivity of T cells of the Lyt-$1,2,3^+$. I-J$^+$ phenotype.[16] Because CB.20 mice differ from BALB/c mice only at a single locus, which includes the *Igh-1* allotype C_H genes, it would appear that this locus, or closely linked genes, regulate the T-cell killing ability of *P. aeruginosa* when the mice are immunized with polysaccharide. However, since C57BL/6 mice can generate a T-cell response to polysaccharide immunization and exhibit *in vitro* bactericidal activity against *P. aeruginosa*, it appears that the *Igh-1* locus may not be the sole determinant of suppressor activity. This conclusion is based on the fact that both C57BL/6 and CB.20 mice are of the *Igh-1*[b] allotype, whereas BALB/c is of the *Igh-1*[a] allotype. Sherman,[17] and Sherman and Riblet[18] have shown that *Igh*-linked genes affected the composition of the $H-2K^b$–specific cytolytic T-lymphocyte–receptor repertoire. In addition, the genes encoding T-cell allo-antigens are found at the distal end of the *Igh* complex.[19-20]

Powderly *et al.*[21-22] subsequently discovered that CB.20 mice can also adoptively transfer protection to granulocytopenic mice with T cells. It was found that polysaccharide immunization generated a greater amount of suppressor activity in CB.20 mice, but that it could be overcome with higher doses of vinblastine (100 μg). The function of vinblastine is to remove a suppressor cell population that normally inhibits T cell-mediated killing of *P. aeruginosa* when the non-responder BALB/c mice are immunized with 10 μg of polysaccharide antigen. In addition, no antibody formation was detected. The cells from CB.20 immunized with 10 μg of polysaccharide and 100 μg of vinblastine failed to kill *P. aeruginosa in vitro*. As previously noted, the CB.20 mice are allotypically congenic with BALB/c mice and differ at loci closely linked to the *Igh-1* locus.

When CB.20 mice were immunized with polysaccharide and vinblastine, they generated T cells that suppressed *in vitro* bactericidal activity of BALB/c T cells. However, T-cell cidal activity in CB.20 mice can be produced by increasing the dose of vinblastine, and the phenotype of the bactericidal T-cell population is identical to that of BALB/c bactericidal cells. Therefore, the difference between BALB/c and CB.20 mice is quantitative differences in suppressor cell activity. The vinblastine role in this system is to eliminate a population of Lyt-1-,2,3+, I-J+ suppressor T lymphocytes that are also induced by polysaccharide immunization. Subsequently, Markham and Powderly[23] were able to inhibit the *in vitro* growth of *P. aeruginosa* and passively protect naive recipient BALB/c mice by infecting BALB/c mice with as few as 100 live bacteria, but without administering vinblastine. This immune response appears to be identical to that generated with vinblastine and polysaccharide immunization. On the other hand, a challenge dose of 10^6 organisms was required to elicit a detectable antibody response. Furthermore, the IT specificity of mouse protection suggests that the bacterial component that bears the IT specificity is the lipopolysaccharide (LPS) component. More recent studies by Markham *et al.*[24] indicate that T suppressor cells that are elicited by polysaccharide immunization can also be generated by immunization with antibacterial T cells. The T suppressor cells are capable of abrogating the *in vivo* induction, as well as *in vitro* and *in vivo* expression of antibacterial T-cell activity. The T suppressor cells are antigen-specific and *H-2* restricted in their suppressor activity. They concluded that the protective T-cell response to *P. aeruginosa* is regulated by a network of T cells that are recognizing idiotypic determinants on *P. aeruginosa*-immune T and B cells. Although the studies described above centered on a non-ocular experimental model, they are reviewed here because of their potential importance and relevance to our ocular studies. Preliminary studies in my laboratory indicate that certain mouse strains intracorneally infected with *P. aeruginosa* may restore corneal clarity independently of a humoral response and that the effect may be mediated by a cellular immune mechanism.

3. CORNEAL INFECTIONS

3.1. Genetic Studies

P. aeruginosa is an opportunistic pathogen that is able to initiate necrotic central corneal ulcerations, although healthy individuals are normally resistant to infection. The keratitis produced is among the most rapidly spreading and destructive bacterial disease of the cornea known and may result in blindness. *Pseudomonas* infections of the cornea commonly occur following corneal trauma or wounds resulting from industrial accidents, in corneal transplants, or cataract extractions. In addition, infection occurs in the absence of corneal injury in those debilitated by age or immunosuppression or by a combination of these factors, as well as in premature infants.[25] At the present time, the more than 20,000,000 persons who use daily wear and extended-wear soft contact lenses may also be at potential risk. Recent studies in several laboratories have employed several experimental models to study *Pseudomonas* infection of the cornea. Many of clinical features of the disease in humans can be reproduced in mice, rats, and rabbits.[26–28] The experimental work to be described below will employ a well-characterized mouse model. In our studies we have established that the murine corneal response is dependent upon both the mouse strain and the bacterial strain.[26]

Early studies with the outbred Swiss–Webster mouse strain indicated that when the corneal surface of young adults (6–8 wk) was abraded and then infected with a topical inoculation of 10^8 *P. aeruginosa* cells, the mice developed a severe corneal infection within 12 to 24 hr. (Corneal infection with *P. aeruginosa* does not occur in adult mice without initial abrasion of cornea.) The eyes were usually sealed for a few days thereafter and the mice subsequently developed a severe keratitis. In most experimental studies, we infected only one eye and used the contralateral eye as an noninfected control for comparative purposes. The infection remained localized to the infected eye and did not spread to the control eye, nor were organisms detected in the bloodstream during the 30-day holding period.[29] However, within 2 to 4 wk post-infection, the mice begin to restore corneal clarity. By 4 wk, the infected eye appeared normal and was macroscopically indistinguishable from the uninfected contralateral control eye. Microscopically, there were remnants of blood vessels (ghosts) still present. (Normally, the central cornea is immunologically privileged in that it is devoid of blood circulation and lymphatic drainage.) To determine whether all mouse strains respond this way, we screened a series of inbred mouse strains. From these we have developed a unique classification of inbred mouse strains that indicates a genetic basis for regulation of the corneal response to infection by *P. aeruginosa* ATCC strain 19660.

During these studies, several different types of corneal response were observed depending on the mouse strain examined, and they constitute the following: Mice that were able to restore corneal clarity within 4 wk or less after infection were classed as naturally resistant.[30-35] Examples of inbred resistant mice were the DBA/1J and DBA/2J strains. On the other hand, most other inbred strains tested were classed as susceptible since corneal infection often led to corneal perforation, shrinkage (phthisis bulbi) and severe ocular destruction and/or cataract formation. Examples of these strains were the BALB/cJ, C57BL/6J, C3H,HeJ, C3H/HeN, AKR, CBA/J, and A/J. In addition, the susceptibility phenotype was seen in 100% of the mice tested. Of particular interest is that the A/J strain seemed to be particularly susceptible to *P. aeruginosa* corneal infection because six of 30 animals died as the result of a systemic infection within 24 to 48 hr post-ocular infection. Whether these deaths are the result of ocular infection or the licking off a lethal amount of the inoculum from other infected mice in the cage is not known; however, we have never seen other strains of mice dying as a result of ocular infection. A third and intermediate response is one of delayed recovery as seen with BALB.B, BALB.K, BALB/cPi, and BALB/cKh mice. With these mice, there is no restoration of corneal clarity at 4 wk and the mice are nominally considered to be susceptible at that time period. However, restoration of corneal clarity developed by 5–6 wk post-infection, thereby indicating a delayed type of recovery that does not usually occur in the other inbred strains classed as susceptible.

Of particular interest with regard to the susceptible BALB/cJ strain is that when athymic, nude mice (nu/nu) derived from them were intracorneally infected with *P. aeruginosa*, the mice exhibited a heightened natural resistance.[36] This response was characterized by little or no corneal opacity within the first 24 hr post-infection with subsequent maintenance of corneal clarity, whereas the heterozygous (nu/+) nude littermates behaved like the parent BALB/c strain and displayed the susceptibility phenotype. The mechanism by which the nude mouse restricts corneal infection is not known. Stereomicroscopic examination of the eyes of the nu/nu mice at 24 hr post-infection revealed slightly cloudy corneas with the iris visible, whereas nu/+ littermates exhibited opaque corneas with the iris not visible. The nu/+

behaved like the parent BALB/c so that the infection resulted in endophthalmitis and shrinkage of the infected eye within 2 wk post-infection. However, the similarly infected nu/nu mice resolved the infection within 24 hr and the eyes appeared identical to their contralateral, control eyes. Histological examination of the corneas of the athymic, nude mice 24 hr post-infection, demonstrated subepithelial capillaries and few neutrophils (with numerous intracellular bacteria in the central cornea). In contrast, the equivalent corneal areas of infected nu/+ littermates showed a striking neutrophilic response similar to that of parent BALB/c mice; however, fewer intracellular bacteria were observed. In addition, the central cornea of the nu/+ mice lacked blood vessels.

We usually observe severe corneal opacity with heavy neutrophil infiltration in all other experimentally infected mouse strains, regardless of whether they are classed as resistant or susceptible.[29–30] However, the cellular response in the nu/nu mice is different in that there is no marked increase in neutrophils at 24 hr post-infection, as observed in nu/+ or the parent BALB/c strain. The specific mechanism(s) of the nude mouse that results in enhanced ocular immunity is unknown at present. An explanation may be that these mice have developed a compensatory protective mechanism as a result of a lack of thymus. Thus, they may be primed for enhanced bactericidal activity unlike their nu/+ littermates, parent BALB/c, or other naturally resistant and susceptible strains.

One of the major advantages in establishing an experimental model encompassing both susceptible and resistant mouse strains is that it allows investigators to dissect the many variables that interact to produce the resistance phenotype. Conceivably, under the right experimental conditions, the resistance phenotype can be replaced temporarily by the susceptibility phenotype. Concomitantly, the identification of susceptible strains permits us to determine the humoral and/or cellular factors that can be transferred or induced, and which may result in the appearance of the resistance phenotype. These types of experiments are described later in this chapter.

To characterize the genetic regulation of the corneal response to infection, we initiated a series of experiments using hybrid animals derived from matings of resistant and susceptible strains.[30] When resistant DBA/2J mice were mated with susceptible BALB/cJ mice, all F1 hybrids (CD2F1) (25 females and 29 males) were uniformly resistant and restored corneal clarity within the 4-wk holding period. The same resistance pattern was also obtained with F_1 hybrids (CD1F1) derived from DBA/1J and BALB/cJ. Again, both males (40) and (33) females restored corneal clarity. In addition, it did not matter whether the parent BALB/cJ mice were males or females when mated to the DBA/2J and DBA/1J mice. These results indicated that the resistance (or susceptibility) phenotype was independent of sex (*i.e.*, autosomal) and that resistance was dominant over susceptibility. However, the latter finding is true only for mating of the resistant DBA/2J or DBA/1J with the susceptible BALB/cJ mice. (A dominant susceptibility phenotype is described later in this chapter.) Also, the fact that BALB/cJ and DBA/2J mice shared the same H-2^d haplotype, indicates that the dominance of an autosomal gene with DBA/2J maps outside the H-2 complex.

Because we have established that there are several dissimilar types of ocular responses to *P. aeruginosa* infection, we next indicated experiments that might shed light on the number of resistance and susceptibility genes present in the resistant DBA/2J and BALB/cJ strains. Therefore, we crossed the two strains with each other and then backcrossed the resultant resistant CD2F1 males to susceptible BALB/cJ females. Conversely, we mated backcrossed resistant CD2F1 females to resistant DBA/2J males. The progeny were then challenged intracorneally at 6–8 wk of age. The results obtained are essentially identical with expected theoretical frequencies for models of either one or two autosomal genes determining resistance. Thus, 68/70 (97.2%) of the CD2F1 × DBA/2J backcrossed mice recovered from corneal infection with an expected recovery of 100%. When BALB/cJ males were mated to CD2F1 females, we observed that 34/65 (52.3%) of the animals expressed the resistance phenotype with an expected recovery rate of 50%. These results strongly support our working hypothesis that either one or two autosomal genes determine corneal resistance to *P. aeruginosa*. In addition, this model is supported by the findings that when the two susceptible strains, BALB/cJ and C57BL/6J, were mated, all the resultant CB6F1 progeny were resistant, regardless of sex (32/32 females, 28/28 males). The resultant resistant F_1 phenotype appears to be an example of genetic complementation between two susceptible strains and suggests that each susceptible strain carries at least one resistant and dissimilar gene and that both genes are necessary for expressing the resistance phenotype.

To study the interaction between these two loci, we examined the F_2 progeny from CB6F1 × CB6F1 (BALB/cJ × C57BL/6J) matings after intracorneal challenge with *P. aeruginosa*. The results of this experiment yielded 67/122 (54.9%) F_2 progeny that were resistant and 55/122 (45.1%) that were susceptible. There was no observable relationship among corneal response, coat color, or sex. For the requirement of a dominant gene at each locus in order to confer resistance, the expected result is a ratio of resistant to susceptible F_2 offspring of 9:7 (56.2%/43.8%). We have therefore provisionally designated the C57BL/6J resistance gene as *PsCR1* (*PsCR* = *Pseudomonas* Corneal Resistance) and the BALB/cJ resistance gene as *PsCR2*. These data do not negate the possibility that more than two genes control resistance; both BALB/cJ and C57BL/6J mice could bear a resistance gene at a third locus.

Other F_1 hybrid studies were conducted between susceptible strains in order to shed further light on the susceptibility/resistance interaction. However, when matings of susceptible C3H/HeJ and BALB/cJ were performed, all of the F_1 mice exhibited the susceptibility phenotype. Because complementation occurred as seen with the CB6F1 hybrids, the results suggest that the C3H/HeJ mice carry the same resistance gene as BALB/cJ (*PsCR2*) at the *PsCR2* locus, and that the *PsCR1* locus carries a susceptibility gene. In addition, when C3H/HeJ mice were mated with C57BL/6J mice, the F_1 progeny all expressed the susceptibility phenotype. From these results, we reasoned that the genotype of C3H/HeJ was *PsCR1*$^{r/r}$, *PsCR2*$^{r/r}$. However, when matings of C3H/HeJ and DAB/2J mice were initiated, the F_1 progeny showed unexpected results. All of these infected animals expressed the susceptibility phenotype and were unable to recover from infection. A dominant susceptibility effect, apparently contributed by the C3H/HeJ parent mice, was the most likely explanation for these results. Thus, there was no longer support for a proposed *PsCR1*$^{r/r}$, *PsCR2*$^{r/r}$ genotype.

To demonstrate that the C3H susceptibility response was under genetic regulation, (C3H/HeJ × DBA/2J)F_2 animals and the progeny of (C3H/H1J × DBA/2J)F_1 males backcrossed with DBA/2J females were screened for their susceptibility to *P. aeruginosa* infection. Of the backcross progeny, we found that 33/94 (35.1%) of the animals recovered from the corneal infection, whereas 61/94 (64.9%) were unable to restore corneal clarity. Since two nonlinked resistant genes, *PsCR1* and *PsCR2*, have been suggested previously, we proposed that a dominant susceptibility gene(s), provisionally designated as *PsCS* (*Pseudomonas* Corneal Susceptibility), is involved. Statistical analysis of the backcross data was performed to determine if one or more dominant susceptibility genes were present. Both one gene ($\chi^2 = 8.32$, $P < 0.01$) and two nonlinked genes ($\chi^2 = 4.53$, $P < 0.05$) were rejected. The expected percentages of resistant backcross progeny are 50% and 25% for the one-gene and two-genes hypotheses, respectively. However, because the observed frequency was 35.1% resistant offspring, it was necessary to consider alternatives to simple Mendelian genetics. One explanation is that two linked dominant susceptibility genes of C3H origin are present. Progeny carrying the recombinant genotypes would then by phenotypically susceptible. In addition, all of the resistant offspring would represent animals that lacked the C3H/HeJ dominant susceptibility alleles. Because the frequency of the resistant offspring (35.1%) represented half of the expected non-recombinant DBA/2J parental genotype, the frequency of animals carrying the parental genotype would be 70.2%. Therefore, the crossover frequency would equal the frequency of recombinant animals, 29.8%.

Using this theory, proper assessment of the F_2 results required determination of the resistance genes in DBA/2J mice. Previous studies between DBA/2J and BALB/cJ mice suggested that a single gene controls resistance.[30-31] Because BALB/cJ carries the *PsCR2* gene, the segregating DBA/2J gene must be at another locus and is presumably *PsCR1*. If DBA/2J mice also carry the *PsCR2* gene (which BALB/cJ presumably carries), then (DBA/2J × C57BL/6J)F_1 animals should be resistant. However, all the F_1 progeny exhibited the susceptibility phenotype. Therefore, it is apparent that the DBA/2J

PsCR2 allele is unlike that of BALB/cJ and the phenotypic expression of the DBA/2J *PsCR2* gene remains to be elucidated. These experiments suggest that DBA/2J mice carry one gene conferring resistance and that this gene can be masked by susceptible gene(s) from either C3H/HeJ or C57BL/6J mice. In the F_2 offspring, the expected frequency of resistant animals can be calculated by squaring the frequency of resistant animals (35.1%) obtained in the backcross experiment. These data predict that 12.3% of the F_2 animals would express the resistance phenotype. F_2 progeny from the (C3H × DBA/2J)F1 × (C3H/HeJ × DBA/2J)F1 matings were then examined for their ability to restore corneal clarity. Of 58 F_2 animals infected we observed that nine (15.5%) were resistant and 49 (84.5%) were susceptible. The supposition of two linked *PsCS* genes was accepted as indicated by the χ^2 value of 0.291 ($0.7 > P > 0.5$). Other possibilities, using both allelic and epistatic interactions, have been considered to explain both the backcross and F_2 data. However, only the working hypothesis presented here appears consistent with previously published data.

These findings are unique in that genetic control of natural resistance to bacterial infections has always been described to be under dominant autosomal genes. This type of host regulation has been described previously in infections involving *Corynebacterium kutscheri*,[37-38] *Mycobacterium lepraemurium*,[39-40] *M. tuberculosis*,[41] *Listeria monocytogenes*,[42-45] *Rickettsia tsutsugamushi*,[46] *R. akari*,[47] *Salmonella typhimurium*,[48-51] and *P. aeruginosa*.[29-31] However, studies described here suggest that two linked dominant susceptibility genes may regulate the natural resistance to *P. aeruginosa* infection.

In a previous report we used (BALB/cJ × DBA/2J)F_2 hybrids to describe the *PsCR1* locus and found that it is not *H-2* linked. In addition, because both mouse strains share the *H-2*^{d} haplotype, it is difficult to determine whether or not *PsCR2* is *H-2* linked. In an attempt to answer this question, we screened several inbred mouse strains. Initially, we examined six congenic lines of C3H with six different haplotypes (C3H/HeJ^k, C3H.SW/Sn^b, C3H.JK/Sn^j, C3H.NB/SnP, C3H.Q^q, and C3H/HeSn^k). All six lines were uniformly susceptible regardless of their *H-2* haplotype. Similar studies were performed with 11 B10 (i.e., C57BL/10) congenic lines and, again, all were uniformly susceptible. These included the following: B10, B10D2, B10M, B10.WB, B10.BR, B10.F, B10.Q, B10.RIII, B10.S, B10.PL, and B10.SM. Congenic lines of the A strain were also tested and three of the four strains exhibited an intermediate response to intracorneal challenge. Thus, 41 of 64 A.BY (*H-2*^{b}) and one of 20 A.SW (*H-2*^{s}) were susceptible. Similar results were obtained with A.CA (*H-2*^{f}) (15/29 susceptible) and A/He (*H-2*^{a}) (8/23 susceptible). Only the A/J (*H-2*^{a}) were all susceptible. These results indicate that the *H-2* locus does not seem to exert an effect on the resistance or susceptibility phenotype.[31]

Because previous studies indicated that the BALB/cJ strain exhibited the susceptibility phenotype, we expected that BALB.B and BALB.K congenic lines would also be uniformly susceptible. However, when these two lines were examined, we found they were uniformly resistant.[31] Thus, 51 of 51 BALB.B mice and 101 of 102 BALB.K mice restored corneal clarity. However, the kinetics of recovery of these two congenic lines differed from that of other naturally resistant strains such as the DBA/1J and DA/2J, which showed gradual and eventually complete recovery within around 3 wk post-challenge. Instead, the BALB.B and BALB.K strains were initially classed as susceptible at 4 wk post-infection, but they began to macroscopically recover and restore corneal clarity by 5–6 wk. This delayed recovery, in comparison with that of the DBA/2J mice, may be due to expression of different alleles, either at one locus or as the result of different intergenic interactions. However, previous studies argue against this type of interpretation. To examine this discrepancy, we initiated studies with F_1 hybrids and backcrossed animals. The first study determined the response of BALB.B × BALB/cJ F1 hybrids as well as BALB.K × BALB/cJ hybrids. However, all the progeny in both cases were resistant. These results suggest that the gene(s) controlling resistance is dominant. The data obtained from reciprocal crosses between males and females indicated that this gene is not sex-linked.

Subsequently, to initiate segregation analyses to determine *H-2* linkage and number of genes involved, we used backcrosses, mating the F_1 hybrids of BALB.B and BALB.K to BALB/cJ with the BALB/cJ parental strain. The phenotypes of the backcross progeny yielded an approximately 1:1:1:1 segregation pattern of the following phenotypes: of 58 BALB.K × BALB/cJ F_1 hybrids mated to BALB/cJ, 12 animals were susceptible and homozygous for the *H-2* complex (i.e. *H-2*$^{d/d}$), 19 animals were resistant and homozygous (*H-2*$^{d/d}$), 12 animals were susceptible and heterozygous (*H-2*$^{k/d}$), and the remaining 15 mice were resistant and heterozygous (*H-2*$^{k/d}$). Similar results were obtained with 54 BALB.B × BALB/cJ hybrids backcrossed to BALB/cJ. Sixteen mice were susceptible and homozygous (*H-2*$^{d/d}$), 11 were resistant and homozygous (*H-2*$^{d/d}$), 15 were susceptible and heterozygous (*H-2*$^{b/d}$), and 12 were resistant and heterozygous (*H-2*$^{b/d}$). The 1:1:1:1 ratio is indicative of two loci segregating independently of each other. Therefore, we conclude that the *H-2* complex and the *PsCR* gene are not linked. Chi-square analyses of these data (χ^2 = 2.43 for [BALB.K × BALB/cJ]F1 × BALB.cJ, and χ^2 = 1.28 for [BALB.B × BALB/cJ]F1 × BALB/cJ) are in agreement with our working hypothesis, which states that *H-2* is not linked to the *PsCR* gene and that only one gene or a group of tightly bound loci control(s) resistance in the BALB.B and BALB.K lines. Because we cannot determine at this time whether this gene is representative of a different allelic form of either the *PsCR1* locus, the *PsCR2* locus, or a third locus, no numbered designation was used or added to the *PsCR* symbol for this gene. In addition, the difference of this *PsCR* locus in the BALB.B and BALB.K strains from the BALB/cJ may be the result of variational differences in sublines of the BALB/cJ strain, since

BALB.B and BALB.K strains were derived from the BALB.cKh sublines (F. Lilly, personal communication).

To determine the location of one or more of the postulated resistance genes, we screened the ocular response of several congenic strains of the BALB/c background carrying one or more genes from the resistant DBA/2 mice. The rationale behind this study was that it would enable us to identify possible chromosomal locations of the *PsCR* gene(s). We examined 13 lines developed by Michael Potter (NIH) and found 5/13 lines were able to restore corneal clarity in 75–100% of the mice.[33-35] These lines were C.D2.Pep-3 (chromosome 1), C.D2. Idh/Pep-3 (chromosome 1), C.D2. Idh-1 (chromosome 1), C.D2. Pgm-1 (chromosome 5), and C.D2.Igh-1c$^{+/+}$ (chromosome 12). Although each line expressed the resistance phenotype, mice carrying the DBA/2 genes on chromosome 1 (*Idh, Pep-3, Idh/Pep-3*) appeared to recover faster than mice carrying the *Pgm-1* and *Igh-1* genes. These observations suggested that a gene or a group of tightly linked genes linked with the *Pep-3* and *Idh-1* isoenzyme loci is the predominant *PsCR* gene(s) in the DBA/2 mouse strain. This resistance gene is located on chromosome 1 between the *Idh-1* and *Pep-3* loci. Within this chromosomal segment several other genes have been identified that regulate resistance to other infectious agents. Of interest is that these other agents are associated only with chronic infections rather than with acute infections and include *Salmonella typhimurium* (*Ity* gene),[52] *Leishmania donovani* (*Lsh*),[53] and *Mycobacterium lepraemurium*.[54] However, recent studies suggest that all three genes are at the same locus and may be one and the same.[55] This gene has been thought to be associated with macrophage function[52] and possible enhanced bactericidal activity.

Our C.D2 congenic data also suggested that two other genes may be involved in regulating resistance to *P. aeruginosa* corneal damage. These were linked to the *Igh-1* and *Pgm-1* genetic markers. The *Igh-1* gene on chromosome 12 is thought to be a structural gene coding for the variable region of heavy-chain immunoglobulin. The *Pgm-1* marker has been associated with phosphoglucomutase activity, but is linked to another macrophage gene termed the *Ric* gene, which is associated with rickettsial immunity. Isoenzyme studies in our laboratory indicated the *Ric* is necessary for corneal resistance in our *P. aeruginosa* model.[35]

To determine if a relationship exists between the *Igh-1* locus and one of the *PsCR* genes, we examined the corneal response to infection in two *Igh-1* congenic lines, BC-8 (*Igh-1*a) and CB-2 (*Igh-1*b). C57BL/Ka (Igh-1b) and BALB/cJ (Igh-1a) were the partner strains, respectively. The *Igh-1*a allele did not change the susceptibility pattern in the CB-20 line, whereas the *Igh-1*b allele caused a significant reduction in prevalence of corneal recovery. This data, along with the C.D2.Igh-1 results, suggested that the *Igh-1* locus does contain a gene(s) that influences natural resistance to corneal infection by *P. aeruginosa*.[33] However, this locus apparently exerts a minor influence.

Based on the results of the chromosomal sites studies, we attempted to determine whether isoenzyme studies would support these studies. Consequently, we mated resistant CD2F1 mice (DBA/2 × BALB/c) to the susceptible BALB/c parent strain and determined the ratio of resistant to susceptible mice. We found that 36/129 of the backcrossed mice were resistant, thereby giving us a 27.9% recovery rate, compared with a postulated recovery value of 25%.[35] This suggests that at least two resistance genes are involved since a one-gene model should have given us a 50% recovery rate, while the theoretical rate for two and three genes should be 25% and 12.5%, respectively. Subsequently, isoenzyme assays of each of 110/129 mice were run on red-blood-cell lysates for two enzyme/markers. These consisted of Pep-3 (peptidase, chromosome 1) and *Pgm-1* (phosphoglucomutase, chromosome 5). The results indicated a loose linkage between a resistance gene (*Ric*) and *Pgm-1* (chromosome 5). It was calculated that the gene was approximately 30.4 centimorgans distal to *Pgm-1*, which places it at or near the *Ric* locus. The latter gene represents a potential site of macrophage function for phagocytosis of intracellular parasites such as rickettsiae. On the other hand, isoenzyme studies with the *Pep-3* gene (peptidase, chromosome 1) did not show correlation with the presence of a second resistance gene as might have been expected from our congenic studies. Because isoenzyme studies did not show a clear correlation between a second resistance gene at chromosome 1, one must ask about the potential role of a gene at this location. One explanation may be that the *Ity* gene location may somehow modulate the resistance response of major genes on other chromosomes (epistasis). In addition, when we mated the resistant C.D2.Idh-1/Pep-3 line with the susceptible BALB/c strain, all the F_1 progeny were resistant, indicating that a resistance gene must be located on chromosome 1 somewhere between *Idh-1* and *Pep-3* loci, possibly at the *Ity/Lsh/Bcg* locus. The result of these mating experiments are analogous to those of the DBA/2 × BALB/c (CD2F1) results, in which DBA/2 expresses dominance over the susceptible BALB/c.

To establish the possibility of susceptibility genes in C57BL/6J mice, we mated them with the resistant DBA/2J mice. However, all the resultant B6D2F1 hybrid mice expressed the susceptibility phenotype. When these F_1 hybrids were backcrossed to the parent DBA/2J strain, 95/106 of these progeny were classed as susceptible. These data suggest that the C57BL/6J mouse strain may be carrying multiple susceptibility genes. Because BALB/cJ mice have been shown previously to complement with C57BL/6J mice to yield 100%-resistant progeny, one possible explanation is that BALB/cJ mice can override the C57BL/6J susceptibility gene(s). If this is true, then one could predict two possible results from crossing B6D2F1 × BALB/cJ progeny. One possibility is that the offspring would express the resistance phenotype. If so, this would be possible if the resistant D2 gene is an allele of *PsCR1*. However, if the D2 gene is not *PsCR1*, then 75% of the offspring should be resistant. Neither was the case. Instead, 52% (26/50) of the animals expressed the resistance phenotype. Thus, the *PsCR2* gene of BALB/cJ mice does not exert an influence on the B6 susceptibility gene(s) as proposed, but only produces resistance in combination with the *PsCR1* allele of B6.

Earlier studies noted that BALB.B, BALB.K, and BALB/cKh strains expressed delayed restoration of corneal clarity and were classed as resistant. Because genetic complementation between BALB/cJ and C57BL/6J resulted in resistant progeny, we wished to determine if this was also true for the progeny of matings between C57BL/6J and BALB.B, BALB.K and BALB/cKh. In all cases, the F_1 progeny expressed the susceptibility phenotype and no genetic complementation. When we extended these studies to determine the segregation pattern of the F_2 progeny, the results showed that 33/97 (34%) of the (BALB.B × C56BL/6J)F2 animals and 9/29 (31%) of (BALB.K × c57BL/6J)F2 animals were resistant. These data suggest a multigenic and/or multiallelic control of both susceptibility and resistance to corneal infection with *P. aeruginosa* and that genetic regulation of natural resistance to infection is multigenic and much more complex than anticipated.

3.2. Humoral Response of Resistant and Susceptible Mice

Because *P. aeruginosa* is an extracellular pathogen, one would expect that the dominant immune response to intracorneal infection would be humoral rather than cellular. Consequently, one possible explanation for the differential responses of resistance and susceptibility is that resistant mouse strains mount a rapid and protective humoral response to infection prior to development of permanent corneal damage. In addition, it is postulated that susceptible mouse strains are immunologically nonresponsive or hyporesponsive. To test this hypothesis, we compared the serum humoral response of the resistant DBA/2J with that of the susceptible C57BL/6J mice over a 30-day holding period.[56] In addition, we also wished to determine whether susceptible C57BL/6J mice can develop protective immunity as the result of both primary and/or secondary corneal infection as well as by the passive transfer of immune serum from animals that have recovered from corneal infection.

Weekly serum samples from 20 mice of each strain were assayed by enzyme-linked immunosorbent assay (ELISA) for IgM, IgG, and IgA directed specifically to *P. aeruginosa*. The results indicate that the DBA/2J mice were able to mount both an IgM and IgG response within 1 wk post-infection. However, no IgA was detected in the serum at any time during the experiment. At the end of 7 days, the IgM titer was 1:800 and the IgG titer was 1:400. The latter titer remained constant for the remainder of the holding period of 4 wk, while the IgM titer dropped to 1:200 and remained constant. At the end of 4 wk post-infection, the recovered mice were reinfected in the contralateral control eye and the serum titers were again monitored for an additional 4 wk. IgM titers did not increase after 7 days, but did rise to 1:400 by week 4. However, the IgG titers rose to 1:400 after 7 days and increased dramatically to 1:6,400 at the end of 4 wk. Concomitantly with the antibody studies, we monitored the ocular response of the animals and found that they restored corneal clarity within 4 wk post–primary infection, although most mice began to do so macroscopically within 7 to 10 days post-infection.

When these studies were repeated with the susceptible C57BL/6J mice, results indicated that the humoral response was of a substantially lower order of magnitude than that obtained with the resistant DBA/2J mice, suggesting that the C57BL/6J mice were humorally hyporesponsive. The IgM and IgG titers at the end of 1 wk were 1:80 and 1:20, respectively, while titers at the end of the 4-wk holding period were 1:10 and 1:200, respectively. However, upon reinfection of the contralateral control eye, the IgM and IgG titers after 1 wk were 1:80 and 1:320, respectively. By the end of the 4-wk holding period these titers had increased to 1:200 and 1:6,400, respectively. At no time during the primary or secondary infection was IgA detected in the serum. As expected, during the primary infection, 23 of 23 infected mice were unable to restore corneal clarity. It should be pointed out that the severity of the infection during the first few days after primary infections was macroscopically indistinguishable from that seen in the resistant DBA/2J mice. However, when the mice were reinfected by using the contralateral control eye, six of 23 C57BL/6J were able to restore corneal clarity of only the contralateral control eye within the next 30-day holding period, but not the primary infected eyes. An additional seven mice showed slight improvement over the response noted with a primary infection. Of particular interest was that if the mice were reinfected at 60 days rather than 30 days post-primary infection, then eight of 28 mice restored complete corneal clarity (grade 0) within 3 days post–secondary infection, while 17 of the 28 mice exhibited a faint corneal opacity (grade 1), respectively. By the end of 6 days, 18 and seven of the 28 mice exhibited grades of 0 and 1, respectively. Only three mice were unable to restore corneal clarity within this period, but these mice recovered and restored corneal clarity within the next 10 days. None of the C57BL/6J mice was able to restore corneal clarity in the eye that received the primary infection even after receiving the secondary corneal infection. The damage in these corneas was permanent, unlike the slow and complete recovery observed previously in BALB.B and BALB.K mice at 5–6 wk after the primary infection, but not at 4 wk post-infection.[56]

To establish that protective antibody was responsible for the recovery of DBA/2J mice after a primary infection, as well as the C57BL/6J mice after a secondary infection, we administered 0.2 ml of immune serum (titer, 1:6,400) obtained from either donor strain after restoration of corneal clarity, to naive C57BL/6J mice 1 hr prior to intracorneal challenge. Also, we tested the efficacy of the serum by challenging the mice with a higher than usual inoculum of 5×10^8 CFU instead of a dose of 10^8 CFU and final evaluation of the results was made at the end of 2 wk rather than at the end of the usual 4-wk holding period. The results obtained showed that six out of 11 mice either recovered completely or showed a moderation in the severity of the ocular damage. However, none of the mice restored corneal clarity when the immune sera was absorbed with heat-inactivated *P. aeruginosa* cells prior to passive transfer to naive recipients. Thus, 12 out of 12 animals exhibited corneal perforation.

3.3. Role of Complement in Corneal Resistance

Other studies from our laboratories indicate that the ability of DBA/2J mice to restore corneal clarity is dependent upon C3 levels; when this complement component is depleted by cobra venom, the mice are unable to restore corneal clarity and subsequently exhibit the susceptibility phenotype.[57] This susceptibility is lost upon reacquisition of normal C3 levels, so that when the mice are reinfected, they restore corneal clarity as expected. However, despite the production of antibodies to *P. aeruginosa* during the primary infection, the mice are unable to recover if their C3 levels are again depleted by cobra venom treatment. It was also demonstrated that C5 was not necessary for restoration of corneal clarity because the naturally resistant DBA/2J strain is C5-deficient.[57] Similar results have been described by others.[58-59] Components of both the classical and alternate complement pathways have been demonstrated previously in infected corneas by others and potentiate phagocytosis of *P. aeruginosa*[57,60-61] and possibly other gram-negative organisms.[62]

3.4. Role of Age in Resistance

Other studies from our laboratories indicate that the natural resistance of Swiss–Webster mice develops with age and that immunocompetency is initially absent at 5 and 10 days post-infection.[63] It is only after the eyes of the animals open at around 15 days that the appearance of immunocompetency begins to develop. In addition, it should be pointed out that 5- and 10-day-old mouse pups do not require corneal abrasion for ocular infection and most of the animals die from a systemic infection within 24–48 hr after injection of the inoculum under the fused eyelid. When 15- to 16-day-old mice whose eyes were opened received *P. aeruginosa* topically onto either unwounded or wounded corneas, it was found that wounding was necessary for initiation of infection. At least 50% of the mice that received corneal wounding and the inoculum exhibited keratitis, endophthalmitis, and subsequent phthisis bulbi, whereas mice without wounded corneas did not exhibit eye infections. In 21-day-old mice, 32% of the mice recovered spontaneously, whereas the remainder exhibited either a complete loss of the eye or microopthalmia and cataracts. The variability of these responses appears to reflect a transitional maturation period of natural resistance to the infecting organisms, because 4- to 6-week-old adult mice normally restore corneal clarity within 3 to 4 wk post-infection. We also observed an age-related susceptibility of mice to ocular challenge with exotoxin A.[64]

3.5. Immunization Studies

Other studies have established that active immunization with *P. aeruginosa* lipopolysaccharide enhances the clearance of the homologous serotypic strain with the concomitant restoration of corneal clarity.[65] However, when active immunization with elastase or passive immunization with antibody to elastase was performed, the mice did not express as much protection as those receiving lipopolysaccharide. This is expected because antibody to lipopolysaccharide aids in the elimination of the bacteria from the cornea, whereas antibody to elastase only neutralizes the potentially deleterious effects of the enzyme, and does not enhance bacterial clearance. Moon *et al.*[66] also demonstrated that passive transfer of monoclonal antibodies directed against *P. aeruginosa* outer membrane proteins such as porin (F) of lipoprotein (H2) conferred protection to the intracorneally infected mice. Corneal and non-corneal studies by other investigators also lend support to the importance of humoral immunity.[67-70] However, the work of Pier *et al.*[12-16] using a non-ocular system indicates that cellular immunity may also play a role in *P. aeruginosa* infections. This depends, however, on the nature and dosage of the immunogen as described earlier in this chapter.

4. DISCUSSION

At the present time it is known that a number of infectious agents to which mice exhibit some form of natural resistance are under genetic control. These include such unrelated organisms as herpes simplex virus,[71] *Coccidioides immitis*,[72] *Salmonella typhimurium*,[50] *Trichinella spiralis*,[73] and *P. aeruginosa*.[9,29] In the case of *P. aeruginosa*, we have implicated at least three genetic loci that may regulate the murine ocular response to infection. These loci are tentatively linked to the *Ity/Lsh/Bcg* gene(s), the *Ric* gene and the *Igh* gene on chromosomes 1, 5, and 12, respectively.[32-35] From the experimental evidence described here, there appears to exist a complex regulatory system of resistance (corneal clarity restored) involving both inter- and intragenic interactions that are associated with the resistant DBA/2J prototype. This gene(s) can be masked by a dominant susceptibility gene(s) carried by C57BL/6J. Concomitantly, the susceptible C57BL/6J mice can undergo genetic complementation with susceptible BALB/cJ mice to produce resistant progeny. Therefore, it is our working hypothesis that the three presently identified loci and their corresponding alleles determine the reported complex genotypic interactions.

The strongest support for this hypothesis comes from the results of the BALB/cKh subline. This line differs from the susceptible BALB/cJ prototype strain, because it can restore corneal clarity when injected intracorneally with *P. aeruginosa* but is unable to complement with C57BL/6J. Segregation analyses have demonstrated that these changes are the result of a single noncomplementing resistance allele that was probably produced by a point mutation. Additional supportive evidence for this hypothesis is provided by examination of the genetic control of the dominant susceptibility and complementing genes. Two dominant susceptible loci are found in both C57BL/6J and C3H/HeJ reference strains, and it is postulated that the presence of either locus will result in corneal injury upon infection.

Segregation studies, CXB recombinant inbred strain analysis,[35] and complementation studies with the C.D2 congenics suggest that BALB/cJ carries two complementation genes, both of which are needed to produce resistant progeny. In contrast, only one of the two C57BL/6J complementing genes are required for resistance. Data from CXB matings (C57BL/6J × BALB/cJ) suggest the following: (1) A *P. aeruginosa* corneal resistance gene is also carried by the C57BL/6J strains, which is masked by the dominant susceptibility loci; (2) the genes responsible for the dominant susceptibility trait in C57BL/6J mice also control complementation with the BALB/cJ strain, which results in resistant F_1 progeny; and (3) the strain distribution pattern and the ratios of susceptible to resistant lines support the control of two genes, the alleles of which determine resistance, complementation, and dominant susceptibility. In addition, there is both inter- and intragenic regulation by three loci in determining the outcome of the corneal infection.

The association of the resistance phenotype with two separate genes regulating macrophage function (*Ity/Lsh/Bcg* loci on chromosome 1 and the *Ric* gene on chromosome 5) was unexpected. These genes have been associated previously only with macrophage function in chronic infection models. In the case of *S. typhimurium*, it is postulated that the role of the macrophage is primarily to function as a bactericidal agent, whereas the function of the *Ric* macrophage gene has not been definitely established, but is thought to regulate the same bactericidal activity toward rickettsia.[74–75] Because neutrophils are the predominant phagocytic cell (98–99%) present in corneal infections during the first 24 to 48 hr of *P. aeruginosa* in mice, it appears that phagocytosis is not the main role of macrophages in our ocular experimental model. This is particularly evident in at least the early infection phase. Consequently, an alternate role for the macrophage in the infectious process must be postulated and may consist of antigen presentation and/or processing prior to T-cell interaction. This is consistent with the congenic data that show the *Igh-1* locus on chromosome 12 also interacts in this system, especially since genes at or near this locus are associated with T-cell function.[17–20] Because *P. aeruginosa* is considered an extracellular agent, one could postulate that the differing susceptibility/resistance phenotypic responses are dependent on the ability to synthesize protective antibody before irreversible ocular damage can occur. Thus, in the case of susceptible strains, it is postulated that the humoral response to ocular immunization by topical infection is nonexistent or hyporesponsive. This hypothesis is supported by non-ocular studies of Markham and Powderly[23] who demonstrated that BALB/c mice can be non-responsive in humoral immunity, depending on dosage and nature of the immunogen. On the other hand, mouse strains that exhibit the resistance phenotype are ostensibly normal in their humoral immune response and therefore synthesize adequate protective antibody within the first week of ocular infection. Further support for this hypothesis is the protection obtained either by immunization with *Pseudomonas* lipopolysaccharide or by passive immunization of mice with monoclonal antibodies to *Pseudomonas* surface proteins, anti-elastase antibody, with immune sera from recovered DBA/2J or secondarily infected C57BL/6J mice.[56] Thus, the role of humoral immunity in ocular infections caused by *P. aeruginosa* is well-established and the differential murine response is under strict genetic control. However, recent preliminary studies from our laboratories suggest that one or more mouse strains may also restore corneal clarity in the absence of a humoral response to the whole organism. Future studies will concentrate on the mechanism by which this phenomenon occurs.

ACKNOWLEDGMENTS. These studies were supported by Public Health Service grant EY-01935 (R. S. Berk) and EY-02986 (L. D. Hazlett), the Core Vision grant P30-EY-04068, training grant T32-EY-07093 and in part by the Michigan Eye Bank.

REFERENCES

1. Berk, R. S., Hazlett, L. D., Potter, M., and Beisel, K. W., 1985, Multigenic regulation of natural resistance of the mouse cornea to *Pseudomonas aeruginosa*, in: *Genetic Control of Host Resistance to Infection and Malignancy, Progress in Leukocyte Biology*, Volume III (E. Skamene, ed.), Alan R. Liss, New York, pp. 367–372.
2. Biozzi, G., Mouton, D., Siqueira, M., and Stiffel, C., 1985, Effect of genetic modification of immune responsiveness on anti-infection and anti-tumor resistance, in: *Genetic Control of Host Resistance to Infection and Malignancy, Progress in Leukocyte Biology*, Volume III (E. Skamene, ed.), Alan R. Liss, New York, pp. 13–18.
3. McPherson, M. A., and Dormer, R. L., 1987, The molecular and biochemical basis of cystic fibrosis, *Biosci. Rep.* **7:**167–185.
4. McPherson, M. A., and Goodchild, M. C., 1988, The biochemical defect in cystic fibrosis, *Clin. Sci.* **74:**337–345.
5. Luzar, M. A., Thomassen, M. J., and Montie, T. C., 1985, Flagella and motility alterations in *Pseudomonas aeruginosa* strains from patients with cystic fibrosis: Relationship to patient clinical condition, *Infect. Immun.* **50:**577–582.
6. Pier, G. B., 1986, Pulmonary disease associated with *Pseudomonas aeruginosa* in cystic fibrosis: Current status of the host-bacterium interaction, *J. Infect. Dis.* **151:**575–580.
7. Houdret, N., Ramphal, R., Scharfman, A., Perini, J. M, Filliat, G., Lamblin, G., and Roussel, P., 1989, Evidence for the *in vivo* degradation of human respiratory mucins during *Pseudomonas aeruginosa* infection, *Biochem. Biophys. Acta.* **992:**96–105.
8. Nelson, J. W., Tredgett, M. W., Sheehan, J. K., Thornton, D. J., Notman, D., and Govan, J. R. W., 1990, Mucinophilic and chemotactic properties of *Pseudomonas aeruginosa* in relation to pulmonary colonization in cystic fibrosis, *Infect. Immun.* **58:**1489–1495.

9. Pennington, J. E., and Williams, R. M., 1979, Influence of genetic factors on natural resistance of mice to *Pseudomonas aeruginosa, J. Infect. Dis.* **139**:396–400.
10. Pier, G. B., 1982, Cross-protection by *Pseudomonas aeruginosa* polysaccharides, *Infect. Immun.* **38**:1117–1122.
11. Markham, R. B., and Pier, G. B., 1983, Characterization of the antibody response in inbred mice to high-molecular-weight polysaccharide from *Pseudomonas aeruginosa* immunotype 1, *Infect. Immun.* **41**:232–236.
12. Pier, G. B., and Markham, R. B., 1982, Induction in mice of cell-mediated immunity to *Pseudomonas aeruginosa* by high molecular weight polysaccharide and vinblastine, *J. Immunol.* **128**:2121–2125.
13. Markham, R. B., Goellner, J. B., and Pier, G. B., 1984, *In vitro* T cell-mediated killing of *Pseudomonas aeruginosa*. I. Evidence that a lymphokine mediates killing, *J. Immunol.* **133**:962–968.
14. Markham, R. B., Pier, G. B., Goellner, J. Y., and Mizel, S. B., 1985, *In vitro* T-cell mediated killing of *Pseudomonas aeruginosa*. II. The role of macrophages and T cell subsets in T cell killing, *J. Immunol.* **134**:4112–4117.
15. Powderly, W. G., Pier, G. B., and Markham, R. B., 1986, T lymphocyte-mediated protection against *Pseudomonas aeruginosa* in granulocytopenic mice. *J. Clin. Invest.* **78**:375–380.
16. Powderly, W. G., Pier, G. B., and Markham, R. B., 1986, *In vitro* T cell-mediated killing of *Pseudomonas aeruginosa*. III. The role of suppressor T cells in nonresponder mice, *J. Immunol.* **136**:299–303.
17. Sherman, L. A., 1982, Genetic linkage of the cytolytic T lymphocyte repertoire and immunoglobulin heavy chain genes, *J. Exp. Med.* **156**:294–299.
18. Sherman, L. A., and Riblet, R., 1985, Comparison of the H-2K^b-specific cytolytic T lymphocyte receptor repertoire in *Igh* recombinant strains, *J. Immunol.* **134**:3569–3573.
19. Owen, F. L., Riblet, R., and Taylor, B. A., 1981, The T suppressor cell alloantigen Tsu^d maps near immunoglobulin allotype genes and may be a heavy chain constant-region marker on a T cell receptor, *J. Exp. Med.* **153**:801–810.
20. Owen, F. L, and Riblet, R., 1984, Genes for the mouse T cell alloantigens Tpre, Tthy, Tind, and Tsu are closely linked near *Igh* on chromosome 12, *J. Exp. Med.* **159**:313–317.
21. Powderly, W. G., Pier, G. B., and Markham, R. B., 1986, *In vitro* T cell-mediated killing of *Pseudomonas aeruginosa*. IV. Nonresponsiveness in polysaccharide-immunized BALB/c mice is attributable to vinblastine-sensitive suppressor cells, *J. Immunol.* **137**:2025–2030.
22. Powderly, W. G., Pier, G. B., and Markham, R. B., 1987, *In vitro* T cell-mediated killing of *Pseudomonas aeruginosa*. V. Generation of bactericidal T cells in nonresponder cells, *J. Immunol.* **138**:2272–2277.
23. Markham, R. B., and Powderly, W. G., 1988, Exposure of mice to live *Pseudomonas aeruginosa* generates protective cell-mediated immunity in the absence of an antibody response, *J. Immunol.* **141**:2039–2045.
24. Markham, R. B., Pier, G. B., and Powderly, W., 1988, Suppressor T cells regulating the cell-mediated immune response to *Pseudomonas aeruginosa* can be generated by immunization with anti-bacterial T cells, *J. Immunol.* **141**:3975–3979.
25. Burns, R. P., and Rhodes, D. H., Jr., 1961, *Pseudomonas* eye infection as a cause of death in premature infants, *Arch. Opthalmol.* **65**:517–525.
26. Hazlett, L. D., Zelt, R., Cramer, C., and Berk, R. S., 1985, *Pseudomonas aeruginosa* induced ocular infection: A histopathological comparison of two strains of different virulence. *Ophthalmic Res.* **17**:289–296.
27. Twining, S. S., Lohr, K. M., and Moulder, J. E., 1986, The immune system in experimental *Pseudomonas* keratitis. Model and early effects, *Invest. Ophthalmol. Vis. Sci.* **27**:507–515.
28. Van Horn, D. L., Davis, S. D., Hyndiuk, R. A., and Pedersen, H. J., 1981, Experimental *Pseudomonas* keratitis in the rabbit: Bacteriological, clinical and microscopic observation, *Invest. Ophthalmol. Vis. Sci.* **20**:213–221.
29. Hazlett, L. D., Rosen, D., and Berk, R. S., 1976, Experimental eye infections caused by *Pseudomonas aeruginosa, Ophthalmic Res.* **8**:311–318.

30. Berk, R. S., Leon, M. A., and Hazlett, L. D., 1979, Genetic control of the murine corneal response to *Pseudomonas aeruginosa*, *Infect. Immun.* **26:**1221–1223.
31. Berk, R. S., Beisel, K. W., and Hazlett, L. D., 1981, Genetic studies of the murine corneal response to *Pseudomonas aeruginosa*, *Infect. Immun.* **34:**1–5.
32. Beisel, K. W., Hazlett, L. D., and Berk, R. S., 1983, Genetic studies on a dominant susceptibility effect on the murine corneal response to *Pseudomonas aeruginosa*, *Proc. Soc. Exp. Biol. Med.* **172:**488–491.
33. Berk, R. S., Hazlett, L. D., Potter, M., and Beisel, K. W., 1985, Multigenic regulation of natural resistance of the mouse cornea to *Pseudomonas aeruginosa*, in: *Genetic Control of Host Resistance to Infection and Malignancy*, Volume III (E. Skamene, ed.), Allan R. Liss, Inc., New York, pp. 367–372.
34. Berk, R. S., Hazlett, L. D., and Beisel, K. W., 1987, Genetic studies on resistant and susceptibility genes controlling the mouse cornea to infection with *Pseudomonas aeruginosa*, in *Antibiotics and Chemotherapy. Basic Research and Clinical Aspects of Pseudomonas aeruginosa*, Volume 39 (G. Döring, I. A. Holder, and K. Botzenhart, eds.), Karger, Basel, pp. 83–91.
35. Berk, R. S., Hazlett, L. D., and Beisel, K. W., 1989, Location of genes regulating resistance of the mouse cornea to *Pseudomonas aeruginosa* infection, in *Modern Trends in Immunology and Immunopathology of the Eye* (A. G. Secchi and I. A. Fregoni, eds.), Masson, Milan, pp. 123–127.
36. Hazlett, L. D., and Berk, R. S., 1978, Heightened resistance of athymic nude (nu/nu) mice to experimental *Pseudomonas aeruginosa* ocular infection, *Infect. Immun.* **22:**926–933.
37. Hirst, R. G., and Wallace, M. E., 1976, Inherited resistance to *Corynebacterium kutscheri* in mice, *Infect. Immun.* **14:**475–482.
38. Pierce-Chase, C. H., Fauve, R. M., and Dubos, R., 1964, Corynebacterial pseudotuberculosis in mice. I. Comparative susceptibility of mouse strains to experimental infection with *Corynebacterium kutscheri*, *J. Exp. Med.* **120:**267–284.
39. Closs, O., and Haugen, O. A., 1973, Experimental murine leprosy. I. Clinical and histological evidence for varying susceptibility of mice to infection with *Mycobacterium lepraemurium*, *Acta Pathol. Microbiol. Scand.* Sect. A, **81:**401–410.
40. Closs, O., and Haugen, O. A., 1974, Experimental murine leprosy. 2. Further evidence for varying susceptibility of outbred mice and evaluation of the response of 5 inbred mouse strains to infection with *Mycobacterium lepraemurium*, *Acta Pathol. Microbiol. Scand.* Sect. A, **82:**459–474.
41. Allen, E. M., Moore, V. L., and Stevens, J. O., 1977, Strain variation in BCG-induced chronic pulmonary inflammation in mice. I. Basic model and possible genetic control by non-H-2 genes, *J. Immunol.* **119:**343–347.
42. Cheers, C., and McKenzie, I. F. C., 1978, Resistance and susceptibility of mice to bacterial infection: Genetics of listeriosis, *Infect. Immun.* **19:**755–762.
43. Cheers, C., McKenzie, I. F. C., Pavlov, H., Waid, C., and York, J., 1978, Resistance and susceptibility of mice to bacterial infection: Course of listeriosis in resistant or susceptible mice, *Infect. Immun.* **19:**763–770.
44. Farr, A. G., Kiely, J.-J., and Unanue, E. R., 1979, Macrophage -T cell interactions involving *Listeria monocytogenes*—Role of the H-2 gene complex, *J. Immunol.* **122:**2395–2404.
45. Skamene, E., Kongshavn, P. A. L., and Sachs, D. H., 1979, Resistance to *Listeria monocytogenes* in mice: Genetic control by genes that are not linked to the H-2 complex, *J. Infect. Dis.* **139:**228–231.
46. Groves, M. G., and Osterman, J. V., 1978, Host defenses in experimental scrub typhus: Genetics of natural resistance to infection, *Infect. Immun.* **19:**583–588.
47. Anderson, Jr., G. W., and Osterman, J. V., 1980, Host defenses in experimental rickettsialpox: Genetics of natural resistance to infection, *Infect. Immun.* **28:**132–136.
48. Gowen, J. W., and Calhoun, M. L., 1943, Factors affecting genetic resistance of mice to mouse typhoid, *J. Infect. Dis.* **73:**40–56.
49. Plant, J., and Glynn, A. A., 1974, Natural resistance to *Salmonella* infection, delayed hypersensitivity and *Ir* genes in different strains of mice, *Nature* **248:**345–347.

50. Plant, J., and Glynn, A. A., 1976, Genetics of resistance to infection with *Salmonella typhimurium* in mice, *J. Infect. Dis.* **133**:72–78.
51. Robson, H. G., and Vas, S. I., 1972, Resistance of inbred mice to *Salmonella typhimurium*, *J. Infect. Dis.* **126**:378–386.
52. Lissner, C. R., Swanson, R. N., and O'Brien, A. D., 1983, Genetic control of the innate resistance of mice to *Salmonella typhimurium*: Expression of the *Ity* gene in peritoneal and splenic macrophages isolated *in vitro*, *J. Immunol.* **131**:3006–3013.
53. Bradley, D. H., Taylor, B. A., Blackwell, J., Evans, E. P., and Freeman, J., 1979, Regulation of leishmania populations within the host. III. Mapping of the locus controlling susceptibility to visceral leishmaniasis in the mouse, *Clin. Exp. Immunol.* **37**:7–14.
54. Brown, I. N., Glynn, A. A., and Plant, J., 1982, Inbred mouse strain resistance to *Mycobacterium lepraemurium* follows *Ity/Lsh* pattern, *Immunol.* **47**:149–156.
55. Skamene, E., Gros, P., Forget, A., Kongshavn, P. A. L., St. Charles, C., and Taylor, B. A., 1982, Genetic regulation of resistance to intracellular pathogens, *Nature* **297**:506–509.
56. Berk, R. S., Montgomery, I. N., and Hazlett, L. D., 1988, Serum antibody and ocular responses to murine corneal infection caused by *Pseudomonas aeruginosa*, *Infect. Immun.* **56**:3076–3080.
57. Cleveland, R. P., Hazlett, L. D., Leon, M. A., and Berk, R. S., 1983, The role of complement in *Pseudomonas* ocular infections, *Invest. Ophthalmol. Vis. Sci.* **24**:237–242.
58. Nilsson, U. R., and Muller-Eberhard, H. J., 1967, Deficiency of the fifth component of complement in mice with an inherited complement defect, *J. Exp. Med.* **125**:1–16.
59. Newman, K., Jr., and Johnson, R. C., 1981, *In vivo* evidence that an intact lytic complement pathway is not essential for successful removal of circulating *Borrelia turicatae* from mouse blood, *Infect. Immun.* **31**:465–469.
60. Mondino, B. J., Ratajczak, H. V., Goldberg, D. B., Schanzlin, D. J., and Brown, S. I., 1980, Alternate and classical pathway components of complement in the normal cornea, *Arch. Ophthalmol.* **98**:346–349.
61. Mondino, B. J., and Hoffman, D. B., 1980, Hemolytic complement activity in normal human donor corneas, *Arch. Ophthalmol.* **98**:2041–2044.
62. Mondino, B. J., Brown, S. I., Rabin, B. S., and Bruno, J., 1978, Alternate pathway activation of complement in a *Proteus mirabilis* ulceration of the cornea, *Arch. Ophthalmol.* **96**:1659–1661.
63. Hazlett, L. D., Rosen, D. D., and Berk, R. S., 1978, Age-related susceptibility to *Pseudomonas aeruginosa* ocular infections in mice, *Infect. Immun.* **20**:25–29.
64. Berk, R. S., Iglewski, B. H., and Hazlett, L. D., 1981, Age-related susceptibility of mice to ocular challenge with *Pseudomonas aeruginosa* exotoxin A, *Infect. Immun.* **33**:90–94.
65. Kreger, A. S., Lyerly, D. M., Hazlett, L. D., and Berk, R. S., 1986, Immunization against experimental *Pseudomonas aeruginosa* and *Serratia marcescens* keratitis: Vaccination with lipopolysaccharide endotoxins and proteases, *Invest. Ophthalmol. Vis. Sci.* **27**:932–939.
66. Moon, M. M., Hazlett, L. D., Hancock, R. E. W., Berk, R. S., and Barrett, R., 1988, Monoclonal antibodies provide protection against ocular *Pseudomonas aeruginosa* infection, *Invest. Ophthalmol. Vis. Sci.* **29**:1277–1284.
67. McMeel, J. W., and Wood, R. M., 1960, Passive immunization against pseudomonas infection of the cornea, *Trans. Am. Acad. Ophthalmol. Otolarnygol.* **64**:486–489.
68. Young, L. S., 1974, Role of antibody in infections due to *Pseudomonas aeruginosa*, *J. Infect. Dis.* **130**:S111–S118.
69. Cryz, S. J., Jr., Furer, E., and Germanier, R., 1983, Protection against *Pseudomonas aeruginosa* infection in a murine burn wound sepsis model by passive transfer of antitoxin A, antielastase, and antilipopolysaccharide, *Infect. Immun.* **39**:1072–1079.
70. Zweerink, H. J., Gammon, M. D., Hutchinson, C. F., Jackson, J. J., Pier, G. B., Puckett, J. M., Sewell, T. J., and Sigal, N. H., 1988, χ-linked immunodeficient mice as a model for testing the protective efficacy of monoclonal antibodies against *Pseudomonas aeruginosa*, *Infect. Immun.* **56**:1209–1214.

71. Lopez, C., 1975, Genetics of natural resistance to herpes virus infections in mice, *Nature* **258:** 152–153.
72. Kirkland, T. N., and Fierer, J., 1983, Inbred mouse strains differ in resistance to lethal *Coccidioides immitis* infection, *Infect. Immun.* **40:**912–916.
73. Wassom, D. L., David, C. S., and Gleich, G. J., 1979, Genes within the major histocompatibility complex influence susceptibility to *Trichinella spiralis* in the mouse, *Immunogenetics* **9:**491–496.
74. Lissner, C. R., Weinstein, D. L., and O'Brien, A. D., 1985, Mouse chromosome 1 *Ity* locus regulates microbicidal activity of isolated peritoneal macrophages against a diverse group of intracellular and extracellular bacteria, *J. Immunol.* **135:**544–547.
75. Groves, M. G., Rosenstreich, D. K., Taylor, B. A., and Osterman, J. V., 1980, Host defenses in experimental scrub typhus: Mapping the gene that controls natural resistance in mice, *J. Immunol.* **125:**1395–1399.

11

Effects of *Pseudomonas aeruginosa* on Immune Functions

MARIO CAMPA, PAOLA MARELLI, and ANTONELLA LUPETTI

1. INTRODUCTION

The ubiquitous distribution of *Pseudomonas aeruginosa* contrasts with its limited colonizing potential for healthy individuals. Despite the fact that *P. aeruginosa* is able to produce a large variety of virulence factors, this microorganism undoubtedly remains an opportunistic pathogen that can infect and eventually cause disease only in patients with defects in local or systemic immunity.

Once given the opportunity to initiate the infectious process, cell-associated and secreted products of the microorganism are capable of impairing host defense mechanisms. This chapter will focus on this aspect of *P. aeruginosa*-host interactions.

MARIO CAMPA, PAOLA MARELLI, and ANTONELLA LUPETTI • Department of Biomedicine, Clinical Microbiology Section, University of Pisa, 56127 Pisa, Italy.

Pseudomonas aeruginosa as an Opportunistic Pathogen, edited by Mario Campa et al. Plenum Press, New York, 1993.

2. INTERFERENCE WITH NONSPECIFIC IMMUNE DEFENSE MECHANISMS

P. aeruginosa can infect virtually any part of the body.[1] To establish infection and eventually cause disease, this microorganism must compete with the autochthonous microflora of the mucosal surface, gain access to susceptible cells, attach to them, persist, multiply, and reach a critical mass to completely express its pathogenic determinants.

P. aeruginosa is one of the earliest microorganisms recognized to produce substances with antibiotic activity on the other bacteria.[2,3] Such substances are the phenazine pigments, of which pyocyanine is the most active and extensively studied. The antibiotic effect of pyocyanine, owing to its interference with bacterial respiration (reviewed in Chapter 3), and that of other phenazine pigments appear to be critically important for *P. aeruginosa* to compete with microorganisms present in its natural environment, the soil.[4] Pyocyanine has also been proven to markedly inhibit the growth of several human pathogens and commensals, as described in detail by Sorensen and Joseph in Chapter 3.

Pyocyanine also slows down the beating of human nasal ciliated epithelial cells *in vitro*[5] and affects the tracheal mucus velocity *in vivo*.[6] Thus, it appears that pyocyanine would favor *P. aeruginosa* colonization by inhibiting the growth of the autochthonous microflora or, as in the case of the respiratory tract, by also inducing a suppression of ciliary beating. The latter is also caused by glycolipids called rhamnolipids,[7] which appear to be secreted only by *P. aeruginosa* among the gram-negative microorganisms.[4,8,9] However, pyocyanine is produced by approximately 50% of all clinical isolates[10] and *in vitro* is secreted extensively only after the exponential phase of growth,[11] although a limited production of the pigment seems to take place throughout bacterial growth.[3] The regulatory mechanisms of phenazine pigment production *in vitro* have been thoroughly investigated,[3,4] (see also Chapter 3), whereas little is known of such mechanisms *in vivo*, at the site of infection. Therefore, at the present time, the role of phenazine pigments in the colonization process by *P. aeruginosa* is largely speculative.

The initial event in infection is the adherence of microorganisms to epithelial cells of mucosal surfaces. *In vitro* and *in vivo* studies have shown that *P. aeruginosa* may adhere to epithelial cells,[12,13] to cilia[14] or to tracheobronchial mucins[15] as described in detail by Irvin in Chapter 2. Although the polar pili are the most extensively studied adhesins of *P. aeruginosa*[12,13] (see also Chapter 2), other bacterial components may play a role in adhesion, such as the glycocalyx, which characterizes the mucoid strains of *P. aeruginosa* often present in the sputum of cystic fibrosis patients. The glycocalyx consists of acetylated heteropolymers of mannuronic and guluronic acid similar to seaweed alginate.[16] Bacterial alginate may mediate the binding of *P. aeruginosa* to human epithelial cells[17] (and Chapter 2) and exoenzyme S (exo-S) has recently been reported to act as an adhesin.[18] Studies regarding epithelial cell receptors mediating *P. aeruginosa* adherence seem to show that they are glycolipids.[19]

A variety of host factors may also influence bacterial adherence. Because *P. aeruginosa* prefers damaged cell surfaces for adhesion, host proteases may favor the bacterium adherence and reduce its clearance by altering the epithelial cell surface through the cleavage of the fibronectin coating[20,21] and/or by inhibiting ciliary beat frequency in the case of mucosal ciliated epithelium.[22] Furthermore, mechanical trauma, acid injury, and foregoing infections significantly enhance *P. aeruginosa* adhesion.[23,24]

P. aeruginosa secretes two distinct proteolytic enzymes termed elastase and alkaline protease, with elastase the more active and abundant. Several studies have documented the ability of purified elastase to degrade a number of biologically important molecules including laminin, fibrin and human collagens, epithelial junctions, transferrin, immunoglobulins, complement components, and receptors on immunocompetent cells (see Chapters 6, 7, 8, and 13). Other substances with enzymatic activity directed mainly against cell membrane components are secreted by *P. aeruginosa*, such as phospholipase C-H, phospholipase C-N, lipase, and alkaline phosphatase (see Chapters 6, 7, 8, and 13). All these exoproducts, acting individually and in concert, in addition to the breakdown of anatomic barriers and the consequent availability of nutrients to the microorganism at the site of infection, may provide denuded cells for *P. aeruginosa* adhesion by altering their surface either directly or through the activation of host proteases, mainly polymorphonuclear leucocyte (PMN) elastase (see Chapters 6 and 13).

Once a pathogen has initiated the infectious process by attaching to a mucosal surface, it must then be capable of replicating on the surface. Nonspecific immune defense mechanisms are the first barrier of the host to the growth of an infectious agent on mucosal surfaces. Iron-binding proteins such as lactoferrin and transferrin are examples of such nonspecific host defenses.[25-27] The body contains iron far in excess, but its availability is restricted by iron-binding compounds. Iron is an essential requirement for bacterial growth. In addition to protease-mediated cleavage of transferrin (see Chapter 13), *P. aeruginosa* can easily overcome the host ability to withhold iron by responding to iron starvation both with the excretion of iron chelators known as siderophores, the best characterized of which are pyochelin and pyoverdin,[28,29] and with the production of a number of surface proteins that seem to be involved in iron uptake[30,31] in the form of iron-siderophore complexes.[32-34] Moreover, alginate may act as an iron-exchange resin allowing concentration of iron and siderophores as well as other essential nutrients around the microorganism[35] and, thus, favoring iron uptake.[34]

Whereas *P. aeruginosa* promotes its attachment and replication on mucosal surfaces through a number of exoproducts, the inflammatory reaction of the host, first by itself and subsequently in concert with the immune response, operates to eliminate the invading microorganism. Recent studies showing that pyocyanine markedly enhances the secretion of interleukin 1 (IL-1) and tumor necrosis factor by human monocytes activated by lipopolysaccharide (LPS)[36] demonstrate that this phenazine pigment contributes to the induction of the inflammatory reaction. Exotoxin A (ETA) may also stimulate the production of IL-1 by murine peritoneal macrophages,[37] and phospholipase C can cause the release of inflammatory mediators from rat peritoneal mast cells and human granulocytes[38] and may induce inflammatory reactions in mice.[39] Furthermore, by triggering the human Hageman factor-dependent activation of kinin cascade, *P. aeruginosa* elastase enhances inflammation.[40,41] However, endotoxin has long been considered the best characterized bacterial component able to elicit host inflammatory response.[42] Such a response might appear to be detrimental to the parasite, because several host defense factors come into play: phagocytic cells, mainly PMN, complement and specific antibodies at later phases of the infectious process. However, it might create a better "milieu" for *P. aeruginosa* to grow and glycolipid receptors mediating the adherence of the microorganism to epithelial cells can be exposed during inflammatory events, thus facilitating bacterial replication and colonization.

Phagocytic cells include PMN and mononuclear phagocytes; the latter consist of circulating monocytes and tissue macrophages. Tissue macrophages represent the first line of defense at local sites, but the inflammatory reaction soon leads to the immigration of PMN into the site of infection. The strongest chemotaxigenic compound of *P. aeruginosa* for PMN is LPS,[43] although activated complement components are also important chemotactins.[44] A prompt recruitment of PMN is of major importance in the case of *P. aeruginosa* infection, because human PMN phagocytose and kill this microorganism more efficiently than macrophages do.[45] Parasites, including *P. aeruginosa*, can be phagocytosed in the absence of opsonins and this phenomenon is known as nonopsonic phagocytosis. Opsonins, the most active and best-characterized of which are complement and specific antibodies, greatly enhance (the so-called opsonic) phagocytosis of *P. aeruginosa*. These and other aspects of *P. aeruginosa*-phagocytic cell interactions have been reviewed by Speert in Chapter 9. Complement plays a central role among the nonspecific host defense mechanisms against *P. aeruginosa*: At the beginning of infection it can be activated via the alternative pathway and may promote phagocytosis and killing of the microorganism in the absence of specific opsonic antibodies (Chapter 9). Additionally, complement may cause direct lysis of *P. aeruginosa* especially of strains expressing a rough type of LPS (see Chapter 9). When the immune response arises, specific antibodies potentiate phagocytosis of the microorganism and polyclonal and monoclonal IgG, IgM, and IgA have all been found to be opsonic. Complement enhances the opsonic activity of IgG but has no effect on IgA activity; IgM requires full complement activity to be effective (see Chapter 9).

Most of the exoproducts of *P. aeruginosa* may aid the microorganism to overcome the host antimicrobial defense mechanisms discussed above. Thus, bacterial proteases have been found to inhibit human PMN chemotaxis;[46] they may further impair *P. aeruginosa* clearance by interfering with opsonic phagocytosis of the microorganism through the proteolytic breakdown of specific antibodies[47-49] and/or complement components.[50] Certain strains of *P. aeruginosa* produce a cytotoxin with specific activity against PMN;[51] this leukocidin, a 27-kD protein having a periplasmic localization,[52] affects motility, phagocytic as well as microbicidal capacity of PMN[51,53] and, at higher concentrations, it lyses such cells.[53,54] A secreted protein of 65 kD has been shown to affect chemotaxis and the uptake and killing activities of rabbit PMN.[55] An extracellular *P. aeruginosa* glycolipoprotein, loosely associated with the cell wall and designed as slime by Liu,[9] also interferes with motility and phagocytic activity of human PMN[56] and causes leukopenia and death when administered intraperitoneally to mice.[57] An antiphagocytic activity has been proposed for alginate as well;[58,59] PMN chemotaxis[60] and the uptake capacity of rabbit and human PMN[59] are strongly impaired by this compound. More recently, it has been suggested that alginate may prevent *P. aeruginosa* elimination by phagocytic cells by enlarging the bacterial volume several times, which would then exceed the size of single PMN.[61] Human PMN exposed *in vitro* to rhamnolipids also exhibit a reduced chemotaxis.[62] Finally, ETA is highly toxic for human macrophages[63] and suppresses granulocyte–macrophage progenitor cells in bone marrow cultures.[64]

Even after ingestion by phagocytes, *P. aeruginosa* is capable of influencing their oxidative metabolism and, therefore, their microbicidal activity. Indeed, bacterial proteases inhibit superoxide anion production[46] and myeloperoxidase-mediated chemiluminescence in human PMN.[65] Inhibitory effects on the PMN generation of reactive oxygen radicals are also exerted by alginate,[66] slime,[56] and rhamnolipids.[62] By contrast, the interference of pyocyanine with the oxidative metabolism of PMN *in vitro* is variable, ranging from inhibition at high concentrations to enhancement at low concentrations (Chapter 3). Assuming that similar variations take place *in vivo* as well, high concentrations of pyocyanine leading to low rate of superoxide generation would prevent *P. aeruginosa* killing and oxygen radical-mediated tissue damage, whereas low concentrations would increase the microbicidal activity of PMN by enhancing the formation of reactive oxygen radicals which may, conversely, give rise to more severe tissue injury. Since no clear-cut data are available demonstrating that oxygen radicals are bactericidal for *P. aeruginosa*, whereas more and more data suggest that *P. aeruginosa* killing is primarily due to lysosomal enzyme activity, pyocyanine may be beneficial or detrimental to the host depending upon its concentration within PMN (see Chapters 3 and 9). Thus, focused studies will be necessary both to firmly establish whether or not oxidative bactericidal mechanisms are important in killing *P. aeruginosa in vitro* and *in vivo* and to develop useful methods to measure pyocyanine concentration inside phagocytic cells during infection. These studies would be of great significance also in view of the fact that pyocyanine may lead to suppression of the immune responsiveness (see section 3) and that this pigment and rhamnolipids are not antigenic owing to their small molecular size; therefore, they are ideal candidates to escape the immune response and to favor *P. aeruginosa* persistence.

From all the results discussed in this section, one can conclude that *P. aeruginosa* is well-equipped to promote its adhesion to mucosal surfaces, to overcome host nonspecific immune defenses, to replicate, and to establish local infection. However, because most of the relevant findings derive from *in vitro* studies, the precise role and relative importance of proteases, cytotoxins, alginate, slime, ETA, exo-S, rhamnolipids, and pyocyanine in tissue invasion are only beginning to be understood.

3. INTERFERENCE WITH SPECIFIC IMMUNE DEFENSE MECHANISMS

It is generally accepted that antibody-mediated opsonophagocytic killing is the major acquired resistance mechanism against *P. aeruginosa*. This view is strongly supported by the markedly increased susceptibility to *P. aeruginosa* infection in patients neutropenic as a result of acute leukemia or other neoplastic diseases and related therapy. Further support of this view comes from the observation that reduced phagocytic cell numbers together with low levels of antibodies are the major determinants of *P. aeruginosa* bacteremia in patients with severe burns. These and other aspects of *P. aeruginosa* infection in burned hosts are described in detail in Chapter 14.

Several *P. aeruginosa* antigens have been claimed to elicit antibodies mediating acquired resistance to infection, but none of those tested so far has proved to be fully "protective", as described in Chapters 15 and 17.

T-cell-mediated immunity (CMI) has long been thought to play a marginal role, if any, in resistance to extracellular parasites. Several studies have been conducted *in vitro* and *in vivo* to establish whether CMI is involved in controlling *P. aeruginosa* infection. Both delayed-type hypersensitivity reactions[67–69] and T-cell-mediated protection (see Chapter 15) have been demonstrated in experimental animals. Recently, such protection has been shown most likely to be mediated by antibody-dependent activation of bactericidal effector T cells.[70] Of particular note in this context is the finding that ETA may act both as a T-cell mitogen and as a polyclonal activator of cytolytic T lymphocytes in mice.[71] No evidence shows that CMI is important against *P. aeruginosa* infection in humans, even though the whole microorganism and its constituents are capable of activating human T lymphocytes[72,73] in an antigenic manner.[74,75] The correlation between increased mortality caused by *P. aeruginosa* and loss of T-cell-mediated immune functions such as skin test responsiveness to tuberculin, mumps, streptokinase–streptodornase, and of mixed lymphocyte culture responsiveness in burn patients[76] support the view that CMI plays a role in acquired resistance to this microorganism in humans.

Collectively, these results indicate that, whereas antibodies to *P. aeruginosa* are undoubtedly relevant to immunoprotection, specific T cells can also limit bacterial growth. However, the actual mechanism underlying protective immunity to *P. aeruginosa* still remains weakly defined.

In the early 1970s, several observations drew attention to the immunosuppressive capacities of *P. aeruginosa*. These include: (1) prolonged survival of skin homografts in patients with extensive burns associated with *P. aeruginosa* sepsis;[77] (2) depression of the tuberculin reaction and delayed rejection of skin homografts in experimental animals given bacterial fractions from *P. aeruginosa*;[77,78] and (3) decline in renal function in a kidney transplant patient when a persistent *P. aeruginosa* urinary tract infection was treated with polymyxin B.[79]

The indications of these early reports have been confirmed and extended by a series of *in vivo* and *in vitro* studies. Thus, it has been shown that the antibody response of mice injected with *P. aeruginosa* can be increased, unmodified, or depressed depending upon the dose of injected bacteria, the time interval between bacterial injection and immunization, and the type of antigen used.[80] Mice experimentally infected with *P. aeruginosa* in the kidney exhibit impaired host versus graft reactions and *in vitro* lymphocyte hyporeactivity to Con A.[81] Moreover, in mice, *P. aeruginosa* infection inhibited contact sensitivity to oxazolone, delayed-type hypersensitivity reaction, when infection is carried out at the same time as sensitization or 24–48 hr before.[82] Simultaneous depression of contact sensitivity to oxazolone and potentiation of antibody production to T-dependent and T-independent antigens has also been observed in *P. aeruginosa*-infected mice.[82,83] Suppression of contact sensitivity was discovered to be mediated by B lymphocytes,[82,84,85] which were found to adoptively transfer such suppression from *P. aeruginosa*-infected mice to syngeneic recipients[84] and to interfere with cell cooperation in the inductive phase of this cellular immune response.[85,86] It has also been suggested that such cells exert their suppressive effect through the production of antibodies that bind to the antigen and, thus, prevent it from reaching antigen-reactive T lymphocytes.[87] Furthermore, since *P. aeruginosa* is a polyclonal B-cell activator,[80] the possibility exists that this microorganism inhibits the development of contact sensitivity to oxazolone by additional cellular mechanisms similar to the ones induced by other polyclonal B-cell activators and shown to mediate the depression of this response in mice. Various types of cells have been described to take part in such a phenomenon. In particular, idiotype-positive anti-oxazolone B lymphocytes arising early after sensitization generate anti-idiotype B lymphocytes. These cells, in turn, activate T suppressor cells, which affect the efferent phase of the immune response.[88–90] The determining factor for the generation of this complex circuit appears to be the ability of the inducing stimulus, be it a microorganism or a bacterial constituent, to bring about polyclonal B-cell activation.[89,90] Cutaneous anergy to the purified protein derivative of tuberculin, and impaired granulomatous response observed in mice infected intravenously with large doses of *Mycobacterium bovis* strain BCG, have been reported to be due, at least in part, to a similar network of interactions among idiotype-positive B lymphocytes, anti-idiotype B lymphocytes and T lymphocytes.[91,92] Interestingly, it has been described that, in mice, the development of T-cell-mediated immunity to *P. aeruginosa* is controlled by complex idiotype network interactions. In particular, antigen-specific B lymphocytes induce contrasuppressor T lymphocytes which, in turn, counteract the effect of T suppressor lymphocytes leading to a potentiation of the antibacterial T-cell response[93] (see also Chapter 15).

Evidence is clear that other types of cells are involved in the *P. aeruginosa*-induced suppression of the host immune reactivity. For example, *P. aeruginosa* can induce monocytes to suppress the *in vitro* proliferative response of human T lymphocytes to the microorganism itself.[94] In mice, *P. aeruginosa* has been found to inhibit two T-cell-mediated responses, anti-*Listeria monocytogenes* immunity, and delayed-type hypersensitivity to sheep erythrocytes, by activating suppressor macrophages.[95] T suppressor cells may also arise during *P. aeruginosa* infection[93,96] (and Chapter 15).

A derangement of the immune response may be brought about by some of the same cell-associated and extracellular products of *P. aeruginosa* that, as discussed above, appear to allow the microorganism to bypass the host nonspecific immune defenses. Indeed, *in vitro* studies have shown that, at certain concentrations, pyocyanine suppresses mitogenic response, interleukin 2 (IL-2) production and expression of IL-2 receptors by human T lymphocytes, and immunoglobulin synthesis by human B lymphocytes[36,97] (see Chapter 3).

P. aeruginosa alkaline protease and elastase inhibit the *in vitro* mitogenic response of human lymphocytes, possibly by causing proteolytic breakdown of IL-2 before it binds to its receptors.[98] In addition, these enzymes selectively cleave CD4 marker on human lymphocytes without exerting any effect on the CD3, CD5, and CD8 markers and on class I and II MHC antigens.[99] Alkaline protease and elastase degrade human interferon-γ which looses its antiviral and macrophage-activating properties; elastase is less active than alkaline protease and in the presence of human serum,[100] in large part because of the serum protease inhibitor α-2-macroglobulin.[100,101] Elastase and alkaline protease also suppress the activity of human natural killer cells *in vitro* by inhibiting their binding to target cells, most likely as a result of proteolytic cleavage of the surface receptors involved.[102] However, the role of such cells in *P. aeruginosa* infection is far from clear.

A direct degradation of specific antibodies[47–49] (see also Chapter 14), represents an additional mechanism whereby proteases may affect host defenses. In a series of articles, Holt and Misfeldt have demonstrated in euthymic *nu/+* mice that ETA, administered before immunization, suppresses *in vitro* and *in vivo* antibody production to both T-dependent and T-independent antigens. T suppressor lymphocytes were implicated in such a phenomenon.[96] By contrast, ETA can enhance these responses in athymic *nu/nu* mice.[96,103] More recently, the interference of ETA with immune reactivity through stimulation of IL-1 production by macrophages has also been reported.[37] Finally, LPS is one of the earliest chemically well-characterized bacterial constituents that have been recognized to dramatically perturb host defense mechanisms (reviewed in ref. 87).

Evidence has been provided that, in mice, *P. aeruginosa* infection may lead to polyclonal activation of B-cell clones, including self-reactive B lymphocytes. The induction of these autoreactive B cells seems to be due to the differentiation of precursor cells into cells actively producing autoantibodies virtually in the absence of cell proliferation.[104] Similar effects are exerted by other polyclonal B-cell activators such as *E. coli* LPS and the purified protein derivative of tuberculin.[105-107] Moreover, it has been shown that three major outer membrane proteins of the bacterium are B-cell mitogens in mice[108] and that slime exerts a mitogenic effect on human lymphocytes.[109] These findings might have great importance in clinical situations such as cystic fibrosis (CF), in which *P. aeruginosa* chronic infections occur. Specific antibodies against antigenic exoproducts and cell-associated antigens of *P. aeruginosa* have been detected in sera of *P. aeruginosa*-infected CF patients (reviewed in ref. 110). Moreover, bacterial elastase and alkaline protease, the involvement of which is well documented in lung pathology, can be detected in the sputum and bronchial lavages of CF patients at early phases of infection before specific antibodies are produced;[111] in later phases, they are no longer detectable as such, but rather as immune complexes.[112] Circulating immune complexes containing antibodies against *P. aeruginosa* have also been found in such patients.[113] These findings clearly indicate that the specific antibody response is not impaired in CF patients. Nonetheless, *P. aeruginosa* infection persists, PMN are stimulated persistently, and consequent PMN-released lysosomal enzymes may cause devastating lung lesions. As a result, a self-antigen might arise and *P. aeruginosa* might potentiate autoantibody production against that antigen, leading to more severe tissue damage.

P. aeruginosa infection has also been shown to disturb the circulation of antigen-reactive lymphocytes in oxazolone-sensitized mice, as a consequence of the enhanced trapping of these cells within the lymph nodes that drain the sites of sensitization.[114,115] Thus, an altered pattern of lymphocyte distribution may represent an additional mechanism by which *P. aeruginosa* interferes with the host immune reactivity.

The results presented in this section suggest that the ability of *P. aeruginosa* to suppress specific immune functions is the outcome of cumulative effects and multiple targets of the bacterial cell-associated and extracellular products. Thus, the immunosuppressive activity figures prominently among the virulence factors of *P. aeruginosa* and it is generally thought to be a key factor allowing the switch from acute to chronic infection and/or the dissemination of the microorganism from a localized infection.

4. CONCLUDING REMARKS

P. aeruginosa is ubiquitous in nature and is able to adapt to changing ecologic circumstances owing to its minimal growth requirements and nutritional versatility. In addition, it is resistant to several antibiotics and, thus, has selective advantages in modern hospital environments (reviewed in ref. 116). Despite these features the extraordinary potential of *P. aeruginosa* to overcome the host-specific and nonspecific immune barriers, the frequency of infection by this microorganism in immunologically intact humans is lower than one would expect. The fact that a variety of agents such as antibiotics, steroids, and interferon are capable of inhibiting the expression of *P. aeruginosa* exoproducts does not seem a sufficient explanation. We must necessarily be missing important elements of the relationship between the host and the parasite. One of these elements might be the host genetic background and susceptibility, which are being explored at present as described in Chapter 10. Modern molecular biology techniques should eventually allow a better understanding of the means whereby *P. aeruginosa* causes human disease.

REFERENCES

1. Pollack, M., 1990, *Pseudomonas aeruginosa*, in: *Principles and Practice of Infectious Diseases* (G.L. Mandell, L.G. Douglas, and J.E. Bennett, eds.), Churchill Livingston, New York, pp. 1673–1691.
2. Schoental, R., 1941, The nature of the antibacterial agents present in *Pseudomonas pyocyanea* cultures, *Br. J. Exp. Pathol.* **22**:137–147.
3. Ingram, J. M., and Blackwood, A. C., 1970, Microbial production of phenazines, *Adv. Appl. Microbiol.* **13**:267–282.
4. Leisinger, T., and Margraff, R., 1979, Secondary metabolites of the fluorescent pseudomonads, *Microbiol. Rev.* **43**:422–442.
5. Wilson, R., Pitt, T., Taylor, G., Watson, D., Mac Dermot, J., Sykes, D., Roberts, D., and Cole, P., 1987, Pyocyanin and 1-hydroxyphenazine produced by *Pseudomonas aeruginosa* inhibit the beating of human respiratory cilia *in vitro*, *J. Clin. Invest.* **79**:221–229.
6. Munro, N., Barker, A., Rutman, A., Taylor, G., Watson, D., Mac Donald-Gibson, W., Towart, R., Taylor, W., Wilson, R., and Cole, P., 1989, Effect of pyocyanin and 1-hydroxyphenazine on *in vivo* tracheal mucus velocity, *J. Appl. Physiol.* **67**:316–323.
7. Hingley, S. T., Hastie, A. T., Kueppers, F., Higgins, M. L., Weinbaum, G., and Shryock, T., 1986, Effect of ciliostatic factors from *Pseudomonas aeruginosa* on rabbit respiratory cilia, *Infect. Immun.* **51**:254–262.
8. Hauser, G., and Karnovsky, M. L., 1954, Studies on the production of glycolipide by *Pseudomonas aeruginosa*, *J. Bacteriol.* **68**:645–654.
9. Liu, P. V., 1974, Extracellular toxins of *Pseudomonas aeruginosa*, *Infect. Dis.* **130**:S94–S99.

10. Knight, M., Hartman, P. E., Hartman, Z., and Young, V. M., 1979, A new method of preparation of pyocyanine and demonstration of an unusual bacterial sensitivity, *Anal. Biochem.* **95**:19–23.
11. Wooley, M. A., and Mc Longhlin, A. S., 1982, The regulation of pyocyanine production in *Pseudomonas aeruginosa*, *Eur. J. Appl. Microbiol. Biotechnol.* **15**:161–166.
12. Woods, D. E., Straus, D. C., Johanson, W. G., Jr, Berry, V. K., and Bass, J. A., 1980, Role of pili in adherence of *Pseudomonas aeruginosa* to mammalian buccal epithelial cells, *Infect. Immun.* **29**:1146–1151.
13. Ramphal, R., Sadoff, J. C., Pyle, M., and Silipigni, J. D., 1984, Role of pili in adherence of *Pseudomonas aeruginosa* to injured tracheal epithelium, *Infect. Immun.* **44**:38–40.
14. Baker, N., and Marcus, H., 1980, Adherence of clinical isolates of *Pseudomonas aeruginosa* to hamster tracheal epithelium *in vitro*, *Curr. Microbiol.* **7**:35–40.
15. Vishwanath, S., and Ramphal, R., 1985, Tracheobronchial mucins receptor for *Pseudomonas aeruginosa*: Predominance of amino sugars in binding sites, *Infect. Immun.* **48**:331–335.
16. Linker, A., and Jones, R. S., 1966, A new polysaccharide resembling alginic acid isolated from pseudomonads, *J. Biol. Chem.* **241**:3845–3851.
17. Doig, P., Smith, N. R., Todd, T., and Irvin, R. T., 1987, Characterization of the binding of *Pseudomonas aeruginosa* alginate to human epithelial cells, *Infect. Immun.* **55**:1517–1522.
18. Baker, N. R., Mino F. V., Deal, C., Shahrabadi, M.S., Simpson, D. A., and Woods, D. E., 1991, *Pseudomonas aeruginosa* exoenzyme-S is an adhesin, *Infect. Immun.* **59**:2859–2863.
19. Baker, N., and Svanborg-Eden, C., 1989, Role of alginate in the adherence of *Pseudomonas aeruginosa*, *Antibiot. Chemother.* **42**:72–79.
20. Woods, D. E., Straus, D. C., Johanson, W. G., Jr., and Bass J. A., 1981, Role of fibronectin in the prevention of adherence of *Pseudomonas aeruginosa* to buccal cells, *J. Infect. Dis.* **143**:784–789.
21. Suter, S., Shaad, U. B., Morgenthaler, J. J., Chevallier, I., and Schnebli, H. P., 1988, Fibronectin-cleaving activity in bronchial secretions of patients with cystic fibrosis, *J. Infect. Dis.* **158**:89–100.
22. Smallman, L. A., Hill, S. L., and Stockley, R. A., 1984, Reduction of ciliary beat frequency *in vitro* by sputum from patients with bronchiectasis: A serine proteinase effect, *Thorax* **39**:663–667.
23. Ramphal, R., Small, P. A., Shands, J. W., Jr., Fischlsweiger, W., and Small, P. A., Jr., 1980, Adherence of *Pseudomonas aeruginosa* to tracheal cells injured by influenza infection or by endotracheal intubation, *Infect. Immun.* **27**:614–619.
24. Ramphal, R., and Pyle, M., 1983, Adhesion of mucoid and non-mucoid *Pseudomonas aeruginosa* to acid-injured tracheal epithelium, *Infect. Immun.* **41**:345–351.
25. Weinberg, E. D., 1978, Iron and Infection, *Microbiol. Rev.* **42**:45–66.
26. Payne, S. M., and Finkelstein, R. A., 1978, The critical role of iron in host-bacterial interactions, *J. Clin. Invest.* **61**:1428–1440.
27. Bullen, J. J., 1981, The significance of iron in infection, *Rev. Infect. Dis.* **3**:1127–1137.
28. Liu, P. V., and Shokrani, F., 1978, Biological activities of pyochelins: Iron-chelating agents of *Pseudomonas aeruginosa*, *Infect. Immun.* **22**:878–890.
29. Cox, C. D., Rinehart, K. L., Moore, M. L., and Cook, J. C., 1981, Pyochelin: Novel structure of an iron-chelating growth promoter for *Pseudomonas aeruginosa*, *Proc. Natl. Acad. Sci USA* **78**:4256–4260.
30. Meyer, J. M., Mock, M., and Abdullah, M. A., 1970, Effect of iron on the protein composition of the outer membrane of fluorescent pseudomonads, *FEMS Microbiol. Lett.* **5**:395–398.
31. Ohkawa, I. Shiga, S., and Kageyama, M., 1980, Effect of iron concentration in the growth medium on the sensitivity of *Pseudomonas aeruginosa* to pyocin S2, *J. Biochem.* **87**:323–331.
32. Sokol, P. A., and Woods, D. E., 1983, Demonstration of an iron-siderophore-binding protein in the outer membrane of *Pseudomonas aeruginosa*, *Infect. Immun.* **40**:665–669.

33. Sokol, P. A., 1984, Production of the ferripyochelin outer membrane receptor by *Pseudomonas* species, *FEMS Microbiol. Lett.* **23**:313–317.
34. Cox, C. D., 1985, Iron transport and serum resistance in *Pseudomonas aeruginosa*, *Antibiot. Chemother.* **36**:1–12.
35. Costerton, J. W., Brown, M. R. W., and Sturgess, J. M., 1979, The cell envelope: Its role in infection, in: *Pseudomonas aeruginosa: Clinical Manifestations of Infection and Current Therapy* (R. G. Doggett, ed.), Academic Press, London, pp. 41–62.
36. Ulmer, A. J., Pryjma, J., Tarnok, Z., Ernst, M., and Flad, H. D., 1990, Inhibitory and stimulatory effects of *Pseudomonas aeruginosa* pyocyanine on human T and B lymphocytes and human monocytes, *Infect. Immun.* **58**:808–815.
37. Misfeldt, M. L., Legaard, P. K., Howell, S. E., Fornella, M. H., and Legrand, R. D., 1990, Induction of interluekin-1 from murine peritoneal macrophages by *Pseudomonas aeruginosa* exotoxin A, *Infect. Immun.* **58**:978–982.
38. Bergmann, U., Scheffer, J., Köller, M., Schönfeld, W., Erbs, G., Müller, F. E., and König, W., 1989, Induction of inflammatory mediators (histamine and leukotrienes) from rat peritoneal mast cells and human granulocytes by *Pseudomonas aeruginosa* strains from burn patients, *Infect. Immun.* **57**:2187–2195.
39. Meyers, D. J., and Berk, R. S., 1990, Characterization of phospholipase C from *Pseudomonas aeruginosa* as a potent inflammatory agent, *Infect. Immun.* **58**:659–666.
40. Holder, I. A., and Neely A. N., 1989, *Pseudomonas* elastase acts as a virulence factor in burned hosts by Hageman factor-dependent activation of the host kinin cascade, *Infect. Immun.* **57**:3345–3348.
41. Yamamoto, T., Shibuya, Y., Nishino, N., Okabe, H., and Kambara, T., 1990, Activation of human Hageman factor by *Pseudomonas aeruginosa* elastase in the presence or absence of negatively charged substances *in vitro*, *Biochim. Biophys. Acta* **1038**:231–239.
42. Pitt, T. L., 1989, Lipopolysaccharide and virulence of *Pseudomonas aeruginosa*, *Antibiot. Chemother.* **42**:1–7.
43. Kharazmi, A., Schiotz, P. O., Høiby, N., Baeck, L., and Döring, G., 1986, Demonstration of neutrophil chemotactic activity in the sputum of cystic fibrosis patients with *Pseudomonas aeruginosa* infection, *Eur. J. Clin. Invest.* **16**:143–148.
44. Schiotz, P. O., Sorensen, H., and H·iby, N., 1979, Activated complement in the sputum from patients with cystic fibrosis, *Acta Pathol. Microbiol. Scand.* (C) **87**:1–5.
45. Peterson, P. K., Verhoef, J., Schmeling, D., and Quie, P. G., 1977, Kinetics of phagocytosis and bacterial killing by human polymorphonuclear leukocytes and monocytes, *J. Infect. Dis.* **136**:502–509.
46. Kharazmi, A., Döring, G., Høiby, N., and Valerius, N.H., 1984, Interaction of *Pseudomonas aeruginosa* alkaline protease and elastase with human polymorphonuclear leukocytes *in vitro*, *Infect. Immun.* **43**:161–165.
47. Döring, G., Obernesser, H. J., and Botzenhart, K., 1981, Extracellular toxins of *Pseudomonas aeruginosa*. II. Effect of two proteases on human immunoglobulins IgG, IgA and secretory IgA, *Zentralbl. Bakteriol. Mikrobiol. Hyg.* (A) **249**:89–98.
48. Fick, R. B., Jr., Baltimore, R. S., Squier, S. U., and Reynolds, H. Y., 1985, IgG proteolytic activity of *Pseudomonas aeruginosa* in cystic fibrosis, 1985, *J. Infect. Dis.* **151**:589–598.
49. Heck, L. W., Alarcon, P. G., Kulhavy, R. M., Morihara, K., Russel, M. W., and Mestecky, J. F., 1990, Degradation of IgA proteins by *Pseudomonas aeruginosa* elastase, *J. Immunol.* **144**:2253–2257.
50. Schultz, D. R., and Miller, K. D., 1974, Elastase of *Pseudomonas aeruginosa*: Inactivation of complement components and complement-derived chemotactic factors, *Infect. Immun.* **10**:128–135.
51. Scharmann, W., Jacob, F., and Porstendorfer, J., 1976, The cytotoxic action of leucocidin from *Pseudomonas aeruginosa* on human polymorphonuclear leukocytes, *J. Gen. Microbiol.* **93**:303–308.

52. Kluftinger, J. L., Lutz, F., and Hancock, R. E. W., 1989, *Pseudomonas aeruginosa* cytotoxin: Periplasmic localization and inhibition of macrophages, *Infect. Immun.* **57**:882–886.
53. Baltch, A. L., Hammer, M. C., Smith, R. P., Obrig, T. G., Conroy J. V., Bishop, M. B., Egy, M. A., and Lutz, F., 1985, Effects of *Pseudomonas aeruginosa* cytotoxin on human serum and granulocytes and their microbicidal, phagocytic and chemotactic functions, *Infect. Immun.* **48**:498–506.
54. Lutz, F., Xiong, G., Jungblut, R., Orlik-Eisel, G., Gobel-Reifert, A., and Leidolf, R., 1991, Pore-forming cytotoxin of *Pseudomonas aeruginosa*: Molecular effects and aspects of pathogenicity, *Antibiot. Chemother.* **44**:54–58.
55. Nonoyama, S., Kojo, H., Mine, Y., Nishida, M., Goto, S., and Kuwahara, S., 1979, Inhibitory effect of *Pseudomonas aeruginosa* on the phagocytic and killing activity of rabbit polymorphonuclear leukocytes: Mechanism of action of a polymorphonuclear leukoyte inhibitor, *Infect. Immun.* **24**:399–403.
56. Laharrague, P. F., Corberand, J. X., Fillola, G., Gleizes, B. J., Fontanilles, A. M., and Gyrard, E., 1984, *In vitro* effect of the slime of *Pseudomonas aeruginosa* on the function of human polymorphonuclear neutrophils, *Infect. Immun.* **44**:760–762.
57. Sensakovic, J. W., and Bartell, P. F., 1974, The slime of *Pseudomonas aeruginosa*: Biological characterization and possible role in experimental infection, *J. Infect. Dis.* **129**:101–109.
58. Baltimore, R. S., and Mitchell, M., 1980, Immunologic investigations of mucoid strains of *Pseudomonas aeruginosa*: comparison of susceptibility to opsonic antibody in mucoid and non mucoid strains, *J. Infect. Dis.* **141**:238–247.
59. Schwarzmann, S., and Boring, J. R. III, 1971, Antiphagocytic effect of slime from a mucoid strain of *Pseudomonas aeruginosa*, *Infect. Immun.* **3**:762–767.
60. Stire, H. G., Zachidniak, K., and Speert, D. P., 1988, Inhibition of polymorphonuclear chemotaxis by the mucoid exopolysaccharide of *Pseudomonas aeruginosa*, *Clin. Invest. Med.* **11**:247–252.
61. Pedersen, S. S., Høiby, N., Epersen, F., and Kharazmi, A., 1991, Alginate in infection, *Antibiot. Chemother.* **44**:68–79.
62. Döring, G., Maier, M., Müller, E., Bibi, Z., Tümmler, B., and Kharazmi, A., 1987, Virulence factors of *Pseudomonas aeruginosa*, *Antibiot. Chemother.* **39**:136–148.
63. Pollack, M., and Anderson, S. E., Jr., 1978, Toxicity of *Pseudomonas aeruginosa* exotoxin A for human macrophages, *Infect. Immun.* **19**:1092–1096.
64. Stuart, R. K., Pollack, M., 1982, *Pseudomonas aeruginosa* exotoxin A inhibits proliferation of human bone marrow progenitor cells *in vitro*, *Infect. Immun.* **38**:206–211.
65. Kharazmi, A., Høiby, N., Döring, G., and Valerius, N. H., 1984, *Pseudomonas aeruginosa* exoproteases inhibit human neutrophil chemiluminescence, *Infect. Immun.* **44**:587–591.
66. Learn, D. B., Brestel, E. P., and Seetharama, S. 1987, Hypochlorite scavenging by *Pseudomonas aeruginosa* alginate, *Infect. Immun.* **55**:1813–1818.
67. Garzelli, C., Colizzi, V., Campa, M., and Falcone, G., 1980, Mouse footpad infection by *Pseudomonas aeruginosa*: Evidence for delayed hypersensitivity to specific bacterial antigen, *Med. Microbiol. Immunol.* **168**:111–118.
68. Colizzi, V., Garzelli, C., Campa, M., Toca, L., and Falcone, G., 1982, Role of specific delayed-type hypersensitivity in *Pseudomonas aeruginosa*-infected mice, *Immunology* **47**:337–344.
69. Campa, M., Toca, L., Lombardi, S., Garzelli, C., Colizzi, V., and Falcone, G., 1982, Cell-mediated immunity and delayed-type hypersensitivity in *Pseudomonas aeruginosa*-infected mice, *Med. Microbiol. Immunol.* **170**:191–199.
70. Markham, R. B., Pier, G. B., and Schreiber, J. R., 1991, The role of cytophilic IgG_3 antibody in T cell-mediated resistance to infection with the extracellular bacterium, *Pseudomonas aeruginosa*, *J. Immunol.* **146**:316–320.
71. Zehavi-Willner, T., 1988, Induction of murine cytolytic T lymphocytes by *Pseudomonas aeruginosa* exotoxin A, *Infect. Immun.* **56**:213–218.
72. Parmely, M. J., Iglewski, B. H., and Horvat, R. T., 1984, Identification of the principal T

lymphocytes-stimulating antigens of *Pseudomonas aeruginosa, J. Exp. Med.* **160**:1338–1349.
73. Parmely, M. J., and Horvat, R. T., 1986, Antigenic specificity of *Pseudomonas aeruginosa* alkaline protease and elastase defined by human T cell clones, *J. Immunol.* **137**:988–994.
74. Munster, A. M., and Leary, A. G., 1977, Cell-mediated immune responses to *Pseudomonas aeruginosa, Am. J. Surg.* **133**:710–712.
75. Porwoll, J. M., Gebel, H. M., Rodey, G. E., and Markham, R. B., 1983, In vitro response of human T cells to *Pseudomonas aeruginosa, Infect. Immun.* **40**:670–674.
76. Munster, A. M., Winchurch, R. A., Burmingham, W. J., and Keeling, P., 1980, Longitudinal assay of lymphocyte responsiveness in patients with major burns, *Ann. Surg.* **192**:772–775.
77. Stone, H. H., Given, K. S., and Martin, J. D., 1967, Delayed rejection of skin homografts in *Pseudomonas* sepsis, *Surg. Gynecol. Obstet.* **124**:1067–1070.
78. Floersheim, G. L., Hopff, W. H., Gasser, M., and Bucker, K., 1971, Impairment of cell-mediated immune responses by *Pseudomonas aeruginosa, Clin. Exp. Immunol.* **9**:241–247.
79. Woodruff, M. F. A., Nolan, B., Robson, J. S., and MacDonald, M. K., 1969, Renal transplantation in man, *Lancet* **i**:6–12.
80. Garzelli, C., Colizzi, V., Campa, M., Bozzi, L., and Falcone G., 1979, Depression of the antibody response in *Pseudomonas aeruginosa*-injected mice, *Infect. Immun.* **24**:32–38.
81. Colizzi, V., Campa, M., Garzelli, C., Toca, L., Bevilacqua, G., and Falcone, G., 1982, Impairment of cell-mediated immunity in *Pseudomonas aeruginosa* pyelonephritis: Lack of supressor cell activity *in vivo, Med. Microbiol. Immunol.* **171**:123–133.
82. Campa, M., Garzelli, C., Ferrannini, E., and Falcone, G., 1976, Evidence for suppressor cell activity associated with depression of contact sensitivity in *Pseudomonas aeruginosa* infected mice, *Clin. Exp. Immunol.* **26**:355–362.
83. Campa, M., Garzelli, C., and Falcone, G., 1975, Depression of contact sensitivity and enhancement of antibody response in *Pseudomonas aeruginosa*-infected mice, *Infect. Immun.* **12**:1252–1257.
84. Colizzi, V., Garzelli, C., Campa, M., and Falcone, G., 1978, Depression of contact sensitivity by enhancement of suppressor cell activity in *Pseudomonas aeruginosa*-injected mice, *Infect. Immun.* **21**:354–359.
85. Campa, M., Colizzi, V., Garzelli, C., Toca, L., and Falcone, G., 1980, *Pseudomonas aeruginosa* infection: activation of B suppressor cells which affect cell cooperation in the induction phase of contact sensitivity to oxazolone in mice, *Curr. Microbiol.* **4**:173–175.
86. Garzelli, C., Colizzi, V., Campa, M., Bozzi, L., and Falcone, G., 1979, Depression of contact sensitivity by *Pseudomonas aeruginosa*-induced suppressor cells which affect the induction phase of immune response, *Infect. Immun.* **26**:4–11.
87. Falcone, G., and Campa, M., 1981, Bacterial interference with the immune response, in: *Microbial Perturbation of Host Defences* (F. O'Grady and H. Smith, eds.), Academic Press, London, pp. 185–210.
88. Benedettini, G., De Libero, G., Mori, L., and Campa, M., 1984, *Staphylococcus aureus* inhibits contact sensitivity to oxazolone by activating suppressor B cells in mice, *Int. Arch. Allergy Appl. Immun.* **73**:269–273.
89. Campa, M., Benedettini, G., De Libero, G., Mori, L., and Falcone, G., 1984, T supressor cells as well as anti-hapten and anti-idiotype B lymphocytes regulate contact sensitivity to oxazolone in mice injected with purified protein derivative from *Mycobacterium tuberculosis, Infect. Immun.* **45**:701–707.
90. Benedettini, G., De Libero, G., Mori, L., Marelli, P., Angioni, M. R., and Campa, M., 1985, *Staphylococcus aureus*-induced suppressor of contact sensitivity in mice. Suppressor cells elicited by polyclonal B-cell activation are regulated by idiotype anti-idiotype interactions, *Cell. Immun.* **93**:508–519.
91. Campa, M., Benedettini, G., and Marelli, P., 1986, B and T lymphocytes regulated by idiotype and anti-idiotype interactions inhibit delayed-type hypersensitivity to BCG in mice, *Cell. Immun.* **98**:93–103.

92. Campa, M., Marelli, P., Ota, F., Zolfino, I., Senesi, S., Malvaldi, G., 1989, B-cell-mediated depression of the granulomatous response to BCG in mice, *Cell. Immun.* **119:**279–285.
93. Powderly, W. G., Schreiber, J. R., Pier, G. B., and Markham, R. B., 1988, T cells recognizing polysaccharide-specific B cells function as contrasuppressor cells in the generation of T cell immunity to *Pseudomonas aeruginosa*, *J. Immunol.* **140:**2746–2752.
94. Issekutz, T. B., and Stoltz, J. M., 1985, Suppression of lymphocyte proliferation by *Pseudomonas aeruginosa*: Mediation by *Pseudomonas*-activated suppressor monocytes, *Infect. Immun.* **48:**832–838.
95. Petit, J.-C., Richard, G., Albert, B., and Daguet, G.-L., 1982, Depression by *Pseudomonas aeruginosa* of two T-cell-mediated responses, anti-*Listeria* immunity and delayed-type hypersensitivity to sheep erythrocytes, *Infect. Immun.* **35:**900–908.
96. Holt, P. S., and Misfeldt, M. L., 1984, Alteration of murine immune response by *Pseudomonas aeruginosa* exotoxin A, *Infect. Immun.* **45:**227–233.
97. Nutman, J., Berger, M., Chase, P. A., Dearborn, D. G., Miller K. M., Waller, R. L., and Sorensen, R. U., 1987, Studies on the mechanism of T cell inhibition by the *Pseudomonas aeruginosa* phenazine pigment pyocyanine, *J. Immunol.* **138:**3481–3487.
98. Theander T. G., Kharazmi, A., Pedersen, B. K., Christensen, L. D., Tvede, N., Poulsen, L. K., Ødum, N., Svenson, M., and Bendtzen, K., 1988, Inhibition of human lymphocyte proliferation and cleavage of interleukin-2 by *Pseudomonas aeruginosa* proteases, *Infect. Immun.* **56:**1673–1677.
99. Pedersen, B. K., Kharazmi, A., Theander, T. G., Odum, N., Andersen, V., and Bendtzen, 1987, Selective modulation of the CD4 molecular complex by *Pseudomonas aeruginosa* alkaline protease and elastase, *Scand. J. Immunol.* **26:**91–94.
100. Horvat, R. T., and Parmely, M. J., 1988, *Pseudomonas aeruginosa* alkaline protease degrades human gamma interferon and inhibits its bioactivity, *Infect. Immun.* **56:**2925–2932.
101. Horvat, R. T., Clabaugh, M., Duval-Jobe, C., and Parmely, M. J., Inactivation of human gamma interferon by *Pseudomonas aeruginosa* proteases: Elastase augments the effects of alkaline protease despite the presence of α_2-macroglobulin, *Infect. Immun.* **57:**1668–1674.
102. Pedersen, B. K., and Kharazmi, A., 1987, Inhibition of human natural killer cell activity by *Pseudomonas aeruginosa* alkaline protease and elastase, *Infect. Immun.* **55:**986–989.
103. Holt, P. S., and Misfeldt, M. L., 1985, Induction of an immune response in athymic nude mice to thymus dependent antigens by *Pseudomonas aeruginosa* exotoxin A, *Cell. Immunol.* **95:**265–275.
104. Garzelli, C., Campa, M., Colizzi, V., Benedettini, G., and Falcone, G., 1982, Evidence for autoantibody production associated with polyclonal B-cell activation by *Pseudomonas aeruginosa*, *Infect. Immun.* **35:**13–19.
105. Garzelli, C., Campa, M., Forlani, A., Colizzi, V., and Falcone, G., 1982, LPS-induced enhancement of plaque-forming cell response to bromelain-treated syngeneic erythrocytes in mouse peritoneal cell cultures, *Int. Arch. Allergy Appl. Immun.* **67:**143–147.
106. Garzelli, C., Forlani, A., Lombardi, S., Colizzi, V., Campa, M., and Falcone, G., 1983, Regulation of the development of plaque-forming cells to bromelain-treated syngeneic mouse erytrocytes in bone marrow cell cultures, *Int. Arch. Allergy Appl. Immun.* **72:**253–259.
107. Campa, M., Garzelli, C., Colizzi, V., Benedettini, G., De Libero, G., and Falcone, G., 1983, Enhancement of the spontaneous development of autoreactive B cells by PPD in mouse peritoneal cell cultures, *Microbiologica* **6:**199–205.
108. Chen, Y-H. U., Hancock, R. E. W., and Mishell, R. I., 1980, Mitogenic effects of purified outer membrane proteins from *Pseudomonas aeruginosa*, *Infect. Immun.* **28:**178–184.
109. Papamichail, M., Dimitracopoulos, G., Tsokos, G., and Papavasiliou, J., 1980, A human lymphocyte mitogen extracted from the extracellular slime layer of *Pseudomonas aeruginosa*, *J. Infect. Dis.* **141:**686–688.
110. Pedersen, S. S., Høiby, N., Shand, G.H., and Pressler, T., 1989, Antibody response to *Pseudomonas aeruginosa* antigens in cystic fibrosis, *Antibiot. Chemother.* **42:**130–153.

111. Döring, G., Obernesser, H. J., Boltzenhart, K., Flehming, B., Høiby, N., and Hofmann, A., 1983, Proteases of *Pseudomonas aeruginosa* in cystic fibrosis, *J. Infect. Dis.* **147**:744–750.
112. Döring, G., Buhl, V., Høiby, N., Schiotz, P. O., and Botzenhart, K., 1984, Detection of proteases of *Pseudomonas aeruginosa* in immune complexes isolated from sputum of cystic fibrosis patients, *Acta Pathol. Microbiol. Immunol. Scand.* (C) **92**:307–312.
113. Moss, R. B., and Hsu, Y-P., 1982, Isolation and characterization of circulating immune complexes in cystic fibrosis, *Clin. Exp. Immunol.* **47**:301–308.
114. Campa, M., Ferrannini, E., Garzelli, C., Colizzi, V., and Falcone, G., 1979, Disturbance of lymphocyte circulation by *Pseudomonas aeruginosa* infection in oxazolone-sensitized mice, *Curr. Microbiol.* **2**:283–286.
115. Campa, M., Toca, L., Garzelli, C., Colizzi, V., Falcone, G., 1980, Reversal of *Pseudomonas aeruginosa*-induced disturbance of lymphocytes circulation in oxazolone-sensitized mice by cyclophosphamide, *Immunol. Lett.* **2**:129–131.
116. Falcone, G., and Campa, M., 1988, Diseases caused by Pseudomonas, in: *Laboratory diagnosis of infectious diseases, Principles and Practice*, (A. Balows, W. J. Hausler, Jr., M. Ohashi, and A. Turano, eds.), Springer-Verlag, New York, pp. 435–442.

Local and Disseminated Diseases Caused by *Pseudomonas aeruginosa*

ANDREW W. ARTENSTEIN and ALAN S. CROSS

1. INTRODUCTION

Pseudomonas aeruginosa is an organism of relatively low virulence that rarely affects those with intact host defenses. In the immunocompromised host, however, it is capable of using a wide array of potential virulence factors to cause a variety of serious infections. *P. aeruginosa* (formerly *Bacillus pyocyaneus*) was originally isolated in pure culture by a French pharmacist named Gessard in 1882.[1] The organism is ubiquitous in nature, has minimal growth requirements, is nutritionally versatile, and thrives in moist environments.[2]

The relative frequency of infections caused by *P. aeruginosa* has increased dramatically over the last 30 years. Two main factors appear to account, in large part, for this change: (1) advances in medical treatments and technologies that have resulted in the prolonged survival of immunologically impaired hosts; and (2) the increased prevalence of gram-negative bacillary nosocomial infections as a consequence of widespread antibiotic use.[3,4] *P. aeruginosa* recently has been noted as the causative agent for ca. 9% of nosocomial infections at all sites.[5,6] Infections with *P. aeruginosa* continue to be associated with a higher mortality than other gram-negative bacillary infections.[7]

ANDREW W. ARTENSTEIN and ALAN S. CROSS • Infectious Disease Service, Department of Medicine, Walter Reed Army Medical Center, and Department of Bacterial Diseases, Walter Reed Army Institute of Research, Washington, D.C. 20307-5001.

Pseudomonas aeruginosa as an Opportunistic Pathogen, edited by Mario Campa *et al.* Plenum Press, New York, 1993.

P. aeruginosa has been associated with a variety of clinical syndromes and can involve nearly every organ system. Many of these manifestations are well-described in the older medical literature whereas some represent the "evolving epidemiology" of this organism.[2] In this chapter we will focus on the clinical manifestations of local and disseminated disease due to *P. aeruginosa*.

2. BACTEREMIA

2.1. Epidemiology

Bacteremia due to *P. aeruginosa* is almost exclusively a nosocomial infection and usually occurs in patients with severe disruptions in their immunocompetence. Predispositions include granulocytopenia, especially in those who become colonized with *Pseudomonas*[8]; hematologic malignancies[9]; previous antibiotic or corticosteroid therapy[10]; prematurity[11]; congenital disease[11]; organ transplants[12]; traumatic injury[13]; or the presence of a serious underlying disease.[14]

Between the first clinical description of bacteremia in 1890 and the first extensive literature review on the subject in 1947, 91 cases had been reported.[15] Since that time, *P. aeruginosa* has accounted for 7–18% of all episodes of gram-negative septicemia[13] and has become an important cause of septicemia in neutropenic patients.[16] The mortality data from several of the major series are shown in Table I. The fatality rate from *Pseudomonas* sepsis, ranging from 38% to 96%, exceeds that from all other causes of gram-negative sepsis.[13] *P. aeruginosa* is also involved in polymicrobial bacteremias in susceptible hosts.[22]

The most important portals of entry for the organism, according to the reports before 1970, were the genitourinary tract in adults, usually related to instrumentation or trauma[19]; and the skin or gastrointestinal tract in chil-

TABLE I
Pseudomonas aeruginosa **Septicemia Mortality Data in Immunocompromised Hosts**

Years	n	Overall mortality	Reference
1954–1957	23	96%	10
1940–1959	91	80%	11
1967–1968	50	78%	17
1971–1972	52	69%	18
1972–1974	108	70%	19
1972–1975	75	63%	20
1972–1981	410	38%	9
1983–1985	133	50%	21

dren.[15] In more recent reports, the respiratory tract is the suspected source in most cases,[23] probably related to oropharyngeal colonization.[24]

2.2. Clinical Presentation

The clinical presentation of *Pseudomonas aeruginosa* septicemia is largely indistinguishable from that of other gram-negative etiologies.[10,19] Fever is usually present, except in premature infants.[11] Ileus, mental status abnormalities, and sudden, refractory hypotension as a preterminal event are common.[10] Jaundice, although a frequent finding in one series,[10] is noted less commonly in others.[19]

2.3. Dermatologic Features

There are a variety of characteristic dermatologic manifestations of disseminated infection with *Pseudomonas aeruginosa*. Skin lesions previously were seen in up to 39% of septicemic patients,[10] but their frequency has decreased in recent series to less than 5% of cases.[9,20] The most characteristic skin lesion of *Pseudomonas* septicemia is ecthyma gangrenosum. This lesion begins with edema and progresses to a painless, round, erythematous macule with or without an adherent vesicle. The macule subsequently becomes indurated, bullous or pustular and ulcerates, forming a black eschar with a surrounding erythematous halo.[25] Lesions may be single or multiple and present in different stages of development.[12] Ecthyma gangrenosum evolves rapidly over 12–24 hr.[13]

Although ecthyma gangrenosum is not pathognomonic for infection with *P. aeruginosa*, it is highly suggestive.[25] Histopathologically, there is evidence of hemorrhagic necrosis with organisms in the media and adventitia of the blood vessels and a relative sparing of the intima.[25] There is a paucity of intraluminal leukocytes and bacterial infiltration and no evidence of thrombosis.[25] *P. aeruginosa* can usually be visualized and cultured from these lesions. Ecthyma gangrenosum most commonly occurs in the gluteal or perineal region, the axillae, or the extremities, although it may be seen at other sites.[25]

Other skin manifestations of disseminated disease include vesicular lesions—inflamed, painful lesions occasionally seen in clusters and containing a bacteria-laden fluid[10]; sharply demarcated cellulitis with areas of hemorrhage and necrosis[10]; diffuse maculopapular truncal eruptions[10,14]; subcutaneous nodules[26] and metastatic abscesses[10]; and grouped petechiae.[27]

2.4. Therapy

The treatment of *Pseudomonas aeruginosa* septicemia is based on clinical experience and principles derived from experimental models: early institution of therapy is critical for optimal survival in the neutropenic host; survival rates are higher in neutropenic patients when combination therapy with an aminoglycoside and a beta-lactam agent is used than when either agent is used alone; and resistance may develop with single drug therapy.[13] Although the initial choice of antimicrobials is evolving, therapy is always begun empirically in the neutropenic patient with fever or other signs of infection. Specific choices, including the possibility of monotherapy with newer agents, should be guided by local antibiotic susceptibility patterns.

2.5. Prognosis

The eventual outcome in cases of disseminated infection with *P. aeruginosa* is largely dependent on the patient's underlying illness.[13] Factors that predict an unfavorable prognosis include a low total leukocyte count, especially less than $100/mm^3$ [9,18,28]; azotemia[20]; a respiratory source of bacteremia[20]; and low serum immunoglobulins.[18]

3. ENDOCARDITIS

3.1. Epidemiology

Prior to the last two decades, infective endocarditis caused by *P. aeruginosa* was extremely rare. It accounted for less than 0.25% of all cases seen at The New York Hospital in the 30-year period preceding 1973.[29] Almost two-thirds of those cases of endocarditis had evidence of underlying heart disease.[29] Since that time, there has been a marked increase in the prevalence of *P. aeruginosa* endocarditis and that caused by gram-negative bacilli in general.[30]

The major predisposition to gram-negative bacillary endocarditis is the illicit parenteral use of drugs, usually heroin, although recent reports have emphasized the role of other illicit drugs.[31,32] Some of these agents, such as pentazocine and tripelennamine, may confer a selective survival advantage to particularly virulent serotypes of *P. aeruginosa*.[33] In 348 cases of gram-negative endocarditis reported in 1980, 32% occurred in intravenous drug users and 10% occurred in patients with prosthetic valves, the other major risk factor for this disease.[30] In that study *P. aeruginosa* accounted for 58% of all addict-associated gram-negative endocarditis, although a marked regional variation in etiologies was noted.[30]

The disease in parenteral drug users usually occurs on native valves, and it has been hypothesized that the valves of these individuals are subject to injury secondary to the foreign materials mixed with the narcotics, or previous bouts of endocarditis. The injury results in fibrotic changes on the valves, creating a potential nidus of infection.[34] This may explain why more than 25% of these cases had no prior history of cardiac abnormalities.[30] The source of the organism has been hypothesized to be tap water or other environmental sources contaminating drug paraphernalia.[31] *P. aeruginosa* may be readily cultured from syringes and other equipment used by addicts.[35]

3.2. Clinical Presentation

Clinically, endocarditis caused by *Pseudomonas aeruginosa* in intravenous drug users usually occurs on the right side of the heart and is usually subacute in nature. The tricuspid valve is involved in more than 50% of addict-associated cases,[30] but biventricular and multi-valve involvement is common.[36] Although fever and heart murmur are consistent findings in these patients,[30,34] peripheral stigmata of infective endocarditis are unusual.[30] The latter is consistent with the findings in endocarditis in non-addicts. Septic pulmonary emboli, as a complication of right-sided endocarditis, occurred in 70% of intravenous drug users in one series.[34] Their usual presentation included cough, pleuritic chest pain, infiltrate on chest Xray, and occasional abscess formation. Left-sided endocarditis occurs less frequently and presents acutely. Congestive heart failure and systemic embolic phenomena may be high-frequency events in this subgroup.[32] Interestingly, there were no cases of ecthyma gangrenosum in one large series.[30]

3.3. Therapy

The treatment of right-sided endocarditis secondary to *P. aeruginosa* usually involves a prolonged course of combination antimicrobials. Most frequently, high doses of an aminoglycoside are combined with an extended-spectrum antipseudomonal penicillin. Individuals who fail this therapy may require a surgical procedure. Tricuspid valvulectomy without valve replacement has been reported to result in cure rates of greater than 80% and is generally well-tolerated.[37] The treatment of left-sided endocarditis due to *P. aeruginosa* also involves combination chemotherapy, although the cure rate remains less than 15% with this treatment alone.[32] This may be improved with early surgical intervention.[32] The overall survival for this disease is nearly 75%, perhaps reflecting the predilection of *P. aeruginosa* endocarditis to affect the right heart and its easier cure there.[30] The relatively young age of most intravenous drug users and the attendant lack of other underlying diseases in this population may also be factors in the favorable survival rate.

4. RESPIRATORY INFECTIONS

4.1. Epidemiology

In the early clinical reviews, *P. aeruginosa* was noted to uncommonly cause pneumonia.[38] Recent data, however, have shown this organism to be an important cause of nosocomial pneumonia, accounting for approximately

15% of these cases, largely in intensive care unit settings.[39] It is usually acquired via endogenous aspiration of organisms from a colonized oropharynx.[24] The susceptibility to colonization is inversely related to the basic health of an individual. *P. aeruginosa* is a rare cause of community acquired pneumonia.[40]

This infection occurs almost exclusively in patients with compromised local or systemic host defenses. Disorders that impair local defenses in the pulmonary system and predispose to *P. aeruginosa* pneumonia include cystic fibrosis (CF), tracheostomy,[13] tracheal intubation,[41] or the use of contaminated respiratory inhalation equipment.[39] Serious underlying diseases such as heart failure and emphysema also appear to predispose patients to this infection. Malignancies, especially of the hematologic variety, appear to predispose the host to the bacteremic form of *Pseudomonas* pneumonia.[42] The mortality rate from the bacteremic form of pneumonia is approximately 80%,[43] higher than that of primary, nonbacteremic pneumonia.

4.2. Clinical Presentation

Clinically, primary *P. aeruginosa* pneumonia is typically characterized by apprehension, toxic appearance, confusion, fever, chills, cough, dyspnea and relative bradycardia.[44] The patient may have an associated pharyngitis, otitis or tracheitis.[44] Leukocytosis is common. Bacteremic *Pseudomonas* pneumonia is frequently a fulminant disease with the characteristics of septicemia.[43] Dermatologic findings, however, appear to be uncommon.[42]

4.3. Radiology

The characteristic radiologic picture of primary *Pseudomonas* pneumonia is that of a diffuse bronchopneumonia, often bilateral and involving multiple lobes, with frequent lower-lobe involvement.[40] The apices are usually spared.[13] Some patients may have nodular infiltrates but lobar consolidation is rare. Small pleural effusions are common[40] and may be hemorrhagic.[44] Empyema is not infrequent,[44] and cavitary lesions may be found.[40] In contrast, the radiologic pattern of the bacteremic form of pneumonia is characterized by the early appearance of pulmonary vascular congestion and interstitial edema, which may progress rapidly to a picture of necrotizing bronchopneumonia.[42] This is correlated pathologically with intraalveolar hemorrhage, minimal inflammatory reaction, necrotic nodules, perivascular hemorrhagic lesions, and evidence of organisms invading the walls of vessels without attendant thrombosis.[13] This latter finding may represent a visceral counterpart to ecthyma gangrenosum.

4.4. Therapy

The treatment of pneumonia caused by *P. aeruginosa* is usually with combination antimicrobials, although the newer beta-lactam agents may offer significant advantages in this disease. Despite appropriate therapy, however, the mortality remains 30–80%.[42]

4.5. Cystic Fibrosis

Respiratory infections caused by *Pseudomonas aeruginosa* are especially prevalent in CF patients and are a major cause of morbidity and mortality in this population.[13] This topic is reviewed extensively in Chapter 13.

5. URINARY TRACT INFECTIONS

5.1. Epidemiology

Primary infection of the urinary tract with *P. aeruginosa* is almost always either a nosocomial or iatrogenic event.[45] Occasionally the genitourinary tract will be infected secondarily from a hematogenous source,[14] but more often will serve as a source of bacteremia.

Whereas *Pseudomonas* accounts for less than 1% of the isolates in populations with recurrent urinary tract infections,[46] it causes approximately 11% of nosocomial genitourinary tract infections.[6] The most important predispositions appear to be the presence of urinary catheters and other foreign bodies[45]; genitourinary tract manipulation[45]; anatomic abnormalities of the urinary tract[45]; and spinal cord injury.[47]

5.2. Clinical Presentation

The clinical manifestations of *P. aeruginosa* urinary tract infections are essentially indistinguishable from those due to other bacteria. Rarely, there have been reports of upper tract infection and renal infarctions secondary to bacterial invasion of renal blood vessels.[14] This is perhaps another example of a visceral equivalent to ecthyma gangrenosum.

5.3. Therapy

The appropriate therapy for these infections depends on many factors, including the chronicity and site of infection (i.e., upper versus lower tract), the presence of foreign bodies or anatomic abnormalities, and the presence or absence of systemic sepsis. Indwelling urinary catheters should be removed if possible and anatomic derangements, e.g. obstruction, should be relieved. Antibiotics should be used if the patient is symptomatic or there is evidence of systemic infection, but should not be used in the presence of a foreign body in an asymptomatic patient.

6. BONE AND JOINT INFECTIONS

6.1. Epidemiology

Musculoskeletal infections caused by *P. aeruginosa* previously had been reported rarely[38] but have been occurring with increasing frequency over the last few decades.[2] These are mostly in the form of nosocomial infections, such as those related to the use of hemodialysis catheters[2] or genitourinary tract manipulation. A significant source of the increased prevalence of these infections, however, is the illicit parenteral use of drugs.

P. aeruginosa osteomyelitis and septic arthritis are acquired via two major routes: spread to bone from a contiguous focus and hematogenous spread to bone, the implicated mechanism in parenteral drug abusers. Vertebral infections may also derive from hematogenous seeding from a genitourinary source via Batson's plexus. Osteomyelitis arising from a contiguous focus may present as a chronic infection. This includes that associated with compound fractures,[13] median sternotomy wounds,[2] decubitus ulcers, and malignant external otitis (see section 11.3.1). In animal models *Pseudomonas* osteomyelitis is more indolent and perhaps less destructive than staphylococcal osteomyelitis.[48]

6.2. Addict-associated Infection

Musculoskeletal infection due to *P. aeruginosa* in heroin addicts is a well-documented syndrome.[49] It usually runs a subacute or chronic course and is marked by the paucity of systemic symptoms. Localized pain is the most common complaint,[50] and the most consistent laboratory finding is an elevated erythrocyte sedimentation rate.[51] The most frequent sites of involvement are the vertebral column,[50,51] symphysis pubis,[50] pelvis,[13] and the sternoclavicular joint.[52] As with endocarditis in these patients, the source of the organism may be contaminated intravenous devices or injectable materials.[13]

6.3. Osteochondritis

Pseudomonas osteochondritis is a clinical syndrome that occurs largely as a complication of puncture wounds of the feet.[53] The source of the organism may be the tennis shoes of the victim or other environmental objects.[54] After an initial period of improvement, the patient presents with persistent pain and swelling of the foot in the absence of systemic signs of infection,[53] which usually delays diagnosis. The treatment of this syndrome is surgical debridement and antimicrobials. Some authors have suggested that a short course of medical therapy, combined with an aggressive surgical approach, may be sufficient.[54] Relapse may occur if an occult septic arthritis is undiagnosed.[54]

7. CENTRAL NERVOUS SYSTEM INFECTIONS

7.1. Meningitis

7.1.1. Epidemiology

P. aeruginosa meningitis is an uncommon disease and, as in other syndromes caused by this agent, usually occurs in a nosocomial setting. It accounted for 9% of central nervous system infections in cancer patients over a 16-year period in one series.[55] The potential routes of infection include direct entry via trauma or neurosurgical manipulation[56]; extension from infectious foci in the head and neck; or hematogenous spread, especially in patients with malignancies.[55] Patients with cerebrospinal fluid shunts or reservoirs and those with tumors of the head and neck are among the patients at greatest risk for *Pseudomonas* meningitis.[57]

7.1.2. Clinical Presentation

Clinically, meningitis caused by *P. aeruginosa* presents similarly to other forms of bacterial meningitis. Fever, headache, mental confusion, and obtundation are common findings. The disease may be fulminant in those with concurrent bacteremia, but it may have a more insidious presentation, with few systemic signs and symptoms, especially in the post-neurosurgical patient.[58] The disease may present in a chronic form in patients with alterations in cranial anatomy, indwelling foreign materials, or cerebrospinal fluid leaks.

7.1.3. Therapy

Because the disease is rare, optimal treatment regimens have not been clearly defined. Systemic aminoglycosides, with their poor penetration into cerebrospinal fluid, are not as useful in *Pseudomonas* meningitis as they are in other diseases due to this organism. Ceftazidime may be the antimicrobial of choice because most strains of *P. aeruginosa* are sensitive to this agent, it achieves adequate drug levels in cerebrospinal fluid, and it is usually well-tolerated.[57] It is unclear whether this agent should be used in conjunction with an intravenous or intrathecal aminoglycoside. The mortality from meningitis due to *P. aeruginosa* appears to be approximately 40% in primary infections, and nearly 70% when infection is acquired hematogenously.[13]

7.2. Brain Abscess

Brain abscess due to *P. aeruginosa* is also a rare event, with only seven cases reported in the literature by 1947.[38] All of these occurred as the result of penetrating head injuries. More recently, this organism was noted to cause

10% of brain abscesses in cancer patients over a 16-year period.[55] Therapy for this disease includes antimicrobials and surgical drainage.

8. WOUND INFECTIONS

Because of its ubiquitous presence in nature, particularly in moist environments, *P. aeruginosa* is a common isolate from wounds. This organism was noted to account for 25% of isolates in the wound infections of Israeli soldiers after the Yom Kippur War,[59] and 67% of the wound isolates in soldiers in Vietnam.[60] *Pseudomonas* was most often isolated after multiple days of hospitalization, reflecting its status as a nosocomial pathogen.[59,60] The field use of antibiotics was felt to have contributed to the presence of *P. aeruginosa* in both studies.[59,60] It should be noted that the presence of *P. aeruginosa* in a wound may only indicate colonization in the absence of clinical infection. *Pseudomonas* wound infection may lead to secondary bacteremia.

P. aeruginosa is also a major cause of burn wound sepsis and a significant cause of morbidity and mortality in these patients.[61] *Pseudomonas* tends to colonize the burn site, and these patients are immunocompromised due to the destruction of their mechanical barrier defense and the variety of immunologic defects related to serious thermal injury.[61] This topic is discussed in detail in Chapter 14.

9. SKIN INFECTIONS

9.1. General Considerations

P. aeruginosa is not an inhabitant of normal, dry skin but flourishes on moist skin or in the presence of topical antibiotics that selectively kill its competitors.[27] It gains access to the host via disruption of the skin by trauma or maceration. A variety of dermatologic manifestations of local disease are due to *P. aeruginosa*. The dermatologic manifestations of disseminated disease are discussed in section 2.3.

9.2. Clinical Syndromes

The green nail syndrome is a paronychial infection with the nail discoloration caused by the diffusion of *Pseudomonas* pigments into the nail plate.[27] It occurs in individuals whose hands are frequently submerged in water. Nail discoloration may persist after the resolution of active infection. The differential diagnosis includes discoloration due to dyes or chemicals and infection by *Aspergillus* species, *P. aeruginosa*, or *Candida albicans*.[62] Treatment includes local measures and incision and drainage of the paronychia.

Toeweb infection occurs primarily in hot, humid climates and in feet with pre-existing tinea pedis infections. The toeweb displays a thick, greenish exudate secondary to scaling or maceration of the stratum corneum.[27] The treatment for this infection includes local measures and systemic antibiotics.

Pseudomonas pyoderma is a purulent, superficial skin infection manifested by a bluish green exudate with a characteristic grapelike odor.[27] It usually arises as a secondary infection in patients with damaged skin due to eczema, tinea pedis, burns or decubitus ulcers. *Pseudomonas* cellulitis is an erythematous lesion with a violaceous, necrotic center. Infection may be deep or associated with subcutaneous nodules.

Ecthyma gangrenosum may rarely occur in the apparent absence of bacteremia. A series of immunosuppressed patients with classic-appearing lesions has been described without accompanying bacteremia.[63] This subgroup may have a better prognosis than their septic counterparts.[63]

Multiple water-associated dermatologic syndromes have recently been described and attributed to infection with *P. aeruginosa*. A diffuse, pruritic, maculopapular and vesiculopustular rash has occurred in epidemic form associated with the use of contaminated spas,[64] hot tubs,[64] whirlpools,[65] swimming pools,[66] and waterslides.[67] Nosocomial outbreaks have been reported as well.

The rash usually occurs in areas covered by bathing suits, but it can occur in a diffuse pattern, sparing only the head and neck.[65] It has been generally noted to occur 8 hr to 5 days after exposure with a mean of 48 hr.[64] Associated symptoms may include headache, dizziness, malaise, otitis externa, mastitis and sore throat.[65] Fever appears to be uncommon.[64] The differential diagnosis includes insect bites, scabies, contact dermatitis, and staphylococcal folliculitis.[64] A serologically identical strain of *P. aeruginosa* can be cultured from the common-source and the skin lesions. Organism entry into the skin may be facilitated by the high temperatures of some water sources and the subsequent dilation of pores.[65] Infection may occur despite adequate chlorination of the water.[68] This syndrome is usually self-limited and resolves after the discontinuation of exposure. However, some previously healthy patients have developed systemic sequelae due to *P. aeruginosa*.[2]

10. OCULAR INFECTIONS

10.1. General Considerations

P. aeruginosa causes a variety of ocular infections and is among the most destructive bacterial pathogens of the human cornea.[38] Although keratitis is the most common ocular infection caused by this organism, it also may cause conjunctivitis,[69] dacryocystitis,[70] orbital cellulitis,[70] ophthalmia neonatorum,[71] endophthalmitis,[72] and a necrotizing infection of the eyelids.[38] Adults rarely disseminate from an ocular focus, although this may occur in premature infants.[70]

10.2. Keratitis

10.2.1. Epidemiology

The initial event in the pathogenesis of keratitis is the induction of a corneal ulcer, usually by some form of trauma that damages the epithelial surface. The trauma is often minor and may even be caused by the use of extended-wear contact lenses.[73] Once the cornea is damaged, certain bacteria tend to invade that site. *P. aeruginosa* is the most common gram-negative bacillus to infect corneal ulcers.[13] The organism may be introduced into the eye by the following routes: contamination of contact lens solution[74]; the use of contaminated mascara[2]; or contamination of ocular medications.

Certain other groups are also susceptible. Burn patients are at risk for these infections secondary to thermal damage to the cornea.[61] Also, there is a high incidence of bacterial keratitis in premature infants and in patients with predisposing ocular conditions, especially if they are using topical steroids.[70]

10.2.2. Clinical Presentation

Clinically, keratitis presents with pain and redness of the eye, often with photophobia and decreased visual acuity. Fever and other systemic symptoms are unusual. On exam a small central ulcer is noted to spread concentrically. This may lead to involvement of the entire cornea and, potentially, to corneal perforation. The presence of gram-negative rods on staining of material taken from the ulcer suggests an etiologic diagnosis.

10.2.3. Therapy

Because *Pseudomonas* keratitis progresses rapidly over hours to days and may lead to panophthalmitis with potential loss of the eye, it should be treated as a medical emergency.[13] Unless an alternative etiology can be discerned readily, immediate anti-pseudomonal therapy is indicated. Topical therapy may be effective in the early stages of this disease but systemic and subtenon aminoglycosides are usually required.[13]

10.3. Endophthalmitis

Endophthalmitis due to *P. aeruginosa* is rare and usually occurs as a complication of intraocular surgery,[72] penetrating injuries, inappropriately treated keratitis, or posterior perforation of a corneal ulcer. Occasionally it may be the result of metastatic infection in septic patients.[70] This disease has a fulminant presentation and may progress to loss of vision over hours.

The clinical features include pain, conjunctival hyperemia, chemosis, decreased visual acuity, hypopyon, or anterior uveitis.[72]

11. OTOLARYNGOLOGIC INFECTIONS

11.1. General Considerations

P. aeruginosa is rarely found in the external auditory canal of healthy persons.[75] However, it may cause a variety of otolaryngologic infections, some of them life-threatening.

11.2. External Otitis

This organism is felt to be the causal agent in approximately 70% of cases of external otitis or "swimmer's ear" when associated with swimming.[27] *P. aeruginosa* tends to inhabit and potentially cause disease in the ear in conditions of injury, maceration, humidity or moistness. External otitis is generally a benign and self-limited disease that is manifested clinically by an itchy or painful, discharging ear.[38] On exam there is an exquisite tenderness on traction of the pinna and an edematous, erythematous external canal. Treatment consists of local measures including topical antibiotics and a drying agent. Recurrences are frequent.

11.3. Malignant External Otitis

Malignant external otitis is a particularly severe form of local disease caused by *P. aeruginosa*; it has been described extensively by Chandler.[76] It begins as an external otitis that fails to respond to topical therapy and becomes locally invasive in a contiguous manner. The disease usually occurs in elderly diabetic patients with evidence of small vessel disease,[77] although it may rarely occur in healthy adults and immunocompromised children.[78]

11.3.1. Pathogenesis

Malignant external otitis is a chronic, indolent infection but can be very destructive. The necrotizing process erodes through the external auditory canal through clefts in the cartilage that forms the floor of the lateral canal.[76] It may subsequently enter the soft tissues of the retromandibular area of the parotid space, resulting in a facial nerve palsy secondary to soft tissue edema.[76] Additionally, the infection may proceed through the mastoid air cells into the temporal bone and result in osteomyelitis of the temporal bone and base of the skull. The latter may lead to a variety of cranial nerve abnormalities[77] as well as spread to contralateral structures via vascular channels. The middle ear is usually spared.[76] Meningitis and brain abscess are uncommon complications.[79]

11.3.2. Clinical Presentation

Malignant external otitis presents as persistent otalgia and purulent otorrhea with exquisite tenderness of the tissues around the ear. Headache and decreased hearing are frequent findings, and trismus may occur if the temporomandibular joint is involved. The early appearance of a facial nerve palsy occurs in 50% of cases.[79] Fever and constitutional symptoms are uncommon, as is leukocytosis. The diagnostic hallmark on physical exam is the presence of persistent granulation tissue on the floor of the external canal near the junction of the cartilaginous and osseous portions.[76] The tympanic membrane usually remains intact.[76] Laboratory findings are few and may include a mild cerebrospinal fluid pleocytosis[77] and a markedly elevated erythrocyte sedimentation rate.[75]

11.3.3. Diagnosis

The diagnosis can be made on clinical grounds with the appropriate use of radiologic and microbiologic techniques. Computerized tomography (CT) scan is currently the imaging modality of choice for defining the anatomic extent of disease,[75] although magnetic resonance imaging (MRI) may prove useful in this regard as well. A precise etiologic diagnosis can be made by the isolation of *P. aeruginosa* from cultures of external auditory canal drainage.

11.3.4. Therapy

Because malignant external otitis is a difficult infection to eradicate and the potential consequences of treatment failure are profound, an aggressive approach to management seems warranted. This usually includes combination antimicrobials and surgical debridement. The precise nature of the surgery is determined by the extent of infection.

11.3.5. Prognosis

The overall mortality from this disease is approximately 20%.[75] Patients who present with neurologic deficits, especially polyneuropathies, tend to have a worse prognosis.[75] This is felt to be a function of the extent of disease.[77] The infection may recur up to 12 months after treatment.[75]

11.4. Other Syndromes

P. aeruginosa may cause a variety of other, less severe otolaryngologic infections. It is a major cause of otitis media in neonates, who present with rhinorrhea, irritability, cough, diarrhea, and difficulty feeding, in the absence of fever.[80] *P. aeruginosa* is the most common bacterial pathogen isolated in cases of chronic, suppurative otitis media in children and adults.[81] Unsuccessful antibiotic therapy for this condition may result in tympanomastoid surgery. It is also a cause of mastoiditis, either associated with malignant external otitis or primary otitis media.[82] This is usually seen in patients with compromised defenses due to underlying illnesses. Other conditions infrequently caused by *P. aeruginosa* include acute suppurative parotitis,[83] chronic sinusitis in hospitalized patients with nasogastric tubes,[84] perichondritis of the auricle,[85] and oropharyngeal ulcerations.[13] These syndromes usually occur as nosocomial infections in the debilitated patient.

12. DIALYSIS INFECTIONS

12.1. General Considerations

P. aeruginosa is the most frequently encountered gram-negative organism in cases of peritonitis in continuous ambulatory peritoneal dialysis (CAPD) patients.[86] Previous catheter exit site infections due to *Pseudomonas*, manifested by pericatheter erythema and/or discharge, may be a risk factor for subsequent peritonitis.[87] There is one report suggesting an increased risk of *Pseudomonas* peritonitis in CAPD patients infected with the human immunodeficiency virus.[88] Also, there have been reports of outbreaks of *P. aeruginosa* peritonitis in CAPD patients associated with the use of contaminated iodine-based cleansing solutions at the catheter site.[89,90]

12.2. Clinical Features

Clinically, this infection is similar to that caused by gram-positive organisms, presenting with cloudy dialysate fluid with or without abdominal pain. CAPD patients with *Pseudomonas* peritonitis may suffer increased morbidity secondary to intraabdominal abscesses[91]; loss of peritoneal space due to scarring[91]; and frequent catheter loss due to persistent infection.[87] Although controversial, most authors recommend early removal of the indwelling Tenckhoff catheter, in addition to antibiotics, to cure this infection.[86,91] This may be especially important when peritonitis is associated with infections of the catheter tunnel or exit site.[92]

13. GASTROINTESTINAL INFECTIONS

13.1. General Considerations

The prevalence of *P. aeruginosa* colonization of the gastrointestinal tract is 3–6% in healthy adults.[93] This rate remains relatively constant despite the relatively large quantity of organisms ingested in uncooked fruits and vegetables. Gastrointestinal carriage rates, however, are known to increase in hospitalized patients,[6] and the organism may cause disease in this setting.

Stanley, in his 1947 monograph, described cases of *P. aeruginosa* infection with ulcerative involvement of the stomach and small intestine with characteristic infiltration of portions of blood vessels, analogous to that seen in ecthyma gangrenosum.[14] He also noted that this organism could cause infections of any portion of the gastrointestinal tract.

P. aeruginosa has been implicated as the causative agent in epidemics of diarrhea in infants[94]; a lethal, necrotizing enterocolitis in newborns[95]; and a rare, enteric feverlike syndrome termed "Shanghai fever."[14] In the latter, patients present with prostration, headache, fever, diarrhea, splenomegaly, and a truncal maculopapular rash.[14] *P. aeruginosa* can be recovered from the skin lesions and is easily cultured from the stool of these patients.[14]

13.2. Typhlitis

13.2.1. Clinical Presentation

Perhaps the most serious gastrointestinal infection caused by *P. aeruginosa* is typhlitis, a necrotizing enterocolitis frequently localized to the cecum, although involvement of the other areas of the colon is not unusual.[13] It is primarily a disease of neutropenic patients and most commonly affects those with hematologic malignancies. This syndrome presents clinically with fever, either generalized or localized (right lower quadrant) abdominal pain, abdominal distention and diarrhea.[96] Other findings may include nausea, vomiting, peritoneal signs and guaiac-positive stool. The differential diagnosis includes acute appendicitis, intraabdominal abscess, and other causes of an acute abdomen. Although other gram-negative bacilli or fungi can cause this disease, *P. aeruginosa* is among the most frequent etiologies.[13]

13.2.2. Therapy

Typhlitis is associated with a high mortality rate, especially in the more severe forms or those associated with bacteremia. The therapy is surgical if the infection is localized. Medical management, to include combination antimicrobials, is probably appropriate for the less severe forms or generalized infection. One series noted symptom resolution in more than 60% of cases with medical therapy alone.[96] Recovery of the granulocyte count appears to be the most important determinant of success with medical management.[96]

13.3. Perirectal Disease

P. aeruginosa is also a frequent cause of perianal and perirectal abscess in neutropenic patients with hematologic malignancies, especially in those with acute leukemia.[97] It accounted for more than 65% of these infections in one series.[97] These abscesses frequently result in hematogenous dissemination, and the prognosis is poor when this occurs. Medical management appears to be the treatment of choice; the role of surgery is controversial.[97,98]

14. MISCELLANEOUS INFECTIONS

Multiple reports have appeared recently of serious *P. aeruginosa* infections following gastrointestinal endoscopic procedures.[99–102] These infections include bacteremia, cholangitis, gangrenous cholecystitis, and liver abscesses. The presumed source of infection was contaminated endoscopes.

A child with the acquired immunodeficiency syndrome (AIDS) was reported recently to present with *Pseudomonas* pneumonia in the absence of neutropenia, hypogammaglobulinemia, or recent hospitalization.[103] The authors speculated whether AIDS patients may be predisposed to this pathogen. A recent series of bacterial infections in AIDS patients, however, did not note the occurrence of *P. aeruginosa* infections except in those who were otherwise predisposed by virtue of intubation, neutropenia or debilitation.[104] Other recently described syndromes caused by *P. aeruginosa* include a case of fatal, nosocomial balanoposthitis in a neutropenic patient[105] and a case report of toxic shock syndrome in a child.[106]

REFERENCES

1. Gessard, C., 1984, On the blue and green coloration that appears on bandages, *Rev. Infect. Dis.* **6:**S775–776.
2. Cross, A. S., 1985, Evolving epidemiology of *Pseudomonas aeruginosa* infections, *Eur. J. Clin. Microbiol.* **4:**156–159.
3. Finland, M., Jones, W. F., and Barnes, M. W., 1959, Occurrence of serious bacterial infections since the introduction of antibacterial agents, *J.A.M.A.* **170:**2188–2197.
4. Rogers, D. E., 1959, The changing pattern of life-threatening microbial disease, *N. Engl. J. Med.* **261:**677–683.
5. Cross, A., Allen, J. R., Burke, J., Ducel, G., Harris, A., John, J., Johnson, D., Lew, M., MacMillan, B., Meers, P., Skalova, R., Wenzel, R., and Tenney, J., 1983, Nosocomial infections due to *Pseudomonas aeruginosa*: Review of recent trends, *Rev. Infect. Dis.* **5:**S837–S845.
6. Morrison, A. J., and Wenzel, R. P., 1984, Epidemiology of infections due to *Pseudomonas aeruginosa*, *Rev. Infect. Dis.* **6:**S627–S642.
7. Bryan, C. S., Reynolds, K. L., and Brenner, E. R., 1983, Analysis of 1,186 episodes of gram-negative bacteremia in non-university hospitals: The effects of antimicrobial therapy, *Rev. Infect. Dis.* **5:**629–638.
8. Schimpff, S. C., Moody, M., and Young, V. M., 1971, Relationship of colonization with *Pseudomonas aeruginosa* to development of *Pseudomonas* bacteremia in cancer patients, in: *Antimicrobial Agents and Chemotherapy—1970* (G. L. Hobby, ed.), Am. Soc. Microbiol., Washington, D.C., pp. 240–244.

9. Bodey, G. P., Jadeja, L., and Elting, L., 1985, *Pseudomonas* bacteremia: Retrospective analysis of 410 episodes, *Arch. Intern. Med.* **145:**1621–1629.
10. Forkner, C. E., Frei, E., Edgcomb, J. H., and Utz, J. P., 1958, *Pseudomonas* septicemia: Observations on twenty-three cases. *Am. J. Med.* **25:**877–889.
11. Curtin, J. A., Petersdorf, R. G., and Bennett, I. L., 1961, *Pseudomonas* bacteremia: Review of ninety-one cases, *Ann. Intern. Med.* **54:**1077–1107.
12. Collini, F. J., Spees, E. K., Munster, A., Dufresne, C., and Millan, J., 1986, Ecthyma gangrenosum in a kidney transplant recipient with *Pseudomonas* septicemia, *Am. J. Med.* **80:** 729–734.
13. Bodey, G. P., Bolivar, R., Fainstein, V., and Jadeja, L., 1983, Infections caused by *Pseudomonas aeruginosa*, *Rev. Infect. Dis.* **5:**279–313.
14. Stanley, M. M., 1947, *Bacillus pyocyaneus* infections: A review, report of cases and discussion of newer therapy including streptomycin, *Am. J. Med.* **2:**253–277.
15. Kerby, B. P., 1947, *Pseudomonas aeruginosa* bacteremia: Summary of literature with report of a case, *Amer. J. Dis. Child.* **74:**610–615.
16. Whimbey, E., Kiehn, T. E., Brannon, P., Blevins, A., and Armstrong, D., 1987, Bacteremia and fungemia in patients with neoplastic disease, *Am. J. Med.* **82:**723–730.
17. Fishman, L. S., and Armstrong, D., 1972, *Pseudomonas aeruginosa* bacteremia in patients with neoplastic disease, *Cancer* **30:**764–773.
18. Tapper, M. L., and Armstrong, D., 1974, Bacteremia due to *Pseudomonas aeruginosa* complicating neoplastic disease: a progress report, *J. Infect. Dis.* **130:**S14–S23.
19. Flick, M. R., and Cluff, L. E., 1976, *Pseudomonas* bacteremia: Review of 108 cases, *Am. J. Med.* **60:**501–508.
20. Baltch, A. L., and Griffin, P. E., 1977, *Pseudomonas aeruginosa* bacteremia: a clinical study of 75 patients, *Am. J. Med. Sci.* **274:**119–129.
21. Bisbe, J., Gateil, J. M., Puig, J., Mallolas, J., Martinez, J. A., Jimenez de Anta, M. T., and Soriano, E., 1988, *Pseudomonas aeruginosa* bacteremia: Univariate and multivariate analysis of factors influencing the prognosis in 133 episodes, *Rev. Infect. Dis.* **10:**629–635.
22. Cooper, G. S., Havilir, D. S., Shlaes, D. M., and Salata, R. A., 1990, Polymicrobial bacteremia in the late 1980's: Predictors of outcome and review of the literature, *Medicine* **69:**114–123.
23. Gallagher, P. G., and Watanakunakorn, C., 1989, *Pseudomonas* bacteremia in a community teaching hospital, 1980–1984, *Rev. Infect. Dis.* **11:**846–852.
24. Johanson, W. G., Pierce, A. K., Sanford, J. P., and Thomas, G. D., 1972, Nosocomial respiratory infections with gram-negative bacilli: The significance of colonization of the respiratory tract, *Ann. Intern. Med.* **77:**701–706.
25. Greene, S. L., Su, W. P. D., and Muller, S. A., 1984, Ecthyma gangrenosum: Report of clinical, histopathologic and bacteriologic aspects of eight cases, *J. Am. Acad. Dermatol.* **11:** 781–787.
26. Bagel, J., and Grossman, M. E., 1986, Subcutaneous nodules in *Pseudomonas* sepsis, *Am. J. Med.* **80:**528–529.
27. Hall, J. H., Callaway, J. L., Tindall, J. P., and Smith, J. G., 1968, *Pseudomonas aeruginosa* in dermatology, *Arch. Dermatol.* **97:**312–323.
28. Whitecar, J. P., Luna, M., and Bodey, G. P., 1970, *Pseudomonas* bacteremia in patients with malignant diseases, *Am. J. Med. Sci.* **260:**216–223.
29. Saroff, A. L., Armstrong, D., and Johnson, W. D., 1973, *Pseudomonas* endocarditis, *Am. J. Cardiol.* **32:**234–237.
30. Cohen, P. S., Maguire, J. H., and Weinstein, L., 1980, Infective endocarditis caused by gram-negative bacteria: A review of literature, 1945–1977, *Prog. Cardiovasc. Dis.* **22:** 205–242.
31. Shekar, R., Rice, T. W., Zierdt, C. H., and Kallick, C. A., 1985, Outbreak of endocarditis caused by *Pseudomonas aeruginosa* setotype 011 among pentazocine and tripelennamine abusers in Chicago, *J. Infect. Dis.* **151:**203–208.

32. Wieland, M., Lederman, M. M., Kline-King, C., Keys, T. F., Lerner, P. I., Bass, S. N., Chmielewski, R., Banks, V. D., and Ellner, J. J., 1986, Left-sided endocarditis due to *Pseudomonas aeruginosa*: A report of 10 cases and review of the literature, *Medicine* **65:**180–189.
33. Botsford, K. B., Weinstein, R. A., Nathan, C. R., and Kabins, S. A., 1985, Selective survival in pentazocine and tripelennamine of *Pseudomonas aeruginosa* serotype O11 from drug addicts, *J. Infect. Dis.* **151:**209–216.
34. Reyes, M. P., Palutke, W. A., Wylin, R. F., and Lerner, A. M., 1973, *Pseudomonas* endocarditis in the Detroit Medical Center 1969–1972, *Medicine* **52:**173–194.
35. Rajashekaraiah, K. R., Rice, T. W., and Kallick, C. A., 1981, Recovery of *Pseudomonas aeruginosa* from syringes of drug addicts with endocarditis, *J. Infect. Dis.* **144:**482.
36. Levine, D. P., Crane, L. R., and Zervos, M. J., 1986, Bactermia in narcotic addicts at the Detroit Medical Center II. Infectious endocarditis: A prospective comparative study, *Rev. Infect. Dis.* **8:**374–396.
37. Robin, E., Belamaric, J., Thoms, N. W., Arbulu, A., and Ganguly, S. N., 1974, Consequences of total tricuspid valvulectomy without prosthetic replacement in treatment of *Pseudomonas* endocarditis, *J. Thoracic. Cardiovasc. Surg.* **68:**461–465.
38. Stanley, M. M., 1947, *Bacillus pyocyaneus* infections: A review, report of cases and discussion of newer therapy including striptomycin (concluded), *Am. J. Med.* **2:**347–367.
39. Hughes, J. M., 1988, Epidemiology and prevention of nosocomial pneumonia, in :*Current Clinical Topics in Infectious Diseases*, Volume 9 (J. S. Remington, M. N. Swartz, eds.), McGraw-Hill, New York, pp. 241–259.
40. Rose, H. D., Heckman, M. G., and Unger, J. D., 1973, *Pseudomonas* pneumonia in adults, *Am. Rev. Respir. Dis.* **107:**416–422.
41. Stevens, R. M., Teres, D., Skillman, J. J., and Feingold, D. S., 1974, Pneumonia in an intensive care unit: A 30-month experience, *Arch. Intern. Med.* **134:**106–111.
42. Iannini, P. B., Claffey, T., and Quintiliani, R., 1974, Bacteremic *Pseudomonas* pneumonia, *J.A.M.A.* **230:**558–561.
43. Pennington, J. E., Reynolds, H. Y., and Carbone, P. P., 1973, *Pseudomonas* pneumonia: A retrospective study of 36 cases, *Am. J. Med.* **55:**155–160.
44. Tillotson, J. R., and Lerner, A. M., 1968, Characteristics of nonbacteremic *Pseudomonas* pneumonia, *Ann. Intern. Med.* **68:**295–306.
45. Strand, C. L., Bryant, J. K., Morgan, J. W., Foster, J. G., McDonald, H. P., and Morganstern, S. L., 1982, Nosocomial *Pseudomonas aeruginosa* urinary tract infections, *J.A.M.A.* **248:**1615–1618.
46. Kunin, C. M., 1970 A ten-year study of bacteriuria in schoolgirls: Final report of bacteriologic, urologic, and epidemiologic findings, *J. Infect. Dis.* **122:**382–393.
47. Montgomerie, J. A., and Morrow, J. W., 1980, Long-term *Pseudomonas* colonization in spinal cord injury patients, *Am. J. Epidemiol.* **112:**508–517.
48. Norden, C. W., and Keleti, E., 1980, Experimental osteomyelitis caused by *Pseudomonas aeruginosa*, *J. Infect. Dis.* **141:**71–75.
49. Tindel, J. R., and Crowder, J. G., 1971, Septic arthritis due to *Pseudomonas aeruginosa*, *J.A.M.A.* **218:**559–561.
50. Salahuddin, N. I., Madhavan, T., Fisher, E. J., Cox, F., Quinn, E. L., and Eyler, W. R., 1973, *Pseudomonas* osteomyelitis: Radiologic features, *Radiology* **109:**41–47.
51. Weissman, G. J., Wood, V. E., and Kroll, L. L., 1973, *Pseudomonas* vetebral osteomyelitis in heroin addicts: Report of five cases, *J. Bone Jt. Surgery* **55-A:**1416–1424.
52. Gifford, D. B., Patzakis, M., Ivler, D., and Swezey, R. L., 1975, Septic artrhritis due to *Pseudomonas* in heroin addicts, *J. Bone Jt. Surgery* **57-A:**631–635.
53. Green, N. E., and Bruno, J., 1980, *Pseudomonas* infections of the foot after puncture wounds, *South. Med. J.* **73:**146–149.
54. Jacobs, R. F., McCarthy, R. E., and Elser, J. M., 1989, *Pseudomonas* osteochondritis complicating puncture wounds of the foot in children: A 10-year evaluation, *J. Infect. Dis.* **160:**657–661.

55. Chernik, N. L., Armstrong, D., and Posner, J. B., 1973, Central nervous system infections in patients with cancer, *Medicine* **52**:563–581.
56. Wise, B. L., Mathis, J. L., and Jawetz, E., 1969, Infections of the central nervous system due to *Pseudomonas aeruginosa*, *J. Neurosurg.* **31**:432–434.
57. Fong, I. W., and Tomkins, K. B., 1985, Review of *Pseudomonas aeruginosa* meningitis with special emphasis on treatment with ceftazidime, *Rev. Infect. Dis.* **7**:604–612.
58. Berk, S. L., and McCabe, W. R., 1980, Meningitis caused by gram-negative bacilli, *Ann. Intern. Med.* **93**:253–260.
59. Klein, R. S., Berger, S. A., and Yekutiel, P., 1975, Wound infection during the Yom Kippur War: Observation concerning antibiotic prophylaxis and therapy, *Ann. Surg.* **182**: 15–21.
60. Tong, M. J., 1972, Septic complications of war wounds, *J.A.M.A.* **219**:1044–1047.
61. Pruitt, B. A., Lindberg, R. B., McManus, W. F., and Mason, A. D., 1983, Current approach to prevention and treatment of *Pseudomonas aeruginosa* infections in burned patients, *Rev. Infect. Dis.* **5**:S889–S897.
62. Shellow, W. V. R., and Koplon, B. S., 1968, Green striped nails: Chromonychia due to *Pseudomonas aeruginosa*, *Arch. Dermatol.* **97**:149–153.
63. Huminer, D., Siegman-Igra, Y., Morduchowicz, G., and Pitlik, S. D., 1987, Ecthyma gangrenosum without bacteremia: Report of six cases and review of the literature, *Arch. Intern. Med.* **147**:299–301.
64. Gustafson, T. L., Band, J. D., Hutcheson, R. H., and Schaffner, W., 1983, *Pseudomonas* folliculitis: An outbreak and review, *Rev. Infect. Dis.* **5**:1–8.
65. Washburn, J., Jacobson, J. A., Marston, E., and Throsen, B., 1976, *Pseudomonas aeruginosa* rash associated with a whirlpool, *J.A.M.A.* **235**:2205–2207.
66. Centers for Disease Control, 1975, Pool-associated rash-illness—North Carolina, *M.M.W.R.* **24**:349–350.
67. Centers for Disease Control, 1983, An outbreak of *Pseudomonas* folliculitis associated with a waterslide—Utah, *M.M.W.R.* **32**:425–427.
68. Khabbaz, R. F., McKinley, T. W., Goodman, R. A., Hightower, A. W., Highsmith, A. K., Tait, K. A., and Band, J. D., 1983, *Pseudomonas aeruginosa* serotype 0:9: New cause of whirlpool-associated dermatitis, *Am. J. Med.* **74**:73–77.
69. Rosenoff, S. H., Wolf, M. L., and Chabner, B. A., 1974, *Pseudomonas* blepharoconjunctivitis: A complication of combination chemotherapy, *Arch. Ophthalmol.* **91**:490–491.
70. Kreger, A. S., 1983, Pathogenesis of *Pseudomonas aeruginosa* ocular diseases, *Rev. Infect. Dis.* **5**:S931–S935.
71. Traboulsi, E. I., Shammas, I. V., Ratl, H. E., and Jarudi, N. I., 1984, *Pseudomonas aeruginosa* ophthalmia neonatorum, *Am. J. Ophthalmol.* **98**:801–802.
72. Ayliffe, G. A. J., Barry D. R., Lowbury, E. J. L., Roper-Hall, M. J., and Walker, W. M., 1966, Postoperative infection with *Pseudomonas aeruginosa* in an eye hospital, *Lancet* **1**:1113–1117.
73. Hassman, G., and Sugar, J., 1983, *Pseudomonas* corneal ulcer with extended-wear soft contact lenses for myopia, *Arch. Ophthalmol.* **101**:1549–1550.
74. Killingsworth, D. W., and Stern, G. A., 1989, *Pseudomonas* keratitis associated with the use of disposable soft contact lenses, *Arch. Ophthalmol.* **107**:795–796.
75. Rubin, J., and Yu, V. L., 1988, Malignant external otitis: Insights into pathogenesis, clinical manifestations, diagnosis, and therapy, *Am. J. Med.* **85**:391–398.
76. Chandler, J. R., 1968, Malignant external otitis, *Laryngoscope* **78**:1257–1294.
77. Doroghazi, R. M., Nadol, J. B., Hyslop, N. E., Baker, A. S., and Axelrod, L., 1981, Invasive external otitis: Report of 21 cases and review of the literature, *Am. J. Med.* **71**:603–614.
78. Sherman, P., Black, S., and Grossman, M, 1980, Malignant external otitis due to *Pseudomonas aeruginosa* in childhood, *Pediatrics* **66**:782–783.
79. Zaky, D. A., Bently, D. W., Lowy, K., Betts, R. F., and Douglas, R. G., 1976, Malignant external otitis: A severe form of otitis in diabetic patients, *Am. J. Med.* **61**:298–302.

80. Bland, R. D., 1972, Otitis media in the first six weeks of life: Diagnosis, bacteriology, and management, *Pediatrics* **49:**187–197.
81. Brook, I., and Finegold, S. M., 1979, Bacteriology of chronic otitis media, *J.A.M.A.* **241:** 487–488.
82. Gates, G. A., Montalbo, P. J., and Meyerhoff, W. L., 1977, *Pseudomonas* mastoiditis, *Laryngoscope* **87:**483–492.
83. Pruett, T. L., and Simmons, R. L., 1984, Nosocomial gram-negative bacillary parotitis, *J.A.M.A.* **251:**252–253.
84. Caplan, E. S., and Hoyt, N. J., 1982, Nosocomial sinusitis, *J.A.M.A.* **247:**639–641.
85. Bassiouny, A.,1981, Perichondritis of the auricle, *Laryngoscope* **91:**422–431.
86. Krothapalli, R., Duffy, W. B., Lacke, C., Payne, W., Patel, H., Perez, V., and Senekjian, H. O., 1982, *Pseudomonas* peritonitis and continuous ambulatory peritoneal dialysis, *Arch. Intern. Med.* **142:**1862–1863.
87. Piraino, B., Bernardini, J., and Sorkin, M., 1987, A five-year study of the microbiologic results of exit site infections and peritonitis in continuous ambulatory peritoneal dialysis, *Am. J. Kidney Dis.* **10:**281–286.
88. Dressler, R., Peters, A. T., and Lynn, R. I., 1989, Pseudomonal and candidal peritonitis as a complication of continuous ambulatory peritoneal dialysis in human immunodeficiency virus-infected patients, *Am. J. Med.* **86:**787–790.
89. Parrott, P. L., Terry, P. M., Whitworth, E. N., Frawley, L. W., Coble, R. S., Wachsmuth, I. K., and McGowan, J. E., 1982, *Pseudomonas aeruginosa* peritonitis associated with contaminated poloxamer-iodine solution, *Lancet* **2:**683–685.
90. Goetz, A., and Muder, R. R., 1989, *Pseudomonas aeruginosa* infections associated with use of povidone-iodine in patients receiving continuous ambulatory peritoneal dialysis, *Infect. Control Hosp. Epidemiol.* **10:**447–450.
91. Juergensen, P. H., Finkelstein, F. O., Brennan, R., Santacroce, S., and Ahern, M. J., 1988, *Pseudomonas* peritonitis associated with continuous ambulatory peritoneal dialysis: A six-year study, *Am. J. Kidney Dis.* **11:**413–417.
92. Bernardini, J., Piraino, B., and Sorkin, M., 1987, Analysis of continuous ambulatory peritoneal dialysis-related *Pseudomonas aeruginosa* infections, *Am. J. Med.* **83:**829–832.
93. Cross, A. S., 1979, *Pseudomonas aeruginosa*, in: *Principles and Practice of Infectious Diseases*, 1st ed. (G. L. Mandell, R. G. Douglas, and J. E. Bennett, eds.), John Wiley and Sons, New York, pp. 1705–1720.
94. Florman, A. L., and Schifrin, N., 1950, Obervations on a small outbreak of infantile diarrhea associated with *Pseudomonas aeruginosa*, *J. Pediatrics* **36:**758–766.
95. Stone, H. H., Kolb, L. D., and Geheber, C. E., 1979, Bacteriologic considerations in perforated necrotizing enterocoloitis, *South. Med. J.* **72:**1540–1544.
96. Starnes, H. F., Moore, F. D., Mentzer, S., Osteen, R. T., Steele, G. D., and Wilson, R. E., 1986, Abdominal pain in neutropenic cancer patients, *Cancer* **57:**616–621.
97. Schimpff, S. C., Wiernik, P. H., and Block, J. B., 1972, Rectal abscesses in cancer patients, *Lancet* **2:**844–847.
98. Shaked, A. A., Shinar, E., and Freund, H., 1986, Managing the granulocytopenic patient with acute perianal inflammatory disease, *Am. J. Surg.* **152:**510–512.
99. Classen, D. C., Jacobson, J. A., Burke, J. P., Jacobson, J. T., and Evans, R. S., 1988, Serious *Pseudomonas* infections associated with endoscopic retrograde cholangiopancreatography, *Am. J. Med.* **84:**590–596.
100. O'Connor, H. J., Babab, J. R., and Ayliffe, G. A. J., 1987, *Pseudomonas aeruginosa* infection during endoscopy, *Gastroenterology* **93:**1451.
101. Davion, T., Braillon, A., Delamarre, J., Delcenserie, R., Joly, J. P., and Capron, J. P., 1987, *Pseudomonas aeruginosa* liver abscesses following endoscopic retrograde cholangiography: report of a case without biliary tract disease, *Dig. Dis. Sci.* **32:**1044–1046.
102. Allen, J. I., Allen, M. O., Olson, M. M., Gerding, D. N., Shanholtzer, C. J., Meier, P. B.,

Vennes, J. A., and Silvis, S. E., 1987, *Pseudomonas* infection of the biliary system resulting from use of a contaminated endoscope, *Gastroenterology* **92:**759–763.
103. Kowal-Vern, A., and McFadden, J., 1989, *Pseudomonas aeruginosa* pneumonia as a presenting entity in an AIDS patient, *Clin. Pediatrics* **28:**403.
104. Witt, D. J., Craven, D. E., and McCabe, W. R., 1987, Bacterial infections in adult patients with the acquired immune deficiency syndrome (AIDS) and AIDS-related complex, *Am. J. Med.* **82:**900–906.
105. Manian, F. A., and Alford, R. H., 1987, Nosocomial infectious balanoposthitis in neurotropenic patients, *South. Med. J.* **80:**909–911.
106. Willems, C. E. D., Jones, B., and Matthew, D. J., 1986, Pseudomonal toxic shock syndrome, *Lancet* **2:**1218–1219.

13

Chronic *Pseudomonas aeruginosa* Lung Infection in Cystic Fibrosis Patients

GERD DÖRING

1. INTRODUCTION

Cystic fibrosis (CF) is the most common lethal genetic disease in white populations, affecting approximately 1 in 2000 to 1 in 4000 live births in Europe and North America.[1] Fifty-three years after it was first described,[2] the gene responsible for the generalized metabolic disorder was identified on chromosome 7.[3–5] It is expressed in a variety of tissues that are affected in CF patients, such as the lungs, pancreas, liver, sweat glands, and nasal epithelia. The gene encodes a membrane protein that most probably regulates ion transport and/or is an ion channel itself, and was therefore named "Cystic Fibrosis Transmembrane Conductance Regulator" (CFTR). The major mutation in CFTR, present in about 70% of the CF mutant chromosomes, is the deletion of a single amino acid residue at position 508. The frequency of ΔF508 varies considerably depending on the geographic location; so far, more than 60 mutations in CFTR differing from ΔF508 have been reported from CF patients.[6]

The mutations in CFTR interfere with the regulation of chloride ion transport through the epithelial cell membrane.[7] Furthermore, sodium

---

GERD DÖRING • Department of General Hygiene and Environmental Hygiene, Hygiene-Institut, University of Tübingen, D-7400 Tübingen, Germany.

Pseudomonas aeruginosa as an Opportunistic Pathogen, edited by Mario Campa *et al.* Plenum Press, New York, 1993.

transport[8] and sulfation of glycoconjugates[9] in CF epithelia are also abnormal. As a result, characteristic changes of the exocrine glands are seen. Secretions from serous glands reveal an increased sodium chloride content, and exocrine glands in the airways, liver, pancreas, intestines and gall bladder produce highly viscous dehydrated secretions. The obstruction of the ducts inhibits the further outflow of secretions and, for example, may lead to pancreatic insufficiency. Hyperplasia and obstruction of the submucosal glands of the trachea and the major bronchi are the earliest histological changes in the respiratory tract; bronchiectasis is already present 6 months after birth.[10] Because of the thickened mucus in the respiratory tract, the disease is called "mucoviscidosis" in some European countries.

Bacterial colonization and infection of the CF respiratory tract occurs soon after birth.[11] Almost invariably, *Staphylococcus aureus* is the first detectable pathogen. Anaerobes, fungi, and a number of gram-positive and gram-negative bacteria may also be found,[12] but *Pseudomonas aeruginosa* is the dominant pathogen.[13,14] Difficult to treat and never eradicated, *P. aeruginosa* remains in the airways of CF patients until their premature death. It is the bacterial lung infection, most notably with *P. aeruginosa*, that causes progressive pulmonary disease and therefore plays a central role in CF, because it is the direct cause of death in the vast majority of these patients.[15–17] Nevertheless, a large heterogeneity exists among CF patients with respect to the severity of the disease, pancreas or liver involvement, and the onset and development of *P. aeruginosa* lung infection, even in patients homozygous for $\Delta 508$.[20]

Major advances in prolonging the lives of CF patients have been made possible by the development of pancreatic enzyme replacement therapy to treat the more or less impaired pancreas function[18] and by improved antibiotic treatment regimes to reduce the number of *P. aeruginosa* organisms in the airways and, as a consequence, to reduce airway obstruction and inflammation.[19] Thus, a median survival of 25–30 years is now common in countries where these drugs are available and are used to treat CF patients, whereas life expectancy is still below 5 years in countries without such treatment. The present review will focus first on the acquisition of *P. aeruginosa* by CF patients from sources inside and outside of hospitals and major transmission routes, second on the host–parasite interactions in this particular *P. aeruginosa* infection type, and last, based on this analysis, on new treatment and prevention strategies for the *P. aeruginosa* lung infection in CF.

2. ACQUISITION

2.1. In Hospitals

Many CF patients attend CF centers for treatment or disease control and there may acquire *P. aeruginosa*, the second most frequent nosocomial gram-negative pathogen after *Escherichia coli*. In hospitals, the sources from which *P. aeruginosa* may be isolated are numerous. In particular, sinks, toilets and showers are often heavily contaminated with persisting *P. aeruginosa* strains. During hand washing, aerosols containing *P. aeruginosa* have been detected in washbasins.[21] The risk of acquiring aerosolized organisms from these sources is highest early in the morning, when the overnight growth of *P. aeruginosa* may yield up to 10^9 organisms per ml. In CF wards, cross-infection between patients may occur, and, finally, the hospital personnel may be responsible for the transmission of *P. aeruginosa* (see also Chapter 1).

A number of epidemiological studies concerning nosocomial cross-colonization and cross-infection between CF patients have been carried out.[21-35] Although cross-infection with *P. aeruginosa* does not seem to be a major problem in some hospitals,[33] cross-colonization and even an epidemic spread of multiresistant *P. aeruginosa* between CF patients has been observed in others.[22,27,29-32,34,35] The improvement of hygienic measures and the separation of infected from non-infected patients have been suggested as ways to decrease the risk of a nosocomial acquisition of *P. aeruginosa*.[36] Epidemiological data indicate that, indeed, a significant reduction in the yearly incidence of newly infected CF patients can be achieved in this manner.[35,36] The reasons why the incidence of chronic *P. aeruginosa* infections in CF varies widely between CF centers and why larger centers seem to have a higher prevalence of *P. aeruginosa* infection than smaller ones[36] are not fully understood and warrant further epidemiological studies.

DNA typing methods for *P. aeruginosa* such as the exotoxin A (ETA) probe[37-39] or whole genome analysis[35] are valuable tools for epidemiological studies in CF, because identical *P. aeruginosa* strains from these patients may differ considerably in their phenotype and thus pose difficulties when older typing methods such as serotyping, phage and pyocine typing are applied.[40] Using such probes it became clear that CF patients normally harbor only a few individual strains that differ genotypically from the strains of other patients.[34-37] Thus, it was possible to answer the question whether new acquisition of *P. aeruginosa*, for example during a summer camp, was due to strain transmission from other infected CF patients or originated from other sources.[34]

2.2. Outside of Hospitals

Most of the time, CF patients are not hospitalized. Infection with the "ubiquitous" *P. aeruginosa* may well occur at home or elsewhere, where sink drains[41] and food[42] may be contaminated. Furthermore, the organism may be transmitted at home between siblings. Indeed, in contrast to nonrelated CF patients, most siblings harbor identical strains.[23,24,30,34-37] The question still arises whether a direct patient-to-patient transmission route is involved or whether the sibling strain is derived from a common source in the environment of the patients. Because *P. aeruginosa*-infected CF patients may spread the bacteria into sinks and toilets,[41] these reservoirs represent possible sources for infection.[43,44]

Acquisition of *P. aeruginosa* during dental treatment seems to be a major risk for CF patients. It has been known for a long time[45] that *P. aeruginosa* can often be isolated from the plastic tubes that contain water used for cooling instruments and reducing pain during dental treatment. Recent investigations showed that such tubing was persistently contaminated with *P. aeruginosa* in 50% of all dental offices (G. Döring, unpublished data). A survey revealed that the large majority of dentists are unaware of the bacterial contamination in the tubing and of CF as a disease. On the other hand, CF patients do not know the risk associated with a dental office.

2.3. Intestinal Colonization

The intriguing question of whether *P. aeruginosa* in CF lungs originates from the patients' own intestines is still open. The basic hypothesis is, first, that the use of *S. aureus*-specific antibiotics increases the risk of the establishment and proliferation of *P. aeruginosa* in the human intestinal tract by disrupting the natural protective flora,[46] as has been shown in animal models.[47] Second, exocrine glands in the intestine may produce an abnormal mucus, leading to obstruction and inflammation, similar to what happens in the respiratory tract.[48] Finally, *P. aeruginosa* is a facultative anaerobic organism[49] and may well colonize the intestinal tract. In three studies on small numbers of CF patients without *P. aeruginosa* lung infections, the incidence of *P. aeruginosa* in stool samples was not higher[27,41,50] than in stool samples of normal healthy individuals.[51] Nevertheless, larger studies are needed to substantiate this result. However, in CF patients with *P. aeruginosa* lung infection, evidence for intestinal colonization was provided in some cases.[41] This is not surprising; sputum with large numbers of *P. aeruginosa* ($>10^8$)[52] may be swallowed and the organisms may survive the acid stomach passage.[53]

3. VIRULENCE AND HOST DEFENSE

3.1. Adhesion

3.1.1. The Role of Inflammation

Colonization of and persistence on epithelial cells are prominent features of successful mucosal pathogens. The ubiquitous distribution of *P. aeruginosa* in the environment and its limited colonizing potential for healthy individuals, however, demonstrates that *P. aeruginosa* needs special conditions to multiply on epithelial cells and cause infection in humans. Whereas *P. aeruginosa* is rapidly eradicated from normal human and animal lungs, pharyngeal clearance mechanisms may be diminished in patients with various diseases.[54–56] A common theme appears to be alteration of cellular surfaces by a variety of mechanisms. Among these mechanisms is inflammation, which may play an important role in facilitating the adherence of *P. aeruginosa* and impairing its clearance. During acute and chronic inflammation, the balance between proteinases and proteinase inhibitors is disturbed and free host proteinases released from neutrophils (polymorphonuclear leukocytes or PMN) may damage epithelial cells by cleaving fibronectin,[57,58] cilia,[59] or immunoglobulins.[60,61] After proteinase injury *P. aeruginosa* adhesion is enhanced.[57] In addition, other factors such as virus infection,[62] or acid injury[63] also significantly increase *P. aeruginosa* adhesion. Furthermore, the effect of host proteinases on *P. aeruginosa* adherence and clearance was demonstrated *in vitro*,[64] and in experimental rat lung infection models *in vivo*.[65] When rat lungs were pretreated with proteinases and then challenged with aerosolized *P. aeruginosa*, tissue damage was correlated with significantly reduced *P. aeruginosa* clearance.[65] Studies in humans postoperatively infected with *P. aeruginosa* show significantly elevated salivary neutrophil elastase levels compared with the noninfected patient group,[60,66] suggesting a relationship between elastase levels and colonization.

In CF, abnormal chest radiographs and macroscopic bronchial casts in lung washings of the majority of noninfected infants less than 3 years old suggest that airway obstruction can develop prior to infection.[11] Is inflammation and hence proteolytic activity present in CF airways before *P. aeruginosa* colonization? The histological detection of inflammatory infiltrates in bronchi, bronchiectasis, and mucopurulent plugging of airways in many patients in the first months of life support this contention.[10,67] More importantly, in most cases *S. aureus* precedes *P. aeruginosa* in CF airways, inducing inflammation and thus facilitating *P. aeruginosa* infection. In contrast to *P. aeruginosa*, *S. aureus* does not prefer injured cell surfaces for adhesion. Furthermore, *S. aureus* shows a significantly higher binding to CF cell lines than to normal control cells, possibly due to the oversulfation of glycoconjugates[9] (G. Döring, unpublished data). Thus *S. aureus* may colonize intact CF respiratory epithelium at an early stage and a premature neutrophil chemotaxis may support this.[68–70]

Evidence that *P. aeruginosa* is associated with inflammation in CF lungs comes from a recent immunohistological study,[71] where mucoid *P. aeruginosa* was detected predominantly in moderately damaged, inflamed airways, mostly at the bronchial level. *P. aeruginosa* was not found in end-stage replaced lung tissue or in relatively well-preserved lung tissue. Similar findings were obtained in a chronic rat lung infection model.[72]

3.1.2. Adhesins and Receptors

Single, nonmucoid *P. aeruginosa* strains most probably are involved in initial adherence. They are thought to spread from the nasal epithelia[73] or via aerosols to the lower respiratory tract. Pili represent one class of adhesins in nonmucoid *P. aeruginosa* strains.[74–77] Adherence to cilia,[78] to tracheobronchial mucins[79,80] and to epithelial cells has been reported *in vitro*. On epithelial cells, glycolipids may represent receptors, since *P. aeruginosa* strains incubated with glycolipids *in vitro* bound to lactosyl ceramide, gangliotriaosyl ceramide, gangliotetraosyl ceramide, and to the gangliosides GM1 and GM3, which contain sialic acid.[81] Such glycolipid receptors may be exposed during inflammatory events. Interestingly, trypsin-treated cells have more receptors for pili than do untreated cells,[76] as suggested early by Woods and co-workers.[74] In mucins the most likely receptors appear to be the type 1 and type 2 disaccharide units.[82]

Later on, mucoid *P. aeruginosa* colonies dominate[71,83–85] and the exopolysaccharide (alginate),[86] which also surrounds nonmucoid strains in low amounts,[87] may mediate binding of *P. aeruginosa* microcolonies.[88] Based on the identical binding of purified pili and a nonpiliated mutant to glycolipids and similar sugar inhibition patterns of nonmucoid and mucoid strains of *P. aeruginosa*, Baker suggested a model in which the putative adhesin molecule may be present on pili or on the outer membrane or distributed in the exopolysaccharide matrix of the bacteria.[81] It has been suggested that exoenzyme S (exo-S) is also strongly involved in *P. aeruginosa* adhesion.[89] Exo-S binds to lactosyl ceramide, gangliotriaosyl ceramide, and gangliosyltetraosyl ceramide as does the whole organism. Binding of *P. aeruginosa* to buccal cells is inhibited by purified exo-S and a monoclonal antibody to exo-S. Finally, exo-S has been detected on the surface of the bacteria by immunogold labeling.[89] Possibly this enzyme also mediates adhesion to mucins in pilin-deficient *P. aeruginosa* mutants.[90] Recently, doubts have been raised over whether the adhesin is indeed exo-S.

Whereas information about *P. aeruginosa* adhesins and eucaryotic cell receptors is accumulating rapidly, the question of whether the organism adheres to CF respiratory cells or to CF mucins remains open. Despite several *in vitro* observations, direct cell adhesion of *P. aeruginosa* has never been demonstrated *in vivo*. Rather, the organism has been found in the mucus.[71,91,92] In bronchial biopsies of CF patients chronically infected with *S. aureus* and *P. aeruginosa*, gram-positive cocci adhering directly to epithelial cells are seen, as well as gram-negative bacterial cells enclosed in mucus and not adhering to epithelial cells (Fig. 1). *In vitro* experiments using a pneumocyte cell line show that *P. aeruginosa* may also persist in intracellular compartments.[93] The different findings clearly reflect the difficulties in defining bacterial adhesion in infection when dealing with a chameleon-like organism such as *P. aeruginosa* which changes its shape and virulence rapidly with respect to its environment (see following).

3.2. Virulence Determinants

The list of potential virulence determinants that may be produced by *P. aeruginosa* during infection and disease is enormous. It is not within the scope of this review to discuss in detail all determinants; the interested reader is

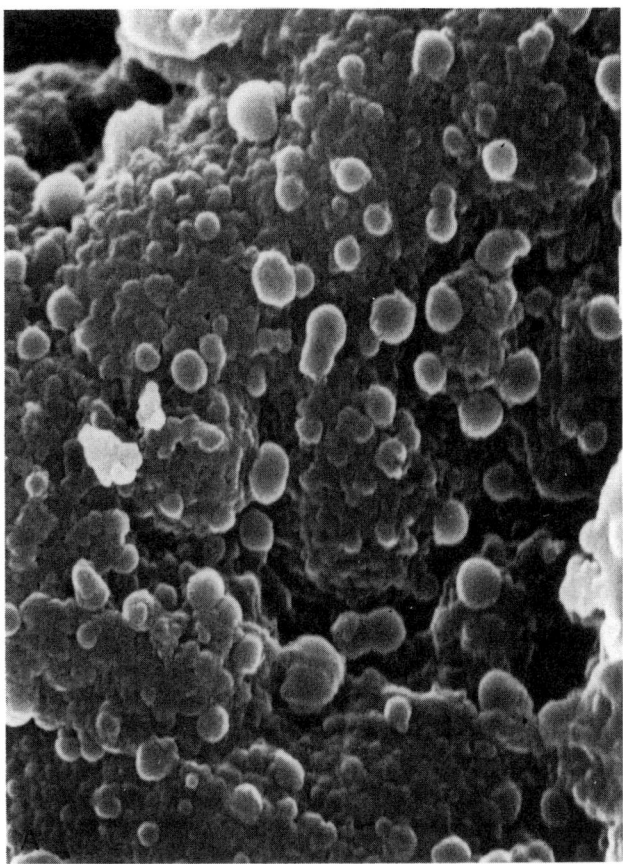

FIGURE 1. Scanning electron micrograph of gram-positive cocci adhering to bronchial epithelial cells (A; ×9000), and transmission electron micrograph of gram-negative bacterial cells enclosed in mucus not adhering to epithelial cells (B; bar = 0.5 μm) from lung biopsies of a CF patient chronically infected with *Staphylococcus aureus* and *Pseudomonas aeruginosa*. Courtesy of C. Dumontel.

referred to excellent reviews on their structure, biochemical function, and putative role in infection.[94–117] They include two protein toxins, exotoxin A (ETA), and exo-S, which enter eucaryotic cells in minute amounts and cause cell death.[94,98,99,101,116] Certain strains also produce enzymes that disintegrate cell membranes and lung surfactants and liberate fatty acids and inorganic phosphate; these are the cytotoxin leukocidin,[103,104] the phospholipases C-H and C-N,[95,105] lipase,[106] and alkaline phosphatase.[96] The proteinase elastase, alkaline proteinase, and the LasA fragment decompose connective tissues[107,108,117] and cleave a variety of biologically important proteins such as immunoglobulins,[109] complement components,[110] transferrin,[111] and recep-

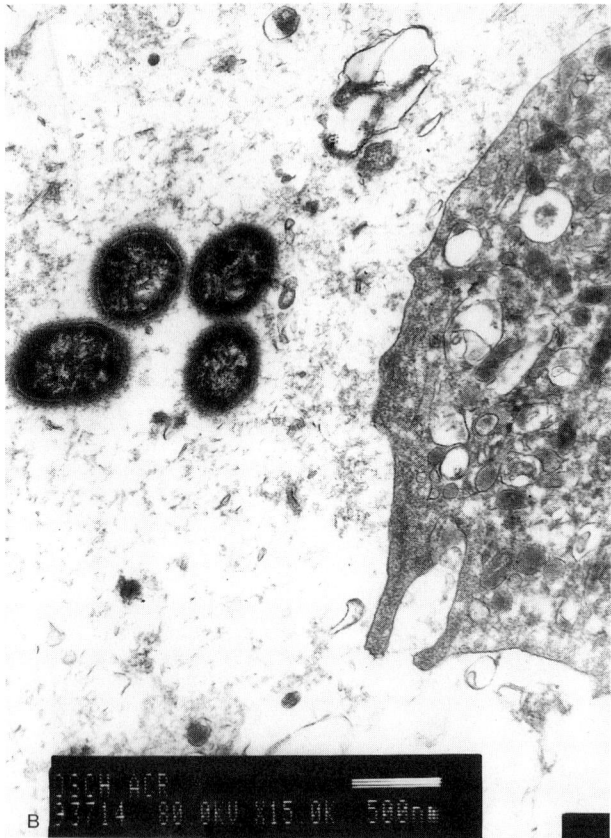

FIGURE 1. (*Continued*)

tors on immunocompetent cells.[112] Secondary metabolites may act as detergents (rhamnolipids),[94,99,100] as siderophores (pyoverdin, pyochelin),[111,113] and as T-cell modulators (phenacin pigments).[114] Exopolysaccharide (alginate) may enlarge the bacterial surface multi-fold and thus prevent elimination by phagocytic cells,[102] and lipopolysaccharide (endotoxin) may activate inflammatory reactions and cause shock.[115]

Despite this impressive list of substances, which is far from complete, *P. aeruginosa* remains an opportunistic pathogen and can infect and eventually cause disease only in compromised hosts.[118] This is in contrast to other pathogens such as, for example, *Corynebacterium diphtheriae*, which causes disease in hosts with an intact defense system. Furthermore, generalized infections with *P. aeruginosa* are seen only in immunocompromised patients, whereas in immunocompetent CF patients[119,120] the opportunistic pathogen can colonize and infect only the respiratory tract. Thus, although we often clearly understand the biochemical basis for toxigenicity and are rapidly accumulating knowledge about toxin genetics, we still have little insight into their roles in infection and in the inanimate environment. Furthermore, as in any discussion about microbial pathogenicity, especially in CF, the complex roles of the host defense mechanisms have to be taken into consideration.

3.2.1. Exotoxin A

The different pathogenic potentials of *C. diphtheriae* and *P. aeruginosa* are especially astonishing with regard to ETA and diphtheria toxin (DT). On a molecular level, the effects of ETA, the "lethal" toxin of *P. aeruginosa*, and DT are strikingly similar.[121] Both proenzymes probably enter eucaryotic cells by receptor-mediated endocytosis,[122] where enzymatically active fragments reach the cytosol and covalently link the ADP-ribosyl moiety of oxidized nicotinamide adenine dinucleotide (NAD) to elongation factor 2 (EL2), terminating protein synthesis.[116,123,124] In patients with diphtheria, the contribution of DT to the disease has been well-established. It reaches the bloodstream from the pseudomembranes in the upper respiratory tract. Damage to internal organs is believed to contribute significantly to rapid death after infection in non-immune individuals.[125] In CF patients, there are no protective antibodies against ETA prior to infection with *P. aeruginosa*, but patients survive the infection a considerably long period of time.[13] Although ETA is produced in the infected CF lungs,[126,127] the toxin does not reach the bloodstream; no toxic effects are observed in parts of the body other than the lungs.[14] One explanation for the different roles of the two enzymes in pathogenicity may be the different nucleotide, and, hence, amino acid sequences.[120,121] Do they differ in their susceptibilities to host proteinases, most notably to neutrophil elastase, which is abundant soon after the initial colonization process in both clinical conditions?[125,130] Indeed, ETA is significantly more sensitive than diphtheria toxin to neutrophil elastase.[131] Thus, the pathogenic importance of ETA, and possibly that of other virulence factors of *P. aeruginosa*, seems to be restricted to the infected airways.

3.2.2. The Humoral Immune Response

In CF, in addition to the inactivating effect of neutrophil enzymes on ETA, a prompt and effective immune response with the production of specific antibodies against bacterial surface components, protein toxins and enzymes takes place. Thus, antibodies against alkaline proteinase,[132,133] elastase,[126,132,133] ETA,[126,127,132,134] phospholipase C,[135] outer membrane proteins,[136,137] lipopolysaccharide,[138,139] a sonicated cell membrane preparations,[133,140] alginate[102,141,142] and exo-S[101] have been detected in the sera of infected CF patients (reviewed in ref. 143). For at least the two proteinases, elastase and alkaline proteinase, it has been shown that specific antibodies from CF patients neutralize their enzymatic activities *in vitro*.[127]

Furthermore, these two enzymes have been detected only in bronchial lavages of CF patients at the beginning of the infection when antibodies were absent.[132] In the chronic course of the infection, the proteinases were not detectable by sensitive radioimmunoassays.[132,144] Rather, immune complexes isolated from bronchial lavages contained both elastase or alkaline proteinase.[144] Thus, the pathogenic importance of the proteinases, if any, seems to be restricted to the early infectious state when specific antibodies have not yet been produced. A longitudinal study on a limited number of patients suggests that specific antibody titers against elastase and alkaline proteinase are detectable 9–12 months after the onset of the infection.[133] Secondary metabolites that escape the immune response, such as pyocyanine, cyanic acid, and rhamnolipids, may well also be active in chronic infectious states. Rhamnolipid has been detected in the sputa of chronically infected CF patients.[145]

3.2.3. The Microenvironment

A permanent and important role of virulence determinants may be the generation of dead tissue in the microenvironment between eucaroytic and adherent bacterial cells. There, proteinases may cleave cell-bound proteins, providing peptides for better growth and denuded cell surfaces for better adherence. Membrane-disintegrating enzymes provide phosphate[96,105] and regulate osmolarity.[105] Toxins enter the cells and terminate protein biosynthesis and cilia beating, thereby inhibiting mucociliary clearance and access of phagocytic cells and antibiotics to the bacterial organism. The dead cell layer probably provokes the growth of *P. aeruginosa*. Such a feature has also been proposed for DT.[146] Similarly, Shiga toxin had no effect on cell invasion, intracellular growth rate or killing of invaded host cells by *Shigella flexneri*, but provoked colonic vascular damage and an increase of neutrophils within the intestinal compartment.[147,148]

Tissue damage seems to be essential for the adherence and persistence of *P. aeruginosa*. Although equipped with potent tools for invading the host and passing through epithelial and endothelial barriers, *P. aeruginosa* remains localized to the respiratory tract in CF, where bacterial macrocolonies are focally distributed in the small airways[71] and bacteremia is seldom seen.[149]

3.2.4. Regulation

The low invasion potential of *P. aeruginosa* in the CF lung might possibly be due to the down-regulation of virulence factor production. There is rapidly growing evidence that bacteria are constantly sensing their environment.[146,150,151] They may turn genes on or off or merely adjust the level to the surroundings. The mechanisms used to control virulence factors share features with other bacterial regulatory systems.[146,150] The signals that are important for gene regulation include osmolarity, temperature, pH, Ca^{2+}, iron, and anaerobicity. In *Salmonella*, these signals act on the *osmZ* gene product, a histone-like protein that rapidly changes the degree of DNA supercoiling, Since transcription is sensitive to supercoiling,[151] this leads to altered gene expression.

Various signals may alter the phenotype of *P. aeruginosa* once it has colonized the airways of CF patients, including high osmolarity due to dehydrated secretions,[152] anaerobicity due to growth on dead tissues, antibiotic treatment that may affect gyrase activity,[153] and nutrient limitation.[154] Although the effects of these stimuli on virulence genes are not completely understood, considerable phenotypic changes have been observed between strains from acute and chronic infections.

The most important phenotypic change in *P. aeruginosa* in CF is a switch from an initially nonmucoid strain to a mucoid variant. The production of exopolysaccharide (alginate) in *P. aeruginosa* is a complex process involving a variety of gene clusters.[155,156] The production of the exopolysaccharide is controlled by at least three *alg*R genes.[155,156] The gene *alg*R1 shows homology with a superfamily of environmentally responsive transcriptional regulators and, indeed, alginate biosynthesis seems to be dependent on environmental conditions.[155,156] Thus, although the mechanism is far from clear, some factors in the CF lung seem to trigger the switch from the nonmucoid to the mucoid phenotype. Clearly, the stimuli are not CF-specific as suggested previously,[155,156] since mucoid *P. aeruginosa* strains have been isolated from other infectious sites such as the skin,[157] urinary tract and ear,[158] cerebrospinal fluid,[159] blood,[160] and lungs[161,162] of non-CF patients. Furthermore, a switch to the mucoid phenotype was demonstrated 6 months after inoculation with a nonmucoid *P. aeruginosa* strain in a chronic lung infection model in rats.[163] The conversion to the mucoid phenotype was associated with a rearrangement of chromosomal DNA upstream of the ETA gene and nonmucoid revertant organisms revealed hybridization patterns identical to the original strain used for inoculation.[163] Finally, the switch from a nonmucoid to a mucoid *P. aeruginosa* phenotype may be induced *in vitro* by culturing the organism in enriched liquid media and under specific aerobic conditions in batch culture.[164,165] Additionally, in phosphate-limited continuous cultures of PAO1, slow growth rates resulted in the appearance of mucoid organisms, and the authors speculate that mucoid variants may first arise during chronic infection in response to nutrient limitation.[154] The application of chemostats to study phenotypic changes in *P. aeruginosa* have been the subject of an excellent review of Brown and Williams.[166] Tissue damage, which is always associated with anaerobicity, may well be one factor explaining the nonmucoid–mucoid switch in the chronic rat lung model. Support for this recently came from heart–lung transplantations in CF where re-infection of the implanted normal lung eventually occurs via *P. aeruginosa* organisms from the upper respiratory tract of the CF patient. The reinfecting strain was nonmucoid and readily eradicated with *P. aeruginosa*-specific antibiotics (P. Helms, personal communication).

In addition to the "alginate switch," other phenotypic changes may be observed in *P. aeruginosa* strains isolated from infected CF or rat lungs: The polysaccharide side chain length of lipopolysaccharide is reduced in mucoid strains[167,168] and iron limitation provokes the production of outer membrane proteins.[169,170] Furthermore, significant decreases in the production of specific virulence determinants such as ETA, exo-S, phospholipase C, and pyochelin levels were demonstrated upon conversion to the mucoid phenotype in the rat lung model, but the elastase level remained unchanged.[163] This is surprising, since *lasB* and *algD* genes showed inverse levels of promoter activity and a see-saw model of co-ordinate regulation of the two virulence factors has been suggested.[171]

In summary, a century-old paradigm in microbial pathogenicity has been abandoned, at least for *P. aeruginosa*: Toxins are no longer held directly responsible for the disease process. Low virulence for survival is the new paradigm.

3.3. Persistence: The Surface Enlargement Strategy

The most dramatic change to occur in the CF airways after colonization with *P. aeruginosa* is the rapid recruitment of neutrophils from the bloodstream. The immigration is rapid and may lead to neutrophil numbers of about 10^7.[52] A major chemotaxigenic compound of *P. aeruginosa* for neutrophils is lipopolysaccharide,[172] whereas important chemotactins are activated complement components,[173] macrophage-derived LTB_4,[174] and *P. aeruginosa*-derived formyl-methionyl oligopeptides.[175] The *P. aeruginosa* macrocolonies, far exceeding the size of a single neutrophil and focally distributed in the small airways of CF patients, are difficult to eliminate by alveolar macrophages or neutrophils,[176] neither of which are impaired in CF. It is the surface enlargement strategy, also used by *S. epidermidis*, for example, that leads to chronic *P. aeruginosa* infection in CF. Its first description *in vitro*[83] and *in vivo*[85] was of major importance.

As *P. aeruginosa* persists, specific antibodies are tailored by the immune system against a variety of antigenic bacterial determinants, and phagocytosis of *P. aeruginosa* becomes much more effective,[177] especially with regard to neutrophils, which are equipped with receptors for the Fc-part of immunoglobulins and activated complement.[178,179] Thus, bacterial opsonization and immune complex formation represents the second approach to eliminating the stimulus. Again, this host strategy also is unsuccessful in CF and, worse, leads to self-destruction and facilitates the further spread of *P. aeruginosa* in the airways. The development of nonopsonizing IgG subclasses such as IgG2 and IgG4 during the chronic course of the infection is only partially understood. Since the first description by Thomassen and co-workers,[180] several groups have reported on total or *P. aeruginosa*-specific IgG subclasses in CF serum.[142,181–187] Because the switch from opsonizing subclasses to nonopsonizing subclasses is also seen in other diseases,[188] it does not seem to be CF-specific.

3.4. Tissue Damage: A Neutrophil Enzyme Effect

The pathogenic events, best described as a type-III hypersensitivity reaction, which lead to tissue damage and ultimately to lung failure and cor pulmonale, have been extensively investigated and reviewed.[120,189–191] Høiby and Axelsen were the first to address the role of the host in tissue damage in CF.[192] The basic observation has been that the occurrence of antibodies against *P. aeruginosa* antigens or immune complexes in CF sera was associated with a poor prognosis.[120,189] Although this correlation was questioned and conflicting results have been obtained on the correlation between the levels of antibodies and immune complexes and the patients' clinical states,[193–202] there is general agreement that the pathological consequences of permanently stimulated neutrophils, in whatever manner, lead to the release of lysosomal enzymes that destroy the lungs.

Neutrophil elastase is by far the best-studied enzyme in this respect. It is released by stimulated neutrophils during successful and frustrated phagocytosis.[203] After the neutrophils have reached the infected lungs from the bloodstream, they do not return to the circulation, but rather decay at the infected site. Thus, lysosomal enzymes are also released after cell death in the airways. Neutrophil elastase, for example, may reach concentrations of more than 100 μg per ml of sputum.[58,130,204–209] Because CF patients may produce 150 ml of sputum per day during acute exacerbations, the total amount of this enzyme is enormous. About 90% of the endogenous inhibitor for neutrophil elastase, α_1-proteinase inhibitor, is locally inactivated by neutrophil elastase[130] and probably also by oxidative attack.[210] Thus, a high imbalance between proteinases and proteinase inhibitors is present in the inflamed lungs of these patients.[130,190,204–207,209] The pathological effects of free neutrophil elastase, demonstrated in a number of *in vitro* and *in vivo* investigations, include cleavage of fibronectin,[58] lung elastin,[46] immunoglobulins and immune complexes,[209] complement,[211,212] complement receptors on neutrophils,[213,214] and other receptors on T cells and B cells.[190] Furthermore, it inhibits ciliary beating[59] and stimulates mucus production from goblet cells.[215] Thus, neutrophil elastase facilitates *P. aeruginosa* adherence by providing denuded epithelial cells with an increased number of receptors for pili. The increased mucin production also may increase *P. aeruginosa* binding in CF lungs.[79,80] Its elimination is prevented by the inhibition of the mucociliary clearance and the impairment of opsonophagocytosis. Finally, by cleaving receptors for interleukin (IL) 1 and IL 2 or the T-cell antigen receptor, it may hypothetically inhibit message transmission and immune recognition. Although high concentrations of IL-1 and tumor necrosis factor have been detected in CF sera[216,217] and bronchial lavages[218] and auto-antibodies to tumor necrosis factor have been found in 72% of all CF patients,[219] their role in the disease process is far from understood.

Is neutrophil elastase a suicide enzyme, killing the host? I propose that it may serve to down-regulate inflammation, after it becomes evident that the bacterial stimulus is impossible to eradicate.[209] Inhibition of message transmission by receptor cleavage, degradation of chemotaxins for PMN, inhibition of the release of lysosomal enzymes and oxygen radicals from PMN by cleavage of immunoglobulins and impairment of immune complex uptake may be involved in this process which has been called a "vicious cycle."[214]

4. NEW STRATEGIES FOR THERAPY AND PREVENTION

4.1. Antibiotics

P. aeruginosa is virtually never eradicated once it has colonized the lungs of CF patients, most probably due to the inaccessibility of the mucoid macrocolonies in anaerobic foci and the effective natural and acquired resistance mechanisms of the pathogen.[220,221] Thus, it is not surprising that the effectiveness of therapy regimes employing antibiotics has been questioned.[222,223] However, there is no doubt that antibiotic therapy has improved significantly the life expectancy in CF. Furthermore, 2-week courses of intensive intravenous treatment given quarterly have greatly slowed the decrease in lung function in these patients and have substantially improved the survival rate in infected CF patients compared with the older treatment "on demand."[19,191] In light of the pathogenic mechanism outlined here, such regular treatment apparently suppresses inflammation more efficiently by reducing the number of bacteria in the airways. In a recent double-blind placebo-controlled trail, antibiotic therapy provided significant additional benefit to bronchodilators and chest physiotherapy in CF patients.[224] Moreover, the degree of improvement correlated with the degree of reduction of *P. aeruginosa* and total bacterial density in the sputum.[224] The different studies on antibiotics in CF are summarized in an excellent review by Michel.[225]

4.2. Anti-Inflammatory Therapy

A better understanding of the pathogenic mechanism of chronic *P. aeruginosa* lung infection, with its key enzyme neutrophil elastase, has led to the strategy of anti-inflammatory therapy in CF. In 1985, a controlled study of prednisone treatment in CF revealed a favorable clinical outcome in the treatment group versus the control group and practically no side effects of the drug.[226] This prompted a double-blind placebo-controlled multicenter study in 1986 with 283 CF patients in the U.S. Careful examination of the patients revealed impairment of growth and several other complications, including diabetes in the treatment group,[227,228] which led to recommendations to stop the trial for all patients in the high-dose prednisone group.[227] These results make it unlikely that the use of steroids will be favored in the long-term treatment of the CF lung infection. Nonsteroidal anti-inflammatory drugs such as piroxicam and ibuprofen, which have been shown to be effective against experimental *P. aeruginosa* lung infection in animals,[229] have also been used in CF patients. Preliminary data from a controlled ibuprofen study do not reveal trends in inflammatory markers.[230] In the piroxicam study, lower frequency of hospitalization was seen of the patients in the treatment group.[231]

The plausible proteinase pathogenesis hypothesis suggests a strategy of increasing the antiproteinase levels in the lung by supplementation with suitable inhibitors. A wide variety of inhibitors has been developed for neutrophil elastase, but only a few may be applied in humans.[232] The α_1-proteinase inhibitor, purified from blood plasma or produced by recombinant DNA technology,[233] and non-immunogenic, small substances such as ICI 200,355[234] may be used. Secretory leukocyte proteinase inhibitor or sulfated polysaccharides[235] are also promising candidates for such a treatment strategy. Clearly, the aerosolized administration of inhibitors is superior to intravenous administration[236] and improved aerosol delivery methods may reduce the amount of inhibitors necessary to neutralize the PMN-elastase burden in the inflamed lungs. Based on several calculations, 175 mg α_1-proteinase inhibitor aerosolized per day will result in α_1-proteinase inhibitor alveolar fluid levels of 1.0 mg/ml.[236,237] A trial using aerosolized α_1-proteinase inhibitor in a small number of CF patients for one week was promising.[238]

Therapy with oxygen radical scavenger is another potential way to reduce inflammation. A combination of superoxide dismutase, which leads to hydrogen peroxide conversion, and catalase, which converts hydrogen peroxide into oxygen and water, is needed to completely reduce the superoxide anion radical. Application of the commercially available superoxide dismutase alone may be harmful, since hydrogen peroxide serves as a substrate for the myeloperoxidase that is present in large amounts in CF sputa.[130] The pathogenic role of myeloperoxidase in CF needs further investigation.

4.3. Immunoprophylaxis and Immunotherapy

Active immunization against *P. aeruginosa* in CF is currently being reconsidered, although previous trials did not yield positive results.[239,240]

New vaccines in various stages of clinical evaluation are composed of *P. aeruginosa* mucoid exopolysaccharide, flagella,[241,242] pili, lipoprotein I,[243] an ETA–polysaccharide conjugate,[244] and an ETA–alginate conjugate.[244] The ETA–polysaccharide conjugate is currently being used to immunize non-infected CF children at an early age.[244] Out of a wish to retain the safety advantage of reversibility, two immunization studies were recently carried out using intravenous gammaglobulin preparations.[245–247] In both studies transient lung function improvement was noticed in the treatment group; larger studies should be carried out to validate these data.

4.4. Disinfection and Hygiene

Another promising strategy for fighting lung infections in CF is the prevention of major transmission routes and the effective disinfection of environmental sources by which CF patients may be infected with these organisms (see also Chapter 1). Epidemiological studies of the transmission of *P. aeruginosa* have revealed that sink drains and toilets in hospitals and at home represent important environmental sources of *P. aeruginosa*. Although it seems impossible to exclude all potential *P. aeruginosa* reservoirs in the environment, disinfection of the major sources might be expected to decrease infection rates. Therefore, a new heating device was developed that inhibits bacterial growth in sink drains and consequently results in *P. aeruginosa*-negative hand cultures after washing.[21] Of considerable importance for potential *P. aeruginosa* infection in CF are also the highly *P. aeruginosa*-contaminated plastic tubes used by dentists to spray a water–air aerosol into the mouth during treatment. Apparently, the usual disinfection method is not sufficient to eradicate the bacteria from such tubes and other procedures have to be used to solve the problem. One possibility is the use of sterile physiological saline for cooling during dental treatment. It should be exciting to observe the results of these measures in the near future.

ACKNOWLEDGMENTS. The author is indebted to C. Dumontel for releasing unpublished material, to N. Baker, R. Ramphal, and N. Høiby for fruitful and stimulating discussions, and to D. Blaurock for language corrections.

REFERENCES

1. Harris, J. H., and Nadler, H. L., 1983, Incidence, genetics, heterozygote, and ante-natal detection of cystic fibrosis, in: *Textbook of Cystic Fibrosis*, (J. D. Lloyd-Still, ed.), John Wright, Boston, pp. 1–7.
2. Fanconi, G., Uehlinger, E., and Knauer, C., 1936, Das Coeliakiesyndrom bei angeborener zystischer Pankreas-Fibromatose und Bronchiektasen, *Wien. Med. Wochensch.* **86:**753–756.
3. Rommens, J. M., Iannuzzi, M. C., Kerem, B., Melmer, G., Drumm, M. L., Melmer, G., Dean, M., Rozmahel, R., Cole, J. L., Kennedy, D., Hidaka, N., Zsiga, M., Buchwald, M.,

Riordan, J. R., Tsui, L.-C., and Collins, F. S., 1989, Identification of the cystic fibrosis gene: Chromosome walking and jumping, *Science* **245**:1059–1065.
4. Riordan, J. R., Rommens, J. M., Kerem, B., Alon, N., Rozmahel, R., Grzelzak, J., Zielenski, J., Silok, S., Plavsic, N., Chou, J.-L., Drumm, M. L., Iannuzzi, M. C., Collins, F. S., and Tsui, L.-C., 1989, Identification of the cystic fibrosis gene: Cloning and characterization of complementary DNA, *Science* **245**:1066–1073.
5. Kerem, B. Rommens, J. M., Buchanan, J. A., Markiewicz, D., Cox, T. K., Chakravarty, A., Buchwald, M., and Tsui, L.-C., 1989, Identification of the cystic fibrosis gene: Genetic analysis, *Science* **245**:1073–1080.
6. Tsui, L.-C., 1991, Molecular genetics of cystic fibrosis and possible mechanisms of protein function, *World Health Organization*, Hereditary diseases program, Report of a joint WHO/ICF(M)A task force on cystic fibrosis, Annex 1, pp. 21–30.
7. Li, M., McCann, J. D., Liedtke, C. M., Nairn, A. C., Greengard, P., and Welsh, M. J., 1988, Cyclic AMP-dependent protein kinase opens chloride channels in normal but not cystic fibrosis airway epithelium, *Nature* **331**:358–360.
8. Boucher, R. C., Stutts, M. J., Knowles, M. R., Cantley, L., and Gatzy, J. T., 1986, Na+ transport in cystic fibrosis respiratory epithelia. Abnormal basal rate and response to adenylate cyclase activation, *J. Clin. Invest.* **78**:1245–1252.
9. Cheng, P.-W., Boat, T. F., Cranfill, K., Yankaskas, I. R., and Boucher, R. C., 1989, Increased sulfation of glycoconjugates by cultured nasal epithelial cells from patients with cystic fibrosis, *J. Clin. Invest.* **84**:68–72.
10. Lloyd-Still, J. D., 1983, Pulmonary manifestations, in: *Textbook of Cystic Fibrosis*, (J. D. Lloyd-Still, ed.), John Wright, Boston, pp. 165–198.
11. Wood, R. E., 1989, Treatment of cystic fibrosis lung disease in the first two years, *Pediatr. Pulmonol.* Suppl. **4**:68–70.
12. Bellon, G., Chomarat, M., and Döring, G., 1991, Bacterial ecology in the airways of cystic fibrosis patients. Abstr. 17th Annu. Meet. E.W.G.C.F.
13. Høiby, N., 1982, Microbiology of lung infections in cystic fibrosis patients, *Acta Paediatr. Scand.* Suppl. **301**:33–54.
14. Myers, M. G., Koontz, F., and Weinberger, M., 1983, Lower respiratory infections in patients with cystic fibrosis, in: *Textbook of Cystic Fibrosis*, (J. D. Lloyd-Still, ed.), John Wright, Boston, pp. 91–107.
15. Wood, R. E., Boat, T. F., and Doershuk, C. F., 1976, Cystic fibrosis: state of the art, *Am. Rev. Respir. Dis.* **113**:833–878.
16. Kulczycki, L. L., Murphy, T. M., and Bellanti, J. A., 1978, Pseudomonas colonization in cystic fibrosis. A study of 160 patients, *J.A.M.A.* **240**:30–34.
17. diSant'Agnese, P. A., and Davis, P. A., 1976, Research in cystic fibrosis, III, *N. Engl. J. Med.* **295**:597–602.
18. Lebenthal, E., and Baswell, D., 1983, The pancreas in cystic fibrosis, in: *Textbook of Cystic Fibrosis*, (J. D. Lloyd-Still, ed.), John Wright, Boston, pp. 293–312.
19. Jensen, T., Pedersen, S. S., Høiby, N., Koch, C., Flensborg, E. W., 1989, Use of antibiotics in cystic fibrosis. The Danish approach, *Antibiot. Chemother.* **42**:237–246.
20. Krogh-Johansen, H., Nir, M., Høiby, N., Koch, C., and Schwartz, M., 1991, Severity of cystic fibrosis in patients homozygous and heterozygous for delta F508 mutation, *Lancet* **337**:631–634.
21. Döring, G., Ulrich, M., Müller, W., Bitzer, J., Schmidt-Koenig, L., Münst, L., Grupp, H., Wolz, C., Stern, M., and Botzenhart, K., 1991, Generation of *Pseudomonas aeruginosa* aerosols during handwashing from contaminated sink drains, transmission to hands of hospital personnel, and its prevention by use of a new heating device, *Zentralbl. Hyg.* **191**:494–505.
22. Høiby, N., and Rosendal, K., 1980, Epidemiology of *Pseudomonas aeruginosa* infections in cystic fibrosis, *Acta Pathol. Microbiol. Scand. Sect [B]* **88**:125–131.

23. Kelly, N. M., Falkiner, F. R., Tempany, E., Fitzgerald, M. X., O'Boyle, C., and Keane, C. T., 1982, Does *Pseudomonas* cross-infection occur between cystic fibrosis patients? *Lancet* **ii**: 688–690.
24. Laraya-Cuasay, L. R., Cundy, K. R., and Huang, N. N., 1976, *Pseudomonas* carrier rates of patients with cystic fibrosis and of members of their families, *J. Pediatrics* **89**:23–26.
25. Seale, T. W., Thirkill, H., Tarpay, M., Flux, M., and Rennert, O. M., 1979, Serotypes and antibiotic susceptibilities of *Pseudomonas aeruginosa* isolates from single sputa of cystic fibrosis patients, *J. Clin. Microbiol.* **9**:72–78.
26. Speert, D. P., Lawton, D., and Damm, S., 1982, Communicability of *Pseudomonas aeruginosa* in a cystic fibrosis summer camp, *J. Pediatrics* **101**:227–229.
27. Speert, D. P., and Campbell, M. E., 1987, Hospital epidemiology of *Pseudomonas aeruginosa* from patients with cystic fibrosis, *J. Hosp. Infect.* **9**:11–21.
28. Thomassen, M. J., Demko, C. A., Doershuk, C. F., and Root, J. M., 1985, *Pseudomonas aeruginosa* isolates: Comparison of isolates from campers and from sibling pairs with cystic fibrosis, *Pediatr. Pulmonol.* **1**:40–45.
29. Zierdt, C. H., and Williams, R. L., 1975, Serotyping of *Pseudomonas aeruginosa* isolates from patients with cystic fibrosis of the pancreas, *J. Clin. Microbiol.* **1**:521–526.
30. Pedersen, S. S., Koch, C., Høiby, N., and Rosendal, K., 1986, An epidemic spread of multiresistant *Pseudomonas aeruginosa* in a cystic fibrosis center, *J. Antimicrob. Chemother.* **17**: 505–516.
31. Zimakoff, J., Høiby, N., Rosendal, K., and Guilbert, J. P., 1983, Epidemiology of *Pseudomonas aeruginosa* infection and the role of contamination of the environment in a cystic fibrosis clinic, *J. Hosp. Infect.* **4**:31–40.
32. Bergan, T., and Høiby, N., 1975, Epidemiological markers for *Pseudomonas aeruginosa*. 6. Relationship between concomitant nonmucoid and mucoid strains from the respiratory tract in cystic fibrosis, *Acta Pathol. Microbiol. Immunol. Scand.* [B] **83**:553–560.
33. Grothus, D., Koopmann, U., von der Hardt, H., and Tümmler, B., 1988, Genome fingerprinting of *Pseudomonas aeruginosa* indicates colonization of cystic fibrosis siblings with closely related strains, *J. Clin. Microbiol.* **26**:1973–1977.
34. Wolz, C., Kiosz, G., Ogle, J. W., Vasil, M. L., Schaad, U., Botzenhart, K., and Döring, G., 1989, *Pseudomonas aeruginosa* cross-colonization and persistence in patients with cystic fibrosis. Use of a DNA probe, *Epidem. Infect.* **102**:205–214.
35. Tümmler, B., Koopmann, U., Grothus, D., Weissbrodt, H., Steinkamp, G., and von der Hardt, H., 1991, Nosocomial acquisition of *Pseudomonas aeruginosa* by cystic fibrosis patients, *J. Clin. Microbiol.* **29**:1265–1267.
36. Høiby, N., and Pedersen, S. S., 1989, Cross-infection with *Pseudomonas aeruginosa* in Danish cystic fibrosis patients, *Antibiot. Chemother.* **42**:124–129.
37. Ogle, J. W., Janda, J. M., Woods, D. E., and Vasil, M. L., 1987, Characterization and use of a DNA probe as an epidemiological marker for *Pseudomonas aeruginosa*, *J. Infect. Dis.* **155**: 119–126.
38. Vasil, M. L., Chamberlain, C., and Grant, C., 1986, Molecular studies of *Pseudomonas* exotoxin A gene, *Infect. Immun.* **52**:538–548.
39. Ojeniyi, B., Wolz, C., Döring, G., Lam, J. S., Rosdahl, V. T., and Høiby, N., 1990, Typing of polyagglutinable *Pseudomonas aeruginosa* isolates from cystic fibrosis patients, *Acta Pathol. Microbiol. Immunol. Scand.* **98**:423–431.
40. Ojeniyi, B., and Høiby, N., 1991, Comparison of different typing methods of *Pseudomonas aeruginosa*, *Antibiot. Chemother.* **44**:13–22.
41. Döring, G., Bareth, H., Gairing, A., Wolz, C., and Botzenhart, K., 1989, Genotyping of *Pseudomonas aeruginosa* sputum and stool isolates from cystic fibrosis patients: Evidence for intestinal colonization and spreading into toilets, *Epidem. Infect.* **103**:555–564.
42. Remington, J. S., and Schimpff, S. C., 1981, Please don't eat the salads, *N. Engl. J. Med.* **304**: 433–435.

43. Gerba, C. P., Wallis, C., and Melnick, J. L., 1975, Microbial hazards of household toilets: Droplet production and the fate of residual organisms, *Appl. Microbiol.* **30:**229–237.
44. Darlow, H. M., and Bale, W. R., 1959, Infective hazards of water-closets, *Lancet* **i:**1196–1200.
45. Exner, M., Vogel, F., and Stelzner, M., 1982, Occurrence of *Pseudomonas aeruginosa* in the oropharynx, *Hyg. Med.* **7:**550–552.
46. Levison, M. E., 1977, Factors influencing colonization of the gastrointestinal tract with *Pseudomonas aeruginosa*, in: *Pseudomonas aeruginosa: Ecological Aspects and Patient Colonization*, (V. M. Young, ed.), Raven Press, New York, pp. 97–109.
47. Hentges, D. J., Stein, A. J., Casey, S. W., and Que, J. U., 1985, Protective role of intestinal flora against infection with *Pseudomonas aeruginosa* in mice: Influence of antibiotics on colonization resistance, *Infect. Immun.* **47:**118–122.
48. Lloyd-Still, J. D., 1983, Growth, nutrition and gastrointestinal problems, in: *Textbook of cystic fibrosis*, (J. D. Lloyd-Still, ed.), John Wright, Bristol, pp. 223–267.
49. Vander Wauven, C., Piérard, A., Kley-Raymann, M., and Haas, D., 1984, *Pseudomonas aeruginosa* mutants affected in anaerobic growth on arginine: Evidence for a four gene cluster encoding the arginine deiminase pathway, *J. Bacteriol.* **160:**928–934.
50. Agnarsson, U., Glass, S., and Govan, J. R. W., 1989, Fecal isolation of *Pseudomonas aeruginosa* from patients with cystic fibrosis, *J. Clin. Microbiol.* **27:**96–98.
51. Kessner, D. M., and Lepper, M. H., 1967, Epidemiologic studies of gram-negative bacilli in the hospital and community, *Am. J. Epidemiol.* **85:**45–60.
52. Bruce, M. C., Poncz, L., Klinger, J. D., Stern, R. C., Tomashefski, J. F., Jr., and Dearborn, D. G., 1985, Biochemical and pathological evidence for proteolytic destruction of lung connective tissue in cystic fibrosis, *Am. Rev. Respir. Dis.* **132:**529–535.
53. Buck, A. C., and Cooke, E. M., 1969, The fate of ingested *Pseudomonas aeruginosa* in normal persons, *J. Med. Microbiol.* **2:**521–525.
54. Pierce, A. K., and Sanford, J. P., 1974, Aerobic gram-negative bacillary pneumonias, *Am. Rev. Respir. Dis.* **110:**647–658.
55. Jackson, A. E., Southern, P. M., Pierce, A. K., Fallis, B. D., and Sanford, J. P., 1967, Pulmonary clearance of gram-negative bacilli, *J. Lab. Clin. Med.* **69:**833–841.
56. Salata, R. A., Lederman, M. M., Shlaes, D. M., Jacobs, M. R., Eckstein, E., Tweardy, D., Toossy, Z., Chielewski, R., Marino, J., King, C. H., Graham, R. C., and Ellner, J. J., 1987, Diagnosis of nosocomial pneumonia in intubated intensive care unit patients, *Am. Rev. Respir. Dis.* **135:**426–432.
57. Woods, D. E., Straus, D. C., Johanson, W. G., Jr., and Bass, J. A., 1981, The role of fibronectin in the prevention of adherence of *Pseudomonas aeruginosa* to buccal cells, *J. Infect. Dis.* **143:**784–790.
58. Suter, S., Schaad, U. B., Morgenthaler, J. J., Chevallier, I., and Schnebli, H. P., 1988, Fibronectin-cleaving activity in bronchial secretions of patients with cystic fibrosis, *J. Infect. Dis.* **158:**89–100.
59. Smallman, L. A., Hill, S. L., and Stockley, R. A., 1984, Reduction of ciliary beat frequency *in vitro* by sputum from patients with bronchiectasis: A serine proteinase effect, *Thorax* **39:**663–667.
60. Niederman, M. S., Merrill, W. W., Polomski, L. M., Reynolds, H. Y., and Gee, J. B. L., 1986, Influence of sputum IgA and elastase on tracheal cell bacterial adherence, *Am. Rev. Respir. Dis.* **133:**255–260.
61. Döring, G., Goldstein, W., Botzenhart, K., Kharazmi, A., Schiøtz, P. O., Høiby, N., and Dasgupta, M., 1986, Elastase from polymorphonuclear leucocytes: A regulatory enzyme in immune complex disease, *Clin. Exp. Immunol.* **64:**597–605.
62. Ramphal, R., Small, P. A., Shands, J. W. Jr., Fischweiger, W., and Small, P. A., Jr., 1980, Adherence of *Pseudomonas aeruginosa* to tracheal cells injured by influenza infection or by endotracheal intubation, *Infect. Immun.* **27:**614–619.

63. Ramphal, R., and Pyle, M., 1983, Adherence of mucoid and nonmucoid *Pseudomonas aeruginosa* to acid-injured tracheal epithelium, *Infect. Immun.* **41:**345–351.
64. Plotkowski, M. C., Beck, G., Tournier, J.M., Bernardo-Filho, M., Marques, E. A., and Puchelle, E., 1989, Adherence of *Pseudomonas aeruginosa* to respiratory epithelium and the effect of leucocyte elastase, *J. Med. Microbiol.* **30:**285–293.
65. Döring, G., and Dauner, H.-J., 1988, Clearance of *Pseudomonas aeruginosa* in different rat lung models, *Am. Rev. Respir. Dis.* **138:**1249–1253.
66. Dal Nogare, A. R., Toews, G. B., and Pierce, A. K., 1987, Increased salivary elastase precedes gram-negative bacillary colonization in postoperative patients, *Am. Rev. Respir. Dis.* **135:**671–675.
67. Bedrossian, C. W. M., Greenberg, S. D., Singer, D. B., Hansen, J. J., and Rosenberg, H. S., 1976, The lung in cystic fibrosis: A quantitative study including prevalence of pathologic findings among different age groups, *Hum. Pathol.* **7:**195–204.
68. Martin, T. R., Rubens, C. E., and Wilson, C. B., 1988, Lung antibacterial defense mechanisms in infant and adult rats: Implications for the pathogenesis of group B streptococcal infections in the neonatal lung, *J. Infect. Dis.* **157:**91–100.
69. Hemming, V. G., Overall, J. C., and Britt, M. R., 1976, Nosocomial infections in a newborn intensive care unit. Results of forty-one months of surveillance, *N. Eng. J. Med.* **294:**1310–1316.
70. Berger, M., 1990, Complement deficiency and neutrophil dysfunction as risk factors for bacterial infection in newborns and the role of granulocyte transfusion in therapy, *Rev. Infect. Dis.* **12:**S401–S409.
71. Baltimore, R. S., Christie, C. D. C., and Smith, G. J. W., 1989, Immunohistopathologic location of *Pseudomonas aeruginosa* in lungs of patients with cystic fibrosis, *Am. Rev. Respir. Dis.* **140:**1650–1661.
72. Cash, H. A., Woods, D. E., McCullough, B., Johanson, W. G., Jr., and Bass, J. A., 1979, A rat model of chronic respiratory infection with *Pseudomonas aeruginosa*, *Am. Rev. Respir. Dis.* **119:**453–459.
73. Römling, U., Grothus, D., and Tümmler, B., 1991, Whole DNA genome typing, *Antibiot. Chemother.* **44:**1–7.
74. Woods, D. E., Straus, D. C., Johanson, W. G., Jr., Berry, V. K., and Bass, J. A., 1980, Role of pili in adherence of *Pseudomonas aeruginosa* to mammalian buccal epithelial cells, *Infect. Immun.* **29:**1146–1151.
75. Ramphal, R., Sadoff, J. C., Pyle, M., and Silipigni, J. D., 1984, Role of pili in adherence of *Pseudomonas aeruginosa* to injured tracheal epithelium, *Infect. Immun.* **44:**38–40.
76. Doig, P., Todd, T., Sastry, P. A., Lee, K. K., Hodges, R. S., Paranchych, W., and Irvin, R. T., 1988, Role of pili in adhesion of *Pseudomonas aeruginosa* to human respiratory epithelial cells, *Infect. Immun.* **56:**1641–1646.
77. Lee, K. K., Doig, P., Irvin, R. T., Paranchych, W., and Hodges, R. S., 1989, Mapping the surface regions of *Pseudomonas aeruginosa* PAK pilin: The importance of the C-terminal region for adherence to human buccal epithelial cells, *Mol. Microbiol.* **30:**285–293.
78. Baker, N., and Marcus, H., 1980, Adherence of clinical isolates of *Pseudomonas aeruginosa* to hamster tracheal epithelium in vitro, *Curr. Microbiol.* **7:**35–40.
79. Vishwanath, S., and Ramphal, R., 1985, Tracheobronchial mucin receptors for *Pseudomonas aeruginosa*. Predominance of amino sugars in binding sites, *Infect. Immun.* **48:**331–335.
80. Ramphal, R., and Pyle, M., 1983, Evidence for mucins and sialic acid as receptors for *Pseudomonas aeruginosa* in the lower respiratory tract, *Infect. Immun.* **41:**339–344.
81. Baker, N., and Svanborg-Eden, C., 1989, Role of alginate in the adherence of *Pseudomonas aeruginosa*, *Antibiot. Chemother.* **42:**72–79.
82. Ramphal, R., Carnoy, C., Fievre, S., Michalski, J.-C., Houdret, N., Lamblin, G., Strecker, G., and Roussel, P., 1991, *Pseudomonas aeruginosa* recognizes carbohydrate chains containing type 1 (Galβ1-3GlcNac) or type 2 (Galβ1-4GlcNac) disaccharide units, *Infect. Immun.* **59:**700–704.

83. Doggett, R. G., Harrison, G. M., Stilwell, R. N., and Wallis, E. S., 1966, An atypical *Pseudomonas aeruginosa* associated with cystic fibrosis of the pancreas, *J. Pediatr.* **68**:628–635.
84. Doggett, R. G., and Harrison, G. M., 1972, *Pseudomonas aeruginosa*: Immune status in patients with cystic fibrosis, *Infect. Immun.* **6**:628–635.
85. Lam, J., Chan, R., Lam, K., and Costerton, J. W., 1980, Production of mucoid microcolonies by *Pseudomonas aeruginosa* within infected lungs in cystic fibrosis, *Infect. Immun.* **28**:546–556.
86. Linker, A., and Jones, R. A., 1964, A new polysaccharide resembling alginic acid from a *Pseudomonas* microorganism, *Nature* **204**:187–188.
87. Pier, G. B., Desjardins, D., Aguilar, T., Barnard, M., and Speert, D. P., 1986, Polysaccharide surface antigens expressed by nonmucoid isolates of *Pseudomonas aeruginosa* from cystic fibrosis patients, *J. Clin. Microbiol.* **24**:189–196.
88. Doig, P., Smith, N. R., Todd, T., and Randall, T. J., 1987, Characterization of the binding of *Pseudomonas aeruginosa* alginate to human epithelial cells, *Infect. Immun.* **55**:1517–1522.
89. Baker, N., Minor, V., Deal, C., Sharabadi, M. S., Simpson, D. A., and Woods, D. E., 1991, *Pseudomonas aeruginosa* exoenzyme-S is an adhesin, *Infect. Immun.*, **59**:2859–2863.
90. Ramphal, R., Koo, L., Ishimoto, K. S., Totten, P. A., Lara, J. C., and Lory, S., 1991, Adhesion of *Pseudomonas aeruginosa* pilin-deficient mutants to mucin, *Infect. Immun.* **59**:1307–1311.
91. Simel, D. L., Masten, B. S., Pratt, P. C., Wisseman, C. L., Shelburne, J. D., and Spock, A., 1984, Scanning electron microscopic study of the airways in normal children and in patients with cystic fibrosis and other lung diseases, *Pediatr. Pathol.* **2**:47–64.
92. Jeffery, P. K., and Brain, A. P. R., 1988, Surface morphology of human airway mucosa: Normal, carcinoma, or cystic fibrosis, *Scanning Electron Microsc.* **2**:553–560.
93. Chi, E., Mehl, T., Nunn, D., and Lory, S., 1991, Interaction of *Pseudomonas aeruginosa* with A549 pneumocyte cells, *Infect. Immun.* **59**:822–828.
94. Liu, P. V., 1974, Extracellular toxins of *Pseudomonas aeruginosa*, *J. Infect. Dis.* **130**:S94–S99.
95. Meyers, D. J., and Berk, R. S., 1990, Characterization of phospholipase C from *Pseudomonas aeruginosa* as a potent inflammatory agent, *Infect. Immun.* **58**:659–666.
96. Husson, M. O., Mielcarek, C., Gavini, F., Caron, C., Izard, D., and Leclerc, H., 1989, Isolation and characterization of monoclonal antibodies against alkaline phosphatase of *Pseudomonas aeruginosa*, *J. Clin. Microbiol.* **27**:1115–1118.
97. Wretlind, B., and Pavlovskis, O. P., 1983, *Pseudomonas aeruginosa* elastase and its role in *Pseudomonas* infections, *Rev. Infect. Dis.* **5**:S998–S1004.
98. Nicas, T. I., and Iglewski, B. H., 1985, The contribution of exoproducts to virulence of *Pseudomonas aeruginosa*, *Can. J. Microbiol.* **31**:387–392.
99. Döring, G., Maier, M., Müller, E., Bibi, Z., Tümmler, B., and Kharazmi, A., 1987, Virulence factors of *Pseudomonas aeruginosa*, *Antibiot. Chemother.* **39**:136–148.
100. Leisinger, T., and Margraff, R., 1979, Secondary metabolites of the fluorescent Pseudomonads, *Microbiol. Rev.* **43**:422–442.
101. Woods, D. E., To, M., and Sokol, P. A., 1989, *Pseudomonas aeruginosa* exoenzyme S as a pathogenic determinant in respiratory infection, *Antibiot. Chemother.* **44**:27–35.
102. Pedersen, S. S., Høiby, N., Espersen, F., and Kharazmi, A., 1991, Alginate in infection, *Antibiot. Chemother.* **44**:68–79.
103. Hayashi, T., and Terawaki, Y., 1991, Molecular approach to *Pseudomonas aeruginosa* cytotoxin: Structure, activation mechanism and phage conversion, *Antibiot. Chemother.* **44**:48–53.
104. Lutz, F., Xiong, G., Jungblut, R., Orlik-Eisel, G., Göbel-Reifert, A., and Leidolf, R., 1991, Pore-forming cytotoxin of *Pseudomonas aeruginosa*: Molecular effects and aspects of pathogenicity, *Antibiot. Chemother.* **44**:54–58.
105. Vasil, M. L., Graham, L. M., Ostroff, R. M., Shortridge, V. D., and Vasil, A. I., 1991, Phospholipase C: Molecular biology and contribution to the pathogenesis of *Pseudomonas aeruginosa*, *Antibiot. Chemother.* **44**:34–47.
106. Jaeger, K.-E., Kharazmi, A., and Høiby, N., 1991, Extracellular lipase of *Pseudomonas*

aeruginosa: Biochemical characterization and effect on human neutrophil and monocyte function in vitro, *Microb. Pathogen.*, in press.
107. Wolz, C., Hellstern, E., Haug, M., Galloway, D. R., Vasil, M. K., and Döring, G., 1991, *Pseudomonas aeruginosa* LasB mutant constructed by insertional mutagenesis reveals elastolytic activity due to alkaline proteinase of LasA fragment, *Mol. Microbiol.* **5**:2125–2131.
108. Steuhl, K. P., Döring, G., Henni, A., Thiel, H. J., and Botzenhart, K., 1987, Relevance of host-derived and bacterial factors in *Pseudomonas aeruginosa* corneal infections, *Invest. Ophthalmol. Vis. Sci.* **28**:1559–1568.
109. Döring, G., Obernesser, H. J., and Botzenhart, K., 1981, Extracellular toxins of *Pseudomonas aeruginosa*. II. Effect of two proteases on human immunoglobulins IgG, IgA and secretory IgA, *Zentralbl. Bakteriol. Mikrobiol. Hyg. (A)* **249**:89–98.
110. Schultz, D. R., and Miller, K. D., 1974, Elastase of *Pseudomonas aeruginosa*: Inactivation of complement components and complement-derived chemotactic and phagocytic factors, *Infect. Immun.* **10**:128–135.
111. Döring, G., Pfestorf, M., Botzenhart, K., and Abdallah, M. A., 1988, Impact of proteases on iron uptake of *Pseudomonas aeruginosa* pyoverdin from transferrin and lactoferrin, *Infect. Immun.* **56**:291–293.
112. Kharazmi, A., 1989, Interactions of *Pseudomonas aeruginosa* proteases with the cells of the immune system, *Antibiot. Chemother.* **42**:42–49.
113. Ankenbauer, R., Sriyosachati, S., and Cox, C. D., 1985, Effects of siderophores on the growth of *Pseudomonas aeruginosa* in human serum and transferrin, *Infect. Immun.* **49**: 132–140.
114. Sorensen, R. U., Fredricks, D. N., and Waller, R. L., 1991, Inhibition of normal and malignant cell proliferation by pyocyanine and 1-hydroxyphenazine, *Antibiot. Chemother.* **44**: 85–93.
115. Pitt, T. L., 1989, Lipopolysaccharide and virulence of *Pseudomonas aeruginosa*, *Antibiot. Chemother.* **42**:1–7.
116. Wick, M. J., Frank, D. W., Storey, D. G., and Iglewski, B. H., 1990, Structure, function and regulation of *Pseudomonas aeruginosa* exotoxin A, *Ann. Rev. Microbiol.* **44**:335–363.
117. Galloway, D. R., *Pseudomonas aeruginosa* elastase and elastolysis, 1991, *Mol. Microbiol.* **5**:2315–2321.
118. Sabath, D. E. (ed.), 1980, *Pseudomonas aeruginosa, the Organism, Diseases it Causes and their Treatment*, Hans Huber Publ., Bern.
119. Moss, R. B., and Lewiston, N. J., 1984, Immunopathology of cystic fibrosis, in: *Immunological Aspects of Cystic Fibrosis* (E. Shapira and G. B. Wilson, eds.), CRC Press, Boca Raton, Florida, pp. 5–28.
120. Döring, G., Albus, A., and Høiby, N., 1988, Immunological aspects of cystic fibrosis, *Chest* **94**:S109–S114.
121. Middlebrook, J. L., and Dorland, R. B., 1984, Bacterial toxins: Cellular mechanisms of action, *Microbiol. Rev.* **48**:199–221.
122. FitzGerald, D., Morris, R., and Saelinger, C., 1980, Receptor-mediated entry of *Pseudomonas* toxin by mouse fibroblasts, *Cell* **21**:867–873.
123. Iglewski, B. H., and Kabat, D., 1975, NAD-dependent inhibitions of protein synthesis by *Pseudomonas aeruginosa* toxin, *Proc. Natl. Acad. Sci. USA* **72**:2284–2288.
124. Collier, R. J., 1975, Diphtheria toxin: Mode of action and structure, *Bacteriol. Rev.* **39**: 54–85.
125. Goldstein, E., and Hoeprich, P. D., 1977, Diphtheria, in: *Infectious diseases* (P. D. Hoeprich, ed.), Harper and Row, San Francisco, pp. 247–258.
126. Klinger, J. D., Straus, D.C., Hilton, C. B., and Bass, J. A., 1978, Antibodies to proteases and exotoxin A of *Pseudomonas aeruginosa* in patients with cystic fibrosis: Demonstration by radioimmunoassay, *J. Infect. Dis.* **138**:49–58.
127. Döring, G., Goldstein, W., Röll, W., Schiøtz, P. O., Høiby, N., and Botzenhart, K., 1985, Role

of *Pseudomonas aeruginosa* exoenzymes in lung infections of patients with cystic fibrosis, *Infect. Immun.* **49**:557–562.
128. Gray, G. L., Smith, D. H., Baldridge, J. S., Hoskins, R. N., Vasil, M. L., Chen, E. Y., and Heyneker, H. L., 1984, Cloning, nucleotide sequence, and expression in *Escherichia coli* of the exotoxin A structural gene of *Pseudomonas aeruginosa*, *Proc. Natl. Acad. Sci. USA* **81**: 2645–2649.
129. Greenfield, L., Bjorn, M. J., Horn, G., Fong, D., Buck, G. A., Collier, R. J., and Kaplan, D. A., 1983, Nucleotide sequence of the structural gene for diphtheria toxin carried by corynebacteriophage β, *Proc. Natl. Acad. Sci. USA* **80**:6853–6857.
130. Goldstein, W., and Döring, G., 1986, Lysosomal enzymes from polymorphonuclear leukocytes and proteinase inhibitors in patients with cystic fibrosis, *Am. Rev. Respir. Dis.* **134**: 49–56.
131. Döring, G., and Müller, E., 1989, Different sensitivity of *Pseudomonas aeruginosa* exotoxin A and diphtheria toxin to enzymes from polymorphonuclear leukocytes, *Microb. Pathogen.* **6**: 287–295.
132. Döring, G., Obernesser, H. J., Botzenhart, K., Flehmig, B., Høiby, N., and Hofmann, A., 1983, Proteases of *Pseudomonas aeruginosa* in patients with cystic fibrosis, *J. Infect. Dis.* **147**: 744–750.
133. Döring, G., and Høiby, N., 1983, Longitudinal study of immune response to *Pseudomonas aeruginosa* antigens in cystic fibrosis, *Infect. Immun.* **42**:197–201.
134. Jagger, K. S., Robinson, D. L., Franz, M. N., and Warren, R. L., 1982, Detection by enzyme-linked immunosorbent assays of antibody specific for *Pseudomonas* proteases and exotoxin A in sera from cystic fibrosis patients, *J. Clin. Microbiol.* **15**:1054–1058.
135. Granström, M., Ericsson, A., Strandvik, B., Wretlind, B., Pavlovskis, O. R., Berka, R., and Vasil, M. L., 1984, Relation between antibody response to *Pseudomonas aeruginosa* exoproteins and colonization/infection in patients with cystic fibrosis, *Acta Paediatr. Scand.* **73**: 772–777.
136. Hancock, R. E. W., Movat, E. C. A., and Speert, D. P., 1984, Quantitation and identification of antibodies to outer membrane proteins of *Pseudomonas aeruginosa* in sera of patients with cystic fibrosis, *J. Infect. Dis.* **149**:220–226.
137. Shand, G. H., Pedersen, S. S., Lam, K., and Høiby, N., 1989, Iron-regulated outer membrane proteins and virulence in *Pseudomonas aeruginosa*, *Antibiot. Chemother.* **42**:15–26.
138. Brett, M. M., Ghoneim, A. T. M., and Littlewood, J. M., 1987, Serum IgG antibodies in patients with cystic fibrosis with early *Pseudomonas aeruginosa* infection, *Arch. Dis. Child.* **62**: 357–361.
139. Moss, R. B., Hsu, Y.-P., Lewiston, N. J., Curd, J. G., Milgrom, H., Hart, S., Dyer, B., and Larrick, J. W., 1986, Association of specific immune complexes, complement activation and antibodies to *Pseudomonas aeruginosa* lipopolysaccharide and exotoxin A with mortality in cystic fibrosis, *Am. Rev. Respir. Dis.* **133**:648–652.
140. Pedersen, S. S., Espersen, R., and Høiby, N., 1987, Diagnosis of chronic *Pseudomonas aeruginosa* infection in cystic fibrosis by enzyme-linked immunosorbent assay, *J. Clin. Microbiol.* **25**:1830–1836.
141. Bryan, L. E., Kureishi, A., and Rabin, H. R., 1983, Detection of antibodies to *Pseudomonas aeruginosa* alginate extracellular polysaccharide in animals and cystic fibrosis patients by enzyme-linked immunosorbent assay, *J. Clin. Microbiol.* **18**:276–282.
142. Albus, A., Saalmann, M., Tesch, W., Pedersen, S. S., and Döring, G., 1989, Increased levels of IgG subclasses, specific for *Pseudomonas aeruginosa* protein and polysaccharide antigens in chronically infected patients with cystic fibrosis, *Acta Pathol. Microbiol. Immunol. Scand.* **97**:1146–1148.
143. Pedersen, S. S., Høiby, N., Shand, G. H., and Pressler, T., 1989, Antibody response to *Pseudomonas aeruginosa* antigens in cystic fibrosis, *Antibiot. Chemother.* **42**:130–153.
144. Döring, G., Buhl, V., Høiby, N., Schiøtz, P.O., and Botzenhart, K., 1984, Detection of

proteases of *Pseudomonas aeruginosa* in immune complexes isolated from sputum of cystic fibrosis patients, *Acta Pathol. Microbiol. Immunol. Scand. (C)* **92**:307–312.
145. Kownatzki, R., Tümmler, B., and Döring, G., 1987, Rhamnolipid of *Pseudomonas aeruginosa* in sputum of cystic fibrosis patients, *Lancet* **i**:1026–1027.
146. Finlay, B. B., and Falkow, S., 1989, Common themes in microbial pathogenicity, *Microbiol. Rev.* **53**:210–230.
147. Clerc, P. L., Ryter, A., Mounier, J., and Sansonetti, P. J., 1987, Plasmid-mediated early killing of eucaryotic cells by *Shigella flexneri* as studied by infection of J774 macrophages, *Infect. Immun.* **55**:521–527.
148. Sansonetti, P. J., and Mounier, J., 1987, Metabolic events mediating early killing of host cells infected by *Shigella flexneri*, *Microb. Pathogen.* **3**:53–61.
149. Colt, H. G., Holden, W. E., and Kaplan, S. S., 1990, On septicemia in an adult with cystic fibrosis: Neutrophil function and serum chemoattractant activity, *Pediatr. Pulmonol.* **6**:63–64.
150. Miller, J. F., Mekalanos, J. J., and Falkow, S., 1989, Coordinate regulation and sensory transduction in the control of bacterial virulence, *Science* **243**:916–922.
151. Higgins, C. F., Hinton, J. C. D., Hulton, C. S. J., Owen-Hughes, T., Pavitt, G. D., and Seirafi, A., 1990, Protein H1: A role for chromatin structure in the regulation of bacterial gene expression and virulence? *Mol. Microbiol.* **4**:2007–2012.
152. Knowles, M. R., Stutts, M. J., Spock, A., Fischer, N., Gutzy, J. J., and Boucher, R. C., 1983, Abnormal ion permeation through cystic fibrosis respiratory epithelium, *Science* **221**:1067–1070.
153. Dalhoff, A., and Döring, G., 1987, Action of quinolones on gene expression and bacterial membranes, *Antibiot. Chemother.* **39**:205–214.
154. Terry, J. M., Pina, S. E., and Mattingly, S. J., 1991, Environmental conditions which influence mucoid conversion in *Pseudomonas aeruginosa* PAO1, *Infect. Immun.* **59**:471–477.
155. Deretic, V., Govan, J. R. W., Konyecsni, W. M., and Martin, D. W., 1990, Mucoid *Pseudomonas aeruginosa* in cystic fibrosis: Mutations in the muc loci affect transcription of the *algR* and *algD* genes in response to environmental stimuli, *Mol. Microbiol.* **4**:189–198.
156. Roychoudhury, S., Zielinski, N. A., DeVault, J. D., Kato, J., Shinabarger, D. L., May, T. B., Maharaj, R., Kimbara, K., Misra, T. K., and Chakrabarty, A. M., 1991, *Pseudomonas aeruginosa* infection in cystic fibrosis: Biosynthesis of alginate as a virulence factor, *Antibiot. Chemother.* **44**:63–67.
157. Schultz, E. W., 1947, A gelatinous variant of *Pseudomonas aeruginosa*, *Proc. Soc. Exp. Biol. Med.* **65**:289–291.
158. McAvoy, M. J., Newton, V., Paull, A., Morgan, J., Gacesa, P., and Russell, N. J., 1989, Isolation of mucoid strains of *Pseudomonas aeruginosa* from non-cystic-fibrosis patients and characterization of the structure of their secreted alginate, *J. Med. Microbiol.* **28**:183–189.
159. Stevens, D., Lieberman, M., McNitt, T., and Price, J., 1984, Demonstration of uronic acid capsular material in the cerebrospinal fluid of a patient with meningitis caused by mucoid *Pseudomonas aeruginosa*, *J. Clin. Microbiol.* **19**:942–943.
160. Anastassiou, E. d., Frangidis, C., and Dimitracopoulos, G., 1986, Nonfatal bacteremia caused by a mucoid, alginate-producing strain of *Pseudomonas aeruginosa*, *Diagn. Microbiol. Infect. Dis.* **5**:277–283.
161. McCarthy, V. P., Rosenberg, G., Rosenstein, B. J., and Hubbard, V. S., 1986, Mucoid *Pseudomonas aeruginosa* from a patient without cystic fibrosis: Implications and review of the literature, *Pediatr. Infect. Dis.* **5**:256–258.
162. Homma, H., Yamanakam, A., Tanimoto, H., Tamura, M., Chijimatsu, Y., Kira, S., and Izumi, T., 1983, Diffuse panbronchiolitis, a disease of the transitional zone of the lung, *Chest* **83**:63–69.
163. Woods, D. E., Sokol, P. A., Bryan, L. E., Storey, D. G., Mattingly, S. J., Vogel, H. J., and Ceri, H., 1991, In vivo regulation of virulence in *Pseudomonas aeruginosa* associated with genetic rearrangement, *J. Infect. Dis.* **163**:143–149.

164. Bayer, A. S., Eftekhar, F., Tu, J., Nast, C. C., and Speert, D. P., 1990, Oxygen-dependent upregulation of mucoid exopolysaccharide (alginate) production in *Pseudomonas aeruginosa*, *Infect. Immun.* **58**:1344–1349.
165. Speert, D. P., Farmer, S. W., Campbell, M. E., Musser, J. M., Selander, R. K., and Kuo, S., 1990, Conversion of *Pseudomonas aeruginosa* to the phenotype characteristic of strains from patients with cystic fibrosis, *J. Clin. Microbiol.* **28**:188–194.
166. Brown, M. R. W., and Williams, P., 1985, The influence of environment on envelope properties affecting survival of bacteria in infections, *Annu. Rev. Microbiol.* **39**:527–556.
167. Hancock, R. E. W., Mutharia, L. M., Chan, L., Darveau, R. P., Speert, D. P., and Pier, G. B., 1983, *Pseudomonas aeruginosa* isolates from patients with cystic fibrosis: A class of serum-sensitive, nontypable strains deficient in lipopolysaccharide O side chains, *Infect. Immun.* **42**:170–177.
168. Ojeniyi, B., Baek, L., and Høiby, N., 1985, Polyagglutinability due to loss of O-antigenic determinants in *Pseudomonas aeruginosa* strains isolated from cystic fibrosis patients, *Acta Pathol. Microbiol. Scand. [B]* **93**:7–13.
169. Anwar, H., Brown, M. r. W., Day, D. A., and Weller, P. H., 1984, Outer membrane antigens of mucoid *Pseudomonas aeruginosa* isolated directly from the sputum of a cystic fibrosis patient, *FEMS Microbiol. Lett.* **24**:235–239.
170. Shand, G. H., Pedersen, S. S., Lam, K., and Høiby, N., 1989, Iron-regulated outermembrane proteins and virulence in *Pseudomonas aeruginosa*, *Antibiot. Chemother.* **42**:15–26.
171. Mohr, C. D., Rust, L., Albus, A. M., Iglewski, B. H., and Deretic, V., 1990, Expression patterns of genes encoding elastase and controlling mucoidy: Co-ordinate regulation of two virulence factors in *Pseudomonas aeruginosa* isolates from cystic fibrosis, *Mol. Microbiol.* **4**:2103–2110.
172. Kharazmi, A., Schiøtz, P. O., Høiby, N., Baek, L., and Döring, G., 1986, Demonstration of neutrophil chemotactic activity in the sputum of cystic fibrosis patients with *Pseudomonas aeruginosa* infection, *Eur. J. Clin. Invest.* **16**:143–148.
173. Schiøtz, P. O., Sørensen, H., and Høiby, N., 1979, Activated complement in the sputum from patients with cystic fibrosis, *Acta Pathol. Microbiol. Scand.[C]* **87**:1–5.
174. Cromwell, O., Morris, H. R., Hodson, M. E., Walport, M. J., Taylor, G. W., Batten, J., and Kay, A. B., 1981, Identification of leukotrienes D and B in sputum of cystic fibrosis patients, *Lancet* **ii**:164–165.
175. Fontan, P. A., Garcia, V. E., Cerquetti, M. C., and Sordelli, D. O., 1989, *Pseudomonas aeruginosa* chemotactins (PAC): Preliminary characterization, *Annu. Meet. Am. Soc. Microbiol.*, B235.
176. Cabral, D. A., Loh, B. A., and Speert, D. P., 1987, Mucoid *Pseudomonas aeruginosa* resists nonopsonic phagocytosis by human neutrophils and macrophages, *Pediatr. Res.* **22**:429–431.
177. Young, L. S., and Armstrong, D., 1972, Human immunity to *Pseudomonas aeruginosa*. In vitro interaction of bacteria, polymorphonuclear leukocytes and serum factors, *J. Infect. Dis.* **126**:257–276.
178. Leslie, R. G. Y., and Alexander, M. D., 1979, Cytophilic antibodies, *Curr. Top. Microbiol. Immunol.* **88**:26–104.
179. Reynolds, H. Y., 1974, Pulmonary host defenses in rabbits after immunization with *Pseudomonas* antigens: The interaction of bacteria, antibodies, macrophages and lymphocytes, *J. Infect. Dis.* **130**:S134–S142.
180. Thomassen, M. J., Boxerbaum, B., Demko, C. A., Kuchenbrod, P. J., Dearborn, D. G., and Wood, R. E., 1979, Inhibitory effect of cystic fibrosis serum on *Pseudomonas* phagocytosis by rabbit and human alveolar macrophages, *Pediatr. Res.* **13**:1085–1088.
181. Shryock, T. R., Mollé, J. S., Klinger, J. D., and Thomassen, M. J., 1986, Association with phagocytic inhibition of anti-*Pseudomonas aeruginosa* immunoglobulin G antibody subclass levels in serum from patients with cystic fibrosis, *J. Clin. Microbiol.* **23**:513–516.

182. Fick, R. B., Olchowski, J., Squier, S. U., Merrill, W. W., and Reynolds, H. Y., 1986, Immunoglobulin G subclasses in cystic fibrosis. IgG2 response to *Pseudomonas aeruginosa* lipopolysaccharide, *Am. Rev. Respir. Dis.* **133**:418–422.
183. Moss, R. B., Hsu, Y.-P., Sullivan, M. M., and Lewiston, N. J., 1986, Altered antibody isotype in cystic fibrosis: Possible role in opsonic deficiency, *Pediatr. Res.* **20**:453–459.
184. Moss, R. B., Hsu, Y.-P., van Eede, P. H., Van Leeuwen, M. V., Lewiston, N. J., and De Lange, G., 1987, Altered antibody isotype in cystic fibrosis. Impaired natural antibody response to polysaccharide antigens, *Pediatr. Res.* **22**:708–713.
185. Pressler, T., Mansa, B., Jensen, T., Pedersen, S. S., Høiby, N., and Koch, C., 1988, Increased IgG2 and IgG3 concentration is associated with advanced *Pseudomonas aeruginosa* infection and poor pulmonary function in cystic fibrosis, *Acta Paediatr. Scand.* **77**:576–582.
186. Eichler, I., Joris, L. Hsu, Y.-P., van Wye, J., Bram, R., and Moss, R., 1989, Nonopsonic antibodies in cystic fibrosis, *J. Clin. Invest.* **84**:1794–1804.
187. Thomassen, M. J., Demko, C. A., and Doershuk, C. F., 1987, Cystic fibrosis: A review of pulmonary infections and interventions, *Pediatr. Pulmonol.* **3**:334–351.
188. Schur, P. H., 1987, IgG subclasses. A review, *Ann. Allergy* **58**:89–99.
189. Høiby, N., Döring, G., and Schiøtz, P. O., 1986, The role of immune complexes in the pathogenesis of bacterial infections, *Ann. Rev. Microbiol.* **40**:29–53.
190. Döring, G., 1989, Polymorphonuclear leukocyte elastase: Its effects on the pathogenesis of *Pseudomonas aeruginosa* infection in cystic fibrosis, *Antibiot. Chemother.* **42**:169–176.
191. Høiby, N., and Koch, C., 1990, *Pseudomonas aeruginosa* infection in cystic fibrosis and its management, *Thorax* **45**:881–884.
192. Høiby, N., and Axelsen, N. H., 1973, Identification and quantitation of precipitins against *Pseudomonas aeruginosa* in patients with cystic fibrosis by means of crossed immunoelectrophoresis with intermediate gel, *Acta Pathol. Microbiol. Scand.* [B] **81**:298–308.
193. Berdischewsky, M., Pollack, M., Young, L. S., Chia, D., Osher, A. B., and Barnett, E. V., 1980, Circulating immune complexes in cystic fibrosis, *Pediatr. Res.* **14**:830–833.
194. Moss, R. B., and Hsiu, Y.-P., 1982, Isolation and characterization of circulating immune complexes in cystic fibrosis, *Clin. Exp. Immunol.* **47**:301–308.
195. Pitcher-Wilmott, R. W., Levinsky, R. J., and Matthew, D. J., 1982, Circulating soluble immune complexes containing *Pseudomonas* antigens in cystic fibrosis, *Arch. Dis. Child.* **57**:577–581.
196. Manthei, U., Taussig, L. M., Beckerman, R. C., and Strunk, R. C., 1982, Circulating immune complexes in cystic fibrosis, *Am. Rev. Respir. Dis.* **126**:253–257.
197. Church, J. A., Jordan, S. C., Keens, T. G., and Wang, C.-I., 1981, Circulating immune complexes in patients with cystic fibrosis, *Chest* **80**:405–411.
198. Wisnieski, J. J., Todd, E. W., Fuller, R. K., Jones, P. K., Dearborn, D. W., Boat, T. F., and Naff, G. B., 1985, Immune complexes and complement abnormalities in patients with cystic fibrosis. Increased mortality associated with circulating immune complexes and decreased function of the alternative complement pathway, *Am. Rev. Respir. Dis.* **132**:770–777.
199. Wheeler, W. B., Williams, M., Matthews, W. J., Jr., and Colten, H. R., 1984, Progression of cystic fibrosis lung disease as a function of serum immunoglobulin G levels: 1 5-year longitudinal study, *J. Pediatr.* **104**:695–699.
200. Dasgupta, M. K., Lam, J., Döring, G., Harley, F. L., Zuberbuhler, P., Lam, K., Reichert, A., Costerton, J. W., and Dossetor, J. B., 1987, Prognostic implications of circulating immune complexes and *Pseudomonas aeruginosa*-specific antibodies in cystic fibrosis, *J. Clin. Lab. Immunol.* **23**:25–30.
201. Disis, M. L., McDonald, T. L., Colombo, J. L., Kobayashi, R. H., Angle, C. R., and Murray, S., 1986, Circulating immune complexes in cystic fibrosis and their correlation to clinical parameters, *Pediatr. Res.* **20**:385–390.
202. Dasgupta, M. K., Zuberbuhler, P., Abbi, A., Harley, F. L., Brown, N. E., Lam, K., Dossetor, J. B., and Costerton, J. W., 1987, Combined evaluation of circulating immune complexes and

antibodies to *Pseudomonas aeruginosa* as an immune profile in relation to pulmonary function in cystic fibrosis, *J. Clin. Immunol.* **7**:51–58.
203. Goldstein, I. M., 1976, Polymorphonuclear leukocyte lysosomes and immune tissue injury, *Prog. Allergy* **20**:301–340.
204. Suter, S., Schaad, U. B., Roux, L., Nydegger, U. E., and Waldvogel, F. A., 1984, Granulocyte neutral proteases and *Pseudomonas* elastase as possible causes of airway damage in patients with cystic fibrosis, *J. Infect. Dis.* **149**:523–531.
205. Tournier, J. M., Jacquot, J., Puchelle, E., and Bieth, J. G., 1985, Evidence that *Pseudomonas aeruginosa* elastase does not inactivate the bronchial inhibitor in the presence of leukocyte elastase, *Am. Rev. Respir. Dis.* **132**:524–528.
206. Suter, S., Schaad, U. B., Tegner, H., Ohlsson, K., Desgrandschamps, D., and Waldvogel, F. A., 1986, Levels of free granulocyte elastase in bronchial secretions from patients with cystic fibrosis: Effect of antimicrobial treatment against *Pseudomonas aeruginosa*, *J. Infect. Dis.* **153**:902–909.
207. Jackson, A. H., Hill, S. L., Afford, S. C., and Stockley, R. A., 1984, Sputum solphase proteins and elastase activity in patients with cystic fibrosis, *Eur. J. Respir. Dis.* **65**:114–124.
208. Fick, R. B., Baltimore, R. S., Squier, S. U., and Reynolds, H. Y., 1985, IgG proteolytic activity of *Pseudomonas aeruginosa* in cystic fibrosis, *J. Infect. Dis.* **151**:589–598.
209. Döring, G., Goldstein, W., Botzenhart, K., Kharazmi, A., Schiøtz, P. O., Høiby, N., and Dasgupta, M., 1986, Elastase from polymorphonuclear leukocytes: A regulatory enzyme in immune complex disease, *Clin. Exp. Immunol.* **64**:597–605.
210. Henson, P. M., and Johnston, R. B., Jr., 1987, Tissue injury in inflammation, *J. Clin. Invest.* **79**:669–674.
211. Johnson, U., Ohlsson, K., and Ohlsson, I., 1976, Effects of granulocyte neutral proteases on complement components, *Scand. J. Immunol.* **5**:421–426.
212. Tosi, M. F., Zakem, H., and Berger, M., 1990, Neutrophil elastase cleaves C3bi on opsonized *Pseudomonas* as well as CR1 on neutrophils to create a functionally important opsonin receptor mismatch, *J. Clin. Invest.* **86**:300–308.
213. Berger, M. Sorensen, R. U., Tosi, M. F., Dearborn, D. G., and Döring, G., 1989, Complement receptor expression on neutrophils at an inflammatory site, the *Pseudomonas*-infected lung in cystic fibrosis, *J. Clin. Invest.* **84**:1302–1313.
214. Berger, M., 1991, Inflammation in the lung in cystic fibrosis. A vicious cycle that does more harm than good? *Clin. Rev. Allergy* **9**:119–142.
215. Sommerhoff, C. P., Nadel, J. A., Basbaum, C. B., and Caughey, G. H., 1990, Neutrophil elastase and cathepsin G stimulate secretions from cultured bovine airway gland serous cells, *J. Clin. Invest.* **85**:682–689.
216. Suter, S., Schaad, U. B., Roux-Lombard, P., Girardin, E., Grau, G., and Dayer, J.-M., 1989, Relation between tumor necrosis factor-α and granulocyte elastase-α1-proteinase inhibitor complexes in plasma of patients with cystic fibrosis, *Am. Rev. Respir. Dis.* **140**:1640–1644.
217. Brown, M. A., Morgan, W. J., Finley, P. R., and Scuderi, P., 1991, Circulating levels of tumor necrosis factor and interleukin-1 in cystic fibrosis, *Pediatr. Pulmonol.* **10**:86–91.
218. Wilmott, R. W., Kassab, J. T., Kilian, P. L., Benjamin, W. R., Douglas, S. D., and Wood, R. E., 1990, Increased levels of interleukin-1 in bronchoalveolar washings from children with bacterial pulmonary infections, *Am. Rev. Respir. Dis.* **142**:365–368.
219. Fomsgaard, A., Svenson, M., and Bendtzen, K., 1989, Auto-antibodies to tumor necrosis factor α in healthy humans and patients with inflammatory diseases and gram-negative bacterial infections, *Scand. J. Immunol.* **30**:219–223.
220. Livermore, D. M., 1989, Role of beta-lactamase and impermeability in the resistance of *Pseudomonas aeruginosa*, *Antibiot. Chemother.* **42**:257–263.
221. Cullmann, W., 1989, Mode of action and development of resistance to quinolones, *Antibiot. Chemother.* **42**:287–300.
222. Gold, R., Carpenter, S., Heuster, H., Corey, M., and Levison, H., 1987, Randomized trial of

ceftazidime versus placebo in the management of acute respiratory exacerbations in patients with cystic fibrosis, *J. Pediatr.* **111:**907–913.
223. Kerem, E., Corey, M., Gold, R., and Levison, H., 1990, Pulmonary function and clinical course in patients with cystic fibrosis after pulmonary colonization with *Pseudomonas aeruginosa*, *J. Pediatr.* **116:**714–719.
224. Regelmann, W. E., Elliott, G. R., Warwick, W. J., and Clawson, C. C., 1990, Reduction of sputum *Pseudomonas aeruginosa* density by antibiotics improves lung function in cystic fibrosis more than do bronchodilators and chest physiotherapy alone, *Am. Rev. Respir. Dis.* **141:**914–921.
225. Michel, B. C., 1988, Antibacterial therapy in cystic fibrosis: A review of the literature published between 1975 and February 1987, *Chest* **94:**S129–S140.
226. Auerbach, H. S., Williams, M., Kirkpatrick, J. A., and Colton, H. R., 1985, Alternate-day prednisone reduces morbidity and improves pulmonary function in cystic fibrosis, *Lancet* **2:**686–688.
227. Rosenstein, B. J., and Eigen, H., 1991, Risks of alternate-day prednisone in patients with cystic fibrosis, *Pediatrics* **87:**245–246.
228. Donati, M. A., Haver, K., Gerson, W., Klein, M., McLaughlin, F. J., and Wohl, M. E. B., 1990, Long-term alternate day prednisone therapy in cystic fibrosis, *Pediatr. Pulmonol.* (Suppl. 5) **9:**A322.
229. Sordelli, D. O., Cerquetti, M. C., Fontan, P. A., and Meiss, R. P., 1989, Piroxicam treatment protects mice from lethal pulmonary challenge with *Pseudomonas aeruginosa*, *J. Infect. Dis.* **159:**232–238.
230. Konstan, M. W., Norvell, T. M., Hilliard, K. A., Shiratsuchi, H., and Berger, M., 1990, Serial bronchoalveolar lavage to evaluate inflammation in cystic fibrosis lung disease, *Pediatr. Pulmonol.* (Suppl. 5) **9:**A309.
231. Sordelli, D. O., Macri, C. N., and Maille, A. J., 1990, A study of the effect of piroxicam treatment to prevent lung damage in CF patients with *Pseudomonas aeruginosa* pneumonia, *Pediatr. Pulmonol.* (Suppl. 5) **9:**A217.
232. Powers, J. C., and Bengali, Z. H., 1986, Elastase inhibitors for treatment of emphysema. Approaches to synthesis and biological evaluation, *Am. Rev. Respir. Dis.* **134:**1097–1100.
233. Crystal, R. G., 1990, α1-antitrypsin deficiency, emphysema, and liver disease. Genetic basis and strategies for therapy, *J. Clin. Invest.* **85:**1343–1352.
234. Sommerhoff, C., Krell, R. D., Williams, J. L., Gomes, B. C., Strimpler, A. M., and Nadel, J. A., 1991, Inhibition of human neutrophil elastase by ICI 200,355, *Eur. J. Pharmakol.* **193:**153–158.
235. Rao, N. V., Kennedy, T. P., Rao, G., Ky, N., and Hoidal, J. R., 1990, Sulfated polysaccharides prevent human leukocyte elastase-induced acute lung injury and emphysema in hamsters, *Am. Rev. Respir. Dis.* **142:**407–412.
236. Smith, R. M., Traber, L. D., Traber, D. L., and Spragg, R. G., 1989, Pulmonary deposition and clearance of aerosolized alpha-1-proteinase inhibitor administered to dogs and to sheep, *J. Clin. Invest.* **84:**1145–1154.
237. Hubbard, R. C., Casolaro, M. A., Mitchell, M., Sellers, S. E., Arabia, F., Matthay, M. A., and Crystal, R. G., 1989, Fate of aerosolized recombinant DNA-produced α_1-antitrypsin: Use of the epithelial surface of the lower respiratory tract to administer proteins of therapeutic importance, *Proc. Natl. Acad. Sci. USA* **86:**680–684.
238. McElvaney, N. G., Hubbard, R. C., Birrer, P., Chernick, M. S., Caplan, D. B., Frank, M. M., and Crystal, R. G., 1991, Aerosol α-1-antitrypsin treatment for cystic fibrosis, *Lancet* **337:** 392–394.
239. Pennington, J. E., Reynolds, H. Y., Wood, R. E., Robinson, R. A., and Levine, A. S., 1975, Use of a *Pseudomonas aeruginosa* vaccine in patients with acute leukemia and cystic fibrosis, *Am. J. Med.* **58:**629–636.

240. Langford, D. T., and Hiller, J., 1984, Prospective, controlled study of a polyvalent *Pseudomonas* vaccine in cystic fibrosis—Three year results, *Arch. Dis. Child.* **59:**1131–1133.
241. Rotering, H., and Dorner, F., 1989, Studies on a *Pseudomonas aeruginosa* flagella vaccine, *Antibiot. Chemother.* **42:**218–228.
242. Crowe, B. A., Enzensberger, O., Schober-Bendixen, S., Mitterer, A., Mundt, W., Livey, I., Pabst, H., Kaeser, R. Eibl, M., Eibl, J., and Dorner, F., 1991, The first clinical trial of Immuno's experimental *Pseudomonas aeruginosa* flagellar vaccines, *Antibiot. Chemother.* **44:**143–156.
243. Finke, M., Muth, G., Reichhelm, T., Thoma, M., Duchene, M., Hungerer, K. D., Domdey, H., and Specht, B.-U., 1991, Protection of immunosuppressed mice against infection with *Pseudomonas aeruginosa* by recombinant *P. aeruginosa* lipoprotein I and lipoprotein I-specific monoclonal antibodies, *Infect. Immun.* **59:**1251–1254.
244. Cryz, S. J., Jr., Fürer, E., Que, J. U., Sadoff, J. C., Brenner, M., and Schaad, U. B., 1991, Clinical evaluation of an octavalent *Pseudomonas aeruginosa* conjugate vaccine in plasma donors and in bone marrow transplants and cystic fibrosis patients, *Antibiot. Chemother.* **44:**157–162.
245. Winnie, G. B., Cowan, R. G., and Wade, N. A., 1989, Intravenous immune globulin treatment of pulmonary exacerbations in cystic fibrosis, *J. Pediatr.* **114:**309–314.
246. Van Wye, J. E., Collins, M. S., Baylor, M., Pennington, J. E., Hsu, Y.-P., Sampanvejsopa, V., and Moss, R. B., 1990, *Pseudomonas* hyperimmune globulin passive immunotherapy for pulmonary exacerbations in cystic fibrosis, *Pediatr. Pulmonol.* **9:**7–18.
247. Winnie, G. B., and Cowan, R. G., Respiratory tract colonization with *Pseudomonas aeruginosa* in cystic fibrosis: Correlation between anti-*Pseudomonas aeruginosa* antibody levels and pulmonary function, *Pediatr. Pulmonol.* **10:**92–100.

14

P. aeruginosa Burn Infections: Pathogenesis and Treatment

IAN ALAN HOLDER

1. INTRODUCTION AND BRIEF HISTORY

Prior to the late 1950s burn deaths related to infection were caused by the gram-positive bacteria *Staphylococcus aureus* and *Streptococcus pneumoniae*.[1,2] Improved methods of fluid therapy introduced between 1950 and 1960 allowed survival of many severely burned patients over the initial period of thermal injury; this increased survival time coupled with the introduction of antibiotics capable of controlling gram-positive sepsis caused a shift in septic complications to those caused by gram-negative bacteria.[3-5] Infections caused by *Pseudomonas aeruginosa* were particularly severe, with high mortality rates.[6] In the intervening years, *P. aeruginosa* continued to cause the most severe, life-threatening infections in burn patients, in spite of the introduction of a wide variety of antibiotics devised specifically for their antipseudomonal activity. One U.S. burn institution reported that from 1959 to 1983, mortality from *P. aeruginosa* infection was 77%; this was 28% higher than the mortality predicted on the basis of severity of injury in the infected patients.[7] Another burn unit reported that between 1969 and 1988, while percent recovery of *Escherichia coli* and *Klebsiella–Enterobacter* from the wounds of burn patients was similar to that of *P. aeruginosa*, *P. aeruginosa* caused more fatal septicemia than the combined deaths from all other gram-negative bacteria.[8] The mortality figures cited in these studies point out the

---

IAN ALAN HOLDER • Shriners Burns Institute, Cincinnati, Ohio 45229-3095.

Pseudomonas aeruginosa as an Opportunistic Pathogen, edited by Mario Campa *et al.* Plenum Press, New York, 1993.

unique host: parasite interaction that is present in *P. aeruginosa* infection in burned individuals; it is an infectious interaction that leads to greater mortality than one would predict and is significantly greater than that caused by other gram-negative bacteria. Today, however, at least in developed countries, modern approaches to patient management (*e.g.*, early, aggressive debridement and excision, enhanced nutritional support, and improved wound care) have reduced septicemia in burn patients. In our unit, for example, in the 5-year period between 1984 and 1988, septicemia was 8% compared with an average of 25% in the three previous 5-year periods, with 25% of septic deaths associated with *P. aeruginosa* in the most current period compared with 41% in previous periods.[8] A recent report from another U.S. burn unit stated that "in this burn center *P. aeruginosa* infection seems to have arisen during the time of development and use of newer antibiotics and improvement of early resuscitative techniques, to have maintained its significance for more than 20 years and then to have suddenly waned."[9] On the other hand, 59% of all wound cultures taken on patients during the first 60 days postburn, and 25% of all positive blood cultures reported during 1987 and 1988 from a French burn unit, were associated with *P. aeruginosa*.[10] In a study from China, the percentage of wound bacterial isolates containing *P. aeruginosa* in a Shanghai burn unit was 12.4% in 1970 and 1971 and remained as high as 10.3% in 1985 and 1986.[11] A study of 96 burn deaths between 1982 and 1987 in a Kuwait burn hospital showed that 49% of the deaths were associated with septicemia and that "commonly the source of sepsis was the burn wound itself and the microorganisms involved most frequently were *P. aeruginosa* . . ."[12] Thus, while *Pseudomonas* infection in burns has diminished in some places, it is still commonly encountered in burn wounds and continues to be a major source of burn infection morbidity and mortality worldwide.

2. ANTIMICROBIAL TREATMENT: PARENTERAL AND TOPICAL

The introduction of the aminoglycoside antibiotic gentamicin in the 1970s opened the modern era of systemic antimicrobial burn infection treatment. Gentamicin was used not only parenterally but also in an ointment base for topical application. Its importance as a treatment modality for the prevention and treatment of *Pseudomonas* burn wound sepsis was such that it was over-used in many institutions with a concomitant increase in the numbers of resistant *P. aeruginosa* strains isolated at various sites.[13–15] A series of newer aminoglycoside-class antibiotics was developed to replace those to which *P. aeruginosa* was resistant. In addition, broad-spectrum penicillin-class antibiotics with antipseudomonal activity were introduced, but the organism also developed resistance to these antibiotics. For example, 40%, 24% and 8% of the strains of *P. aeruginosa* isolated at this institution in 1988 were resistant to gentamicin, tobramycin and amikacin, respectively; during the same time resistance to extended-spectrum penicillins ranged from 38% for ticarcillin to 12% for piperacillin. Because of this, combinations of these two classes of antibiotics are currently used to treat severe *P. aeruginosa* infections.[16,17]

The introduction of 0.5% silver nitrate and mafenide acetate in the mid-1960s heralded the modern age of topical antimicrobial treatment of burn wounds. Since that time a wide variety of antimicrobials for topical use in burns has been suggested;[18–20] the most commonly used topical today is silver sulfadiazine.[21] No topical antimicrobial agent is without potential use problems,[21] and none is uniformly effective against *P. aeruginosa*.[19–21] In addition, solutions of parenteral antimicrobials and antibiotics have been suggested as topical soaks for the prevention and treatment of burn wound infections.[22–24] However *in vitro* testing suggests that strains of *P. aeruginosa* are resistant to many of these formulations as well.[25]

3. IMMUNOTHERAPY

Numerous studies have tried immunological treatment or immunoprophylaxis against *P. aeruginosa* infection. A variety of lipolysaccharide (LPS) 0 serotype-specific antigens, cell-wall polysaccharides, LPS core antigen, "original endotoxin protein," and cell-wall extracts have been used to study active immunization of burned patients or experimental animals or to prepare antiserum to examine the effects of passive immunization on the prevention or treatment of *P. aeruginosa* infections. These studies have been reviewed recently[26] and will not be covered here (see also Chapter 17).

4. PSEUDOMONAS VIRULENCE-ASSOCIATED FACTORS: THEIR ROLE IN PATHOGENESIS IN BURNED HOSTS

In the 1960s, Liu and co-workers described a variety of exoproducts elaborated by *P. aeruginosa* strains and ascribed virulence-associated characteristics to them.[27–29] Among these products were proteases[28] and exotoxin A (ETA).[29] Prior to these studies, the two major proteases produced by *P. aeruginosa*, alkaline protease and elastase, had been purified, crystallized, and characterized[30,31] but ETA was a newly described virulence-associated factor. Subsequently ETA was purified and characterized[32–34] and shown to cause shock when injected into dogs.[35] A series of studies by Pavlovskis and colleagues demonstrated that ^{14}C-labeled ETA was taken up in a dose–response-related manner in Vero cells in culture.[36] ETA uptake correlated with decreases in ^{14}C-uridine or ^{14}C-amino-acid uptake in the ETA-treated cells, suggesting an effect on the cells' synthetic apparatus; adding mixtures of ETA plus specific antitoxin to the cultured cells did not affect uptake of

^{14}C-uridine indicating that antibody to ETA could nullify its toxic action. When ^{125}I-labeled ETA was injected intravenously into mice, most of the label was found in the kidney; however, within 4-hr post-injection, 50% of the protein-synthetic capacity of the liver was inhibited and shortly before death of the mice protein synthesis in the liver was almost completely inhibited.[37] Decreased protein synthesis occurred to a significantly lesser degree in other major organs, suggesting the liver, rather than the kidney, as the "target" organ for ETA. In addition, intravenous injection of two LD_{50} doses of ETA into mice caused necrotic lesions and fatty changes in the livers of the intoxicated mice with concomitant increases in the serum levels of the liver-associated enzymes aspartate amino transferase, alanine amino transferase, and alkaline phosphatase.[38] The results of these studies were put into perspective when the mechanism of action of ETA was demonstrated.[39] ETA is an adenosine-diphosphate-ribosylating (ADPR) enzyme that is a potent inhibitor of mammalian cell protein synthesis. It inhibits protein synthesis by catalyzing the transfer of the ADP ribosyl moiety of nicotinamide adenine dinucleotide to elongation factor 2 (EF2), essential to protein synthesis. The ADP–ribose:EF2 complex is nonfunctional, and protein synthesis ceases as functional EF2 is depleted. Inhibition of protein synthesis in intact cells and *in vitro* measurement of ADPR activity have become standard methods to determine the presence of ETA in bacterial culture filtrates and in serum of infected animals. In addition, the fact that ETA inhibits protein synthesis by inactivation of mammalian cell EF2 would suggest the use of measurements of EF2 in the organs of burned animals infected by various strains of *P. aeruginosa* as an assay of ETA activity.

The role(s) that these *Pseudomonas* virulence-associated factors, especially ETA, played in *P. aeruginosa* burn infections could not be elucidated in the absence of an animal model relevant to their study. While other burned rodent: *Pseudomonas* infection models have shown that burned animals become highly susceptible to *P. aeruginosa* infection,[40,41] the Stieritz and Holder burned mouse model (BMM)[42] is the most commonly used model to study the pathogenesis of *P. aeruginosa* infections.

In this model, a 15% total body surface, partial thickness burn is imposed on the shaven back of anesthetized mice. The injection of low numbers (10^2 colony-forming units, CFU) of fully virulent *P. aeruginosa* into the burned area causes an 80–100% lethal infection within 5 days, compared with 10-day LD_{50} of $>10^6$ CFU using the same strain to challenge non-burned mice. Thus, the increased susceptibility of the burned mouse to lethal *Pseudomonas* infection reflected observations in burned patients. Whereas the model did not fully mimic the burned patient circumstance because the organisms were injected into the burned wound rather than having to penetrate from surface colonization, their growth in the burned tissues was logarithmic and no systemic spread occurred from the burned site until 10^5 CFU/gm of burned tissue was present. These data showed that the progression of infection from burned skin to systemic invasion followed the same course as defined clinically for burn wound sepsis. Thus, the model appeared relevant to study the pathogenesis of *P. aeruginosa* infections in burns and was adopted with slight modifications by many research groups. Unless otherwise indicated, all results presented below have been obtained using the BMM.

4.1. Exotoxin A

The first evidence that toxemia was associated with *P. aeruginosa* burn infections *in vivo* was obtained from experiments using the BMM.[43] In this study it was shown that low numbers of *P. aeruginosa* (100 CFU), when injected into the partial-thickness 15% total body surface burned site on the shaven back of a mouse, proliferated rapidly at the site of inoculation. When the organisms in the burned skin tissue reached a critical concentration, generalized toxemia resulted, with subsequent mortality; the process was not reversible at this stage, even when the numbers of infecting organisms were reduced substantially by aggressive antibiotic treatment. However, when the reduction was accompanied by administration of rabbit serum prepared against filter-sterilized extracts of infected burned tissues, approximately 40% of the animals survived for at least 96 hr. This was not true with the use of antiserum prepared against uninfected burned tissue extracts. These data suggested that the antiserum afforded protection by inactivating a "toxin" produced by the organisms growing in the infected burned tissues rather than by reducing the numbers of infecting organisms.

Bartell *et al.*[44] demonstrated that a "toxic event" occurred *in vivo* as part of the pathogenic process of *P. aeruginosa* infection in unburned mice. Significant reduction in the *P. aeruginosa* population by treatment of the infected mice using specific lytic bacteriophage did not reduce mortality when treatment was withheld until a critical number of infecting bacteria was surpassed. This suggested to the authors that, by that time, a sufficient amount of a "lethal factor" had been produced to kill the mice in the absence of continued increase in the infecting bacterial load.

Using measurements of ADPR activity as evidence of ETA in serum and reduction in liver EF2 levels as evidence of the action of ETA, Saelinger *et al.*[45] provided direct evidence that ETA is produced in *P. aeruginosa* burn infections. They demonstrated that ADPR enzyme activity was present in saline extracts of burned *P. aeruginosa*-infected skin tissue, but not in the uninfected burned tissue. Further, enzyme activity increased in the serum of burned infected mice as the infection progressed, and this was followed by concomitant decreases in the levels of liver EF2. Antitoxin treatment of burned mice infected using two median lethal doses of *P. aeruginosa* strain PA-103 showed enhanced long-term survival compared with controls.[46] It must be noted, however, that strain PA-103, a high-ETA-producing but low-protease-producing strain, was not virulent in the BMM; LD_{50} of $>10^6$ compared with LD_{100} of

10^2 for fully virulent strains.[47] When burned mice infected with *fully* virulent *P. aeruginosa* strains were treated with antitoxin, an increase in the mean time to death was noted, but there was no long-term survival.[46] Studies from another laboratory showed similar results[48]; antitoxin treatment of burned mice infected with a fully virulent *P. aeruginosa* strain extended the mean time to death of the animals and blocked depletion of liver EF2, but no long-term survival was seen. An additional study confirmed that antitoxin treatment did not increase long-term survival in burned *P. aeruginosa*-infected mice,[49] but these authors did not comment on the effect of this treatment on mean time to death. Active immunization, using ETA toxoid in adjuvant, induced high serum levels of antitoxin antibody that protected mice from at least 100 LD_{50} challenge doses of purified ETA.[50] However, immunized mice that were burned and infected with *P. aeruginosa* showed increased survival time but no significant increases in long-term survivorship. In this study, as well as in a study where passive antitoxin therapy was given,[48] immunological therapy plus treatment using a dose of gentamicin which alone did not add significantly to survival provided substantial increases in the numbers of long-term survivors. These results indicate that in the face of continued microbial growth in the host, toxin neutralization alone is not sufficient to enhance long-term survival. These data suggest, also, that perhaps other virulence-associated factors play a role in lethal *P. aeruginosa* burn infections.

In contrast to results of active ETA immunization experiments in the BMM that showed enhanced survival rates,[50] ETA toxoid immunization of rats subsequently burned and infected using the scalded rat model[51] resulted in no improvement.[52] The reason for this disparity is not clear; however, it has been shown that burned rats are significantly less susceptible than burned mice to infection by *P. aeruginosa* strains isolated from septic burn patients.[53] Therefore, the rat may not be an appropriate animal in which to study some pathogenic and virulence-associated factors of *P. aeruginosa* infections in burns. In any case, experimental data from studies using the BMM suggested that ETA might be a virulence-associated factor in *P. aeruginosa* burn infections in humans. Clearly, however, this suggestion was inferential because no ETA studies had been done in burned *P. aeruginosa*-infected patients. On the other hand, studies showing a rising titer of antibody to ETA in the serum of *P. aeruginosa*-infected patients who were not burned suggested that ETA was produced *in vivo* during a variety of human infections.[53–56] In cancer patients, antibodies to ETA were found in patients colonized or infected by *P. aeruginosa*.[57] Titers in colonized patients were significantly higher than those in uninfected patients, while titers in infected patients were significantly higher than in patients who were only colonized by the organism. Passive antitoxin treatment of mice using various high-titer patient sera was fully or partially protective to mice intoxicated with four LD_{50} doses of ETA. Antibody to ETA also was found in the serum of *P. aeruginosa*-infected cystic fibrosis (CF) patients.[58] Results from another study showed that deaths from

Pseudomonas bacteremia were significantly associated with, among other things, infection with ETA-producing strains and antitoxin levels <2 μg/ml of patient serum.[59] It is clear from these diverse studies that ETA is elaborated *in vivo* in a wide variety of patient populations infected by *P. aeruginosa*. Based on these facts, the assumption seems warranted that ETA is elaborated in human burn patient *P. aeruginosa* infections and that this exoproduct plays a part in the pathogenic process.

4.2. Proteolytic Enzymes

As mentioned earlier, Morihara purified and characterized *Pseudomonas* elastase and alkaline protease in the 1960s.[30,31] These enzymes were implicated as responsible for hemorrhages in internal organs,[60,61] especially the lung,[62] and were shown to cause the destruction of corneal tissue in *P. aeruginosa* eye infections.[63–65]

The idea that proteases in addition to ETA may play a part in the pathogenesis of *P. aeruginosa* burn infections came from studies in which the toxigenic but protease-deficient strain PA-103 was used to examine the role of ETA in these infections.[46] The LD_{50} in burned mice for this strain was 10^6 CFU whereas fully virulent strains were 100% lethal when 10^2 CFU were injected into the burn site.[47] Supplementing low-dose (10^2 CFU) PA-103 burn wound injections with non-lethal amounts of *Pseudomonas* elastase or alkaline protease reduced the LD_{50} of PA-103-infected burned mice to that of burned mice infected with fully virulent *P. aeruginosa* strains.[47] A non-*Pseudomonas* protease—thermolysin—could substitute for the *Pseudomonas* enzymes. In addition to increased mortality observed in burned low-dose PA-103 infected mice supplemented with protease injections, liver EF2 levels were depleted by 42% compared with essentially no depletion in low-dose PA-103-infected mice without protease supplementation.[48] Conversely, when burned mice infected with fully virulent *P. aeruginosa* strains were treated with protease inhibitors infection mortality was reduced. That protease inhibitor treatment enhanced survival in *P. aeruginosa*-infected burned mice was substantiated by other studies.[66,67] These results provided reinforcing evidence that proteases are important factors in the pathogenesis of *P. aeruginosa* burn infections.[47] A study using fully virulent wild-type *P. aeruginosa* strains and their protease-deficient mutants to cause infections in the BMM further confirmed the role of proteases in lethality of *Pseudomonas* burn infection.[68] In this study, the LD_{50} of infections with the protease-deficient strains was at least one log higher than that of the wild-type parent. Although all strains used had the same generation time *in vitro*, fewer bacteria were found in the blood of burned mice infected with the mutant strain than in the blood of burned mice infected with the wild-type strain. Survival of mice infected with the protease-producing strain was enhanced by antiprotease serum; this treatment had no effect in mice infected with protease-deficient mutants.

Results of these studies implicated *Pseudomonas* proteolytic enzyme production as a contributing factor in the virulence of *P. aeruginosa* in infections in burned hosts, but did not provide information on how the enzymes act in this regard. That injections of purified *Pseudomonas* enzymes into skin caused the generation of hemorrhagic, necrotic lesions was known for many years[28,69] before it was shown that these enzymes specifically cleaved human type III and IV collagens[70] and degraded tissue-associated basement laminin.[71] These studies implied that at least one way in which these enzymes served as virulence factors was to enhance the invasive potential of the protease-producing versus the protease-deficient infecting strain. In the case of infections in burns, it was shown that a fully virulent *P. aeruginosa* strain (ETA- and protease[s]-producing) grew in extracts of burned tissue at a rate twice as fast as a protease-deficient strain.[72] This was true even though both strains grew at the same rate in extracts of normal tissue. Thus, it seemed that burned tissue was nutritionally poor for rapid *Pseudomonas* growth and required the presence of protease(s) to reduce local proteins into more usable substrates for the organisms' growth. Inhibition of protease elaboration by inclusion of ammonium salts in the burned skin extract in which the virulent strain was grown reduced the growth rate of the virulent strain to that seen in the protease-deficient strain, whereas the addition of protease (or amino acids, the products of protease activity) increased the growth rate of the protease-deficient strain to that of the virulent strain, supporting the foregoing. The dual features of increased growth of protease-producing *P. aeruginosa* strains in burned tissue and the direct skin-protein degrading capacity of the enzymes make protease production a potent virulence-associated factor in burns by increasing both the bacterial load as well as the invasive potential of such strains.

In addition, *Pseudomonas* proteases, either elastase, alkaline protease or both, have been shown to degrade or inactivate numerous host proteins that are important in host homeostatic and defense mechanisms. Among these proteins are plasma α_1-proteinase inhibitor,[73,74] C1-inhibitor and α_1-antichymotrypsin,[75] interleukin-2 (IL-2),[76] complement,[77] gamma interferon[78] and immunoglobulin G (IgG).[79–81] Plasma IgG levels in burned mice infected with a virulent *P. aeruginosa* declined as the infection progressed, until death of the animals.[81] The plasma IgG decline seen post-infection was superimposed on the decline in plasma IgG caused by the burn injury itself. Treatment of burned infected mice using the broad-spectrum serum protease inhibitor α_2-macroglobulin prevented the infection-associated plasma IgG decline. This was correlated with increased survival in the treated animals. Infection-related plasma IgG decline was not observed when the burned mice were infected using a protease-defective strain. These data suggested an alternative or additional mechanism by which protease(s) production by a *P. aeruginosa* strain served as a virulence factor in the pathogenesis of burn infections, that is, direct degradation of important host defense proteins.

Another means by which *P. aeruginosa* protease(s) may act as a virulence factor in burn infections is suggested from studies that show *Pseudomonas* proteases activate host Hageman factor.[82,83] This, plus the fact that thermal injury itself activates Hageman factor,[84] may influence how the *Pseudomonas* enzymes act to enhance lethality of burn infections more than infections in other susceptible patient populations. Hageman factor occupies a position at the apex of a number of interrelated protease-activated and protease-generating cascade pathways (kininogen–kinin, coagulation, fibrinolytic, complement), the under- or uncontrolled activation of which have negative immunological consequences.[85] Under normal circumstances these systems are kept in delicate balance and are activated appropriate to the needs of the host, followed by inhibition when the needs of the host are met. In severe thermal injury, under-controlled Hageman factor-mediated activation of down-line cascades causes increase in the total serum protease level plus proteolytic consumption or degradation of many host defense proteins. This contributes to various immunological alterations that occur following thermal injury[84,85] which make the burned host susceptible to infection. As pointed out in section 1, however, although recovery of gram-negative bacteria other than *P. aeruginosa* from burn wounds occurs in approximately the same percentage as *P. aeruginosa*, mortality from *Pseudomonas* infections is significantly higher.[6–8] Superimposition of a *P. aeruginosa* virulent strain infection, with its ability to add to host proteolytic load per se, and also by its protease-associated ability to activate Hageman factor further in the burned host, may push the host's proteolysis control beyond the "straw that broke the camel's back" threshold. In this case, the host is rendered almost defenseless against the infecting *P. aeruginosa*, and without strenuous therapeutic intervention the infection proceeds to lethality.

4.3. Pili

The adherence of *P. aeruginosa* to epidermal cells, and its relationship to colonization of burned skin surfaces, has been investigated using a flagellated (F+):piliated (P+) wild-type parent and combinations of non-flagellated (F−):non-piliated (P−) mutants.[86] P+ strains adhered to epidermal cells isolated from mouse skin in equal amounts, whether the P+ strain was F+ or F−. These results showed that pili, not flagella, were necessary for epidermal cell adherence. Anti-pilus serum blocked epidermal binding by the P+ strains. No significant differences in numbers of adherent bacteria were found in adherence studies that used epidermal cells prepared from normal mouse skin or skin taken from the burned site on mice using the BMM. No reduction in adherence was seen when normal epidermal cell suspensions, killed *in vitro* by heating, were used, suggesting that *P. aeruginosa* pilus-associated adherence would not be lost in cells killed by burning.

The same F+ and P+ strains and their mutants were used for *in vivo* experiments using the BMM.[87] In these studies the LD_{50} for the P− strain was ten-fold higher than for the P+ strain. Also, P+ organisms were isolated from the blood, liver, lungs, and kidney of mice infected with that strain, whereas this was not true for mice infected with the P− strain. The LD_{50} for F+ strains was 10^5 higher than for F− strains. Therefore, it appeared that both pili and flagella are important in *P. aeruginosa* burn infections. The virulence aspects of pili and flagella appeared independent since the P+F+ strain was the most virulent ($LD_{50} = \log_{10} 1.7-2.3$ CFU), followed within one log by the P−F+ strain. The P+F− strain LD_{50} was, however, several logs higher ($\log_{50} 7.2-7.5$ CFU) whereas the P−F− strain was essentially avirulent with $\log_{10} LD_{50} = 9$.

4.4. Flagella, Motility, and Chemotaxis

In 1980, McManus *et al.*,[88] using the Walker scalded rat model,[51] found that nonmotile mutants of a fully virulent strain of *P. aeruginosa* were of reduced virulence. Whereas the motile wild-type parent strain and the mutants were not prepared by a mutagenesis procedure that assured the mutants were isogenic with the parent, results of biochemical testing, growth characteristics, serotypes, and antibiogram were the same for parent and mutants, suggesting that the strains differed only in their motility characteristics. Thus, an association was suggested between motility and virulence of *P. aeruginosa* in burn infections. Supporting this were results from a BMM study, which showed that a nonmotile mutant of *P. aeruginosa* strain M-2, fully virulent in the BMM, lost its virulence in this model.[89] More important, perhaps, was the fact that spontaneous reversion of the mutant to motility restored full virulence to the strain. In testing three *P. aeruginosa* strains shown to vary in virulence in the BMM, others found that the virulent strain ($LD_{100} = 10^2$ CFU) was both motile and showed positive chemotaxis toward several chemoattractant substances.[90] One of the two less virulent strains was nonmotile and the second strain, although fully motile, did not show positive chemotactic capacity toward the chemoattractants. The nonmotile strain used in this study was nonmotile because it lacked flagella (fla−) rather than having nonfunctional flagella (mot−).[91] Its low virulence could have been associated with its lack of motility. Alternatively, it is possible that flagella play a nonmotility role in *Pseudomonas* burn wound infections, *e.g.* attachment, but, infection with the strain lacking flagella would not allow this aspect of virulence to be expressed. In either case, the experimental results would have been the same.

That the role of the flagellum in virulence is associated with directed motility of the strain was demonstrated in a study that generated mot− and fla− isogenic mutant strains from a virulent wild-type parent.[91] Virulence was reduced 100–100,000 times in both the mot− mutant with its nonfunctioning flagella and the strain that lacked flagella (fla−).

A schema for the antigenic composition of *P. aeruginosa* flagella was published in 1978.[92] Two major antigenic flagella types, "a" and "b," were described. The b flagella appeared to be antigenically homogeneous while the a flagella had a major a antigenic component and several minor a antigenic determinants. Antiserum prepared against either a or b flagella inhibited motility of the respective flagella-antigen-containing *P. aeruginosa* strains when assayed, *in vitro* with a soft-agar motility plate.[93,94] In addition, active immunization with a or b flagella enhanced survival in mice subsequently burned and infected with a *P. aeruginosa* strain with a flagella antigen homologous to the antigen used for immunization.[94,95] Divalent immunization with flagella antigen provided protection when the mice were subsequently burned and infected with *P. aeruginosa* strains containing flagella of either antigenic type.[95] Quantitative bacterial counts in the infected burned skin tissue and livers of infected immunized versus nonimmunized mice showed that whereas bacterial counts from the skin in both groups were the same, counts from the liver were significantly lower in the immunized mice. This led the authors to speculate that anti-flagella immunization was protective in burn wound infections because the organisms were "immobilized" within the skin tissue and were not able to spread systemically. Passive transfer of anti-flagella serum was also shown to enhance survival of burned mice infected with a *P. aeruginosa* strain with flagella antigen type homologous to the antiserum used for treatment.[96] These authors also counted high numbers of bacteria in skin of control and treated animals but reduced numbers in the liver of animals treated passively with anti-flagella serum. They came to the same conclusion about the mechanism of action of anti-flagella therapy. In this study, however, anti-flagella treatment was not protective in neutropenic mice. This posed another explanation for survival, namely that anti-flagella antibody enhanced opsonophagocytic activity in the immunized mice. This was shown to be the case by a study in which the addition of anti-flagella serum to mouse peritoneal macrophages grown *in vitro* resulted in increased uptake of radiolabeled *P. aeruginosa* of the flagella type homologous to the serum.[97]

5. SPECULATIONS ON THE ROLE(S) OF *PSEUDOMONAS* VIRULENCE-ASSOCIATED FACTORS ON THE PATHOGENIC PROCESS OF BURN WOUND INFECTIONS AND NOVEL TREATMENT APPROACHES

All the studies cited in previous sections have provided some insight into the role(s) of the individual *P. aeruginosa* virulence-associated factors in *P. aeruginosa* infection in a burned host. I now propose a theoretical scenario concerning the continuum involved in human *Pseudomonas* burn infections from initial colonization of the burned skin to the point at which septic death is inevitable. Although the hypothetical events described have not necessarily been shown to occur in burned patients infected with *P. aeruginosa*, they provide an integrated sequence of events to account for most of the results obtained from pathogenesis studies of *P. aeruginosa* infection in burned animals, using primarily the BMM.

This scenario can provide a basis for discussion among microbiologists, clinicians, and others involved in the care and treatment of burned patients. Furthermore, I hope this hypothesis points out the justification for and value of basic pathogenesis research studies, which if taken individually, may not make an immediate impact on understanding human disease but which taken as a whole may provide that understanding. In addition, I will endeavor to show that along with understanding part of the pathogenic process under investigation, these studies frequently suggest novel ways in which to interrupt the disease process. From this information may come the treatments of the future.

Before describing the sequence of events involved in *Pseudomonas* infections in burns, some understanding of the burned host is needed. Thermal injury of any magnitude causes immunosuppression in the burned host. Whereas the genesis of post-burn immunosuppression is complex, part of the "post-burn immunosuppression syndrome" is caused by host protease-activated and protease-generating cascade system activation initiated by thermal injury. Additionally, proteases released from injured cells enter the circulation. Normal serum protease inhibitors are used up in trying to control this trauma-related influx of proteases. Thus, host protease inhibitor levels are also reduced. This sets up a circumstance in the host whereby proteolytic activity is undercontrolled and there is a net increase in host total serum protease activity.[98] It is into this burned host environment that subsequent infection is superimposed. Compared with other bacteria, the various virulence-factors associated with *P. aeruginosa* make it better adapted to take advantage of the burned host's physiological environment, and this explains why these infections are so much more severe and life-threatening in burn patients than are others.

With this is prologue, the following section is a theoretical description of how the individual *P. aeruginosa* virulence-associated factors may interrelate with each other and the burned host and lead from initial colonization of the burn wound to burn-wound infection, burn-wound sepsis and finally death, due to multiple organ failure. It assumes that initial colonization is with a *P. aeruginosa* strain containing the full array of virulence features described in previous sections.

First, colonization of the burned skin surface by *P. aeruginosa* must occur. The colonizing organisms, usually in low numbers, are acquired through contamination of the wound by the patient's own flora or transferred from environmental sources to the wound, frequently by treatment personnel.[99–101] A few pseudomonads penetrate into subcutaneous soft tissue via hair follicles, trauma-induced "breaks" in the burned skin tissue, or, alternatively, are aided in their penetration by the production of tissue-destructive proteolytic enzymes.

Once adherent to the cells of the subcutaneous tissue by their pili, the organisms grow and at the same time, produce more protease(s) and also ETA. Protease degradation of host proteins in the immediate growing area of the microorganisms causes local tissue destruction as well as providing simple nutritional substances—amino acids—to the bacteria and this, in turn, enhances their growth.

In addition to causing damage to the soft tissue in which the pseudomonads are growing, the protease(s) may cleave host defense proteins that enter the infected area, making this local burn plus infection site more immunosuppressed than from the burn alone and therefore, even less able to clear the infection. As the growth rate and number of organisms in the local site increase, the nutrients in the immediate area of microbial growth become diminished. This creates a nutrient gradient: low nutrient content immediate to the growing site of the bacteria with increasing concentrations farther away. This gradient is "sensed" by the chemotactically competent *P. aeruginosa*. Fully motile (Fla+Mot+) strains can move to the area of higher nutritional availability and begin this process again. At some point in their movement to areas of higher nutrition, they encounter blood vessels where, perhaps through proteolytic destruction of the vessel walls, the organisms are picked up in the circulation. Burn wound sepsis has occurred! Via hematogenous spread, small local foci of infection are established in other host organs where the growth and spread process described for skin tissue continues to occur. While these local "infection spreading" processes are proceeding, the pseudomonads are continuously elaborating additional protease and ETA. These exoproducts become absorbed into the circulation where the protease(s) may cleave many host serum proteins involved in immunoresistance. Some of the host proteins degraded are protease inhibitors. This decreases further the host's control of increased circulating proteolytic activity, caused by the initial thermal trauma. Coupled with this is the capacity of the *P. aeruginosa* elastase to cause additional activation of the host Hageman factor with more protease activity being generated by added host cascade system activation. In this manner, the host becomes even less capable of defending itself against the infecting *P. aeruginosa*.

Concomitantly, ETA makes its way through the circulation to its major target organ, the liver, where it inhibits protein synthesis. At the same time that host homeostatic and defense proteins are reduced severely due to consumption and/or massive proteolytic cleavage, the major resupply organ for many of these proteins is becoming more and more dysfunctional. The liver is a major source for the synthesis of a number of proteins essential both to the well-being of the host and to its resistance to infection. Thus, the *P. aeruginosa* virulence-associated factors, protease(s) and ETA, may work in concert not only to deprive the host of the action of defense substances already present in the circulation and local body fluids but to reduce the host capacity to replenish these substances as well. At this point, the host is poorly equipped to fight the infection, and death, probably from multiple organ system failure, is likely to ensue.

This scenario presents the unique pathogenic process of *P. aeruginosa* infection in burn patients as a continuous and related temporal sequence of events starting with the initial colonization of the burn wound and ending with the eventual death of the infected host. The role that *Pseudomonas* virulence-associated factors may play at each point in this pathogenic process is hypothesized. Although there is no clinical or microbiological documentation to prove that this sequence of events occurs in burn infections in patients, the description takes into account research studies associating certain biological activities of each virulence factor with its potential role in the pathogenesis of burn wound infections. Furthermore, the specific point in the continuous pathogenic process at which different virulence-associated activities of *P. aeruginosa* are expressed, to provide for their maximum virulence-enhancing capacities, is considered. In this way, the pathogenic events as outlined provide a cohesive, integrated account of the role(s) that various virulence-associated factors might play.

Some of the studies used to put this account together have suggested ways in which the *P. aeruginosa* burn infection processes may be interrupted. These are outlined in Fig. 1. Early intervention at the initial colonization/penetration and burned skin growth phase of events, using antipilus serum, might interfere with *P. aeruginosa* adherence to burned tissue cells. Antiflagella immunotherapy might be applicable at this point as well. These treatments could be used alone or in conjunction with antibiotics to help further reduce initial microbial load. Antitoxin treatment has been shown to have a salutary effect on survival in *Pseudomonas* burn infections. Antitoxin treatment may help by allowing the host to resupply itself with homeostatic and immunoregulatory proteins which would not be provided by a liver whose protein synthetic capacity is inhibited due to ETA activity. This therapy would be most useful in conjunction with concomitant treatment directed toward reducing total antimicrobial load, *e.g.* antibiotic treatments[48,66,102] or in combination with antibody directed against specific *Pseudomonas* LPS.[67,102] Therapy using various protease inhibition treatments has been successful in enhancing survival from *Pseudomonas* burn infections. Treatment could be directed toward the *Pseudomonas* proteases using specific antisera,[68] against circulating host-derived protease activity[66,67] or both[48,81]; collective data suggest that as long as total protease activity in the host is brought under control, regardless of the source(s) of the protease activity, survival appears enhanced.

As discussed previously, both thermal injury and *Pseudomonas* proteases activate host Hageman factor with corresponding activation of down-line

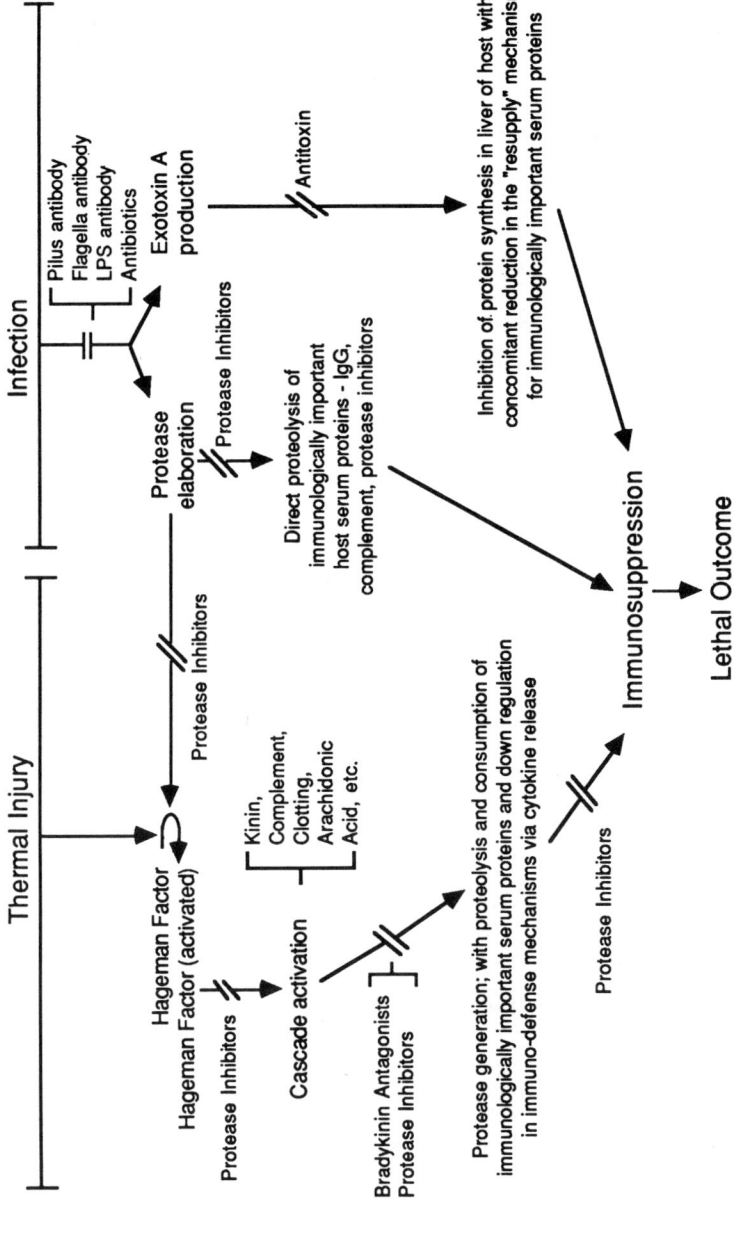

FIGURE 1. Burned host–*Pseudomonas* interactions leading to lethal infection. Novel multiple treatment approach.

host protease-related cascade systems. An intermediate product of activation of one of these systems—the kininogen–kinin cascade—is bradykinin. Bradykinin causes further activation of several additional down-line cascades with the attendant negative immunologic consequences.[85] This fact suggests a possible alternative therapeutic approach: inhibition of the activity of bradykinin by the use of bradykinin antagonists.[103] Although no studies have been done in this regard, on a theoretical basis this treatment approach may provide a salutary effect in burned *P. aeruginosa* infected hosts.

None of the therapies described above provided uniform long-term survival for burned *P. aeruginosa*-infected animals. In fact, antitoxin treatment required concomitant therapy to reduce total microbial load to be most effective.[43,48,50] Multifactoral treatment for *Pseudomonas* infections is not a new concept. Homma and colleagues in the late 1970s demonstrated that immunization (active or passive) using original endotoxin protein—a common *Pseudomonas* LPS-associated antigen plus toxoids of elastase and alkaline protease—was more successful in treating hemorrhagic pneumonia in mink or corneal infections in mice than immunization with the individual components of the "vaccine."[104,105] A multifactor therapy approach will probably be the most efficacious approach in *Pseudomonas* infections in burns also. Support for this idea comes from results of a recent study where combined treatment using the protease inhibitor α-1-proteinase inhibitor to reduce total proteolytic load in the host, antitoxin to reduce the effects of ETA, and *Pseudomonas* hyperimmune globulin to reduce host microbial load, was more successful than treatments that used a single-component approach.[67]

REFERENCES

1. Langohr, J. L., Owen, C. R., and Cope, O., 1947, Bacteriologic study of burn wounds, *Ann. Surg.* **125**:452–455.
2. Lynch, J. B., Kim, K. A., Larson, D. L., Doyle, J. E., and Lewis, S. R., 1971, Changing patterns of mortality in burns, *Plast. Reconstr. Surg.* **48**:329–332.
3. Yow, E. M., 1952, Development of *Proteus* and *Pseudomonas* infections during antibiotic therapy, *J.A.M.A.* **149**:1184–1186.
4. Tumbusch, W. T., Vogel, E. H., Butkiewicz, J. V., Graber, C. D., Larson, D. L., and Mitchell, E. T., 1961, Septicemia in burn injury, *J. Trauma* **1**:22–27.
5. Stone, H. H., 1966, Review of *Pseudomonas* sepsis in thermal burns, *Ann. Surg.* **163**:297–301.
6. Moncrief, J. A., and Rivera, J. A., 1958, The problem of infection in burns by resistant micro-organisms with a note on the use of bacitracin, *Ann. Surg.* **147**:295–299.
7. Speller, D. E. E., 1980, Hospital infection by multi-resistant gram-negative bacilli, *J. Antimicrob. Chemother.* **6**:168–170.
8. Holder, I. A., 1990, Microbiology of the burn compromised patient, in: *Pathogenesis of Wound and Biomaterial Associated Infections* (T. Wadstrom, I. Eliasson, I. A. Holder, and A. Ljungh, eds.), Springer-Verlag, London, pp. 91–100.
9. McManus, A. T., 1989, *Pseudomonas aeruginosa*: A controlled burn pathogen? in: *Pseudomonas aeruginosa Infection*, Antibiotics Chemotherapy, Volume 42 (N. Høiby, S. S. Pederson, G. Shand, G. Döring, and I. A. Holder, eds.), Karger, Basel, Switzerland, pp. 103–108.

10. Wasserman, D., Schlotterer, M., Lebreton, F., Levy, J., and Guelfi, M. D., 1989, Use of topically applied silver sulphadiazine plus cerium nitrate in major burns, *Burns* **15:** 257–260.
11. Koo, D. S., Gu, X. M., Zhen, S., DeZhen, Z., Shi, S. W., and Xiang, S. J., 1989, Assessment of topical therapy of the burn wound with silver sulphadiazine after its use for 15 years in a burn unit, *Burns* **15:**193–196.
12. Bang, R. L., and Saif, J. K., 1989, Mortality from burns in Kuwait, *Burns* **15:**315–321.
13. Shulman, J. A., Terry, P. M., and Hough, C. E., 1971, Colonization with a gentamicin resistant *Pseudomonas aeruginosa* pyocine type 5 in a burn unit, *J. Infect. Dis.* **124:**S18–S23.
14. Sogaard, H., Zimmerman-Nielsen, C., and Siboni, K., 1974, Antibiotic-resistant gram-negative bacilli in a urological ward for male patients during a nine-year period: Relationship to antibiotic consumption, *J. Infect. Dis.* **130:**646–650.
15. Holder, I. A., 1976, Gentamicin resistant *Pseudomonas aeruginosa* in a burns unit, *J. Antimicrob. Chemother.* **2:**309–316.
16. LeFrock, J. L., Molavi, A., and Smith, B. R., 1984, Current use of aminoglycosides, *Infect. Surg.* **3:**57–65.
17. Pruitt, B. A., 1983, Treating burn and soft tissue infections, *Infect. Surg.* **2:**625–650.
18. Holder, I. A., Vanderpool, L., and Wesselman, J., 1985, Para-chloro-meta-xylenol (PCMX): A new, potential topical antimicrobial agent, *J. Burn Care Rehab.* **6:**58–61.
19. Holder, I. A., Schwab, M., and Jackson, L., 1979, Eighteen months of routine topical antimicrobial susceptibility testing of isolates from burn patients: Results and conclusions, *J. Antimicrob. Chemother.* **5:**455–463.
20. Fox, C. L., Vyasa Rao, T. N., Azmeth, R., Gandhi, S. S., and Modak, S., 1990, Comparative evaluation of zinc sulfadiazine and silver sulfadiazine in burn wound infection, *J. Burn Care Rehab.* **11:**112–117.
21. Wachtel, T. L., 1987, Topical antimicrobials, in: *Burns in Children* (H. F. Carvajal, D. H. Parks, eds.), Year Book Medical Publishers, Inc., Chicago, pp. 106–118.
22. Waisbren, B. A., 1976, Treatment of severe burns, *Compr. Ther.* **2:**33–42.
23. Moyer, C. A., Brentano, L., Gravens, D. L., Margraf, H. W., and Monafo, W. W., 1965, Treatment of large human burns with 0.5% silver nitrate solution, *Arch. Surg.* **90:**812–867.
24. Shuck, J. M., Einfeldt, L. E., and Trainor, M. P., 1972, Sulfamylon solution dressings in the management of burn wounds: Preliminary clinical report, *J. Trauma* **12:**999–1002.
25. Holder, I. A., 1989, The wet disc antimicrobial solution assay: An *in vitro* method to test efficacy of antimicrobial solutions for topical use, *J. Burn Care Rehab.* **10:**203–208.
26. Holder, I. A., 1988, *Pseudomonas* immunotherapy, *Serodiag. Immunother.* **2:**7–16.
27. Liu, P. V., Abe, Y., and Bates, J. L., 1961, The roles of various fractions of *Pseudomonas aeruginosa* in its pathogenesis, *J. Infect. Dis.* **108:**218–227.
28. Liu, P. V., 1966, The roles of various fractions of *Pseudomonas aeruginosa* in its pathogenesis: II. Effects of lecithinase and protease, *J. Infect. Dis.* **116:**112–116.
29. Liu, P. V., 1966, The roles of various fractions of *Pseudomonas aeruginosa* in its pathogenesis: III. Identity of the lethal toxins produced *in vitro* and *in vivo*, *J. Infect. Dis.* **116:**481–489.
30. Morihara, K., 1963, *Pseudomonas aeruginosa* proteinase: I. Purification and general properties, *Biochem. Biophys. Acta* **73:**113–124.
31. Morihara, K., Tsuzuki, H., Oka, T., Inoue, H., and Ebata, M., 1965, *Pseudomonas aeruginosa* elastase. Isolation, crystallization, and preliminary characterization, *J. Biol. Chem.* **240:** 3295–3304.
32. Liu, P. V., Yoshii, S., and Hsieh, H., 1973, Exotoxins of *Pseudomonas aeruginosa*. II. Concentration, purification, and characterization of exotoxin A, *J. Infect. Dis.* **128:**514–519.
33. Liu, P. V., and Hsieh, H., 1973, Exotoxins of *Pseudomonas aeruginosa*. III. Characteristics of antitoxin A, *J. Infect. Dis.* **128:**520–526.
34. Callahan, L. T., III, 1974, Purification and characterization of *Pseudomonas aeruginosa* exotoxin, *Infect. Immun.* **9:**113–118.

35. Atik, M., Liu, P. V., Hanson, B. A., Amini, S., and Rosenberg, C. F., 1968, *Pseudomonas* exotoxin shock. A preliminary report of studies in dogs, *J.A.M.A.* **205**:134–140.
36. Pavlovskis, O. R., and Gordon, F. B., 1972, *Pseudomonas aeruginosa* exotoxin: Effect on cell cultures, *J. Infect. Dis.* **125**:631–636.
37. Pavlovskis, O. R., and Shackelford, A. H., 1974, *Pseudomonas aeruginosa* exotoxin in mice: Localization and effect on protein synthesis, *Infect. Immun.* **9**:540–546.
38. Pavlovskis, O. R., Voelker, F. A., and Shackelford, A. H., 1976, *Pseudomonas aeruginosa* exotoxin in mice: Histopathology and serum enzyme changes, *J. Infect. Dis.* **133**:253–259.
39. Iglewski, B. H., and Kabat, D., 1975, NAD-dependent inhibition of protein synthesis by *Pseudomonas aeruginosa* toxin, *Proc. Natl. Acad. Sci. U.S.A.* **72**:2284–2288.
40. McRipley, R. J., and Garrison, D. W., 1964, Increased susceptibility of burned rats to *Pseudomonas aeruginosa*, *Proc., Soc. Exp. Biol. Med.* **115**:336–338.
41. Liedberg, C. F., 1960, Antibacterial resistance in burns. I. The effect of intraperitoneal infection on survival and the frequency of septicemia. An experimental study in the guinea pig, *Acta Chir. Scand.* **120**:88–94.
42. Stieritz, D. D., and Holder, I. A., 1975, Experimental studies of the pathogenesis of infections due to *Pseudomonas aeruginosa*: Description of a burned mouse model, *J. Infect. Dis.* **131**:668–691.
43. Stieritz, D. D., and Holder, I. A., 1978, Experimental studies of the pathogenesis of *Pseudomonas aeruginosa* infection: Evidence for the *in vivo* production of a lethal toxin, *J. Med. Microbiol.* **11**:101–109.
44. Bartell, P. F., Orr, T. E., and Garcia, M., 1968, The lethal events in experimental *Pseudomonas aeruginosa* infection in mice, *J. Infect. Dis.* **118**:165–172.
45. Saelinger, C. B., Snell, K., and Holder, I. A., 1977, Experimental studies on the pathogenesis of infections due to *Pseudomonas aeruginosa*: Direct evidence of toxin production during *Pseudomonas* infection of burned host tissues, *J. Infect. Dis.* **136**:555–561.
46. Pavlovskis, O. R., Pollack, M., Callahan, L. T., III, and Iglewski, B. H., 1977, Passive protection by antitoxin in experimental *Pseudomonas aeruginosa* burn infections, *Infect. Immun.* **18**:596–602.
47. Holder, I. A., and Haidaris, C. G., 1979, Experimental studies of the pathogenesis of infections due to *Pseudomonas aeruginosa*: Extra-cellular protease and elastase as *in vivo* virulence factor. *Can. J. Microbiol.* **45**:593–599.
48. Snell, K., Holder, I. A., Leppla, S. A., and Selinger, C. B., 1978, Role of exotoxin and protease as possible virulence factors in experimental infections with *Pseudomonas aeruginosa*, *Infect. Immun.* **19**:839–845.
49. Cryz, S. J., Furer, E., and Germanier, R., 1983, Protection against *Pseudomonas aeruginosa* infection in a murine burn wound sepsis model by transfer of antitoxin A, anti-elastase, and anti-lipopolysaccharide, *Infect. Immun.* **39**:1072–1079.
50. Pavlovskis, O. R., Edman, D. C., Leppla, S. H., Wretlind, B., Lewis, L. R., and Martin, K. E., 1981, Protection against experimental *Pseudomonas aeruginosa* infection in mice by active immunization with exotoxin A toxoids, *Infect. Immun.* **32**:681–689.
51. Walker, H. L., and Mason, Jr., A. D., 1968, A standard animal burn, *J. Trauma* **8**:1049–1051.
52. Walker, H. L., McLeod, C. G., Jr., Leppla, S. H., and Mason, Jr., A. D., 1979, Evaluation of *Pseudomonas aeruginosa* toxin A in experimental rat burn wound sepsis, *Infect. Immun.* **25**:828–830.
53. Fox, C. L., Jr., Sampath, A. C., and Stanford, J. W., 1970, Virulence of *Pseudomonas* infection in burned rats and mice, *Arch. Surg.* **101**:508–512.
54. Pollack, M., Callahan, III, L. T., and Taylor, N. S., 1976, Neutralizing antibody to *Pseudomonas aeruginosa* exotoxin in human sera: Evidence for *in vivo* toxin production during *Pseudomonas* infection of burned skin tissues, *J. Infect. Dis.* **136**:555–561.
55. Pollack, M., and Taylor, N. S., 1977, Serum antibody to *Pseudomonas aeruginosa* exotoxin measured by a passive hemagglutination assay, *J. Clin. Microbiol.* **6**:58–61.

56. Pollack, M., and Young, L. S., 1979, Protective activity of antibodies to exotoxin A and lipopolysaccharide at the onset of *Pseudomonas aeruginosa* septicemia in man, *J. Clin. Microbiol.* **63**:276–286.
57. Crowe, K. E., Bass, J. A., Young, V. M., and Straus, D. C., 1982, Antibody response to *Pseudomonas aeruginosa* exoproducts in cancer patients, *J. Clin. Microbiol.* **15**:115–122.
58. Klinger, J. D., Straus, D. C., Hilton, C. F., and Bass, J. A., 1978, Antibodies to protease and exotoxin A of *Pseudomonas aeruginosa* in patients with cystic fibrosis: Demonstration by radioimmunoassay, *J. Infect. Dis.* **138**:49–58.
59. Cross, A. S., Sadoff, J. C., Iglewski, B. H., and Sokol, P. A., 1980, Evidence for the role of toxin A in the pathogenesis of infection with *Pseudomonas aeruginosa* in humans, *J. Infect. Dis.* **142**:538–546.
60. Kawaharajo, K., Homma, J.Y., Aoyama, Y., Okada, E., and Morihara, K., 1975, In vivo studies on protease and elastase from *Pseudomonas aeruginosa*, *Jpn. J. Exp. Med.* **45**:89–100.
61. Meinke, G., Barum, J., Rosenberg, B., and Berk, R., 1970, In vivo studies with the partially purified protease (elastase) from *Pseudomonas aeruginosa*, *Infect. Immun.* **2**:583–589.
62. Fetzer, A. E., Werner, A. S., and Hagstrom, J. W. C., 1967, Pathologic features of *Pseudomonas* pneumonia, *Am. Rev. Resp. Dis.* **96**:1121–1130.
63. Kawaharajo, K., Abe, C., Homma, J. Y., Kawane, M., Gotoh, T., Tanaka, N., and Morihara, K., 1974, Corneal ulcers caused by protease and elastase from *Pseudomonas aeruginosa*, *Jpn. J. Exp. Med.* **44**:435–442.
64. Gray, L. D., and Kreger, A. S., 1975, Rabbit corneal damage produced by *Pseudomonas aeruginosa* infection, *Infect. Immun.* **12**:419–432.
65. Kreger, A. S., Griffin, I. K., 1974, Physiochemical fractionation of extracellular cornea-damaging proteases of *Pseudomonas aeruginosa*, *Infect. Immun.* **9**:828–834.
66. Neely, A. N., and Holder, I. A., 1987, Experimental studies of the pathogenesis of infections due to *Pseudomonas aeruginosa*: Treatment using *Pseudomonas* hyperimmune globulin plus minocycline and effects of minocycline on protease elaboration, *Serodiag. Immunother.* **1**:193–200.
67. Holder, I. A., and Neely, A. N., 1989, Combined host and specific anti-*Pseudomonas*-directed therapy for *Pseudomonas aeruginosa* infections in burned mice: Experimental results and theoretic considerations, *J. Burn Care Rehab.* **10**:131–137.
68. Pavlovskis, O. R., and Wretlind, B., 1979, Assessment of protease (elastase) as a *Pseudomonas aeruginosa* virulence factor in experimental mouse burn infection, *Infect. Immun.* **24**:181–187.
69. Kawaharajo, K., Homma, J. Y., Aoyama, Y., and Morihara, K., 1975, In vivo studies on protease and elastase from *Pseudomonas aeruginosa*, *Jpn. J. Exp. Med.* **45**:89–100.
70. Heck, L. W., Morihara, K., McRae, W. B., and Miller, E. J., 1986, Specific cleavage of human type III and IV collagens by *Pseudomonas aeruginosa* elastase, *Infect. Immun.* **51**:115–118.
71. Heck, L. W., Morihara, K., and Abrahamson, D. R., 1986, Degradation of soluble laminin and depletion of tissue-associated basement membrane laminin by *Pseudomonas aeruginosa* elastase and alkaline protease, *Infect. Immun.* **54**:149–153.
72. Cicmanec, J. F., and Holder, I. A., 1979, Growth of *Pseudomonas aeruginosa* in normal and burned skin extract: Role of extracellular proteases, *Infect. Immun.* **25**:477–483.
73. Morihara, K. Tsuzuki, H., and Oda, K., 1979, Protease and elastase of *Pseudomonas aeruginosa*: Inactivation of human plasma α_1-proteinase inhibitor, *Infect. Immun.* **24**:189–193.
74. Morihara, K., Tsuzuki, H., Harada, M., and Iwata, T., 1984, Purification of human plasma α_1-proteinase inhibitor and its inactivation by *Pseudomonas aeruginosa* elastase, *J. Biochem.* **95**:795–804.
75. Catanese, J., and Kress, L. F., 1984, Enzymatic inactivation of human plasma C1-inhibitor and α_1-antichymotrypsin by *Pseudomonas aeruginosa* proteinase and elastase, *Biochim. Biophys. Acta* **789**:37–43.
76. Theander, T. G., Kharazmi, A., Pedersen, B. K., Christensen, L. D., Tvede, N., Poulsen,

L. K., Odum, N., Svenson, M., and Bendtzen, K., 1988, Inhibition of human lymphocyte proliferation and cleavage of interleukin-2 by *Pseudomonas aeruginosa* proteases, *Infect. Immun.* **56:**1673–1677.
77. Schultz, D. R., and Miller, K. D., 1974, Elastase of *Pseudomonas aeruginosa*: Inactivation of complement components and complement-derived chemotactic and phagocytic factors, *Infect. Immun.* **10:**128–135.
78. Horvat, R., and Parmely, M. J., 1988, *Pseudomonas aeruginosa* alkaline protease degrades human gamma interferon and inhibits its bioactivity, *Infect. Immun.* **56:**2925–2932.
79. Döring, G., Obernesser, H. J., and Botzenhart, K., 1981, Extra-cellular toxins of *Pseudomonas aeruginosa*. II. Effect of two proteases on human immunoglobulin IgG, IgA and secretory IgA, *Zentralbl. Bakteriol. Parasitenkd. Infektionskr. Hyg. Abt. 1. Orig. Reihe A.* **249:** 89–98.
80. Döring, G., Dalhoff, A., Vogel, O., Brunner, H., Droge, U., and Botzenhart, K., 1984, *In vivo* activity of proteases of *Pseudomonas aeruginosa* in a rat model, *J. Infect. Dis.* **149:**532–537.
81. Holder, I. A., and Wheeler, R., 1984, Experimental studies of the pathogenesis of infections owning to *Pseudomonas aeruginosa*: Elastase, an IgG protease, *Can. J. Microbiol.* **30:**1118–1124.
82. Holder, I. A., and Neely, A. N., 1989, *Pseudomonas* elastase acts as a virulence factor in burned hosts by Hageman factor-dependent activation of the host kinin cascade, *Infect. Immun.* **57:**3345–3348.
83. Molla, A., Yammamoto, T., Akaike, T., Miyoshi, S., and Maeda, H., 1989, Activation of Hageman factor and prekallikrein and generation of kinin by various microbial proteases, *J. Biol. Chem.* **264:**10589–10594.
84. Holder, I. A., and Neely, A. N., 1990, Hageman factor dependent kinin activation in burns and its theoretical relationship to post burn immunosuppression syndrome and infection, *J. Burn Care Rehab.*, in press.
85. Bjornson, A. B., and Bjornson, H. S., 1984, Theoretical interrelationship among immunologic and hematologic sequelae of thermal injury, *Rev. Infect. Dis.* **6:**704–714.
86. Sato, H., and Okinaga, K., 1987, Role of pili in the adherence of *Pseudomonas aeruginosa* to mouse epidermal cells, *Infect. Immun.* **55:**1774–1778.
87. Sato, H., Okinaga, K., and Saito, H., 1988, Role of pili in the pathogenesis of *Pseudomonas aeruginosa* burn infection, *Microbiol. Immunol.* **32:**131–139.
88. McManus, A. T., Moody, E. E., and Mason, A. D., 1980, Bacterial motility: A component in experimental *Pseudomonas aeruginosa* burn wound sepsis, *Burns* **6:**235–239.
89. Montie, T. C., Doyle-Huntzinger, D., Craven, R. C., and Holder, I. A., 1982, Loss of virulence associated with absence of flagellum in an isogeneic mutant of *Pseudomonas aeruginosa* in the burned mouse model, *Infect. Immun.* **38:**1296–1298.
90. Craven, R. C., and Montie, T. C., 1981, Motility and chemotaxis of three strains of *Pseudomonas aeruginosa* used for virulence studies, *Can. J. Microbiol.* **27:**458–460.
91. Drake, D., and Montie, T. C., 1988, Flagella, motility and invasive virulence of *Pseudomonas aeruginosa*, *J. Gen. Microbiol.* **134:**43–52.
92. Ansorg, R., 1978, Flagella specific H antigenic schema of *Pseudomonas aeruginosa*, *Zentralbl. Bakteriol. Parasitenkd. Infektionskr. Hyg. Abt. 1. Orig. Reihe A.* **242:**228–238.
93. Montie, R. C., Craven, R. C., and Holder, I. A., 1982, Flagellar preparations from *Pseudomonas aeruginosa*: Isolation and characterization, *Infect. Immun.* **35:**281–288.
94. Holder, I. A., and Naglich, J. G., 1986, Experimental studies of the pathogenesis of infections due to *Pseudomonas aeruginosa*: Immunization using divalent flagella preparations, *J. Trauma* **26:**118–122.
95. Holder, I. A., Wheeler, R., and Montie, T. C, 1982, Flagellar preparations from *Pseudomonas aeruginosa*: Animal protection studies, *Infect. Immun.* **35:**276–280.
96. Drake, D., and Montie, T. C., 1987, Protection against *Pseudomonas aeruginosa* infection by passive transfer of anti-flagellar serum, *Can. J. Microbiol.* **35:**755–763.

97. Anderon, T. R., and Montie, T. C., 1989, Flagellar antibody stimulated opsonophagocytosis of *Pseudomonas aeruginosa* associated with response to either a- or b-type flagellar antigen, *Can. J. Microbiol.* **35**:890–894.
98. Neely, A. N., Nathan, P., and Highsmith, R. F., 1988, Plasma proteolytic activity following burns, *J. Trauma* **28**:362–367.
99. Edmonds, P., Suskind, R. R., MacMillan, B. G., and Holder, I. A., 1972, Epidemiology of *Pseudomonas aeruginosa* in a burns hospital: Evaluation of serological, bacteriophage and pyocin typing methods, *Appl. Microbiol.* **24**:213–218.
100. Edmonds, P., Suskind, R. R., MacMillan, B. G., and Holder, I. A., 1972, Epidemiology of *Pseudomonas aeruginosa* in a burns hospital: Surveillance by a combined typing system, *Appl. Microbiol.* **24**:219–225.
101. Holder, I. A., 1977, Epidemiology of *Pseudomonas aeruginosa* in a burns hospital, in: *Pseudomonas aeruginosa: Ecological Aspects and Patient Colonization* (V. M. Young, ed.), Raven Press, New York, pp. 77–95.
102. Collins, M. S., Tsay, G. C., Hector, R. F., Roby, R. E., and Dorsey, J. H., 1986, Immunoglobulin G: Potentiation of tobramycin and azlocillin in the treatment of *Pseudomonas aeruginosa* sepsis in neutropenic mice and neutralization of exotoxin A in vivo, *Rev. Infect. Dis.* **8**:S420–S425.
103. Burch, R. M., Farmer, S. C., and Steranka, L. R., 1990, Bradykinin receptor antagonists, *Med. Res. Rev.* **10**:237–269.
104. Honda, E., Homma, J. Y., Abe, C., Tanamoto, K., Noda, H., and Yanagawa, R., 1977, Effects of the common protective antigen (OEP) and toxoids of protease and elastase from *Pseudomonas aeruginosa* on protection against hemorrhagic pneumonia in mink, *Zentralbl. Bakteriol. Parasitenkd. Infektionskr. Hyg. Abt. a Orig. Reihe A.* **237**:297–309.
105. Hirao, Y., and Homma, J. Y., 1978, Therapeutic effect of immunization with OEP, protease toxoid and elastase toxoid on corneal ulcers in mice due to *Pseudomonas aeruginosa* infection, *Jpn. J. Exp. Med.* **48**:41–51.

15

Acquired Resistance to *P. aeruginosa*

GERALD B. PIER

1. INTRODUCTION

Infections due to *Pseudomonas aeruginosa* are difficult to acquire without a basic underlying condition such as immunosuppression or cystic fibrosis (CF). Innate resistance to this organism is high. Community-acquired infection is rare, limited mostly to non-life-threatening conditions such as folliculitis from a hot tub or whirlpool and otitis externa. Eye infections due to *P. aeruginosa* can be problematic, particularly for individuals who wear soft contact lenses,[1] but again, trauma or some other predisposing ocular condition must usually be present for this organism to cause infection. In the presence of an underlying condition, *P. aeruginosa* can be a formidable pathogen. *P. aeruginosa* first gained notoriety as an opportunistic pathogen in burn patients and individuals undergoing chemotherapy that resulted in neutropenia.[2] Over the 20–30 years, it has become the dominant pathogen in the lungs of CF patients, accounting for most of the morbidity and mortality in these individuals.[3,4,5] *P. aeruginosa* can infect virtually any part of the body,[6] causing endocarditis, respiratory infections, bacteremia, central nervous system infections, ear and eye infections, bone and joint infections, and infections of the urinary tract, soft tissues and skin, and gastrointestinal tract.

GERALD B. PIER • Channing Laboratory, Department of Medicine, Brigham and Women's Hospital, Harvard Medical School, Boston, Massachusetts 02115-5899.

Pseudomonas aeruginosa as an Opportunistic Pathogen, edited by Mario Campa *et al.* Plenum Press, New York, 1993.

When given the opportunity, *P. aeruginosa* can evade many different types of host defenses to colonize and infect a human host.

Therefore, to understand the immunologic mechanisms of acquired resistance to *P. aeruginosa* infection, one must identify the principal host immunologic effectors and bacterial antigenic targets. Both of these areas are broad, and a plethora of publications can be reviewed on immunity to *P. aeruginosa* and on the bacterial antigens provoking that immunity. However there are some major recurrent themes in the mechanisms of acquired resistance. Opsonic antibody-mediated immunity to respiratory and disseminated infection is often documented, and serotype-specific antibodies to the lipopolysaccharide (LPS) O–side chain predominate as immune effectors against infections caused by LPS-smooth strains. Cell-mediated immunity has received attention, and T-cell-mediated protection in mice has been well-documented.[7,8,9,10] Complement and phagocytic cells participate in antibody-mediated immunity, and thus play important roles in acquired resistance. Many other antigens besides LPS O–side chains have received attention as targets of protective antibody, including outer membrane proteins[11,12,13] and lipoproteins[14,15,16]; LPS core antigens[17]; original endotoxin protein[18,19,20]; flagella[21,22]; ribosomal antigens[23,24]; and extracellular toxins and proteins.[25,26,27] This review will focus on the major themes of antibody and cellular immune effectors participating in acquired resistance and the antigenic targets these effectors recognize.

2. IMMUNITY TO INFECTION

Acquired resistance implies a permanent or transient acquisition of specific immunologic effectors, usually acquired via active or passive immunization. *Active immunization* may occur naturally following exposure to the pathogen and development of clinical or inapparent infection or artificially following vaccination with the bacterium or purified antigens. *Passive immunity* is a temporary state resulting from transfer to a recipient of immune effectors, most often antibody. (In inbred animals, lymphocytes can also be used.) Naturally acquired immune effectors often are specific to bacterial antigens that are key to eliciting immune resistance. Identification of these effectors and their antigenic specificity is often helpful in defining the mechanisms of acquired resistance to infection.

Several important studies have defined critical aspects of immunity to *P. aeruginosa* infection in animals and humans. In the analyses of immunity to *P. aeruginosa* infection, important distinctions in antigen expression have emerged between strains causing acute infections in compromised hosts and chronic infections in CF patients. Linker and Jones[28] described the exopolysaccharide produced by mucoid strains of *P. aeruginosa* isolated from CF patients as similar to seaweed alginate. This bacterial alginate was initially thought to be non-immunogenic,[29,30] but Pier et al. first demonstrated animal[31] and human[32] immune responses to this antigen, and designated it mucoid exopolysaccharide (MEP). Other investigators rapidly confirmed their findings.[33,34,35] In addition, 80% of these mucoid isolates were found by Hancock et al.[36] to express a rough type of LPS, lacking O–side chains. Again, other investigators soon confirmed this finding.[37,38] The CF-associated isolates produced large quantities of MEP and few-to-no O–side chains (i.e., rough LPS), whereas isolates from immunocompromised hosts produced little MEP[39] and smooth LPS. These distinctions figure prominently in differences in acquired resistance to P. aeruginosa infection in these markedly divergent clinical situations.

3. ACQUIRED RESISTANCE TO INFECTION IN NON-CF HUMANS

3.1. Naturally Acquired Active Immunity to Non-CF-Associated P. aeruginosa Infections

Young et al.[40] and Crowder et al.[41] demonstrated that in non-CF-infected humans, the principal antibody to arise following P. aeruginosa infection is directed against LPS serotype determinants. Pollack and Young[42] documented that bacteremic patients with high levels of antibody to P. aeruginosa LPS O–side chains in acute-phase serum samples were more likely to survive infection than were patients with low antibody levels. Baltch et al.[43] recently provided supporting data from a study involving 42 bacteremic patients. These studies consistently indicate that naturally acquired immunity to LPS serotype determinants is associated with survival after P. aeruginosa bacteremia and recovery from infection.

Other studies have suggested that antibody to exotoxin A (ETA) is important in immune resistance. In the study noted above, Pollack and Young[42] suggested that antibody to ETA was associated with survival after bacteremia, but patients with antibody to ETA tended to have antibody to LPS as well. There were insufficient patients with high levels of antibody only to ETA to evaluate its protective role. Cross et al.[26] showed protection associated with high levels of antibody to ETA, but they did not control for the covariance of these antibodies with antibodies to LPS. On the basis of Pollack and Young's findings,[42] it is likely that most of these patients also had high levels of antibody to LPS. Baltch et al.[43] did not observe any relationship between patient outcome and levels of antibody to ETA, elastase or protease. Animal studies designed to assess the protective role of antibody to ETA in protection have been equivocal,[44,45,46,47] with most investigators unable to demonstrate effective protection against fully virulent strains. In addition, Wretlind et al.[48] showed that isogenic derivatives of strain PAO deficient in ETA and elastase production are as virulent as the parental strain in experimental burn infections. Since the major pathologic role of ETA is likely intoxication of liver cells due to ADP-ribosylation of elongation factor-2 (EF2),[49] anti-ETA may augment protection by decreasing liver damage during infection.

3.2. Vaccine-Induced Immunity to Non-CF-Associated *P. aeruginosa* Isolates

Vaccine-induced immunity is the ultimate test of the efficacy of a particular acquired resistance effector. Such immunity involves purification of antigens in an immunogenic nontoxic form, demonstration of an appropriate immune response, and determination of protective efficacy against either infection or death. Passive therapy using the induced effector certifies its efficacy. In the case of *P. aeruginosa* such therapies usually require passive transfer of polyclonal or monoclonal antibody to the target antigen. Passive protection not only serves to verify experimentally the vaccine's mode of action but also demonstrates the potential usefulness of passive therapy. It is unlikely that any antigen that induces effective immunity will have a widespread prophylactic use as an active vaccine, except perhaps in CF patients before the onset of colonization. Passive therapy in at-risk patients or in patients with established *P. aeruginosa* infection is likely to be more common once an effective therapy is developed.

3.2.1. Antigens Eliciting Effective Immunity to Non-CF-Associated P. aeruginosa *Isolates*

Fisher *et al.*[50] classified *P. aeruginosa* into seven immunotypes based upon cross-protection studies in mice. Hanessian *et al.*[51] showed that the active bacterial antigen eliciting immunity was LPS. Many other studies in humans and animals have indicated that the highest level of immunity to *P. aeruginosa* is obtained with LPS serotype-specific antibody. On the basis of the work by Fisher *et al.*,[50] a heptavalent LPS vaccine was prepared and tested for active and passive efficacy in a variety of patient populations.[52,53,54] Although clinical efficacy was not clearly demonstrated, there were indications that the vaccine was effective. However, the toxicity encountered in immunized patients discouraged further use. Miler *et al.*[55] developed a polyvalent vaccine that offered active and passive protection against *P. aeruginosa* infections in burn patients.[56,57,58,59] The active component of this vaccine was shown to be LPS.[60,61] Cryz *et al.*[44] demonstrated in mice that antibody to LPS offered significant protection against infection. Pier and co-workers prepared nontoxic, immunogenic derivatives of the LPS O–side chain, known as high-molecular-weight polysaccharides (HMW-PS),[62,63,64,65] which elicit antibody-mediated protection against a variety of infections in animals.[62,66,67] Taken together, these studies provide strong evidence for a predominant role of antibody to *P. aeruginosa* serotype antigens in acquired immunity to LPS-smooth isolates.

Non-O-side chain antigens have also been reported to be targets of protective antibody, although there is little information supporting these claims from naturally acquired human immunity; most of these studies come from animal experimentation. Hancock *et al.* did report on the immune response of CF patients to outer membrane proteins (OMP) during infection.[68] However, like all other immune responses made by CF patients during infection, the failure of these antibodies to participate in bacterial clearance questions their protective role. Animal studies showed that active and passive immunization to OMP F can protect against *P. aeruginosa* intraperitoneal infection,[13] ocular infection,[69] burn infection,[11] and pulmonary infection induced in rats[12] by the agar bead method.[70] Von Specht and colleagues demonstrated that lipoprotein I in the outer membrane can also serve as a target for protective antibodies[14,16] to intraperitoneal infection of mice, and antibodies to OMP H2 protected mice against ocular infection.[69] Recent studies using cloned protein F and lipoprotein I[16,71] demonstrated protective efficacy in animals, indicating that contamination of OMP preparations with *P. aeruginosa* LPS does not explain protective efficacy. However, these studies routinely failed to make adequate comparisons of the protective efficacy to OMP with that to LPS, and generally used low challenge doses (routinely 1–30 LD_{50} doses) to demonstrate efficacy. In a study by Matthews-Greer and Gilleland[11] in which they demonstrated protection against burn infection, control mice required immunization with 7 μg of LPS from strain PAO1 to mimic the level of LPS contaminating the 10 μg dose of OMP F used to immunize the animals. Whereas challenge of OMP F-immunized mice with strains of *P. aeruginosa* heterologous to the PAO1 LPS serotype demonstrated protective efficacy against doses of 2×10^5 to 2×10^6 (1 to 3 LD_{50} doses), mice challenged with strain H296, expressing a LPS serologically identical to PAO1, required a dose of 3×10^{11} to show no difference in protection between LPS- and OMP F-immune animals. Thus, it takes a dose of bacteria at least five to six orders of magnitude greater to overcome LPS immunity than OMP F immunity, a fact indicating the highly efficacious nature of serotype-specific immunity. In general, the argument for using OMP antigens as protective immunogens is their lack of serologic variability. However, the value of this argument diminishes when one considers the much lower level of protection to *P. aeruginosa* infection that immunity to OMP stimulates compared with immunity to LPS O–side chains, the cost of producing OMP versus serotype vaccines, and the limited serotype diversity of pathogenic *P. aeruginosa* strains (seven to 10 serotypes account for >90% of infecting strains[72,73]). Another argument for use of OMP vaccines is the toxicity of LPS-based vaccines, but both HMW-PS[63,64,65] and O–side chain protein conjugates[74,75] have been tested as human vaccines with no apparent toxicity problems. Given these concerns for OMP vaccines, and the current testing in humans of vaccines using some form of O–side chains, the future of OMP to elicit acquired resistance to *P. aeruginosa* seems limited.

Recently there has been interest in the protective efficacy of immunity directed to LPS core antigens. It is argued that these antigens display limited serologic diversity, thereby enhancing the value of their vaccine potential. However, quantitative studies have not been performed to compare the level of protection achieved by antibodies to core epitopes with antibodies to O–side chain epitopes. Yokoto *et al.*[17] examined the reactivity of LPS core epitopes with human monoclonal antibodies. Although reactivity occurred across serotypes, limited serologic diversity among core epitopes has not been established. Several investigators have described neutral polysaccharides associated with LPS preparations,[76,77,78] although their exact relatedness to LPS is not clear. Two of these structures, both containing α 1-3 linked rhamnose,[78,79] have been shown to react with a monoclonal antibody, E87,[80] which also reacts with a fraction of LPS designated "A bands."[81,82] The A bands reportedly can be separated from the "B bands," which are to serologically diverse O–side chains by chromatography in deoxycholate buffers; A band LPS differs chemically from B band LPS by the lack of phosphate and the presence of sulfate in the lipid A. However, Goldberg *et al.*[83] recently reported that the E87 reactive antigen (*i.e.*, A bands) is not carried on a different molecule than the O–side chains (*i.e.*, B bands). They used an enzyme-linked immunoabsorbent assay (ELISA) wherein fractions from the deoxycholate column were used to inhibit the binding of monoclonal antibody E87 to both LPS and purified D-rhamnan. These workers indicated that the results of Rivera and McGroarty[82] could be explained by the lack of sensitivity of the immunoblotting procedures that were used to detect E87-reactive antigen. Immunoblotting apparently is not sensitive enough to detect A bands in the same fractions as the O–side chain. The value of antibody to these neutral polysaccharides in protection has not been fully determined, although Skalla and Pier[84] found that polyclonal antibodies to these antigens were neither opsonic nor protective in animals.

Homma and colleagues demonstrated the protective efficacy in animals of an antigen designated original endotoxin protein.[18,19,20,85] This vaccine protects mink against hemorrhagic pneumonia due to *P. aeruginosa*[18] and mice against burn and corneal infections when combined with toxoids of elastase and protease.[20,86] However, the biochemical properties of original endotoxin protein are not well established nor is the immunologic basis for the vaccine's efficacy. It has also been shown that normal humans respond immunologically to this antigen in the first few years of life.[87]

Motility of *P. aeruginosa* has been found to be important in virulence,[88,89,90] and a number of investigations have looked at the potential of acquired resistance specific to the flagella antigen in protective immunity. Flagella are classified into two major types, a and b, with type a having five subtypes (a0–a4). Antibodies specific to either type b or a cross reactive epitope shared among all subtypes of type a promotes uptake of bacteria by phagocytes,[91] but no intracellular killing was observed. This was attributed to the absence of fresh serum as a complement source in the assays. Immunization of animals with purified flagella has been shown to protect against infection of burn wounds.[21,22,88,92] CF patients were found to have elevated titers of antibodies to flagella epitopes;[93] however, normal humans also had good ELISA titers to this antigen. It is not known if these titers are elevated in the acute phase sera of patients who survive *P. aeruginosa* infection, as was shown for antibodies to LPS,[42] if antibodies to flagella are decreased in patients who die from infection, or if the levels of antibody present in normal individuals are sufficient for protection. A human vaccine has been developed[94] and is currently undergoing evaluation.

Lieberman and co-workers have tested the efficacy of ribosomal vaccines against *P. aeruginosa* infection,[23,24] but the antigenic target of the protective antibody is not known. These workers claim LPS is not detectable in the ribosomal preparation, although Gonggrijp *et al.*[95] demonstrated its presence. The fact that the ribosomal vaccines show serotype-specific protection indicates with near certainty that the active component is LPS, and the immunity is specific to these antigens. It seems unlikely that there is a ribosomal antigen that covaries completely with LPS serotype antigens.

In summary, the best-documented acquired-resistance mechanism against *P. aeruginosa* infection is antibody-mediated immunity to LPS O–side chains. Other antigenic targets have slight advantages as potential targets of protective immunity, but until they are shown to elicit antibodies with a protective efficacy close to that of antibody to O–side chains, their value may be considered minimal. Antibodies to extracellular toxins have not convincingly been shown to participate in acquired resistance, although the possibility exists that they may augment immune effectors directed to cell surface antigens. Antibodies to flagella seem to offer solid protection in burn-wound models, and may provide immunity at a level comparable to antibody to LPS. However, it is not known if motility is important in non-burn-wound infections, and if phase variants of *P. aeruginosa* lacking flagella could be virulent in these other clinical settings.

3.3. Antibody Isotype, Complement, and Phagocytes in Acquired Resistance to Non-CF-Associated *P. aeruginosa* Infection

Phagocytic killing of *P. aeruginosa* is thought to be the principal mediator of acquired resistance,[96,97] an idea strongly supported by the heightened susceptibility of neutropenic patients to *P. aeruginosa* infection. Occasional observations of bactericidal antibody (*i.e.*, non-phagocyte-mediated) have been reported,[98] although growth conditions were found to affect the susceptibility of *P. aeruginosa* to serum bactericidal activity. In general, LPS-smooth strains of *P. aeruginosa* are thought to be serum-resistant.

Antibody isotype has not been found to have a major effect on protective immunity. Polyclonal and monoclonal human IgG, IgM, and IgA have all been found to be opsonic and protective in animals,[32,99,100,101] but the activity of IgM required full complement activity. Some studies suggested suboptimal protection by murine monoclonal and rabbit polyclonal IgM[102,103] whereas others recently showed protective efficacy against infection in neutropenic mice by human monoclonal IgM.[100,101,104] Monoclonal human IgG$_2$ antibodies to the O–side chain were found to be extremely protective against infection in mice[99,105]; other IgG subclasses have not been tested.

As noted above, complement has been found to be important in protection mediated by IgM antibody because of a lack of Fc receptors for IgM on phagocytic cells, which necessitates the deposition of opsonic fragments of C3 onto the bacterial surface. Complement was found to enhance the opsonic activity of IgG antibodies but had no effect on IgA-antibody activity.[99,106] Complement deficiency is not generally considered to be a predisposing factor for *P. aeruginosa* infection. Cerquetti *et al.*[107] showed that C5-deficient mice do not clear *P. aeruginosa* from the lungs as well as C5-sufficient animals after aerosol exposure. Complement is best seen as an auxiliary immune effector in protection against non-CF-associated *P. aeruginosa* infection, but it appears to be less critical than sufficient numbers of phagocytes, particularly polymorphonuclear leukocytes (PMN).

3.4. T-cell Immunity to Non-CF-Associated Isolates of *P. aeruginosa*

The possible role of T cells in controlling *P. aeruginosa* infection has been examined. Colizzi *et al.*[108] reported on the development of T-cell-mediated delayed hypersensitivity in mice immunized with *P. aeruginosa* cells, but this immunity did not protect animals against live-cell challenge at a local site. These workers also found[109] that injection of *P. aeruginosa* could depress the development of contact sensitivity to oxazolone when the bacterial cells were injected with this agent. Pier and Markham[7] demonstrated the development of protective cell mediated immunity in mice given a low dose of HMW-PS antigen and vinblastine, which was also shown to effectively protect neutropenic mice from infection.[9] This immunity was transferable by CD8+ (Ly 2,3+) T cells. The role of the vinblastine was to eliminate a suppressor cell interfering with the activity of the bactericidal T cell.[8] T-cell immunity could also be elicited by high doses of HMWP or sublethal infection with live bacterial cells.[110] *In vitro* experiments indicated that the protective T cells were capable of killing the *P. aeruginosa* cells.[8,10,111,112] To achieve both *in vitro* bacterial killing and *in vivo* protection the T cells needed to be exposed to the immunizing antigen. However, *in vitro* killing and *in vivo* protection against serologically diverse strains of *P. aeruginosa* was noted, indicating that a bactericidal lymphokine was responsible for the T-cell protection.[9,111] Transfer of immunity did not require matching at the major histocompatibility

(MHC) locus; however, the suppressor cell that interfered with the bactericidal effector T cell functioned in an MHC-restricted fashion.[113] Recently Markham et al.[114] reported that murine IgG$_3$ antibodies bound to the bactericidal effector T cell mediate recognition of the bacterial polysaccharide, an indication that T-cell protection is most likely accomplished by an antibody-dependent cellular cytotoxicity mechanism. Whether there is a role for cell-mediated immunity to *P. aeruginosa* infection in humans is not clear. No direct demonstration of such immunity has been reported, although human T cells reactive to extracellular *P. aeruginosa* proteins have been characterized.[115,116] Porwell et al.[117] and Munster and Leary[118] showed that normal human T cells responded in an antigenic fashion to killed whole *P. aeruginosa* cells. Other reports indicate that *P. aeruginosa* phenazine pigments suppress lymphocyte proliferation,[119,120] suggesting an inhibition of cellular immune function that participates in the progression of disease. Markham and Powderly[110] showed that as few as 10^2 live *P. aeruginosa* cells could elicit T-cell protection in neutropenic mice, and suggested that exposure to low doses of live bacteria could provoke T-cell immunity in normal humans. Although the data for a role for T-cell immunity in humans is circumstantial, the studies in mice have gone a long way toward elucidating a possible mechanism for that immunity.

4. ACQUIRED RESISTANCE TO INFECTION IN CF PATIENTS

The acquisition of *P. aeruginosa* infection by CF patients is nearly inevitable: 85% acquire pulmonary infection by age 15 years,[121,122] and more than 90% die of direct pulmonary complications from chronic *P. aeruginosa* infection.[4] The emergence of the LPS-rough, mucoid phenotype has been noted here. Antibodies to LPS O–side chains would not be expected to play an important role in protective immunity to chronic infection. Potent immune responses to these antigens have been documented during infection,[29,123,124,125] but they apparently do little to stop the progression of infection. Eichler et al.[126] claimed that chronically infected CF patients have poor antibody response to LPS and a selective defect in opsonic activity. However, ignoring for the moment the fact that O–side chain antigens are poorly expressed among CF isolates, this study showed that CF patients have high overall opsonic activity against a mucoid, LPS-smooth strain, and the "defect" was present only if the opsonic activity was "corrected" by the overall antibody titer. A trial of an LPS-based vaccine failed to demonstrate protective efficacy,[127] but no data were presented regarding the potency of the immune response among the vaccinates or the occurrence of "non-vaccine" serotypes among the infecting strains. This limits interpretation of these results. The predominant expression of the A band neutral polysaccharides by the rough LPS of CF isolates has also been reported, and an association has been shown between poor clinical condition and elevated antibody activity using dot blots to A band antigen.[128] Immune responses of CF patients to many *P. aeruginosa* antigens have been demonstrated, although most appear not to show any association with resistance to infection.

4.1. Naturally Acquired Resistance Among CF Patients to *P. aeruginosa* Infection

Pier *et al.*[129] reported on the resistance to infection among CF patients, showing that 14 of 16 older (>12 years) CF patients without *P. aeruginosa* infection had opsonic-killing antibody specific to the MEP antigen. Tosi *et al.*[130] also showed the presence of opsonic antibodies to MEP among older, non-colonized patients. In the study by Pier *et al.*[129] these opsonic antibodies were lacking in younger, non-colonized patients and normal humans and, in chronically colonized patients, were present only at low levels. Thus, under natural exposure or chronic infection the immune response to MEP consists principally of non-opsonic-killing antibody. Opsonization of mucoid *P. aeruginosa* requires the classical pathway of complement[131,132]; even when high levels of factor B or C5-deficient sera are used along with sera containing nonopsonic antibody to MEP, there is still no phagocytic killing (Fig. 1). Opsonic antibodies protected mice and rats against chronic *P. aeruginosa* infection in the agar bead model, whereas the nonopsonic antibodies provided no protection.[133] Opsonic and nonopsonic antibodies are directed at different epitopes as shown by experiments where these antibodies do not compete for binding to the antigen.[129] Immunization of mice with low doses of MEP elicits opsonic-killing antibody, while high doses elicit non-opsonic-killing antibody,[134] a finding suggesting a dose-dependent response to the different epitopes on this antigen. Opsonic antibodies deposit high levels of ester-linked C3bi onto the bacterial surface, whereas nonopsonic antibodies do not,[132] facts that explain their differing biologic activities. Unfortunately, purified MEP has been poorly immunogenic in healthy humans,[135] and in the search for more immunogenic forms of the antigen, conjugates of MEP and carrier proteins hold some promise.[132]

4.2. Vaccine-Induced Immunity and Prospective Immunotherapeutic Strategies

Trials of vaccines to prevent infection in CF patients have not been successful. Pennington *et al.*[54,136] showed that a heptavalent LPS-based vaccine had no efficacy in already colonized patients. These studies preceded general recognition that most isolates of *P. aeruginosa* from chronically colonized CF patients express little or no O–side chain antigen. CF patients are thought to be initially colonized with LPS-smooth, nonmucoid strains,[39] and a LPS-based vaccine, PEV-01, was given to uncolonized patients in an attempt to prevent colonization by these LPS-smooth strains.[127] Yet no efficacy was

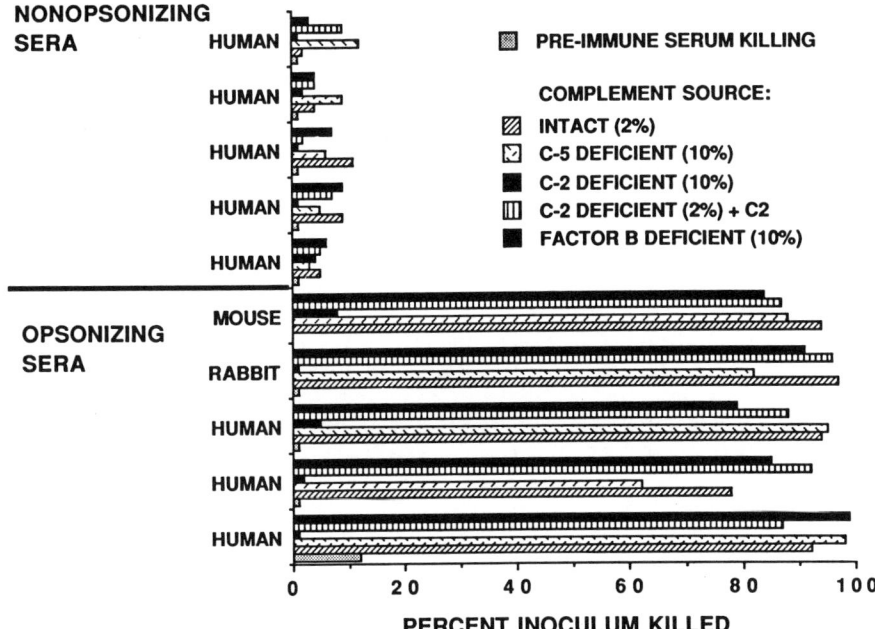

FIGURE 1. Opsonic killing of mucoid *P. aeruginosa* strain 2192 in the presence of the indicated complement source by five human sera containing only nonopsonic antibody to mucoid exopolysaccharide (MEP) and by five human and animal sera containing opsonizing antibody to MEP. Pre-immune serum killing was measured with intact complement. Note inability of nonopsonizing sera to kill regardless of complement source, and loss of killing activity by opsonizing sera only when C2 is depleted.

demonstrated by this trial. Recently, Schaad et al.[137] immunized noncolonized CF patients with a conjugate vaccine consisting of the O polysaccharide linked to ETA as a carrier. They noted a good immune response to most of the O–side chain antigens, an indication of the vaccine's immunogenicity, but as there is no appropriate control group for comparison, this can not be considered an efficacy study.

Immunotherapeutic strategies for preventing or treating *P. aeruginosa* infection in CF patients are on the horizon. Passive therapy using intravenous IgG is being considered for colonized patients, with the goal of reducing the bacterial load in the lungs and diminishing the damage caused by bacterial products and the host's inflammatory response to infection. This therapy likely will use antibody to MEP and/or O–side chains, the latter preparation potentially effective against strains expressing residual amounts of O–side chain antigens. Active vaccination of patients either before or early into colonization might be feasible once appropriate antigens and immunologic effectors are known. Supplementation of these vaccines to provide protection against bacterial elastase, protease and ETA and exotoxin S (exo-S) might make the therapy more effective. Experimental evidence has been generated for a role for all of these products in infection. Grimwood et al.[138,139] showed that subinhibitory concentrations of antibiotics down-regulate the production of P. aeruginosa extracellular toxins; this therapy effectively limits pathologic damage in rat lungs infected with P. aeruginosa encased in agar beads. In recent years the life expectancy of CF patients has stabilized, and immunotherapy offers a potential new means for helping to extend and improve their quality of life.

4.3. Antibody Isotype, Complement, and Phagocytes in Acquired Resistance to Infection in CF Patients

Some controversy has arisen over the contribution of antibody isotype to progressive infection. Moss and colleagues[126,140,141] suggested that poorly opsonic IgG_2 and IgG_4 antibodies to P. aeruginosa LPS arise during chronic colonization of CF patients and contribute to the poor ability to clear organisms. However, as noted above, these antibodies are specific to O–side chains that are not produced at high levels by most isolates.[36,37,142] Furthermore, these workers, along with others,[129,130] report consistently that colonized CF patients have high levels of opsonic activity against P. aeruginosa strains, yet these antibodies do not facilitate bacterial clearance or halt progression of infection. Thus, the overall biological activity of the serum, and not the presence of specific immunoglobulin isotypes, should determine the serum's protective efficacy. The only qualitative difference in antibody reported to date is by Pier et al., regarding the opsonic activity of the antibody to the MEP antigen.[129]

Why opsonic antibody to MEP would be protective, while opsonins against other bacterial antigens are not, is not clear. On the surface, it appears that opsonic activity should be the prime determinant of protection, and not the specificity of the surface antigens to which the opsonins bind. However, it has been reported that P. aeruginosa in the lungs of CF patients grows in microcolonies, embedded in the bacterial glycocalyx.[30,143,144] This glycocalyx is composed mostly of MEP[144] which reportedly has antiphagocytic effects[145,146,147] in vitro. Antibodies to non-MEP antigens might be expected to bind below the outer MEP layer, activating complement and promoting deposition of C3 fragments close to the bacterial surface. These bound opsonins could not bind to Fc and C3 receptors on phagocytes, which is necessary for bacterial uptake and killing. In support of this theory, Pier et al. recently reported that antibodies to MEP deposit 81 ± 11% of bound C3 fragments in ester linkages to the bacteria, whereas non-MEP-specific opsonins deposit only 27 ± 14% of the C3 in easter linkages. The rest is amide-linked to the bacterium. Presumably the ester-bound fragments deposited by antibody to MEP are linked to the abundant hydrozyl groups on the MEP, thereby locating them on the outer bacterial surface and making them available for interaction with phagocytes. The non-MEP antibodies bind the C3 mostly to amide groups that are present only close to or in the bacterial outer membrane, where they are less accessible to receptors on phagocytes. Using a modified Robbins chamber to mimic *in vitro* bacterial microcolony growth in a biofilm, Jensen et al.[148] showed that human PMN have reduced chemiluminescence responses to the embedded organisms compared with free-floating or planktonic organisms. MEP-specific opsonins were not used in these experiments, so their potential effect on organisms in a biofilm is not known. Overall, these data suggest that MEP-specific opsonins are potentially valuable because they can promote deposition of fragments of the critical opsonin, C3, onto the outer bacterial surface where they are more readily available for binding to receptors on phagocytes. It is interesting that no difference exists in the activation of complement by opsonic and nonopsonic antibody to MEP in the presence of the purified antigen (Fig. 2). Thus, the

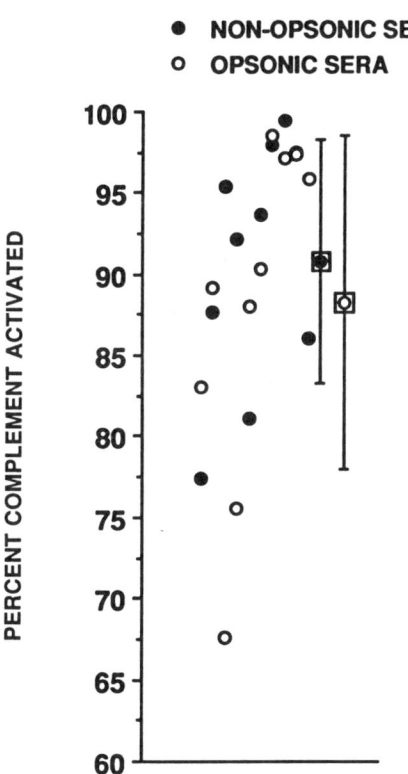

● NON-OPSONIC SERA
○ OPSONIC SERA

FIGURE 2. Ability of both opsonic and nonopsonic human sera to activate complement in the presence of purified mucoid exopolysaccharide (MEP). Purified antigen (25 μg/ml) was incubated with 1:10 serum dilutions and 10% human serum as a complement source for 30 min at 37°C. The residual complement activity was then measured by addition of rabbit red blood cells (0.1%) and measurement of the hemoglobin released after 30 min at 37°C. Nonopsonic sera came from normal humans and opsonic sera from both immunized humans and cystic fibrosis patients with MEP-specific opsonic-killing antibody.

differing biologic activities of these antibodies are accounted for in their ability to promote C3 deposition, not their ability to activate complement. Such an explanation would be consistent with the finding that both opsonic and nonopsonic antibody to MEP comprise IgM, IgG_1 and IgG_2 antibody isotypes (unpublished observation).

Because the isolates of *P. aeruginosa* recovered from chronically infected CF patients have a rough LPS, they are sensitive to the bactericidal effects of low levels of complement in normal human serum.[36] We must assume, *a priori*, that the levels of active complement in the lungs of patients are insufficient to control the infection. Furthermore, complement is apparently degraded into fragments by the activity of bacterial and host elastase,[140,149,150,151] but whether these fragments figure prominently in the initial phases of infection is not known. Baltimore and colleagues[147,152] showed that some mucoid strains of *P. aeruginosa* are more resistant to opsonization and phagocytosis than are nonmucoid strains, a finding that implicated MEP as a classic antiphagocytic capsule. However, this finding applies only to a minority of mucoid strains tested. Pier and Ames[153] reported that most isolates of mucoid *P. aeruginosa* are killed by the alternative pathway of complement, whereas Schiller[154] demonstrated a role for both the alternative and classical pathways in bactericidal activity. If the alternative pathway predominates, then it may not be present at high enough levels in the lung milieu to be effective. Schiller *et al.*[155] showed that the LPS-rough strains activate less complement than the LPS-smooth strains, even though they are susceptible to its bactericidal activity. Reduced activation of complement may contribute to chronic infection by down-regulating the host inflammatory response. Overall, complement is important in both phagocyte-dependent and -independent killing of mucoid *P. aeruginosa*, and the ability to activate complement and direct the deposition of opsonic and cidal fragments to the appropriate targets will be important to the success of immunotherapy.

One promising aspect of opsonic antibodies to MEP is their ability to opsonize bacteria for phagocytosis in the presence of low levels of complement.[129,131] Whether antibodies to other bacterial antigens function as well in limited concentrations of complement is not known. However, once infection is established, it may be difficult for any immunotherapy to be effective. In the infected CF lung, the inflammatory response results in high levels of neutrophil elastase,[156] and possibly bacterial elastases and proteases,[151,157,158] although the latter may be neutralized by host antibodies.[159] Not only are antibody and complement degraded by these enzymes, but the receptors on phagocytes for C3bi, CR3, as well as bacterial-bound C3bi, are degraded.[160,161] Thus, once infection is established at a sufficient level to maintain adequate levels of elastolytic and proteolytic activity in the inflamed lung, the immune effectors, no matter how appropriate, have an uphill battle against these destructive enzymes. Whether the immune system can overcome this negative aspect of inflammation remains to be seen.

5. SUMMARY

Many mechanisms of acquired resistance to *P. aeruginosa* infection have been described. Antibody-mediated opsonophagocytosis appears to be the main effector, although a role for T-cell immunity has been demonstrated in animals. Antibodies specific to cell-surface polysaccharides appear to be the most effective, yet evidence for immunity to OMP, flagella, and original endotoxin protein, as well as enhanced resistance from antibody to extracellular toxins, have been reported. LPS-smooth isolates that generally cause acute infections in immunocompromised hosts will likely be the targets of immunotherapy using active vaccination or passive therapy with intravenous IgG directed to O–side chain antigens. LPS-rough, mucoid isolates from chronically infected CF patients will likely be treated with opsonic antibody to MEP, or possibly to residual O–side chains, and active vaccination prior to colonization may be feasible with an appropriately immunogenic vaccine. Phagocytic cells, particularly PMN, play the predominant role in bacterial killing, and complement usually augments phagocytic uptake and killing. In the case of the LPS-rough strains, there is an absolute requirement for complement in bacterial killing. Substantiation of the value of these immune effectors will come from clinical trials documenting efficacy. Several are already underway and more are planned.

REFERENCES

1. Wilson, L. A., 1978, Bacterial corneal ulcers, in: *Clinical Ophthalmology* (T. D. Duane, ed.), Harper and Row, New York, pp. 1–40.
2. Morrison, A. J., and Wenzel, R. P., 1984, Epidemiology of infections due to *Pseudomonas aeruginosa*, *Rev. Infect. Dis.* **6**:S627–S640.
3. Fick, R. B., 1989, Pathogenesis of the *Pseudomonas* lung lesion in cystic fibrosis, *Chest* **96**: 158–164.
4. di Sant'Agnese, P. A., and Davis, P. B., 1979, Cystic fibrosis in adults: 75 cases and a review of 232 cases in the literature, *Am. J. Med.* **66**:121–132.
5. Hornick, D. B., 1988, Pulmonary host defense: Defects that lead to chronic inflammation of the airway, *Clin. Chest. Med.* **9**:669–678.
6. Pollack, M., 1990, *Pseudomonas aeruginosa*, in: *Principles and Practices of Infectious diseases* (G. L. Mandell, R. G. Douglas, J. E. Bennett, eds.), Churchill Livingstone, New York, pp. 1673–1691.
7. Pier, G. B., and Markham, R. B., 1982, Induction in mice of cell mediated immunity to *Pseudomonas aeruginosa* by high molecular weight polysaccharide and vinblastine, *J. Immunol.* **128**:2121–2125.
8. Powderly, W. G., Pier, G. B., and Markham, R. B., 1986, In vitro T cell-mediated killing of *Pseudomonas aeruginosa*. IV. Nonresponsiveness of polysaccharide-immunized BALB/c mice is attributable to vinblastine-sensitive suppressor T cell, *J. Immunol.* **137**:2025–2030.
9. Powderly, W. G., Pier, G. B., and Markham, R. B., 1986, T lymphocyte-mediated protection against *Pseudomonas aeruginosa* infection in granulocytopenic mice, *J. Clin. Infest.* **78**: 375–380.

10. Powderly, W. G., Pier, G. B., and Markham, R. B., 1986, In vitro T cell-mediated killing of *Pseudomonas aeruginosa*. III. The role of suppressor T cells in non-responder mice, *J. Immunol.* **136:**299–303.
11. Matthews-Greer, J. M., and Gilleland, H. E., Jr., 1987, Outer membrane protein F (porin) preparation of *Pseudomonas aeruginosa* as a protective vaccine against heterologous immunotype strains in a burned mouse model, *J. Infect. Dis.* **155:**1282–1291.
12. Gilleland, H. E., Jr., Gilleland, L. B., and Matthews-Greer, J. M., 1988, Outer membrane protein F preparation of *Pseudomonas aeruginosa* as a vaccine against chronic pulmonary infection with heterologous immunotype strains in a rat model, *Infect. Immun.* **56:**1017–1022.
13. Hancock, R. E. W., Mutharia, L. M., and Mouat, E. C., 1985, Immunotherapeutic potential of monoclonal antibodies against *Pseudomonas aeruginosa* protein F, *Eur. J. Clin. Microbiol.* **4:**224–227.
14. von Specht, B. U., Strigl, G., Ehret, W., and Brendel, W., 1987, Protective effect of an outer membrane vaccine against *Pseudomonas aeruginosa* infection, *Infection* **15:**408–412.
15. Marget, M., Eckhardt, A., Ehret, W., von Specht, B. U., Duchene, M., and Domdey, H., 1988, Cloning and characterization of cDNAs coding for the heavy and light chains of a monoclonal antibody specific for *Pseudomonas aeruginosa* outer membrane protein I, *Gene* **74:**335–345.
16. Finke, M., Duchene, M., Eckhardt, A., Domdey, H., and von Specht, B. U., 1990, Protection against experimental *Pseudomonas aeruginosa* infection by recombinant *P. aeruginosa* lipoprotein I expressed in *Escherichia coli*, *Infect. Immun.* **58:**2241–2244.
17. Yokota, S., Ochi, H., Ohtsuka, H., Kato, M., and Noguchi, H., 1989, Heterogeneity of the L-rhamnose residue in the outer core of *Pseudomonas aeruginosa* lipopolysaccharide, characterized by using human monoclonal antibodies, *Infect. Immun.* **57:**1691–1696.
18. Shimizu, T., Homma, J. Y., Abe, C., Tanamoto, T., Aoyama, Y., Yanagawa, R., Fujimoto, Y., Noda, H., Takashima, I., Honda, E., and Minamide, S., 1976, Effect of common protective antigen vaccination to protect mink from challenge exposure with *Pseudomonas aeruginosa*, *Am. J. Vet. Res.* **37:**1441–1444.
19. Aoi, Y., Noda, H., Yanagawa, R., Homma, J. Y., Abe, C., Morihara, K., Goda, A., Takeuchi, S., and Ishihara, T., 1979, Protection against hemorrhagic pneumonia of mink by *Pseudomonas aeruginosa* multicomponent vaccine, *Jpn. J. Exp. Med.* **49:**199–207.
20. Hirao, Y., and Homma, J. Y., 1978, Therapeutic effect of immunization with OEP, protease toxoid and elastase toxoid on corneal ulcers in mice due to *Pseudomonas aeruginosa* infection, *Jpn. J. Exp. Med.* **48:**41–51.
21. Drake, D., and Montie, T. C., 1987, Protection against *Pseudomonas aeruginosa* infection by passive transfer of anti-flagella serum, *Can. J. Microbiol.* **33:**755–763.
22. Montie, T. C., Drake, D., Sellin, H., Slater, O., and Edmonds, S., 1987, Motility, virulence, and protection with a flagella vaccine against *Pseudomonas aeruginosa* infection, *Antibiot. Chemother.* **39:**233–248.
23. Lieberman, M. M., and Ayala, E., 1983, Active and passive immunity against *Pseudomonas aeruginosa* with a ribosomal vaccine and antiserum in C3H/HeJ mice, *J. Immunol.* **131:**1–3.
24. Lieberman, M. M., and Allen, R. C., 1986, Opsonic activity of antisera to ribosomal vaccine fractions with live and formalinized *Pseudomonas aeruginosa*, *Can. J. Microbiol.* **32:**531–533.
25. Pollack, M., 1983, The role of exotoxin A in *Pseudomonas* disease and immunity, *Rev. Infect. Dis.* **5:**S979–S984.
26. Cross, A. S., Sadoff, J. C., Iglewski, B. H., and Sokol, P. A., 1980, Evidence for the role of toxin A in the pathogenesis of infection with *Pseudomonas aeruginosa* in humans, *J. Infect. Dis.* **142:**538–546.
27. Nicas, T. I., Bradley, J., Lochner, J. E., and Iglewski, B. H., 1985, The role of exoenzyme S in infections with *Pseudomonas aeruginosa*, *J. Infect. Dis.* **152:**716–721.
28. Linker, A., and Jones, R. S., 1966, A new polysaccharide resembling alginic acid isolated from pseudomonads, *J. Biol. Chem.* **241:**3845–3851.

29. Høiby, N., Andersen, V., and Bendixen, G., 1975, *Pseudomonas aeruginosa* infection in cystic fibrosis, *Acta Pathol. Microbiol. Scand. [Section C]* **83:**459–468.
30. Lam, J., Chan, R., Lam, K., and Costerton, J. W., 1980, Production of mucoid microcolonies by *Pseudomonas aeruginosa* within infected lungs in cystic fibrosis, *Infect. Immun.* **28:** 546–556.
31. MaCone, A., Pier, G. B., Pennington, J. E., Matthews, W. M., Jr., and Goldmann, D., 1981, Mucoid *Escherichia coli* in cystic fibrosis, *N. Engl. J. Med.* **304:**1445–1449.
32. Pier, G. B., Matthews, W. J., and Eardley, D. D., 1983, Immunochemical characterization of the mucoid exopolysaccharide of *Pseudomonas aeruginosa*, *J. Infect. Dis.* **147:**494–503.
33. Bryan, L. E., Kureishi, A., and Rabin, H. R., 1983, Detection of antibodies to *P. aeruginosa* alginate extracellular polysaccharide in animals and cystic fibrosis patients by enzyme-linked immunosorbent assay, *J. Clin. Microbiol.* **18:**276–282.
34. Speert, D. P., Lawton, D., and Mutharia, L., 1984, Antibody to *P. aeruginosa* mucoid exopolysaccharide and to sodium alginate in cystic fibrosis sera, *Pediatr. Res.* **8:**431–434.
35. Pedersen, S. S., Espersen, F., Høiby, N., and Jensen, T., 1990, Immunoglobulin-A and Immunoglobulin-G antibody responses to alginates from *Pseudomonas aeruginosa* in patients with cystic fibrosis, *J. Clin. Microbiol.* **28:**747–755.
36. Hancock, R. E. W., Mutharia, L. M., Chan, L., Darveau, R. P., Speert, D. P., and Pier, G. B., 1983, *Pseudomonas aeruginosa* isolates from patients with cystic fibrosis: A class of serum-sensitive, nontypable strains deficient in lipopolysaccharide O side-chains, *Infect. Immun.* **42:**170–177.
37. Ojeniyi, B., Baek, L., and Høiby, N., 1985, Polyagglutinability due to loss of O-antigenic determinants in *Pseudomonas aeruginosa* strains isolated from cystic fibrosis patients, *Acta Pathol. Microbiol. Scand. Sect. B* **93:**7–13.
38. Pitt, P. L., MacDougall, J., Penketh, A. R. L., and Cooke, E. M., 1986, Polyagglutinating and non-typable strains of *Pseudomonas aeruginosa* in cystic fibrosis, *J. Med. Microbiol.* **21:** 179–186.
39. Pier, G. B., DesJardins, D., Aguilar, T. Barnard, M., and Speert, D. P., 1986, Polysaccharide surface antigens expressed by non-mucoid isolates of *Pseudomonas aeruginosa* from cystic fibrosis patients, *J. Clin. Microbiol.* **24:**189–196.
40. Young, L. S., Yu, B. H., and Armstrong, D., 1970, Agar-gel precipitating antibody in *Pseudomonas aeruginosa* infections, *Infect. Immun.* **2:**495–503.
41. Crowder, J. G., Fisher, M. W., and White, A., 1972, Type-specific immunity in *Pseudomonas* disease, *J. Lab. Clin. Med.* **79:**47–54.
42. Pollack, M., and Young, L. S., 1979, Protective activity of antibodies to exotoxin A and lipopolysaccharide at the onset of *Pseudomonas aeruginosa* septicemia in man, *J. Clin. Invest.* **63:**276–286.
43. Baltch, A., Williams, S., Franke, M., Smith, R., Lutz, F., Asperilla, M., Griffin, P., and Michelsen, P., 1990, Survival and serum antibody (Ab) concentration to cytotoxin, toxin A, lipopolysaccharide (LPA), protease & elastase in patients with *Pseudomonas aeruginosa* (PA) bacteremia, *Annu. Meet. Am. Soc. Microbiol.*, Abstract E20, 122.
44. Cryz, S. J., Jr., Furer, E., and Germanier, R., 1984, Protection against fatal *Pseudomonas aeruginosa* burn wound sepsis by immunization with lipopolysaccharide and high-molecular-weight polysaccharide, *Infect. Immun.* **43:**795–799.
45. Pavlovskis, O. R., Pollack, M., Callahan, L. T., III, and Iglewski, B. H., 1979, Passive protection by antitoxin in experimental *Pseudomonas aeruginosa* burn infections, *Infect. Immun.* **18:**596–602.
46. Pavlovskis, O. R., Edman, D. C., Leppla, S. H., Wretlind, B., Lewis, L. R., and Martin, K. E., 1981, Protection against experimental *Pseudomonas aeruginosa* infection in mice by active immunization with exotoxin A, *Infect. Immun.* **32:**681–689.
47. Snell, K., Holder, I. A., Leppla, S. H., and Saelinger, C. B., 1978, Role of exotoxin and protease as possible virulence factors in experimental infections with *Pseudomonas aeruginosa*, *Infect. Immun.* **19:**839–845.

48. Wretlind, B., Bjorklind, A., and Pavlovskis, O. R., 1987, Role of exotoxin A and elastase in the pathogenicity of *Pseudomonas aeruginosa* strain PAO experimental mouse burn infection, *Microb. Pathogen.* **2:**397–404.
49. Iglewski, B. H., and Kabat, D., 1975, NAD-dependent inhibition of protein synthesis by *Pseudomonas aeruginosa* toxin, *Proc. Natl. Acad. Sci. USA* **72:**2284–2288.
50. Fisher, M. W., Devlin, H. B., and Gnabasik, F., 1969, New immunotype schema for *Pseudomonas aeruginosa* based on protective antigens, *J. Bacteriol.* **98:**835–836.
51. Hanessian, S., Regan, W., Watson, D., and Haskell, T. H., 1971, Isolation and characterization of antigenic components of a new heptavalent *Pseudomonas* vaccine, *Nature New Biol.* **229:**209–210.
52. Alexander, J. W., and Fisher, M. W., 1974, Immunization against *Pseudomonas* infection after thermal injury, *J. Infect. Dis.* **130:**S152–S158.
53. Young, L. S., Meyer, R. D., and Armstrong, D., 1973, *Pseudomonas aeruginosa* vaccine in cancer patients, *Ann. Intern. Med.* **79:**518–527.
54. Pennington, J. E., Reynolds, H. Y., Wood, R. E., Robbins, R. A., and Levine, A. S., 1975, Use of a *Pseudomonas aeruginosa* vaccine in patients with acute leukemia and cystic fibrosis, *Am. J. Med.* **58:**629–636.
55. Miler, J. M., Spilsbury, J. F., Jones, R. J., Roe, E. A., and Lowbury, E. J. L., 1977, A new polyvalent *Pseudomonas* vaccine, *J. Med. Microbiol.* **10:**19–27.
56. Jones, R. J., Roe, E. A., and Gupta, J. L., 1978, Low mortality in burned patients in a *Pseudomonas* vaccine trial, *Lancet* **2:**401–403.
57. Jones, R. J., Roe, E. A., and Gupta, J. L., 1979, Controlled trials of a polyvalent *Pseudomonas* vaccine in burns, *Lancet* **2:**977–982.
58. Jones, R. J., Roe, E. A., and Gupta, J. L., 1980, Controlled trial of *Pseudomonas* immunoglobulin and vaccine in burn patients, *Lancet* **2:**1263–1265.
59. Roe, E. A., and Jones, R. J., 1983, Immunization of burned patients against *Pseudomonas aeruginosa* infection at Safdarjang Hospital, New Delhi, *Rev. Infect. Dis.* **5:**S922–S930.
60. MacIntyre, S., McVeigh, T., and Owen, P., 1986, Immunochemical and biochemical analysis of the polyvalent *Pseudomonas aeruginosa* vaccine PEV, *Infect. Immun.* **51:**675–686.
61. MacIntyre, S., Lucken, R., and Owen, P., 1986, Smooth lipopolysaccharide is the major protective antigen for mice in the surface extract from IATS serotype 6 contributing to the polyvalent *Pseudomonas aeruginosa* vaccine PEV, *Infect. Immun.* **52:**76–84.
62. Pier, G. B., Pollack, M., and Cohen, M., 1984, Immunochemical characterization of high-molecular weight polysaccharide from Fisher immunotype 3 *Pseudomonas aeruginosa*, *Infect. Immun.* **45:**309–313.
63. Pier, G. B., and Pollack, M., 1989, Isolation, structure, and immunogenicity of *Pseudomonas aeruginosa* immunotype 4 high-molecular-weight polysaccharide, *Infect. Immun.* **57:**426–431.
64. Pier, G. B., Sidberry, H. F., Zolyomi, S., and Sadoff, J. C., 1978, Isolation and characterization of a high-molecular-weight polysaccharide from the slime of *Pseudomonas aeruginosa*, *Infect. Immun.* **22:**908–918.
65. Pier, G. B., Sidberry, H. F., and Sadoff, J. C., 1981, High-molecular-weight polysaccharide antigen from *Pseudomonas aeruginosa* immunotype 2, *Infect. Immun.* **34:**461–468.
66. Pollack, M., Pier, G. B., and Prescott, R. K., 1984, Immunization with *Pseudomonas aeruginosa* high-molecular-weight polysaccharides prevents death from *Pseudomonas* burn infections in mice, *Infect. Immun.* **43:**759–760.
67. Pier, G. B., and Bennett, S. E., 1986, Structural analysis and immunogenicity of *Pseudomonas aeruginosa* immunotype 2 high molecular weight polysaccharide, *J. Clin. Invest.* **77:**491–495.
68. Hancock, R. E. W., Mouat, E. C., and Speert, D. P., 1984, Quantitation and identification of antibodies to outer-membrane proteins of *Pseudomonas aeruginosa* in sera of patients with cystic fibrosis, *J. Infect. Dis.* **149:**220–226.

69. Moon, M. M., Hazlett, L. D., Hancock, R. E. W., Berk, R. S., and Barrett, R., 1988, Monoclonal antibodies provide protection against ocular *Pseudomonas aeruginosa* infection, *Invest. Opthalmol. Vis. Sci.* **29**:1277–1284.
70. Cash, H. A., Woods, D. E., McCullough, B., Johanson, W. G., Jr., and Bass, J. A., 1979, A rat model of chronic respiratory infection with *Pseudomonas aeruginosa*, *Am. Rev. Respir. Dis.* **119**:453–459.
71. Matthews-Greer, J. M., Robertson, D. E., Gilleland, L. B., and Gilleland, H. E., 1990, *Pseudomonas aeruginosa* outer membrane protein-F produced in *Escherichia coli* retains vaccine efficacy, *Curr. Microbiol.* **20**:171–175.
72. Schaad, U. B., Lang, A. B., Wedgwood, J., Buehlamnn, U., and Fuerer, E., 1990, Serotype-specific serum IgG antibodies to lipopolysaccharides of *Pseudomonas aeruginosa* in cystic fibrosis: Correlation to disease, subclass distribution, and experimental protective capacity, *Pediatr. Res.* **27**:508–513.
73. Pier, G. B., and Thomas, D. M., 1982, Lipopolysaccharide and high molecular weight polysaccharide serotypes of *Pseudomonas aeruginosa*, *J. Infect. Dis.* **145**:217–223.
74. Cryz, S. J., Jr., Sadoff, J. C., and Fürer, E., 1989, Octavalent *Pseudomonas aeruginosa* O-polysaccharide-toxin A conjugate vaccine, *Microb. Pathogen.* **6**:75–80.
75. Cryz, S. J., Jr., Sadoff, J. C., and Que, J. U., 1989, Conjugate vaccines against *Pseudomonas aeruginosa* and malaria, *Contrib. Microbiol. Immunol.* **10**:166–189.
76. Yokota, S., Kaya, S., Sawada, S., Kawamura, T., Araki, Y., and Ito, E., 1987, Characterization of a polysaccharide component of lipopolysaccharide from *Pseudomonas aeruginosa* IID 1008 (ATCC 27584) as D-rhamnan, *Eur. J. Biochem.* **167**:203–209.
77. Kocharova, N. A., Knirel, Y. A., Shashkov, A. S., Kochetkova, N. K., and Pier, G. B., 1988, Structure of an extracellular, cross reactive polysaccharide from *Pseudomonas aeruginosa* immunotype 4, *J. Biol. Chem.* **263**:11291–11295.
78. Kocharova, N. A., Hatano, K., Shashkov, A. S., Knirel, Y. A., Kochetkov, N. K., and Pier, G. B., 1989, The structure and serologic distribution of an extracellular neutral polysaccharide from *Pseudomonas aeruginosa* immunotype-3, *J. Biol. Chem.* **264**:15569–15573.
79. Yokota, S., Kaya, S., Araki, Y., Ito, E., Kawamura, T., and Sawada, S., 1990, Occurrence of D-rhamnan as the common antigen reactive against monoclonal antibody-E87 in *Pseudomonas aeruginosa* IFO-3080 and other strains, *J. Bacteriol.* **172**:6162–6164.
80. Sawada, S., Kawamura, T., Masuho, Y., and Tomibe, K., 1985, A new common polysaccharide antigen of strains of *Pseudomonas aeruginosa* detected with a monoclonal antibody, *J. Infect. Dis.* **152**:1290–1299.
81. Rivera, M., Bryan, L. E., Hancock, R. E. W., and McGroarty, E. J., 1988, Heterogeneity of lipopolysaccharide from *Pseudomonas aeruginosa*: Analysis of lipopolysaccharide chain length, *J. Bacteriol.* **170**:512–521.
82. Rivera, M., and McGroarty, E. J., 1989, Analysis of a common-antigen lipopolysaccharide from *Pseudomonas aeruginosa*, *J. Bacteriol.* **171**:2244–2248.
83. Goldberg, J. B., Hatano, K., and Pier, G. B., 1990, *Pseudomonas aeruginosa* produces a single lipopolysaccharide (LPS) species comprised of both serologically variant O-side chains and common neutral polysaccharide antigens, *Pediatr. Pulmonol. Suppl.* **5**:239.
84. Skalla, M., and Pier, G. B., 1988, Structural determinations and immunologic properties of two small polysaccharides from *Pseudomonas aeruginosa* lipopolysaccharide (LPS), *Annu. Meet. Am. Soc. Microbiol.* Abstract B-118, 49.
85. Sasaki, M., Ito, M., and Homma, J. Y., 1975, Immunological studies on the original endotoxin protein (OEP) of *Pseudomonas aeruginosa*. Adjuvant effect of OEP *in vivo*, *Jpn. J. Exp. Med.* **45**:335–343.
86. Kawaharajo, K., and Homma, J. Y., 1977, Effects of elastase, protease and common antigen (OEP) from *Pseudomonas aeruginosa* on protection against burns in mice, *Jpn. J. Exp. Med.* **47**:495–500.
87. Shinozaki, T., Fujii, R., Sanai, Y., and Homma, J. Y., 1981, Development of antibodies

to OEP, exotoxin A and exoenzymes of *Pseudomonas aeruginosa* in man, *Jpn. J. Exp. Med.* **51:** 165–170.
88. Drake, D., and Montie, T. C., 1988, Flagella, motility and invasive virulence of *Pseudomonas aeruginosa*, *J. Gen. Microbiol.* **134:**43–52.
89. Montie, T. C., Doyle-Huntzinger, D., Craven, R. C., and Holder, I. A., 1982, Loss of virulence associated with absence of flagellum in an isogenic mutant of *Pseudomonas aeruginosa* in the burned-mouse model, *Infect. Immun.* **38:**1296–1298.
90. Sato, H., Okinaga, K., and Saito, H., 1988, Role of pili in the pathogenesis of *Pseudomonas aeruginosa* burn infection, *Microbiol. Immunol.* **32:**131–139.
91. Anderson, T. R., and Montie, T. C., 1989, Flagellar antibody stimulated opsonophagocytosis of *Pseudomonas aeruginosa* associated with response to either a-type or b-type flagellar antigen, *Can. J. Microbiol.* **35:**890–894.
92. Holder, I. A., and Naglich, J. G., 1986, Experimental studies of the pathogenesis of infections due to *Pseudomonas aeruginosa*: Immunization using divalent flagella preparations, *J. Trauma* **26:**118–122.
93. Anderson, T. R., Montie, T. C., Murphy, M. D., and McCarthy, V. P., 1989, *Pseudomonas aeruginosa* flagellar antibodies in patients with cystic fibrosis, *J. Clin. Microbiol.* **27:**2789–2793.
94. Rotering, H., and Dorner, F., 1989, Studies on a *Pseudomonas aeruginosa* flagella vaccine, *Antibiot. Chemother.* **42:**218–228.
95. Gonggrijp, R., Volleberg, M. P. W., Lemmens, P. J. M. R., and van Boven, C. P. A., 1981, Evidence for the presence of lipopolysaccharide in a ribonuclease-sensitive ribosomal vaccine of *Pseudomonas aeruginosa*, *Infect. Immun.* **31:**896–905.
96. Young, L. S., 1972, Human immunity to *Pseudomonas aeruginosa*. II. Relationship between heat-stable opsonins and type-specific lipopolysaccharides, *J. Infect. Dis.* **126:**277–284.
97. Young, L. S., 1974, Role of antibody in *Pseudomonas aeruginosa* infections, *J. Infect. Dis.* **130:** S111–S116.
98. DeMatteo, C. S., Hammer, M. C., Baltch, A. L., Smith, R. P., Sutphen, N. T., and Michelsen, P. B., 1981, Susceptibility of *Pseudomonas aeruginosa* to serum bactericidal activity. A comparison of three methods with clinical correlations, *J. Lab. Clin. Med.* **98:**511–518.
99. Pier, G. B., Thomas, D., Small, G., Siadak, A., and Zweerink, H., 1989, *In vitro* and *in vivo* activity of polyclonal and monoclonal human immunoglobulin G, M and A against *Pseudomonas aeruginosa* lipopolysaccharide, *Infect. Immun.* **57:**174–179.
100. Zweerink. H. J., Gammon, M. C., Hutchinson, C.F., Jackson, J. J., Pier, G. B., Puckett, J. M., Sewell, T. J., and Sigal, N. H., 1988, X-linked immunodeficient mice as a model for testing the protective efficacy of monoclonal antibodies against *Pseudomonas aeruginosa*, *Infect. Immun.* **56:**1209–1214.
101. Zweerink, H. J., Gammon, M. C., Hutchinson, C. F., Jackson, J. J., Lombardo, D., Miner, K. M., Puckett, J. M., Sewell, T. J., and Sigal, N. H., 1988, Human monoclonal antibodies that protect mice against challenge with *Pseudomonas aeruginosa*, *Infect. Immun.* **56:**1873–1879.
102. Bjornson, A. B., and Michael, J. G., 1972, Biological activities of rabbit immunoglobulin M and immunoglobulin G antibodies to *Pseudomonas aeruginosa*, *Infect. Immun.* **2:**453–461.
103. Barclay, G. R., Yap, P. L., McClelland, D. B. L., Jones, R. J., Roe, E. A., McCann, M. C., Micklem, L. R., and James, K., 1986, Characterisation of mouse monoclonal antibodies produced by immunisation with a single serotype component of a polyvalent *Pseudomonas aeruginosa* vaccine, *J. Med. Microbiol.* **21:**87–90.
104. Zweerink, H. J., Detolla, L. J., Gammon, M. C., Hutchinson, C. F., Puckett, J. M., and Sigal, N. H., 1990, A human monoclonal antibody that protects mice against *Pseudomonas*-induced pneumonia, *J. Infect. Dis.* **162:**254–257.
105. Sawada, S., Kawamura, T., and Masuho, Y., 1987, Immunoprotective human monoclonal antibodies against five major serotypes of *Pseudomonas aeruginosa*, *J. Gen. Microbiol.* **133:** 3581–3590.

106. Pier, G. B., and Thomas, D. M., 1983, Characterization of the human immune response to a polysaccharide vaccine from *Pseudomonas aeruginosa*, *J. Infect. Dis.* **148**:206–213.
107. Cerquetti, M. C., Sordelli, D. O., Bellanti, J. A., and Hooke, A. M., 1986, Lung defenses against *Pseudomonas aeruginosa* in C5-deficient mice with different genetic backgrounds, *Infect. Immun.* **52**:853–857.
108. Colizzi, V., Garzelli, C., Campa, M., Toca, L., and Falcone, G., 1982, Role of specific delayed-type hypersensitivity in *Pseudomonas aeruginosa*-infected mice, *Immunology* **47**:337–344.
109. Colizzi, V., Garzelli, C., Campa, M., and Falcone, G., 1978, Depression of contact sensitivity by enhancement of suppressor cell activity in *Pseudomonas aeruginosa*-infected mice, *Infect. Immun.* **21**:354–359.
110. Markham, R. B., and Powderly, W. G., 1988, Exposure of mice to live *Pseudomonas aeruginosa* generates protective cell-mediated immunity in the absence of an antibody response, *J. Immunol.* **140**:2039–2045.
111. Markham, R. B., Goellner, J., and Pier, G. B., 1984, In vitro T cell mediated killing of *Pseudomonas aeruginosa*. 1. Evidence that a lymphokine mediates killing, *J. Immunol.* **133**:962–968.
112. Powderly, W. G., Pier, G. B., and Markham, R. B., 1987, *In vitro* T cell-mediated killing of *Pseudomonas aeruginosa*. V. Generation of bactericidal T cells in nonresponder mice, *J. Immunol.* **138**:2272–2277.
113. Markham, R. B., Pier, G. B., and Powderly, W. G., 1988, Suppressor T cells regulating the cell-mediated immune response to *Pseudomonas aeruginosa* can be generated by immunization with anti-bacterial T cells, *J. Immunol.* **141**:3975–3979.
114. Markham, R. B., Pier, G. B., and Schreiber, J. R., 1991, The role of cytophilic IgG3 antibody in T-cell-mediated resistance to infection with the extracellular bacterium *Pseudomonas aeruginosa*, *J. Immunol.* **146**:316–320.
115. Parmely, M. J., and Horvat, R. T., 1986, Antigenic specificities of *Pseudomonas aeruginosa* alkaline protease and elastase defined by human T cell clones, *J. Immunol.* **137**:988–994.
116. Parmely, M. J., Iglewski, B. H., and Horvat, R. T., 1984, Identification of the principal T lymphocyte-stimulating antigens of *Pseudomonas aeruginosa*, *J. Exp. Med.* **160**:1338–1349.
117. Porwell, J. M., Gebel, H. M., Rodey, G. E., and Markham, R. B., 1983, In vitro response of human T cells to *Pseudomonas aeruginosa*, *Infect. Immun.* **40**:670–674.
118. Munster, A. M., and Leary, A. G., 1977, Cell-mediated immune responses to *Pseudomonas aeruginosa*, *Am. J. Surg.* **133**:710–712.
119. Nutman, J., Chase, P. A., Dearborn, D. G., Berger, M., and Sorensen, R. U., 1988, Suppression of lymphocyte proliferation by *Pseudomonas aeruginosa* phenazine pigments, *Isr. J. Med. Sci.* **24**:228–232.
120. Sorensen, R. U., Klinger, J. D., Cash, H. A., Chase, P. A., and Dearborn, D. G., 1983, *In vitro* inhibition of lymphocyte proliferation by *Pseudomonas aeruginosa* phenazine pigments, *Infect. Immun.* **41**:321–330.
121. Demko, C. A., and Byard, P. J., 1988, Long-term effect of *Pseudomonas aeruginosa* colonization of pulmonary function in patients with cystic fibrosis, *Pediatr. Pulmonol. Suppl.* **2**:115.
122. Kerem, E., Corey, M., Gold, R., and Levison, H., 1990, Pulmonary function and clinical course in patients with cystic fibrosis after pulmonary colonization with *Pseudomonas aeruginosa*, *J. Pediatr.* **116**:714–719.
123. Kronborg, G., Fomsgaard, A., Shand, G. H., and Høiby, N., 1989, Determination of the components of immune complexes made *in vitro* with antigens derived from *Pseudomonas aeruginosa*, *J. Immunol. Meth.* **122**:51–57.
124. Fomsgaard, A., Høiby, N., Shand, G. H., Conrad, R. S., and Galanos, C., 1988, Longitudinal study of antibody response to lipopolysaccharide during chronic *Pseudomonas aeruginosa* lung infection in cystic fibrosis, *Infect. Immun.* **56**:2270–2278.
125. Fomsgaard, A., Dinesen, B., Shand, G.H., Pressler, T., and Høiby, N., 1989, Antilipo-

polysaccharide antibodies and differential diagnosis of chronic *Pseudomonas aeruginosa* lung infection in cystic fibrosis, *J. Clin. Microbiol.* **27:**1222–1229.
126. Eichler, I., Joris, L., Hsu, Y. P., Vanwye, J., Bram, R., and Moss, R., 1989, Nonopsonic antibodies in cystic fibrosis: *Pseudomonas aeruginosa* lipopolysaccharide-specific immunoglobulin-G antibodies from infected patient sera inhibit neutrophil oxidative responses, *J. Clin. Invest.* **84:**1794–1804.
127. Langford, D. T., and Hiller, J., 1984, Prospective, controlled study of a polyvalent *Pseudomonas* vaccine in cystic fibrosis–Three year results, *Arch. Dis. Child.* **59:**1131–1134.
128. Lam, M. Y., McGroarty, E. J., Kropinski, A. M., MacDonald, L. A., Pedersen, S. S., Høiby, N., and Lam, J., 1989, Occurrence of a common lipopolysaccharide antigen in standard and clinical strains of *Pseudomonas aeruginosa*, *J. Clin. Microbiol.* **27:**962–967.
129. Pier, G. B., Saunders, J. M., Ames, P., Edwards, M. S., Auerbach, H., Goldfarb, J., Speert, D.P., and Hurwitch, S., 1987, Opsonophagocytic killing antibody to *Pseudomonas aeruginosa* mucoid exopolysaccharide in older, non-colonized cystic fibrosis patients, *N. Engl. J. Med.* **317:**793–798.
130. Tosi, M., Berger, M., Zakem, H., and Schreiber, J., 1990, Opsonic activity of antibodies (Ab) to MEP and non-MEP antigens of *P. aeruginosa* (PA) in serum from CF patients with chronic PA lung infection vs. older non-colonized CF patients, *Pediatr. Pulmonol. Suppl.* **5:**276.
131. Ames, P., DesJardins, D., and Pier, G. B., 1985, Opsonophagocytic killing activity of rabbit antibody to *Pseudomonas aeruginosa* mucoid exopolysaccharide, *Infect. Immun.* **49:**281–285.
132. Pier, G. B., Skalla, M., Grout, M., DesJardins, D., and Collier, R. J., 1990, Opsonic and complement deposition properties of antibodies elicited by *P. aeruginosa* mucoid exopolysaccharide (MEP) and conjugates of MEP and a non-toxic exotoxin A deletion mutant (tAdm), *Annu. Meet. Am. Soc. Microbiol.*, Abstract E22, 123.
133. Pier, G. B., Small, G. J., and Warren, H. B., 1990, Protection against mucoid *Pseudomonas aeruginosa* in rodent models of endobronchial infection, *Science* **249:**537–540.
134. Garner, C. V., DesJardins, D., and Pier, G. B., 1990, Immunogenic properties of *Pseudomonas aeruginosa* mucoid exopolysaccharide, *Infect. Immun.* **58:**1835–1842.
135. Garner, C. V., and Pier, G. B., 1988, Human immune response to *Pseudomonas aeruginosa* mucoid exopolysaccharide vaccine, *Clin. Res.* **36:**465A.
136. Pennington, J. E., 1974, Preliminary investigations of *Pseudomonas aeruginosa* vaccine in patients with leukemia and cystic fibrosis, *J. Infect. Dis.* **130:**S159–S162.
137. Schaad, U. B., Lang, A. B., Wedgwood, J., Ruedberg, A., Fürer, E., Que, J. U., and Cryz, S. J., Jr., 1990, Immunization of non-colonized cystic fibrosis patients with a *Pseudomonas aeruginosa* O-polysaccharide-toxin A conjugate vaccine, *Pediatr. Pulmonol. Suppl.* **5:**91–92.
138. Grimwood, K., To, M., Rabin, H. R., and Woods, D. E., 1989, Inhibition of *Pseudomonas aeruginosa* exoenzyme expression by subinhibitory antibiotic concentrations, *Antimicrob. Agents Chemother.* **33:**41–47.
139. Grimwood, K., To, M., Rabin, H. R., and Woods, D. E., 1989, Subinhibitory antibiotics reduce *Pseudomonas aeruginosa* tissue injury in the rat lung model, *J. Antimicrob. Chemother.* **24:**937–945.
140. Moss, R. B., Hsu, Y. P., Lewiston, N. J., Curd, J. G., Milgrom, H., Hart, S., Dyer, B., and Larrick, J. W., 1986, Association of systemic immune complexes, complement activation, and antibodies to *Pseudomonas aeruginosa* lipopolysaccharide and exotoxin A with mortality in cystic fibrosis, *Am. Rev. Respir. Dis.* **133:**648–652.
141. Moss, R. B., Hsu, Y. P., Sullivan, M. M., and Lewiston, N. J., 1986, Altered antibody isotype in cystic fibrosis: Possible role in opsonic deficiency, *Pediatr. Res.* **20:**453–456.
142. Penketh, A., Pitt, T., Roberts, D., Hodson, M., and Batten, J. C., 1983, The relationship of phenotype changes in *Pseudomonas aeruginosa* to the clinical condition of patients with cystic fibrosis, *Am. Rev. Respir. Dis.* **172:**605–608.
143. Baltimore, R. S., Christie, C. D. C., and Smith, G. J. W., 1989, Immunohistopathologic localization of *Pseudomonas aeruginosa* in lungs from patients with cystic fibrosis: Implica-

tions for the pathogenesis of progressive lung deterioration, *Am. Rev. Respir. Dis.* **140**:1650–1661.
144. Speert, D. P., Dinmick, J. E., Pier, G. B., Saunders, J. M., Hancock, R. E. W., and Kelly, N., 1987, An immunohistological evaluation of *Pseudomonas aeruginosa* pulmonary infection in two patients with cystic fibrosis, *Pediatr. Res.* **22**:743–747.
145. Schwarzmann, S., and Boring, J. R., II, 1971, Antiphagocytic effect of slime from a mucoid strain of *Pseudomonas aeruginosa*, *Infect. Immun.* **3**:762–767.
146. Ruhen, R. W., Holt, P. G., and Papadimitriou, J. M., 1980, Antiphagocytic effect of *Pseudomonas aeruginosa* exopolysaccharide, *J. Clin. Pathol.* **33**:1221–1222.
147. Baltimore, R. S., and Mitchell, M., 1980, Immunologic investigations of mucoid strains of *Pseudomonas aeruginosa*: Comparison of susceptibility to opsonic antibody in mucoid and nonmucoid strains, *J. Infect. Dis.* **141**:238–247.
148. Jensen, E. T., Kharazmi, A., Lam, K., Costerton, J. W., and Høiby, N., 1990, Human polymorphonuclear leukocyte response to *Pseudomonas aeruginosa* grown in biofilms, *Infect. Immun.* **58**:2383–2385.
149. Hann, S., and Holsclaw, D. S., 1976, Interactions of *Pseudomonas aeruginosa* with immunoglobulins and complement in sputum, *Infect. Immun.* **14**:114–117.
150. Fick, R. B., Robbins, R. A., Squier, S. U., Schoderbek, W. E., and Russ, W. D., 1986, Complement activation in cystic fibrosis respiratory fluids: *In vivo* and *in vitro* generation of C5a and chemotactic activity, *Pediatr. Res.* **20**:1258–1268.
151. Schultz, D. R., and Miller, K. D., 1974, Elastase of *Pseudomonas aeruginosa*: Inactivation of complement and complement-derived chemotactic and phagocytic factors, *Infect. Immun.* **10**:128–135.
152. Baltimore, R. S., and Shedd, D. G., 1983, The role of complement in the opsonization of mucoid and non-mucoid strains of *Pseudomonas aeruginosa*, *Pediatr. Res.* **17**:952–958.
153. Pier, G. B., and Ames, P., 1984, Mediation of the killing of rough, mucoid isolates of *Pseudomonas aeruginosa* from patients with cystic fibrosis by the alternative pathway of complement, *J. Infect. Dis.* **150**:223–228.
154. Schiller, N. L., 1988, Characterization of the susceptibility of *Pseudomonas aeruginosa* to complement-mediated killing: Role of antibodies to the rough lipopolysaccharide on serum-sensitive strains, *Infect. Immun.* **56**:632–639.
155. Schiller, N. L., Hatch, R. A., and Joiner, K. A., 1989, Complement activation and C3 binding by serum-sensitive and serum-resistant strains of *Pseudomonas aeruginosa*, *Infect. Immun.* **57**:1707–1713.
156. Suter, S., Schaad, U. B., Roux, L., Nydegger, U. E., and Waldvogel, F. A., 1984, Granulocyte neutral proteases and *Pseudomonas* elastase as possible causes of airway damage in patients with cystic fibrosis, *J. Infect. Dis.* **149**:523–531.
157. Bainbridge, T., and Fick, R. B., 1989, Functional importance of cystic fibrosis immunoglobulin-G fragments generated by *Pseudomonas aeruginosa* elastase, *J. Lab. Clin. Med.* **114**:728–733.
158. Jones, M. M., Seilheimer, D. K., Pier, G. B., and Rossen, R. D., 1990, Increased elastase secretion by peripheral blood monocytes in cystic fibrosis patients, *Clin. Exper. Immunol.* **80**:344–349.
159. Döring, G., Obernesser, H.-J., Botzenhart, K., Flehmig, B., Høiby, N., and Ofman, A., 1983, Proteases of *Pseudomonas aeruginosa* in patients with cystic fibrosis, *J. Infect. Dis.* **147**:744–750.
160. Berger, M., Sorensen, R. U., Tosi, M. F., Dearborn, D. G., and Döring, G., 1989, Complement receptor expression on neutrophils at an inflammatory site, the *Pseudomonas*-infected lung in cystic fibrosis, *J. Clin. Invest.* **84**:1302–1313.
161. Tosi, M. F., Zakem, H., and Berger, M., 1990, Neutrophil elastase cleaves C3bi on opsonized *Pseudomonas* as well as CR1 on neutrophils to create a functionally important opsonin receptor mismatch, *J. Clin. Invest.* **86**:300–308.

16

Susceptibility and Resistance of *Pseudomonas aeruginosa* to Antimicrobial Agents

FRANCIS BELLIDO and ROBERT E. W. HANCOCK

1. INTRODUCTION

The treatment of *Pseudomonas aeruginosa* infections is a constant challenge for physicians. A combination of features such as ability to survive and spread in hostile environments, multiple virulence determinants, and intrinsic resistance to commonly used antibiotics and disinfectants makes this bacterium a major life-threatening pathogen. Particularly susceptible are those patients with altered host defenses or those who are debilitated by cystic fibrosis (CF), major surgery, traumatic wounds, severe burns, or neoplastic diseases. Indeed, *P. aeruginosa* is the third most common cause of nosocomial infections after *Escherichia coli* and *Staphylococcus aureus*, accounting for approximately 10% of all hospital-acquired infections. *P. aeruginosa* strains are not susceptible to many of the conventionally used antibiotics (Table I). This high intrinsic resistance has been ascribed to low outer-membrane permeability, due to certain structural features that distinguish *P. aeruginosa* from other common gram-negative bacteria (see section 2). In addition, *P. aeruginosa* may develop several mechanisms of resistance to oppose the action of antibiotics,

---

FRANCIS BELLIDO • Eli Lilly, 1214 Geneva, Switzerland.   ROBERT E. W. HANCOCK • Department of Microbiology, University of British Columbia, Vancouver, British Columbia, Canada V6T 1W5.

Pseudomonas aeruginosa as an Opportunistic Pathogen, edited by Mario Campa *et al.* Plenum Press, New York, 1993.

TABLE I
Comparison of *P. aeruginosa* and *E. coli* Susceptibilities to Antibiotics

Antibiotic class	Representative antibiotics	MIC (μg/ml)[a]	
		E. coli	*P. aeruginosa*
β-lactams			
Aminopenicillins	Ampicillin	4	>128
α Carboxypenicillins	Carbenicillin/Ticarcillin	4	32–64
Acylureirodopenicillins	Piperacillin	2	2
	Azlocillin	16	4
Carbapenems	Imipenem	0.25	2
Cephems	Cefoperazone	0.1	4
	Cefsulodin	64	2
	Cefotaxime	0.03	32
	Ceftazidime	0.12	2
	Cefepime	0.04	2.5
Monobactams	Aztreonam	0.03	2–8
Aminoglycosides	Gentamicin	0.5	2
	Tobramycin	0.5	0.5
	Amikacin	2	4
Polymyxins	Colistin	1	4
Quinolones	Ciprofloxacin	0.025	0.1
Others	Tetracycline	2	32
	Chloramphenicol	4	64
	Erythromycin	64	200

[a]Normal MIC of strains lacking resistance transfer plasmids, derepressed chromosomal β-lactamase or increased intrinsic resistance due to porin alterations.

including modifications of the outer-membrane entry pathways, production of antibiotic-inactivating enzymes, and alterations of target-structures. The main antibiotics showing antipseudomonal activity belong to the β-lactam and aminoglycoside families. However, recently, fluoroquinolones such as ciprofloxacin have also proved to be useful against *P. aeruginosa*. Due to space limitations, no attempt will be made here to present an exhausting analysis of the complexity and the numerous facets of antibiotic action against *P. aeruginosa*. Instead emphasis will be placed on the main determinants of antibiotic activity and bacterial resistance for the above commonly used antibiotics.

2. β-LACTAMS

2.1. Antipseudomonal β-Lactams

During the last two decades, rigorous efforts of the pharmaceutical industry to improve on the properties of the first penicillin derivatives have led to a profusion of new β-lactams. Considering the diversity of their chemical structure, the traditional distinction between penicillins and cephalosporins has become inappropriate for the classification of these new products. In this review we have adopted the nomenclature suggested by Brown[1] which is based on chemical structure. The only classes of β-lactams discussed here will be those presenting consistent, therapeutically relevant antipseudomonal activity.

The first commercially available β-lactam to show activity against *P. aeruginosa* was carbenicillin. Another α-carboxypenicillin, ticarcillin, was from two to four times more active, allowing administration of lower doses and, accordingly, reduced platelet dysfunction and hypokalemia.[2] Despite this breakthrough in antibiotherapy, the clinical use of these two compounds against *P. aeruginosa* was limited by their moderate activity and high sensitivity to β-lactamase inactivation (Table I). Consequently, the emergence of resistant strains was rapid and led to frequent therapeutic failures. Subsequently, newer penams, with an extended spectrum of activity, were developed. The minimum inhibitory concentration (MIC) of the acylureidopenicillins, mezlocillin, piperacillin and azlocillin against *P. aeruginosa* were 20-fold lower than those of α-carboxypenicillins. However, these antibiotics still remained susceptible to hydrolysis by β-lactamases. This problem seems to have been overcome by development of a new generation of penams such as alpacillin and foramidocillin. Like the α-carboxypenicillins, ureidopenicillins show excellent synergy with aminoglycosides against *P. aeruginosa*.

Another class of β-lactams exhibiting excellent activity against *P. aeruginosa* are the carbapenems. These molecules have a double bond at the 2–3 position and a carbon atom instead of sulfur in the penem ring. While preserving the efficacy of penams against gram-positive bacteria, these substitutions extend the spectrum of activity to a level unmatched by any other class of antibiotic. The only commercially available compound of this group is imipenem, a semi-synthetic derivative of thienamycin. Its wide range of activity includes *Psedomonas* spp. with the exception of *P. maltophilia* and *P. cepacia*.

The name cephem refers to all the cephalosporins and cephamycins. The latter differ from cephalosporins by the presence of a methoxy moiety in the 7α position. None of the cephamycins shows good antipseudomonal activity and therefore, they will not be discussed here. The main cephems that are active against *P. aeruginosa* are the so-called third- and fourth-generation cephalosporins. Cefotaxime and ceftriaxone were the first (third-generation) cephalosporins to exhibit moderate antipseudomonal activity. However, cefoperazone, and especially ceftazidime, are the only third-generation agents with excellent activity against *P. aeruginosa*. New investigational products such as cefepime, cefpirome, E-1040, and BO-1341, called fourth-generation cephalosporins because they are all characterized by a quaternary nitrogen moiety at the 3 position, have proved to be promising antipseudomonal agents.[4-6] Cefsulodin, a cephem that, like piperacillin, has a piperazine side chain, is a unique cephalosporin in that its activity is limited to *P. aeruginosa*.

Azthreonam, a monobactam containing also the aminothiazole oxime side chain of the third- and fourth-generation cephalosporins, is exclusively active against gram-negative bacteria.[7] However, its efficacy against *P. aeruginosa* is moderate and clearly lower than that of the best antipseudomonal cephalosporins (Table I).

Although most of the newer cephalosporins also show *in vitro* synergy with aminoglycosides, physicians prefer to combine an aminoglycoside with a carboxy- or ureidopenicillin because this combination is potentially less nephrotoxic and less expensive.[8]

2.2. Determinants of Efficacy

The efficacy of each β-lactam molecule depends on its ability to access and subsequently inhibit essential inner membrane-bound enzymes, the penicillin-binding-proteins (PBP), which are necessary for the biosynthesis of peptidoglycan.[9] In gram-positive bacteria, β-lactams have relatively free access to these enzymes. However, in gram-negative microorganisms, the outer membrane is a major obstacle any antibiotic must overcome before reaching its target(s) (Fig. 1). In the case of β-lactams, once in the periplasm they must also resist the hydrolytic inactivation of β-lactamases. Thus, the efficacy of β-lactams in gram-negative bacteria results from the interplay of at least three factors: the rate of permeation across the outer membrane, the kinetic parameters of the β-lactamase–β-lactam interaction, and the affinity of the PBP for the β-lactam (Fig. 1). Zimmermann and Rosselet proposed a model to describe this complex interplay.[10] These authors postulated that the penetration of β-lactams into bacterial cells equilibrates at a steady state in which the rate of diffusion of β-lactams through the outer membrane is balanced by the hydrolysis of β-lactamase in the periplasmic space. These events can be described by the Fick's first law of diffusion and the Michaelis-Menten equation, respectively, in the following equation

$$V = C \cdot (S_o - S_p) = Vmax \cdot S_p / S_p + Km \qquad (1)$$

in which V = the rate of hydrolysis by intact cells, C = outer membrane permeability constant specific for the given microorganism and β-lactam, $Vmax$ and Km are the Michaelis constants, S_o = the external concentration of the antibiotic, and S_p = the periplasmic concentration of the β-lactam.

2.2.1. Outer Membrane Permeability

The structure of the outer membrane of *P. aeruginosa* (Fig. 1) and its role in resistance to β-lactam antibiotics have been documented extensively in recent reviews.[11–14] Briefly, the outer membrane of gram-negative bacteria consists of an asymmetric lipid bilayer in which proteins are associated with an external leaflet of lipopolysaccharide (LPS) molecules and an internal phospholipid monolayer[15]. The outer membrane is the structure that controls the trafficking of nutrients and metabolites between the bacterium and its environment. Because LPS molecules are negatively charged, and tightly bound to each other by cross-bridging with Mg^{2+} cations, the outer membrane acts as a permeability barrier for hydrophobic compounds.[11] To gain access to its internal targets, any antibiotic molecule must cross the outer membrane. A large number of hydrophobic or amphiphilic antibiotics such as macrolides, rifamycins, lincosamides, fusidic acid, and novobiocin are thought to be inactive against many gram-negative pathogens because of their slow penetration through the outer membrane.[11] In *P. aeruginosa*, two main pathways allow antipseudomonal antibiotics to enter into the cell.[11] Polycationic antibiotics such as aminoglycosides and polymyxin have been shown to promote their own uptake through the outer membrane by destroying the stabilizing effect of Mg^{2+}–crossbridging of the adjacent LPS molecules (see section 3.2). In contrast, β-lactams are thought to penetrate to the periplasm through channel-forming proteins, named porins. Several lines of evidence have shown that most porins form nonspecific water-filled pores, which act as a sieving barrier allowing the free passage of molecules with a molecular size lower than the exclusion limit.[15]

Protein F or OprF,[13] the major outer membrane protein of *P. aeruginosa*, has been suggested as the entry pathway for β-lactam antibiotics.[12–14] In addition, OprF plays an important role in outer membrane stability and bacterial cell shape.[16,17] However, as discussed in several recent reviews,[12,14,18] the role of this protein is currently a source of controversy. Several authors[11–13] have produced a variety of evidence that OprF functions as a porin with a large channel, although only a small proportion of the total OprF molecules per cell seem to form such channels (with the bulk of OprF molecules forming small, antibiotic-impermeable channels).[12] Conversely, Nakae and collaborators, using the same liposome swelling methods as used by one of the authors above,[11] have suggested OprF does not function as a porin.[17,19] The same authors, using the same methodology, *i.e.* the liposome swelling assay, proposed OprC, OprE and OprD function as general porins and as the major routes of entry for β-lactams in *P. aeruginosa*.[19] However, the data produced by this laboratory have been criticized for lack of internal consistency.[13,14] Recently, Bellido *et al.*[19a] cloned the *E. coli* raffinose into wild-type and OprF-deficient *P. aeruginosa* strains to allow the study of polysaccharides' penetration through the outer membrane. Their results strongly suggest that OprF is the most prominent porin for compounds larger than disaccharides in *P. aeruginosa*.

Protein D2 (OprD) has been shown to be a saturable, substrate-specific channel for imipenem and basic amino acids.[20] This selectivity for imipenem over the other β-lactams seems due to the presence in OprD channels of a specific binding site for positively charged penems and carbapenems. Other, investigational β-lactam antibiotics seem also to take advantage of specific transport systems across the gram-negative bacterial outer membrane. For example, the catechol-cephalosporins are able to chelate ferric iron and

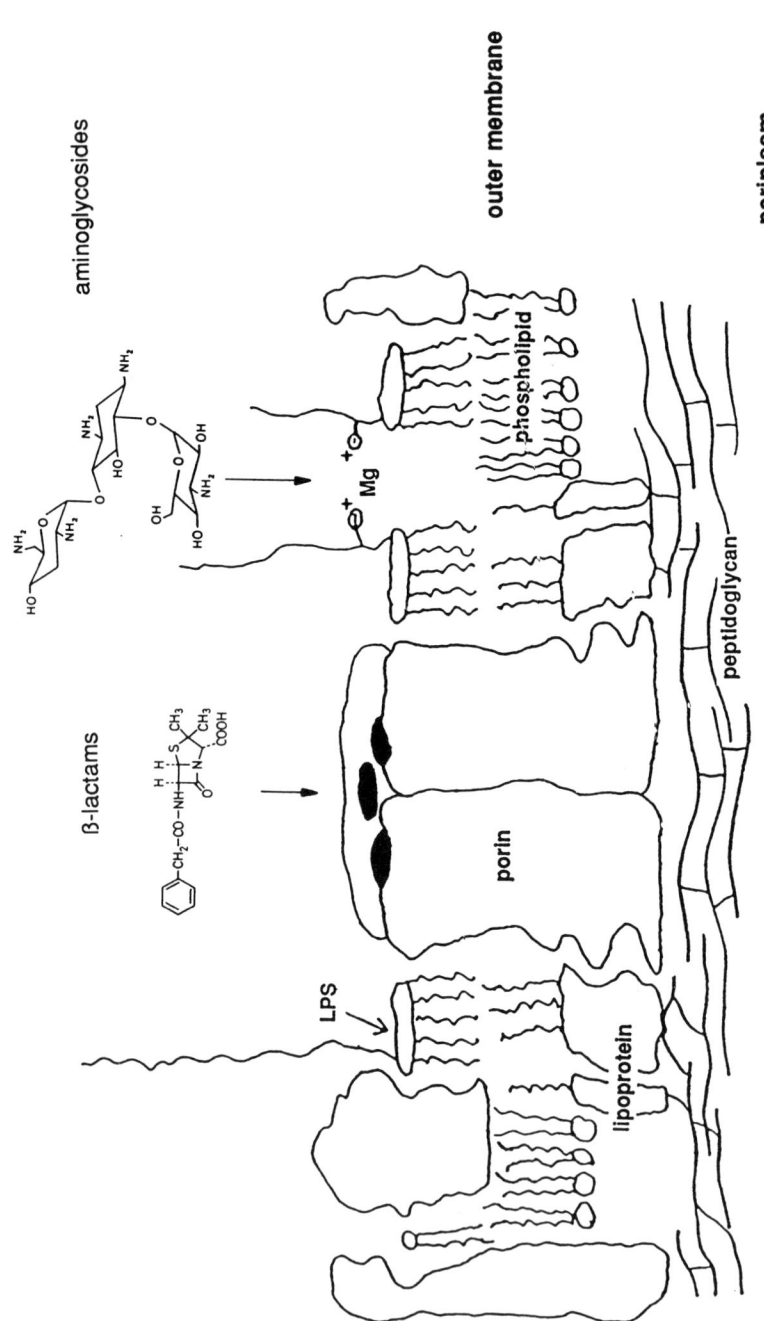

EFFECTS OF MICROBIAL AGENTS ON *P. AERUGINOSA* 327

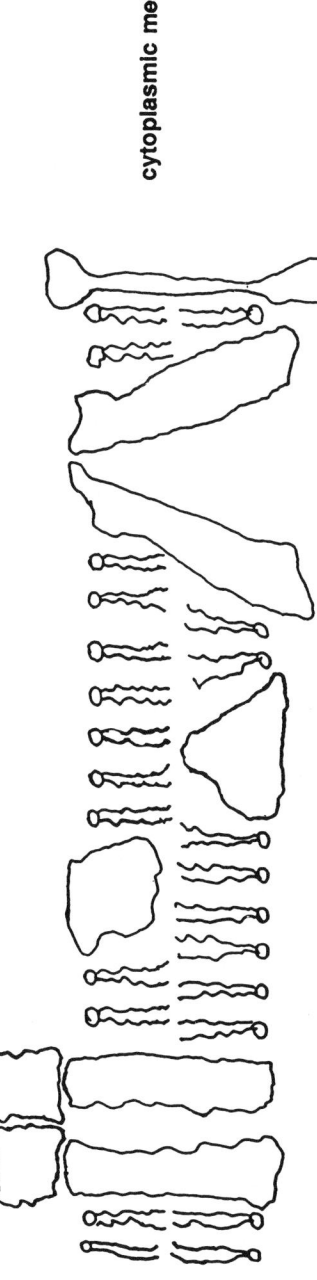

FIGURE 1. Schematic representation of the cell envelope showing the two major antibiotic uptake pathways through the outer membrane of *P. aeruginosa*, namely the porin pathway (left arrow) for β-lactams and the self-promoted uptake pathway (right arrow) for aminoglycosides. The asymmetric outer membrane consist of an external leaflet of lipopolysaccharide (LPS) molecules and an internal phospholipid monolayer. The β-lactam targets are located in the cytoplasmic membrane layer which is orientated towards the periplasm. Aminoglycosides have to cross this inner membrane to reach their cytoplasmic targets.

penetrate the *P. aeruginosa* outer membrane through the siderophore-scavenger pathways.[21]

Outer membrane permeability of β-lactams in intact *P. aeruginosa* cells have been measured by the Zimmermann and Rosselet method.[11] Results for easily β-lactamase-hydrolysed β-lactams such as nitrocefin[22], cephacetrile, and cephaloridine[23] showed outer membrane permeability coefficients to be 12 to 500-fold lower than the values obtained for *E. coli*. Data for the newer β-lactams are not available from intact *P. aeruginosa* cells because of several methodological limitations.[24] Indeed, the Zimmermann and Rosselet method can only be applied if the β-lactam is a good substrate for the β-lactamase. Most of the recently developed β-lactams exhibit too high a stability to β-lactamase hydrolysis for their outer membrane permeability to be accurately determined under the same experimental conditions. Another source of difficulty in applying the Zimmermann and Rosselet method to *P. aeruginosa* has been illustrated by the work of Hewinson *et al.*[25] These authors found that the permeability coefficient of cephalosporin C varied according to external antibiotic concentration, whereas Fick's law states that it should be a constant under normal conditions. Such a puzzling effect likely may be ascribed to the presence of outer membrane-bound β-lactamase that considerably limits the applicability of Zimmermann and Rosselet method to *P. aeruginosa*.[14,24] The study of the diffusion of β-lactams through porin-reconstituted vesicles is also difficult because of the problem of controlling charge and counter-ion effects that obscure actual permeation rates of the β-lactam studied and because the low total permeability of *P. aeruginosa* porins limits assay sensitivity. However, this method has been applied in *P. aeruginosa* to newer zwitterionic β-lactams such as the fourth-generation cephalosporins.[26] These molecules penetrate the outer membrane at rates about 300-fold lower than *E. coli* and 10-fold lower than *E. cloacae*. Results with these latter two bacteria also suggest that their outer membranes are much more permeable to zwitterionic compounds than to negatively charged β-lactams. However, the extrapolation of these findings to *P. aeruginosa* does not necessarily follow because the outer membrane of *P. aeruginosa* seems to be relatively indifferent to the physicochemical properties of the β-lactams,[11,44] a result that is predictable given the proposed large channel size of the major porin.

2.2.2. β-Lactamase

P. aeruginosa strains can produce both chromosomal and plasmid-mediated β-lactamases. Sabath *et al.*[27] first reported in 1965 the discovery of an inducible chromosomal cephalosporinase. Since then this enzyme has been reported in all wild-type strains of *P. aeruginosa* and has been further classified as Class Id in the scheme of Richmond and Sykes.[28] The amino-acid sequence around the active site ser of *P. aeruginosa* cephalosporinase showed a high degree of homology with the chromosomal β-lactamase of *Enterobacteriaceae*.[29] Therefore, this enzyme belongs to the molecular class C in the scheme of Amber, extended by Knott-Hunziker.[29] Based on analytical isoelectric focusing studies, *P. aeruginosa* seems to produce four distinct subgroups of cephalosporinase corresponding to four alkaline pIs.[30] Several β-lactams are capable of inducing the *P. aeruginosa* cephalosporinase. This property diminishes the efficacy of inducing β-lactams. For example, it has been reported that self-induced β-lactamase production decreased imipenem susceptibility of *P. aeruginosa*, although insufficiently to elevated MIC beyond the clinical range.[31,36] Constitutive high levels of cephalosporinase may also be observed in *P. aeruginosa* after a double mutation that results in a stably derepressed β-lactamase.[29] Consequently, the bacteria become resistant to multiple β-lactams.

In addition to the chromosomal cephalosporinase, at least 15 plasmid-borne β-lactamases have been isolated from *P. aeruginosa*.[29] These enzymes include broad-spectrum β-lactamases (TEM-1, TEM-2, SHV-1, HMS-1, LCR-1, NPS-1), oxallinases (OXA-2, OXA-3, OXA-4, OXA-5, OXA-6), and carbenicillinases (CARB-3, CARB-4, PSE-1, PSE-2, PSE-3, PSE-4).

New β-lactams such as the third-generation cephalosporins, monobactams and carbapenems were thought to completely resist β-lactamase inactivation since several authors were unable to detect hydrolysis with β-lactamase crude extracts[32]. Nevertheless, cephalosporinases exhibited high affinity for all of these compounds. To explain the resistance to new β-lactams in β-lactamase-overproducing gram-negative strains, Then and Angerhn[32] proposed the "trapping" model, involving non-hydrolytic binding of β-lactams to β-lactamase. However, several authors have pointed out that this concept was mistakenly based on inappropriate measurements of β-lactamase hydrolysis.[14,33,42] Two newer antibiotics, *i.e.*, cefpirome and cefepime, remain effective against β-lactamase-overproducing gram-negative strains that are resistant to third-generation cephalosporins. The reason of this efficacy has been ascribed to high β-lactamase stability and low affinity for the enzyme, although higher rates of outer membrane permeability are also involved.[26,33]

2.2.3. Penicillin-Binding Proteins (PBP)

P. aeruginosa has been shown to possess a PBP pattern equivalent to that of *E. coli*.[34] Seven PBP have been described with molecular weights ranging from 118,000 to 350,000 Da. However, the functions of these enzymes are not as well known as in *E. coli*. Thus, only PBP-5 has been described as a D-alanine carboxypeptidase.[35] Some PBP of *P. aeruginosa* also may not be totally similar to their *E. coli* counterparts. For example, a modified PBP-4 was associated with a clinical case of resistance to imipenem whereas the equivalent protein in *E. coli* is a non-essential carboxypeptidase.[36] Inhibition of *P. aeruginosa*

PBP by β-lactams results in morphological changes comparable to those observed in *E. coli*. However, differences in affinity are also noticeable (Table II). For example, low concentrations of sulfocephalosporins such as cefsulodin inhibit *P. aeruginosa* PBP-3, whereas its *E. coli* counterpart is insensitive. Further, in *P. aeruginosa*, to a greater extent than in *E. coli*, the affinity of PBP for given β-lactams seems not to be correlated with their efficacy (cf. Tables I and II). This is probably due to the role played by other factors in *P. aeruginosa* such as low outer-membrane permeability and inducible β-lactamase.

Recently, a possible correlation between the affinity of β-lactamase and the affinity of PBP for the new β-lactams has been suggested in *E. cloacae*.[33] We feel that this finding probably can be extrapolated to other bacteria and might have considerable implications in the design of new β-lactam molecules.

2.3. Resistance

As mentioned before, *P. aeruginosa* is intrinsically resistant to a wide range of β-lactams. Low outer-membrane permeability by itself cannot account for this resistance because even slower-penetrating β-lactams equilibrate their external and periplasmic concentrations within 1 minute.[37,38] Therefore, an additional mechanism must be associated with low outer-membrane permeability to achieve high intrinsic resistance.[37,38] This mechanism may involve the inducible type-Id chromosomal cephalosporinase in the case of easily hydrolyzed β-lactams or those that are strong inducers of β-lactamase.[39]

Initially susceptible strains can develop resistance during β-lactam therapy. In some cases, this can involve acquisition of a plasmid-borne β-lactam-

TABLE II
Affinity of β-Lactams for the Essential PBP[a] of *P. aeruginosa* and *E. coli*[51,52]

	I_{50} for PBP (βg/ml)							
	P. aeruginosa				*E. coli*			
β-lactam	1A	1B	2	3	1A	1B	2	3
Ampicillin	0.25	0.9	0.5	1.3	1.4	3.9	*0.7*	*0.9*
Carbenicillin	0.07[b]	0.5	0.3	*0.1*	2.1	5.0	4.0	*2.1*
Azlocillin	0.1	0.5	ND[c]	*0.02*	0.8	1.6	0.4	*0.05*
Cefsulodin	19	2	>250	*0.3*	*0.5*	3.7	>250	>250
Cefoperazone	1.0	2.0	>200	*<0.02*	0.5	1.5	0.9	*<0.02*
Cefotaxime	0.04	0.2	ND	*0.01*	*0.02*	0.4	4.0	*0.01*
Ceftazidime	0.8	6.0	25	*0.1*	0.9	3.4	240	*0.06*
Imipenem	0.3	0.6	<0.6	4.0	*0.2*	0.6	*<0.1*	9.8
Aztreonam	8.4	2.6	ND	*0.04*	1.7	310	>500	*0.17*

[a]Three other PBP (PBP4, 5 and 6) are not included here since they were shown to be nonessential in *E. coli*.
[b]Numbers in italics represent I_{50} values for the PBP with the highest affinity.
[c]ND = not determined.

ase. A recent survey has revealed emergence of resistance and therapeutic failure may occur in approximately 15% of patients suffering from *P. aeruginosa* infections and treated with one of the new β-lactams.[40] The mechanisms responsible for the emergence of resistance in *P. aeruginosa* may involve overproduction of chromosomal cephalosporinase, diminished outer membrane permeability, and modified PBP affinity. The first one has been incriminated in the emergence of resistance during ceftazidime therapy in CF patients[41] and in experimental *P. aeruginosa* endocarditis in rabbits.[42] It is likely that *in vivo* selection of stably derepressed β-lactamase-producing *P. aeruginosa* strains can account in most cases for the rapid emergence of β-lactam resistance in CF patients.[43] Fortunately, the future use of newer agents such as fourth-generation cephalosporins, which are effective even against such derepressed strains, could considerably decrease the risk of emergence of resistance in chronic infections. Indeed, a recent study has shown that spontaneous *in vitro* mutation to cefepime-resistance is extremely low in *P. aeruginosa*.[44] Emergence of resistance to β-lactams has also been linked to *P. aeruginosa* outer-membrane modifications. Godfrey *et al.* observed a correlation between β-lactam resistance and changes in LPS structure[45] or in OprF structure.[46] However, the role of the latter in β-lactam resistance is a source of controversy (see section 2.2.1.). Outer membrane protein D2 (OprD) of *P. aeruginosa* has been unequivocally associated with the emergence of resistance to one class of β-lactams. Several authors have reported the emergence of resistant strains during imipenem therapy.[36,47,48] Interestingly, this resistance affects only imipenem and not other β-lactams and is associated with the loss of outer-membrane porin protein OprD. This is probably because OprD contains a specific binding site for imipenem and its loss substantially reduces uptake across the outer membrane (see section 2.2.1.)

Several studies have associated resistance to β-lactams with modified PBP in different clinical isolates of *P. aeruginosa*.[36,49,50] However, it seems that the emergence of clinical resistance due to changes in PBP affinity is rare in gram-negative bacteria. This is consistent with the idea that these alterations may impair the viability of cells.[36] However, with the clinical use of newer β-lactams, such as the fourth-generation cephalosporins, showing high β-lactamase resistance and rapid uptake through the gram-negative outer membrane, there is the possibility that bacteria will develop such resistance mechanisms more commonly in the future.

3. AMINOGLYCOSIDES

3.1. Determinants of Efficacy

Aminoglycosides remain one of the most valuable tools possessed by physicians to combat serious gram-negative infections. They are especially effective in treatment of urinary tract infections due to their high excretion in urine, however their major use against life-threatening *P. aeruginosa* infections is in combination with an anti-pseudomonal penicillin or cephalosporin.[53] One severe limitation in combating infections in specific tissues is their limited and at times unpredictable penetration.[54] Attempts to overcome this problem in *P. aeruginosa* infections of the lungs of CF patients include aerosolization and inhalation therapy[55] and use of doses up to 10 times the normal human dose.[55] Antagonism by divalent cations (see section 3.2.) and polyanions can also decrease aminoglycoside effectiveness.

A major factor that limits the usage of aminoglycosides is their strong reputation as toxic antibiotics. The word "reputation" is used advisedly because the frequency of aminoglycoside nephrotoxicity varies from 2–10%. Futhermore it appears to be dose-related and somewhat restricted to specific patient groups, especially those who are elderly and debilitated.[54] Nephrotoxicity is usually mild and reversible, although aminoglycoside ototoxicity, which occurs with a similar frequency, is irreversible.

Of the many known aminoglycosides, only gentamicin, amikacin, and tobramycin (Fig. 2) are commonly used against *P. aeruginosa* infections. The MIC_{90} of gentamicin and tobramycin for *P. aeruginosa* is approximately 6 μg/ml, which is close to the achievable peak serum levels at the usual human dose (5 mg/kg/day).[54] For this reason, these antibiotics are usually combined with an anti-pseudomonal penicillin.[56] In contrast, the peak serum concentration of amikacin following the standard intravenous dose is approximately 25–35 μg/ml, or nearly double the MIC_{90} for *P. aeruginosa* (16 μg/ml). Despite this, amikacin is usually also combined with anti-pseudomonal penicillin (*e.g.* ticarcillin) with which it is often synergistic and most effective.[53]

Forty-six years have elapsed since the first reported isolation of the aminoglycoside streptomycin, and numerous prominent scientists have attempted to uncover details of the mode of action and uptake of aminoglycosides.[51,58–60] However, the precise molecular details of the mode of uptake or action are still not known and we refer the reader to the above review articles. In general terms, aminoglycoside action against susceptible *P. aeruginosa* can be described as follows: Cationic aminoglycosides initially interact electrostatically with the negatively charged cell surface, followed by disruption of the outer membrane and self-promoted uptake across the outer membrane. This is followed by two energized uptake steps across the outer membrane, the slow-phase EDPI and the rapid-phase EDPII. Killing of cells apparently

---

FIGURE 2. Structure of the major anti-*Pseudomonas* aminoglycosides and the points of action of the aminoglycoside-modifying agents found in *Pseudomonas*. Abbreviations: AAC = acetylating enzyme; AAD = adenylating enzyme (the number in brackets represents the carbon at which the enzyme acts: *N.B.* there are three types of AAC(6′) and two types of AAC(3)(with differing activity spectra); R1 and R2 in the gentamicin structure each represent H or CH_3 depending on which of the three forms of gentamicin (C1, C1a or C2) present as a mixture in commercial gentamicin preparations, is represented.

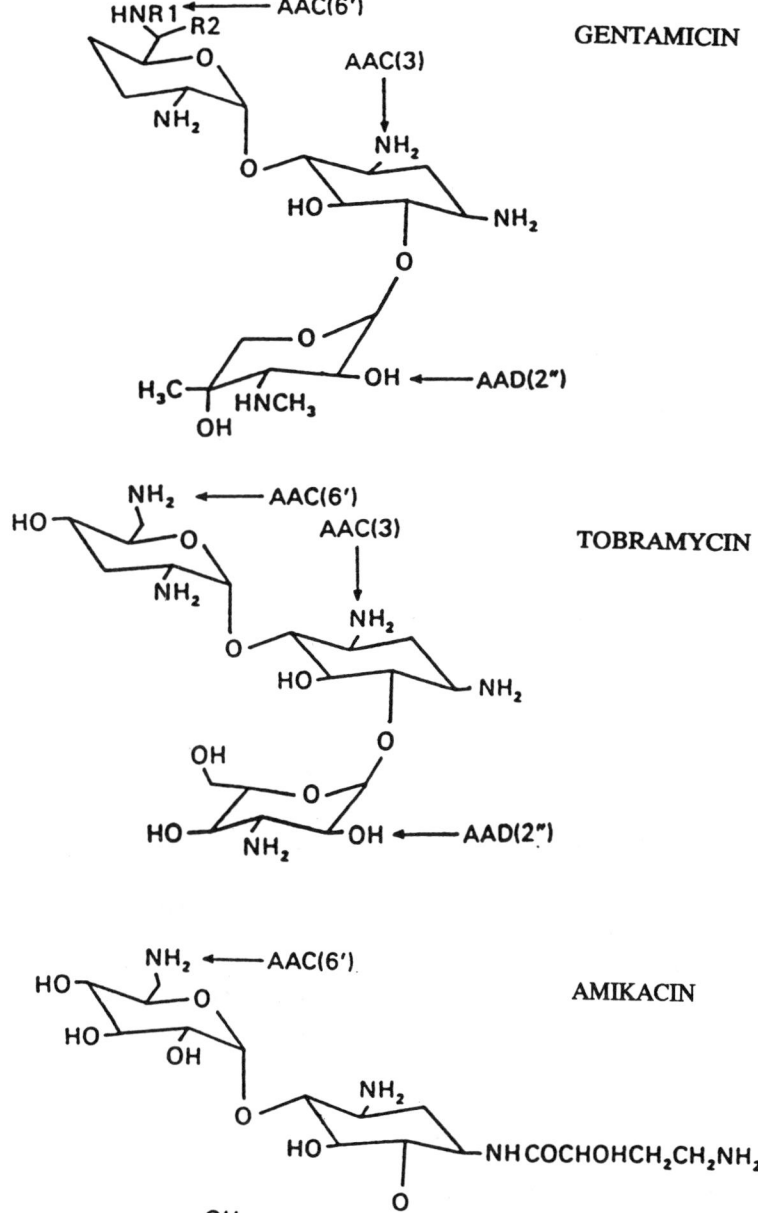

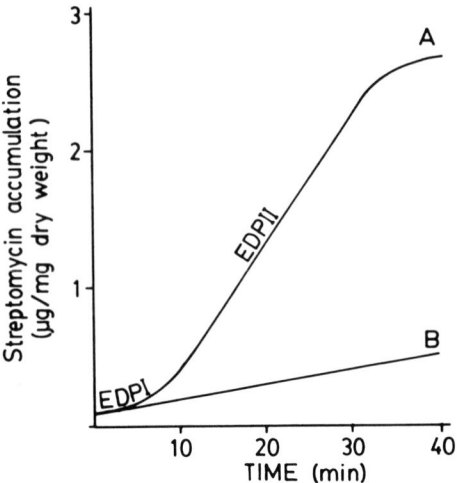

FIGURE 3. Kinetics of aminoglycoside uptake in *Pseudomonas aeruginosa* wild-type, susceptible strains (curve A) and strains resistant to aminoglycosides by virtue of possession of an R-plasmid specifying an aminoglycoside-modifying enzyme (curve B). Data are shown for streptomycin, but similar kinetics are seen with tobramycin. EDPI, EDPII = energy-dependent phases I and II, respectively.

occurs at or near the time of initiation of EDPII (Fig. 3).[59] The actual mechanism of killing remains unknown and recently has been proposed to involve either inhibition of the initiation of DNA replication[59,62] or creation of membrane channels by induced errors during protein synthesis.[61] Nevertheless, it is apparent that the ability of aminoglycosides to interact with ribosomes is involved since, e.g., *rpsL* mutants altered in ribosomal protein S12 do not initiate EDPII and are resistant to streptomycin (which has a high affinity binding site on S12). Because such mutants occur at low frequency in the laboratory, and are apparently not found in the clinic,[63] we will not discuss further the interaction of aminoglycosides with ribosomes. Instead we will concentrate on those stages of aminoglycoside interaction with cells that can be altered to cause clinically significant resistance.

3.2. Outer Membrane Permeation

It is now well-established that aminoglycosides cross the outer membrane, using the self-promoted uptake mechanism in *P. aeruginosa* (see ref. 64 for review and original references). Thus laboratory mutants with a defect in this pathway (due to overproduction of an outer-membrane protein OprH = H1, which apparently blocks the pathway) are resistant to killing by aminoglycosides. Such mutants have no alteration in the porin pathway. Conversely, a *tolA* mutant, which demonstrated enhanced outer membrane interaction with aminoglycosides, was supersusceptible to aminoglycosides.

The self-promoted uptake pathway involves sites in the outer membrane at which divalent cations (usually Mg^{2+} or Ca^{2+}) crossbridge adjacent lipopolysaccharide molecules on the surface of the bacterium (Fig. 1). Such sites have been shown to be important in maintaining the barrier function of the outer membrane. These sites have an affinity that is at least two orders of magnitude higher for polycationic aminoglycosides than for these divalent cations. Thus aminoglycosides can interact with such sites in a cooperative fashion to competitively displace the divalent cations, as shown in studies using fluorescent or spin label probes. Due to the bulky nature and higher positive charge of aminoglycosides relative to the displaced cations, the packing order of the LPS in the outer membrane is disturbed, as assessed using spin-label probes, and this can be observed electron microscopically as morphologial distortions (*e.g.*, blebs, cracks) at higher concentrations. This results in an increase in outer-membrane permeability toward at least three different probes: a chromogenic β-lactam nitrocefin; a hydrophobic fluorophor NPN; and lysozyme, an enzyme that digests the peptidoglycan. Such increased outer-membrane permeability is dependent upon the aminoglycoside concentration in a sigmoidal fashion and is blocked by excess divalent cations, suggesting that it is due to cooperative interactions at divalent cation binding sites. Consistent with this, LPS from the aminoglycoside supersusceptible *tolA* mutant binds aminoglycosides better than does wild-type LPS, and the *tolA* mutant is more susceptible to the effect of aminoglycosides on permeability. Furthermore, the relative ability of eight aminoglycosides to make permeable the outer membrane was found to be related to their MIC. For these reasons we have proposed[58,64] that aminoglycosides make permeable the outer membrane to other molecules of aminoglycoside, *i.e.* promote their own uptake.

3.3. Cytoplasmic Membrane Penetration

Aminoglycosides cross the cytoplasmic membrane of *P. aeruginosa* by two energy-dependent steps, the slow-EDPI and accelerated-EDPII phases. Bryan and collaborators[57,65] showed that both steps had similar features in both *P. aeruginosa* and *E. coli*, *i.e.* inhibition by divalent cations, uncouplers, and inhibitors of electron transport. In addition, streptomycin-resistant *rpsL* mutants of both bacteria did not initiate the EDPII phase of streptomycin uptake. Thus we can assume that aminoglycosides use similar pathways of energized uptake in both bacteria. Whereas the precise mechanism is unclear even in *E. coli* where it has been better studied, several features seem evident. First, aminoglycoside uptake in EDPII is kinetically unusual in that it is irreversible. Second, the major driving force for aminoglycoside uptake appears to be the electrical potential gradient (which is oriented interior negative) across the cytoplasmic membrane,[24,25,27] and uptake requires a threshold value of this potential. Third, there is an apparent requirement for electron transport independent of this electrical potential gradient. Bryan and Kwam[57] have proposed that this reflects the use, by aminoglycosides, of oxidized respiratory quinones as carriers.

3.4. Plasmid-Mediated Resistance

Plasmid-mediated resistance to aminoglycosides has been discussed in several excellent reviews[66,67] and we concern ourselves here with only those mechanisms that influence the widely-used anti-pseudomonal aminoglycosides gentamicin, tobramycin, and amikacin. The incidence of plasmid-mediated resistance is difficult to assess due to the existence in some cases of significant levels of non-plasmid-mediated low-level resistance.[66,68] In addition, there are large differences in reported incidences from study to study, possibly due to local outbreaks and/or poor antibiotic management.[69] Nevertheless the incidence of plasmid-mediated resistance usually ranges between 5 and 12% of all isolates.[69–71]

Plasmid-mediated aminoglycoside resistance in *P. aeruginosa* is often due to aminoglycoside-modifying enzymes. Such enzymes can transfer phosphate, acetyl, or nucleotidyl groups to specific sites on the aminoglycosides.[66,67] The sites of action of enzymes that specifically affect MIC for gentamicin, tobramycin, and/or amikacin in *Pseudomonas* are shown in Fig. 2. Other enzymes are specified in *P. aeruginosa* but do not affect resistance to these aminoglycosides.[72] In addition, a chromosomal gene can be amplified by mutation to result in aminoglycoside resistance although not to the above commonly used aminoglycosides.[73] Aminoglycoside-modifying enzymes apparently are located in the periplasm[74] and interact with aminoglycosides to reduce affinity for ribosomes and prevent the onset of EDPII.

3.5. Clinical Resistance Development

Three large published studies (Table III) have indicated that the frequency of gentamicin resistance among *P. aeruginosa* isolates is *ca.* 5–10%,[69,70] whereas a task force study from 13 centers worldwide indicated levels of

TABLE III
Aminoglycoside Resistance in *Pseudomonas aeruginosa*[69,70]

Date of survey	Location	Number of isolates examined	% isolates resistant to gentamicin
1981	Switzerland	2235	5.9
1984	U.K.	1866	5.5
1983–84	Netherlands	2635	10.1

resistance from 9–20%.[73] However, higher resistance levels were observed in some centers.[67,69,71] There are two major causes of resistance. These include high-level enzymatic resistance, as described above, and so-called permeability or non-enzymatic resistance. The former high-level resistance is specific (Fig. 2); Thus often it can be overcome by merely changing the aminoglycoside administered. However, nonenzymatic resistance, although it causes lower level resistance, is still clinically significant and is of substantial concern because it results in cross-resistance to all aminoglycosides.[67,68] Either mechanism can predominate in a given center for unknown reasons.[67–69] It should be noted, however, that aminoglycoside resistance apparently can be reduced when a β-lactam is co-administered.[75]

Nonenzymatic (impermeability-mediated) resistance has been studied by Bryan and colleagues in some detail. It was found to be associated with diminished energized uptake of streptomycin[76] and gentamicin[74] but no evidence was found for resistant ribosomes, enzymatic inactivation, slower growth rate, or R factors. It was shown in one isolate that impermeability-type resistance was associated with a smooth-to-rough transition in the LPS (*i.e.* loss of O antigen).[77] On the basis of the known mechanism of uptake of aminoglycosides across the *P. aeruginosa* outer membrane, we propose that this LPS alteration decreases the affinity of LPS for aminoglycosides, resulting in lower levels of uptake due to reduced self-promoted uptake across the outer membrane. Such resistance has not been modeled in the laboratory. When serial subcultures of *P. aeruginosa* are exposed to increasing levels of aminoglycosides, isolates are obtained with high levels of resistance to all aminoglycosides, markedly slower growth rates, reduced virulence in mice, and acquisition of undefined growth requirements.[78] Some of these properties were shown by a mutant isolated by Bryan *et al.*[79] This mutant proved to have a decrease in the activity of cytochrome C_{552} a component of nitrate reductase. This in turn led to a specific alteration in energized aminoglycoside transport. Although such a resistance mechanism has not been shown *in vivo* it seems to fit with the proposals of Bryan with regard to phenotypic adaptation (persistence) in the CF lung.[63]

Animal models have been used to demonstrate another type of resistance, adaptive resistance.[80–82] In these studies it was shown that inoculum and time of initiation of treatment after infection substantially influenced the ability of aminoglycosides to inhibit the growth of *P. aeruginosa*. A delay in the initiation of aminoglycoside therapy of as little as 2 hr, had an enormous effect on the rate of recovery of organisms.[81] Such resistance was phenotypic rather than due to mutation and reversed *in vitro*.[81,82] One potential cause was oxygen limitation, since the presence of *Pseudomonas in vivo* at a localized infection site led to decreased oxygen tension, a factor that increased the MIC *in vitro* 16-fold.[82] Such a phenotypic resistance mechanism could result in the dissociation of *in vivo* and *in vitro* antibiotic susceptibility of *P. aeruginosa*, a phenomenon observed previously.[63,80] Similar considerations may apply to the observed high resistance of *P. aeruginosa* associated with catheter materials.[83] Reduced oxygen tensions within the thick adherent biofilm and/or reduced metabolic capacity could in this instance explain the observed aminoglycoside resistance (and consequently the failures of antibiotic chemotherapy in catheter-associated urinary tract infections).

4. QUINOLONES

4.1. Determinants of Efficacy

One of the major hopes for chemotherapy of *P. aeruginosa* infections in recent years has been the introduction of fluoroquinolones. Although a large variety of related antibiotics have been introduced, we will largely restrict our discussion here to ciprofloxacin, which remains the quinolone with the lowest MIC for *P. aeruginosa* (Table I); as the first such compound introduced into clinical practice, it is the most-used in therapy. Despite the low MIC[90] for *P. aeruginosa in vitro* (*ca.* 0.25–1 μg/ml), therapeutic results have sometimes been disappointing, in large part due to resistance development.[84–89] Nevertheless, in CF patients, despite a rarity of bacteriological cures and high incidence of resistance development, there is often an improvement in lung function with ciprofloxacin therapy.[87,88] Combinations of ciprofloxacin with other agents usually has an additive, rather than synergistic effect,[90] and resistance to ciprofloxacin can develop in CF patients.

The probable target of ciprofloxacin, as with other quinolones, appears to be the A subunit of DNA gyrase. Thus the concentration of ciprofloxacin causing 50% inhibition of DNA synthesis in *P. aeruginosa* made permeable by EDTA[91] equates well with the MIC, whereas *gyr A* mutants with alterations in DNA gyrase subunit A (Table IV) have eight-fold or greater increases in MIC. However, the binding site still remains a source of controversy. Whether quinolones bind directly to DNA gyrase or to the tertiary DNA gyrase–DNA complex remains to be determined.[95] The involvement of SOS DNA repair response in quinolone action is also under active investigation.[95]

A point of major concern is whether MIC performed *in vitro* on normal media accurately reflect *in vivo* susceptibility. Similar concerns were previously expressed for aminoglycoside antibiotics. For example, it has been demonstrated that cation supplementation,[91,92] in addition to low pH,[92] increased the MIC of ciprofloxacin and other quinolones about two- to eight-fold depending on the medium. This might substantially increase the MIC for clinical isolates to a level outside the clinically achievable range.

4.2. Uptake Across the Outer Membrane

Several studies have shown that the outer membrane of *P. aeruginosa* is a significant barrier to quinolone uptake. In particular, Kubesch *et al.*[93] dem-

TABLE IV
Genetically Mapped Quinolone-Resistant Mutants of *P. aeruginosa* Strain PAO[96,104,105]

Mutation	Genetic Map Position (min)	Altered Phenotype	Times increase in MIC relative to wild-type[a]						
			CIP	NOR	NAL	CB	CAP	GM	IMP
gyr A (= *nalA,cfxA nfxA*)	39	DNA gyrase subunit A	8×	8×	64×	1×	1×	1×	ND
nalB (= *cfxB*)	20	Transport; OM protein over-produced	8×	4×	8×	4×	8×	0.5×	1×
nfxB	0	Transport; OM protein over-produced	8×	16×	2×	0.25×	1×	0.25×	0.5×
nfxC	46	Transport; OM altered	16×	32×	16×	0.5×	>2×	0.25×	8×

[a]CIP = ciprofloxacin; NOR = norfloxacin; NAL = nalidixic acid; CB = carbanicillin; CAP = chloramphenicol; GM = gentamicin; IMP = imipenem.

onstrated that the outer membrane permeabilizer polymyxin B nonapeptide decreased the MIC, for *P. aeruginosa* strains, of ciprofloxacin, norfloxacin and ofloxacin by two- to 40-fold whereas nalidixic-acid MIC were decreased more than 100-fold. In addition, Bedard et al.[91] demonstrated that the permeabilizer EDTA lowered the ciprofloxacin concentration required to observe inhibition of DNA synthesis by five-fold. Our own data has shown that overexpression of outer-membrane protein OprH in the regulatory mutant strain H181 or from the cloned gene decreased quinolone MIC eight to 16-fold when compared with the isogenic wild-type strain H103 (R.E.W. Hancock and M. Bains, unpublished data). In contrast to these data, there is considerably less evidence that the outer membrane of wild-type *E. coli* strains forms a substantial barrier to fluoroquinolones.[91,94] Although, the IC_{50} of ciprofloxacin for *E. coli* NT525[95] and *P. aeruginosa* MP-001[96] DNA gyrase in supercoiling assays is similar, the MIC are 100-fold higher for *P. aeruginosa*, demonstrating the importance of low permeability in this species. Also *gyr A* mutants of these strains have similar IC_{50} values but MIC that are 100-fold different.[95,96]

The mechanism of uptake of fluoroquinolones across the outer membrane of *P. aeruginosa* remains a mystery. Several mechanisms have been suggested. These include self-promoted uptake (divalent cations antagonize killing and uptake).[91,93,97] However, our own studies (unpublished data) have shown that quinolones cause none of the increases in outer-membrane permeability that are symptomatic of interaction of aminoglycosides with the outer membrane, whereas outer-membrane mutants, resistant to aminoglycosides by virtue of OprH overproduction,[64] are supersusceptible to fluoroquinolones. Other researchers have suggested that *P. aeruginosa* outer-membrane protein OprF is responsible for fluoroquinolone uptake, based on the fact that clinical resistant mutants lacking OprF have been demonstrated in some studies.[98–100] This has been contradicted by Chamberland et al.[101] who showed no correlation between quinolone resistance and OprF deficiency in one clinical isolate and its derivatives, whereas Woodruff and Hancock[102] concluded that OprF-deficient strains had such severe structural defects that they did not permit definitive conclusions to be made regarding antibiotic permeation. Nevertheless, it seems possible that OprF deficiency does give rise to fluoroquinolone resistance *in vivo*; otherwise it is difficult to understand why fluoroquinolone therapy should give rise to such mutants. This scenario would be appropriate if we assume that *in vitro* experiments do not accurately reflect *in vivo* conditions and susceptibility; one problem with clinical mutants is that one often observes multiple alterations.[100] Thus the association between any one alteration and quinolone resistance should rely on a series of isogenic strains. In this regard, the relationship (or lack of relationship) between LPS phenotype and ciprofloxacin resistance[101,103] requires further study. Three other genetically defined ciprofloxacin-resistant mutants, *nalB*, *nfxB* and *nfxC*, have been ascribed to outer membrane alterations[96,103,104] (Table IV). In the former two, which map separately, outer-membrane proteins with different molecular weights (51kDa and 54 kDa) have been reported to be overproduced.[96,104] However, no formal proof exists that this overproduction of an outer-membrane protein directly results in the observed decrease in quinolone uptake and quinolone resistance. For example, a regulatory mutation giving rise to ciprofloxacin resistance and overexpression of a 60-kDa GroEL-like protein has been observed in *E. coli*.[106] Other authors have demonstrated alterations in minor outer-membrane proteins that correlate with ciprofloxacin resistance[105,107,108]; one of these, *nfxC*, is well characterized genetically.[105] These authors have suggested the involvement of outer-membrane proteins OprG and a 40-kDa minor outer-membrane protein,[107] OprC, OprD, and OprE[108] or underexpression of OprD (and OprG) but overexpression of a 50-kDa outer-membrane protein.[105] These alterations are not consistent either with one another or with the other mutants described above. Thus we conclude that current data is insufficient to define the mechanism of uptake of quinolones across the outer membrane. If the critical alterations are indeed in the outer membrane, a major possibility would be the involvement of LPS in quinolone uptake since (1) LPS structure can be altered by numerous individual gene mutations; and (2) LPS mutants of *P. aeruginosa* show alterations in outer-membrane protein profiles.[109]

4.3. Assays of Quinolone Uptake

The literature on quinolone uptake both in *P. aeruginosa* and *E. coli* is remarkably inconsistent[e.g. 91,94,105,110] Examples include: the substantial backgrounds (*i.e.* zero time values although these can be partly suppressed by increasingly vigorous washing); frequent lack of observed time kinetics; variable effects of CCCP and other inhibitors; differences in uptake conditions required to show transport defects in ciprofloxacin-resistant mutants; lack of correlation between whole-cell inhibitory concentrations in intact cells and MIC in *P. aeruginosa* (cf. *E. coli*); inconsistencies between concentrations resulting in DNA-gyrase inhibition and MIC in *E. coli*,[95] suggesting concentrative uptake, and the linearity of uptake levels as a function of ciprofloxacin concentration, that is more consistent with simple or facilitated diffusion; disparities in one study between Mg^{2+} effects on MIC and lack of Mg^{2+} inhibition of uptake; lack of correlation in *P. aeruginosa* cf. *E. coli* of MIC with measured rates of uptake. Detailed studies have been performed in *P. aeruginosa* by Bedard *et al.*[91] and in *E. coli* by Diver *et al.*[94] However, we do not feel that it has been clearly demonstrated that productive ciprofloxacin uptake (leading to internalization and target inhibition) has been demonstrated or measured. Clearly this awaits the isolation of strains with mutations specifically influencing trans-cytoplasmic membrane uptake. Nevertheless, it is difficult to see how hydrophilic molecules such as quinolones could be taken up by simple diffusion across the cytoplasmic membrane, as suggested by some authors.

4.4. Mechanisms of Resistance

The common occurrence of quinolone resistance during clinical therapy of *P. aeruginosa* infections by quinolones, has led to a large number of *in vivo* studies attempting to define resistance mechanisms. These are summarized in Table V, where we have attempted to correlate findings with the genetically well-characterized mutants. The most complete study was recently presented by Yoshida *et al.*[100] who used the *E. coli gyrA* or *gyrB* genes in an attempt to complement mutants with alterations in these genes in *P. aeruginosa* quinolone-resistant mutants isolated after clinical therapy. Among 17 resistant clinical strains, 12 bore a *gyrA* mutation and one a *gyrB* mutation. At least two of the *gyrA*-altered mutant strains and the *gyrB* mutant apparently had other underlying mutations.

Whereas many well-defined mutants exist, it is not uncommon for resistant isolates to revert, post-therapy, to susceptibility levels similar to or at least closer to those of pre-therapy isolates.[63,101] Two explanations are possible. One is that such resistant isolates (termed persisters by Bryan[63]) have phenotypic adaptations (as opposed to mutations) that allow them to resist

TABLE V
Analysis of Other Quinolone-Resistant Mutants of *Pseudomonas aeruginosa*

Isolation[a]	Selecting quinolone[b]	Tentative identification[c]	Other properties	Ref.
Clinic	CIP	gyrA[d]	rough LPS	110
Clinic	—[e]	gyrA[d,f]	—	100
Clinic	CIP	gyrA[d,f]	OprF−	101
Clinc	ENOX	gyrA[f]	OprF−	98
Clinic	—[e]	gyrB[d,f]	—	100
Animals	PER	gyrA[d]	rough LPS	107
Animals	VAR	gyrA	—	111
Animals	PER/CIP	nfxC[f]	—	112
In vitro	NAL/ENOX	gyrA[d]	—	100
In vitro	CIP/NOR	gyrA	—	113
In vitro	CIP	gyrA	—	103
In vitro	CIP	nalB[f]	rough LPS	103
In vitro	NAL	nalB	—	100
In vitro	CIP	nalB	= Qr2	107
In vitro	CIP	nfxC	= Qr1; OprG reduced; 40 K minus	207
In vitro	ENOX	nfxB[f]	—	100

[a]Clinic = isolates arising during clinical therapy; animals = isolate arising during experimental therapy of animals; *In vitro* = laboratory selected isolates.
[b]Abbreviations as per Table IV; PER = pefloxacin; ENOX = enoxacin; VAR = various quinolones used.
[c]Identification based on MIC and phenotypic descriptions in ref. 63, 70, 71, and Table IV.
[d]Confirmed genetically or by DNA gyrase assays.
[e]Not described.
[f]One or two MIC differences for non-quinolone antibiotics observed.

killing by the quinolone. Withdrawal of the adaptive pressure causes the organism to return to the pre-therapy state. An alternative explanation is that these are true genetic mutants that, upon therapeutic failure and subsequent discontinuation of the therapy, could revert. The revertant would then overgrow the mutant as long as it could grow more rapidly *in vivo* (as suggested by Bryan[63]). The high frequency of selection of quinolone-resistant mutants *in vitro* (10^{-5} to 10^{-7} in two studies[99,111]) and an expected similar frequency of back mutations, make this a distinct possibility.

ACKNOWLEDGEMENTS. The authors wish to acknowledge the Canadian Cystic Fibrosis Foundation, who financially supported most of the authors' work described herein, and who are providing support in the form of a fellowship to F.B.

REFERENCES

1. Brown, A. G., 1982, β-lactam nomenclature, *J. Antimicrob. Chemother.* **10**:365–372.
2. Parry, M. F., and Neu, H. C. 1976, Ticarcillin for treatment of serious infections with gram-negative bacteria, *J. Infect. Dis.* **134**:476–480.

3. Bryan, L. E. (ed.), 1989, *Microbial Resistance to Drugs*, Springer-Verlag, Berlin.
4. Neu, H. C., 1989, Penicillins, in: *Principles and Practice of Infectious Diseases*, (G.L. Mandell, ed.), Churchill Livingstone, New York, pp. 230–246.
5. Neu, H. C., Chiu, N.-X., and Novelli, A., 1988, In vitro activity of E-1040, a novel cephalosporin with potent activity against *Pseudomonas aeruginosa, Antimicrob. Agents Chemother.* **32:**1666–1675.
6. Nakagawa, S., Sanada, M., Matsuda, K., Hashizume, T., Asahi, Y., Ushijima, R., Ohtake, N., and Tanaka, N., 1979, *In vitro* and *in vivo* antibacterial activities of BO-1341, a new antipseudomonal cephalosporin, *Antimicrob. Agents Chemother.* **33:**1423–1427.
7. Rolinson, G. N., 1986, β-lactam antibiotics, *J. Antimicrob. Chemother.* **17:**5–36.
8. Ristuccia, A. M., and Cunha, B. A. (eds.), 1984, *Antimicrobial Therapy*, Raven Press, New York.
9. Nikaido, H., and Normark, S., 1987, Sensitivity of *Escherichia coli* to various β-lactams is determined by the interplay of outer membrane permeability and degradation by periplasmic β-lactamases: A quantitative predictive treatment, *Mol. Microbiol.* **1:**29–36.
10. Zimmermann, W., and Rosselet, A., 1977, Function of the outer membrane of *Escherichia coli* as a permeability barrier to β-lactam antibiotics, *Antimicrob. Agents Chemother.* **12:** 368–372.
11. Nikaido, H., and Hancock, R. E. W., 1986, Outer membrane permeability of *Pseudomonas aeruginosa*, in: *The Bacteria*, Vol. 10 (J. R. Sokatch, ed.), Academic Press, Orlando, pp. 145–193.
12. Hancock, R. E. W., 1987, Role of porins in outer membrane permeability, *J. Bacteriol.* **169:** 929–933.
13. Hancock, R. E. W., Siehnel, R., and Martin, N., 1990, Outer membrane proteins of *Pseudomonas, Mol. Microb.* **4:**1069–1075.
14. Nikaido, H., 1989, Role of the outer membrane of gram-negative bacteria in antimicrobial resistance, in: *Microbial Resistance to Drugs* (L. E. Bryan, ed.), Springer-Verlag, Berlin, pp. 1–34.
15. Nikaido, H., and Vaara, M., 1985, Molecular basis of bacterial outer membrane permeability, *Microbiol. Rev.* **49:**1–32.
16. Woodruff, W., and Hancock, R. E. W., 1989, *Pseudomonas aeruginosa* outer membrane protein F: Structural role and relationship to the *E. coli* OmpA protein, *J. Bacteriol.* **171:** 3304–3309.
17. Gotoh, N., Wakebe, H., Yoshihara, E., Nakae, T., and Nishino, T., 1989, Role of protein F in maintaining structural integrity of the *P. aeruginosa* outer membrane. *J. Bacteriol.* **171:** 983–990.
18. Siehnel, R. J., Martin, N. L., and Hancock, R. E. W., 1990, Function and structure of the porin proteins OprF and OprP of *P. aeruginosa*, in: *Pseudomonas* (S. Silver, ed.), Am. Soc. Microbiol., Washington, pp. 328–342.
19. Yoshihara, E., and Nakae, T., 1989, Identification of porins in the outer membrane of *P. aeruginosa* that form small diffusion pores, *J. Biol. Chem.* **264:**6297–6301.
19a. Bellido, F., Martin, N. L., Siehnel, R. J., and Hancock, R. E. W., 1992, Reevaluation, using intact cells, of the exclusion limit and role of porin OprF in *Pseudomonas aeruginosa* outer membrane permeability. *J. Bacteriol.* **174:**5196–5203.
20. Trias, J., and Nikaido, H., 1990, Diffusion of antibiotics via specific pathways across the outer membrane of *P. aeruginosa*, in: *Pseudomonas* (S. Silver, ed.), Am. Soc. Microbiol., Washington, pp. 319–327.
21. Watanabe, N., Nagasu, T., Katsu, K., and Kitoh, K. 1987, E-0702, a new cephalosporin, is incorporated into *E. coli* cells via the *ton-b*-dependent iron transport system. *Antimicrob. Agents Chemother.* **31:**497–504.
22. Angus, B. L., Carey, A. M., Caron, D. A., Kropinski, A. M. B., and Hancock, R. E. W., 1982, Outer membrane permeability of *Pseudomonas aeruginosa* comparison of a wild-type with an antibiotic-supersusceptible mutant, *Antimicrob. Agents Chemother.* **21:**299–309.

23. Yoshimura, F., and Nikaido, H., 1982, Permeability of *Pseudomonas aeruginosa* outer membrane to hydrophilic solutes, *J. Bacteriol.* **152**:636–642.
24. Bellido, F., Pechère, J. C., and Hancock, R. E. W., 1990, Novel method for measurement of outer membrane permeability in intact *Enterobacter cloacae* strains cells, *Antimicrob. Agents Chemother.*, in press.
25. Hewinson, R. G., Lane, D. C., Slack, M. P. E., and Nichols, W. W., 1986, The permeability parameter of outer membrane of *P. aeruginosa* varies with the concentration of a test substrate cephalosporin C, *J. Gen. Microbiol.* **132**:27–33.
26. Nikaido, H., Liu, W., and Rosenberg, E. Y., 1990, Outer membrane permeability and β-lactamase stability of dipolar ionic cephalosporins containing methoxyimino substituents, *Antimicrob. Agents Chemother.* **34**:337–342.
27. Sabath, L. D., Jago, M., and Abraham, E. P., 1965, Cephalosporinase and penicillinase activities of a β-lactamase from *Pseudomonas pyocyanea*, *Biochem. J.* **96**:739–752.
28. Richmond, M. H., and Sykes, R. B., 1973, The β-lactamases of Gram-negative bacteria and their possible physiological role, *Adv. Microbiol. Physiol.* **9**:31–88.
29. Sanders, C. C., 1989, The chromosomal β-lactamases, in: *Microbial Resistance to Drugs* (L. E. Bryan, ed.), Springer-Verlag, Berlin, pp. 129–149.
30. Matthew, M., and Harris, A. M., 1976, Identification of β-lactamases by analytical isoelectric focusing: Correlation with bacterial taxonomy, *J. Gen. Microbiol.* **94**:55–67.
31. Livermore, D. M., and Yang, Y. J., 1987, β-lactamase lability and inducer power of newer β-lactam antibiotics in relation to their activity against β-lactamase-inducibility mutants of *Pseudomonas aeruginosa*, *J. Infect. Dis.* **155**:775–782.
32. Then, R. L., and Angehrn, P., 1982, Trapping of nonhydrolyzable cephalosporins in *Enterobacter cloacae* and *Pseudomonas aeruginosa* as a possible resistance mechanism, *Antimicrob. Agents Chemother.* **21**:711–717.
33. Bellido, F., Pechère, J. C., and Hancock, R. E. W., 1990, Reevaluation of the factors involved in the efficacy of new β-lactams in *Enterobacter cloacae*, *Antimicrob. Agents Chemother.*, in press.
34. Noguchi, M. H., Matsuhashi, M., and Mutsuhashi, S., 1979, Comparable studies of penicillin-binding proteins in *Pseudomonas aeruginosa* and *Escherichia coli*, *Eur. J. Biochem.* **100**:41–49.
35. Noguchi, H., Fukasawa, M., Komatsu, T., Mitsuhashi, S., and Matsuhashi, M., 1985, Mutation in *P. aeruginosa* causing simultaneous defects in PBP-5 and in enzyme activities of penicillin release and D-alanine carboxy peptidase, *J. Bacteriol.* **162**:849–851.
36. Bellido, F., Veuthey, C., Blaser, J., Bauernfeind, A., and Pechère, J. C., 1990, Novel resistance to imipenem associated with an altered PBP-4 in a *Pseudomonas aeruginosa* clinical isolate, *J. Antimicrob. Chemother.* **25**:57–68.
37. Hancock, R. E. W., 1986, Intrinsic antibiotic resistance of *Pseudomonas aeruginosa*, *J. Antimicrob. Chemother.* **18**:653–656.
38. Hancock, R. E. W., and Woodruff, W. A., 1988, Roles of porin and β-lactamase in β-lactam resistance of *Pseudomonas aeruginosa*, *Rev. Infect. Dis.* **10**:770–775.
39. Pitt, T. L., Livermore, D. M., Miller, G., Vatopoulos, A., and Legakis, N. J., 1990, Resistance mechanisms of multiresistant serotype 012 *Pseudomonas aeruginosa* isolated in Europe, *J. Antimicrob. Chemother.* **26**:319–328.
40. Milatovic, D., and Braveny, A., 1987, Development of resistance during antibiotic therapy, *Eur. J. Clin. Microbiol.* **6**:234–244.
41. Schryvers, A. B., Ogunariwo, J., Chamberland, S., Godfrey, A. J., Rabin, H. R., and Bryan, L. E., 1987 Mechanism of *Pseudomonas aeruginosa*, persistence during treatment with broad-spectrum cephalosporins of lung infections in patients with cystic fibrosis, *Antimicrob. Agents Chemother.* **31**:1438–1439.
42. Bayer, A. S., Peters, J., Parr, T. R., Jr., Chan, L., and Hancock R. E. W., 1987, Role of β-lactamase in *in vivo* development of ceftazidime resistance in experimental *Pseudomonas aeruginosa* endocarditis, *Antimicrob. Agents Chemother.* **31**:253–258.

43. Giwercman, B., Lambert, P. A., Rosdahl, V. T., Shand, G. H., and Høiby, N., 1990, Rapid emergence of resistance to *Pseudomonas aeruginosa* in cystic fibrosis patients due to *in vivo* selection of stable partially derepressed β-lactamase producing strains, *J. Antimicrob. Chemother.* **26**:247–259.
44. Fung-Tomc, J., Huczko, E., Pearce, M., and Kessler, R. E., 1988, Frequency of *in vitro* resistance of *Pseudomonas aeruginosa* to cefepime, ceftazidime and cefotaxime, *Antimicrob. Agents Chemother.* **32**:1443–1445.
45. Godfrey, A. J., Hatlelid, L., and Bryan, L. E., 1984, Correlation between lipopolysaccharide structure and permeability resistance in β-lactam-resistant *P. aeruginosa*, *Antimicrob. Agents Chemother.* **26**:181–186.
46. Godfrey, A. J., and Bryan, L. E., 1987, Penetration of β-lactams through *Pseudomonas aeruginosa* porin channels. *Antimicrob. Agents Chemother.* **31**:1216–1221.
47. Quinn, J. P., Dudeck, E. J., Di Vincenzo, C. A., Lucks, D. A., and Lerner, S. A., 1986, Emergence of resistance of imipenem during therapy for *Pseudomonas aeruginosa* infections, *J. Infect. Dis.* **154**:289–294.
48. Büscher, K.-H., Cullmann, W., Dick, W., and Opferkuch, W., 1987, Imipenem resistance in *Pseudomonas aeruginosa* resulting from diminished expression of an outer membrane proteins, *Antimicrob. Agents Chemother.* **31**:703–708.
49. Mirelman, D., Nuchamowitz, Y., and Rubinstein, E., 1981, Insensitivity of peptidoglycan biosynthetic reactions to β-lactam antibiotics in a clinical isolate of *Pseudomonas aeruginosa*, *Antimicrob. Agents Chemother.* **19**:681–695.
50. Godfrey, A. J., Bryan, L. E., and Rabin, H. R., 1981, β-lactam-resistant *Pseudomonas aeruginosa* with modified penicillin-binding proteins emerging during cystic fibrosis treatment, *Antimicrob. Agents Chemother.* **19**:705–711.
51. Lorian, V. (ed.), 1986, *Antibiotics in Laboratory Medicine*, Williams & Wilkins, Baltimore.
52. Then, R. L., and Kohl, I., 1985, Affinity for penicillin-binding proteins, *Chemotherapy* **31**:246–254.
53. Young, L. S., Wenzel, R. P., Sabath, L. D., Pollack, M., Pennington, J. E., and Platt, R., 1984, The outlook for prevention and treatment of infections due to *Pseudomonas aeruginosa*, *Rev. Infect. Dis.* **6**:S769–S774.
54. Ristuccia, A. M., and Cunha, B. A., 1982, The aminoglycosides. *Med. Clin. N. Am.* **66**:303–312.
55. Stephens, D., Garey, N., and Isels, A. F., 1983, Efficacy of inhaled tobramycin in the treatment of pulmonary exacerbations in children with cystic fibrosis, *Pediatr. Infect.* **2**:209–211.
56. Rabin, H. R., Harley, F. L., Bryan, L. E. and Elfring, G., 1980, Evaluation of a high dose tobramycin and ticarcillin treatment protocol in cystic fibrosis based on improved susceptibility criteria and antibiotic pharmacokinetics, in: *Perspectives in Cystic Fibrosis* (J. Sturgess, ed.), Canadian Cystic Fibrosis Foundation, Toronto, pp. 370–375.
57. Bryan, L. E., and Kwan, S., 1983, Roles of ribosomal binding, membrane potential, and electron transport in bacterial uptake of streptomycin and gentamicin, *Antimicrob. Agents Chemother.* **23**:835–845.
58. Hancock, R. E. W., 1981, Aminoglycoside uptake and mode of action—with special reference to streptomycin and gentamicin. I. Antagonists and mutants, *J. Antimicrob. Chemother.* **8**:249–276.
59. Hancock, R. E. W., 1981, Aminoglycoside uptake and mode of action—with special reference to streptomycin and gentamicin. II. Effects of aminoglycosides on cells, *J. Antimicrob. Chemother.* **8**:429–445.
60. Taber, H. W., Mueller, J. P., Miller, P. F., and Arrow, A. S., 1987, Bacterial uptake of aminoglycoside antibiotics, *Microbiol. Rev.* **51**:439–457.
61. Davis, B. D., Chen, L., and Tai, P. C., 1986, Misread protein creates membrane channels: An essential step in the bactericidal action of aminoglycosides, *Proc. Natl. Sci. USA* **83**:6164–6168.

62. Matsunaga, K., Yamaki, H., Nishimura, T., and Tanaka, N., 1986, Inhibition of DNA replication initiation by aminoglycoside antibiotics, *Antimicrobiol. Agents Chemother.* **30**:468–474.
63. Bryan, L. E., 1990, Microbial persistence or phenotypic adaptation to antimicrobial agents, cystic fibrosis as an illustrative case. in: *Microbial Resistance to Drugs* (L. E. Bryan, ed.), Springer-Verlag KG, Berlin, pp. 411–420.
64. Hancock, R. E. W., and Bell, A., 1988, Antibiotic uptake into gram-negative bacteria, *Europ. J. Clin. Microbiol. Infect. Dis.* **7**:713–720.
65. Bryan, L. E., and van den Elzen, H. M., 1977, Effects of membrane-energy mutations and cations or streptomycin and gentamicin accumulation by bacteria: A model for entry of streptomycin and gentamicin in susceptible and resistant bacteria, *Antimicrob. Agents Chemother.* **12**:163–177.
66. Phillips, I., and Shannon, K., 1984, Aminoglycoside resistance, *Brit. Med. Bull.* **40**:28–35.
67. Miller, G. H., Sabatelli, F. J., Hare, R. S., and Waitz, J. A., 1980, Survey of aminoglycoside resistance patterns, *Dev. Indust. Microbiol.* **21**:91–104.
68. Bryan, L. E., Shahrabadi, M. S., and van den Elzen, H. M., 1974, Gentamicin resistance in *Pseudomonas aeruginosa*: R-factor-mediated resistance, *Antimicrob. Agents Chemother.* **6**:191–199.
69. Williams, R. J., 1988, Epidemiology of antibiotic resistance in gram-negative bacteria, *J. Hosp. Infect.* (Suppl. A) **22**:130–134.
70. de Neeling, A. J., Rutgers, A., Schot, C. S., van Klingeren, B., 1987, Survey of resistance of *Pseudomonas aeruginosa* to aminoglycosides and β-lactam antibiotics in the Netherlands, *J. Antimicrob. Chemother.* **19**:703–706.
71. O'Brien, T. F., 1987, Resistance of bacteria to antibacterial agents: Report of task force 2, *Rev. Infect. Dis.* **9**:S244–S260.
72. Phillips, I., King, B. A., and Shannon, K. P., 1978, The mechanisms of resistance to aminoglycosides in the genus *Pseudomonas*, *J. Antimicrob. Chemother.* **4**:121–129.
73. Okii, M., Iyobe, S., and Mitsuhashi, S., 1983, Mapping of a gene specifying aminoglycoside 3'-phosphotransferase II in the *Pseudomonas aeruginosa* chromosome, *J. Bacteriol.* **155**:643–649.
74. Dickie, P., Bryan, L. E., and Pickard, M. A., 1978, Effect of enzymatic adenylation on dihydrostreptomycin accumulation in *Escherichia coli* carrying an R-factor model explaining aminoglycoside resistance by inactivating mechanisms, *Antimicrob. Agents Chemother.* **14**:569–580.
75. Johnson, D., 1985, Use of discriminative models of *Pseudomonas aeruginosa* bacteremia in granulocytopenic rats for testing antimicrobial efficacy, *Eur. J. Clin. Microbiol.* **4**:207–212.
76. Tseng, J. T., Bryan, L. E., and van den Elzen, H. M., 1972, Mechanisms and spectrum of streptomycin resistance in a natural population of *Pseudomonas aeruginosa*, *Antimicrob. Agents Chemother.* **2**:136–141.
77. Bryan, L. E., O'Hara, K., and Wong, S., 1984, Lipopolysaccharide changes in impermeability-type aminoglycoside resistance in *Pseudomonas aeruginosa*, *Antimicrob. Agents Chemother.* **26**:250–255.
78. Weinstein, M. J., Drube, C. G., Moss, E. L. Jr., and Waitz, J. A., 1971, Microbiologic studies related to bacterial resistance to gentamicin, *J. Infect. Dis.* **124**:S11–S17.
79. Bryan, L. E., Nicas, T., Holloway, B. W., and Crowther, C., 1980, Aminoglycoside-resistant mutation of *Pseudomonas aeruginosa* defective in cytochrome C_{552} and nitrate reductase, *Antimicrob. Agents Chemother.* **17**:71–79.
80. Davis, S. D., 1974, Dissociation between results of *in vitro* and *in vivo* antibiotic susceptibility tests for some strains of *Pseudomonas aeruginosa*, *Antimicrob. Agents Chemother.* **5**:281–288.
81. Kelly, N. M., Rawling, E. G., and Hancock, R. E. W., 1989, Determinants of the efficacy of tobramycin therapy against isogenic non mucoid and mucoid derivatives of *Pseudomonas aeruginosa* PAO1 growing in peritoneal chambers in mice, *Antimicrob. Agents Chemother.* **33**:1207–1211.

82. Davey, P., Barza, M., and Stuart, M., 1988, Tolerance of *Pseudomonas aeruginosa* to killing by ciprofloxacin, gentamicin and imipenem *in vitro* and *in vivo*, *J. Antimicrob. Chemother.* **21:** 395–404.
83. Nickel, J. C., Wright, J. B., Ruseska, I., Marrie, T. J., Whitfield, C., and Costerton, J. W., 1985, Antibiotic resistance of *Pseudomonas aeruginosa*, *Eur. J. Clin. Microbiol.* **4:**213–218.
84. Malinverni, R., and Glauser, M. P., 1988, Comparative studies of fluoroquinolones in the treatment of urinary tract infections, *Rev. Infect. Dis.* **10:**S153–S163.
85. Desplaces, N., and Acar, J. F., 1988, New quinolones in the treatment of join and bone infections, *Rev. Infect. Dis.* **10:**S179–S183.
86. Wolfson, J. S., and Hooper, D. C., 1989, Bacterial resistance to quinolones: Mechanisms and clinical importance, *Rev. Infect. Dis.* **11:**S960–S968.
87. Raeburn, J. A., Govan, J. R. W., McCrae, W. M., Greening, A. P., Collier, P. S., Hodson, M. E., Goodchild, M. C., 1987, Ciprofloxacin therapy in cystic fibrosis, *J. Antimicrob. Chemother.* **20:** 295–296.
88. Grenier, B., 1989, Use of the new quinolones in cystic fibrosis, *Rev. Infect. Dis.* **11:**S1245–S1252.
89. Davies, B. I., and Maesen, F. P. V., 1986, Quinolones in chest infections, *J. Antimicrob. Chemother.* **18:**296–299.
90. Neu, H. C., 1989, Synergy of fluoroquinolones with other antimicrobial agents, *Rev. Infect. Dis.* **11:**S1025–S1025.
91. Bedard, J., Chamberland, S., Wong, S., Schollaardt, T., and Bryan, L. E., 1989, Contribution of permeability and sensitivity to inhibition of DNA synthesis in determining susceptibilities of *Escherichia coli*, *Pseudomonas aeruginosa* and *Alcaligenes faecalis* to ciprofloxacin, *Antimicrob. Agents Chemother.* **33:**1457–1464.
92. Blaser, J., and Lüthy, R., 1988, Comparative study on antagonistic effects of low pH and cation supplementation on *in vitro* activity of quinolones and aminoglycosides against *Pseudomonas aeruginosa*, *J. Antimicrob. Chemother.* **22:**15–22.
93. Kubesch, P., Wehsling, M., and Tümber, B., 1987, Membrane permeability of *Pseudomonas aeruginosa* to 4-quinolones, *Zentralbl. Bakteriol. Hyg. A* **265:**197–202.
94. Diver, J. M., Piddock, L. J. V., and Wise, R., 1990, The accumulation of 5-quinolone antibacterial agents by *Escherichia coli*, *J. Antimicrob. Chemother.* **25:**319–333.
95. Hooper, D. C., Wolfson, J. S., Ng, E. Y., and Swartz, M. N., 1989, Mechanisms of action of and resistance to ciprofloxacin, *Amer. J. Med.* (suppl 4A) **82:**12–20.
96. Robillard, N. J., and Scarpa, A. L., 1988, Genetic and physiological characterization of ciprofloxacin resistance in *Pseudomonas aeruginosa* PAO, *Antimicrob. Agents Chemother.* **32:** 535–539.
97. Chapman, J. S., and Georgopapadakou, N. H., 1988, Routes of quinolone permeation into *Escherichia coli*, *Antimicrob. Agents Chemother.* **32:**438–442.
98. Piddock, L. J. V., Wijnands, W. J. A., and Wise, R., 1987, Quinolone/ureidopenicillin cross-resistance, *Lancet* **ii:**907.
99. Diakos, G. L., Lolans, V. T., and Jackson, G. G., 1988, Alterations in outer membrane proteins of *Pseudomonas aeruginosa* associated with selective resistance to quinolones, *Antimicrob. Agents Chemother.* **32:**785–787.
100. Yoshida, H., Nakamura, M., Bogaki, M., and Nakamura, S., 1990, Proportion of DNA gyrase mutants among quinolone-resistant strains of *Pseudomonas aeruginosa*, *Antimicrob. Agents Chemother.* **34:**1273–1275.
101. Chamberland, S., Malouin, F., Rabin, H. R., Schollaardt, T., Parr, T. R., and Bryan, L. E., 1990, Persistence of *Pseudomonas aeruginosa* during ciprofloxacin therapy of a cystic fibrosis patient: Transient resistance to quinolones and protein F-deficiency, *J. Antimicrob. Chemother.* **25:**995–1010.
102. Woodruff, W. A., and Hancock, R. E. W., 1988, Construction and characterization of *Pseudomonas aeruginosa* protein F-deficient mutants after *in vitro* and *in vivo* insertion mutagenesis of the cloned gene, *J. Bacteriol.* **170:**2592–2598.

103. Legakis, N., Tzouvelekis, L. S., Makris, A., and Kotsifaki, M., 1989, Outer membrane alterations of *Pseudomonas aeruginosa* selected by ciprofloxacin, *Antimicrob. Agents Chemother.* **33:**124–127.
104. Hirai, K., Suzue, S., Irikura, T., Iyobe, S., and Mitsuhashi, S., 1987, Mutations producing resistance to norfloxacin in *Pseudomonas aeruginosa, Antimicrob. Agents Chemother.* **31:**582–586.
105. Fukuda, H., Hosaka, M., Hirai, K., and Iyobe, S., 1990, New norfloxacin resistance gene in *Pseudomonas aeruginosa* PAO, *Antimicrob. Agents Chemother.* **34:**1757–1761.
106. Hallett, P., Mehlert, A., and Maxwell, A., 1990, *Escherichia coli* cells resistant to the DNA gyrase inhibitor, ciprofloxacin, overproduce a 60 kD protein homologous to GroEL, *Mol. Microbiol.* **4:**345–353.
107. Chamberland, S., Bayer, A. S., Schollaardt, T., Wong, S. A., and Bryan, L. E., 1989, Characterization of mechanisms of quinolone resistance in *Pseudomonas aeruginosa* strains isolated *in vitro* and *in vivo* during experimental endocarditis, *Antimicrob. Agents Chemother.* **33:**624–634.
108. Yamano, Y., Nishikawa, T., and Komatsu, Y., 1990, Outer membrane proteins responsible for the penetration of β-lactams and quinolones in *Pseudomonas aeruginosa, J. Antimicrob. Chemother.* **26:**175–184.
109. Hancock, R. E. W., and Carey, A. M., 1979, Outer membrane of *Pseudomonas aeruginosa*: Heat- and 2-mercaptoethanol-modifiable proteins, *J. Bacteriol.* **140:**902–910.
110. Masecar, B. L., Celesk, R. A., and Robillard, N. J., 1990, Analysis of acquired ciprofloxacin resistance in a clinical strain of *Pseudomonas aeruginosa, Antimicrob. Agents Chemother.* **34:**281–286.
111. Fernandes, P. B., Hanson, C. W., Stamm, J. M., Vojtko, C., Shipowitz, N. L., and St. Martin, E., 1987, The frequency of *in vitro* resistance development to fluoroquinolones and the use of a murine pyelonephritis model to demonstrate selection of resistance *in vivo, J. Antimicrob. Chemother.* **19:**449–465.
112. Michea-Hamzehpour, M., Auckenthaler, R., Regamey, P., and Pechère, J.-C., 1987, Resistance occurring after fluoroquinolone therapy of experimental *Pseudomonas aeruginosa* peritonitis, *Antimicrob. Agents Chemother.* **31:**1803–1808.
113. Sanders, C. C., Sanders, W. E., Goering, R. V., and Werner, V., 1984, Selection of multiple antibiotic resistance by quinolones, β-lactams and aminoglycosides with special reference to cross-resistance between unrelated drug classes, *Antimicrob. Agents Chemother.* **26:**797–801.

17

Immunochemical Prophylaxis against *Pseudomonas aeruginosa*

MICHAEL S. COLLINS

1. INTRODUCTION

Healthy people are rarely infected by *Pseudomonas aeruginosa*. Consequently, serious *P. aeruginosa* infections are rarely community-acquired. However, in the hospital setting, *P. aeruginosa* causes about 7–15% of life-threatening bacterial infections such as bacteremia and pneumonia.[1-5] In cystic fibrosis (CF), *P. aeruginosa* is the predominant pathogen.[6,7] *P. aeruginosa* merits special attention as a common bacterial nosocomial pathogen, for the mortality rate is significantly higher than that seen in infections caused by other common gram-negative bacilli and staphylococci.[8-10] Thus, in the host compromised by extreme youth or age, trauma, cancer, immunosuppressive therapy, or mechanical ventilation, *P. aeruginosa* can be a highly virulent pathogen.[1,2,8-10] In the compromised patient *P. aeruginosa* has several attributes that contribute to its high virulence. *P. aeruginosa* is innately less sensitive than other common gram-negative bacilli to modern antimicrobials such as semisynthetic penicillins, third-generation cephalosporins, aminoglycosides, and fluorinated carboxyquinolones.[11-15] Resistance can emerge during antimicrobial therapy, resulting in treatment failure.[16-20] Also, it is insensitive to frequently used agents such as trimethoprim-sulfamethoxazole, tetracycline, ampicillin, and first- and second-generation cephalosporins. The use of these

---

MICHAEL S. COLLINS • Miles Pharmaceutical Division, Miles Inc., West Haven, Connecticut 06516-4175.

Pseudomonas aeruginosa as an Opportunistic Pathogen, edited by Mario Campa *et al.* Plenum Press, New York, 1993.

latter oral antimicrobials for infection prophylaxis profoundly alters normal flora and can promote colonization of the host.[21–23] Whereas enteric bacilli and staphylococci that are usually found as normal flora, only about 4–12% of healthy people are colonized by *P. aeruginosa*.[24] However, when hospitalization exceeds several days, the incidence of colonization in debilitated patients can exceed 40%.[25,26] An increased incidence of colonization in debilitated patients is strongly associated with an increased incidence of infection. Finally, *P. aeruginosa* elaborates an array of virulence factors that are directly toxic to host tissue and thus promote dissemination from sites of local infection.[27–29] Although *P. aeruginosa* was first described as a human pathogen in 1892,[30] infections were infrequently described until the 1950s. Its emergence at that time as a significant pathogen was due to at least two reasons: Advances in medical care allowed patients with severe underlying disease to live longer, thus increasing the time available for colonization and eventual infection. Also, the widespread use of penicillin G and sulfa drugs greatly reduced the number of streptococcal and staphylococcal infections. The elimination of gram-positive cocci by antimicrobials with little or no anti-*Pseudomonas* activity allowed *P. aeruginosa* and other gram-negative bacilli to flourish. During this time the only antibiotic available with anti-*Pseudomonas* activity was polymyxin B. A few reports describe its effectiveness in severe infections, but overall, polymyxin B therapy usually failed.[31] Antibiotic management of severe *P. aeruginosa* infections became possible with the introduction of gentamicin and carbenicillin in the 1960s.[32] Even then there were many treatment failures, especially in patients with serious underlying disease.[2,33,34] During the 1960s the high rate of treatment failure with antibiotics and the high mortality rate associated with *P. aeruginosa* infections prompted numerous attempts to improve treatment outcome by immunotherapy. These efforts continue to this day.

2. ACTIVE IMMUNOTHERAPY

A vaccine can be broadly classified into one of two types. Complex vaccines contain an array of high-molecular-weight components, and the protective antigen(s) may remain undefined. They include killed or attenuated whole-cell preparations, autolysates, and various extracts. Commercially available complex vaccines include those against *Bordetella pertussis*, *Salmonella typhi*, *Vibrio cholerae*, and *Yersinia pestis*. Defined vaccines contain a purified antigen or a mixture of antigens and lack extraneous microbial components. Commercially available defined vaccines include *Haemophilus influenzae* b, *Streptococcus pneumoniae* and *Neisseria meningitidis* polysaccharides, and toxoids of *Corynebacterium diphtheriae* and *Clostridium tetani*. Both complex and defined vaccines have been widely studied for induction of active immunity against *P. aeruginosa* and for generation of antiserum or purified immunoglobulin for passive immunotherapy.

2.1. Complex Vaccines, LPS-based

Millican et al.[35] prepared formalinized and heated (100°C × 3 hr) whole-cell vaccines of a clinical isolate of *P. aeruginosa*. In scalded mice, both vaccines were equally protective against the vaccine strain, indicating that the protective antigen was heat-stable. Markley and Smallman[36] prepared vaccines from culture supernatant of 12 serotypes of *P. aeruginosa*. Protection in mice was serotype-specific when vaccines were administered ≥7 days before burning and challenge. A marked degree of nonspecific protection was seen when vaccines including those prepared from *Escherichia coli* and *Proteus mirabilis* were given 3 and 2 days prior to burn and challenge. In 1968 Jones[37] began a series of studies with vaccines prepared from culture filtrates of *P. aeruginosa*. A vaccine prepared from strain P14 given 4 days before challenge conferred protection against nine of 15 serotypes.[38] However, when given 14 days prior to challenge, protection waned to three of 15 serotypes. In 1976 Miller and colleagues[39] described a new cell-free vaccine prepared from EDTA–glycine extracts of viable cells of 16 International Antigen Typing Scheme (IATS) serotypes of *P. aeruginosa*. Monospecific vaccines conferred excellent protection against homologous serotypes. The 16-valent vaccine was termed PEV by Wellcome Research Laboratories. In a small study in India, immunization of burned patients with PEV was associated with lowered mortality.[40] Recent studies indicate that the protective antigen in PEV vaccine is lipopolysaccharide (LPS).[41,42] MacIntyre et al.[42] demonstrated that protection was correlated with the LPS fraction possessing 10 or more O-antigen repeating units. LPS with three or less O-antigen repeating units was 50- to 100-fold less protective in mice. PEV contains a large amount of antigenic protein. Removal of protein by hydrophobic absorption had no effect on PEV protection,[42] confirming that protection afforded by PEV is entirely LPS-mediated.

2.2. Defined Vaccines, LPS-based

Serotype schemata for *P. aeruginosa* are usually based upon bacterial-cell agglutination reactions in antisera.[43] In 1969 Fisher and colleagues[44] prepared killed whole-cell vaccines of each of the 10 Verder and Evans[45] serotypes. Challenge of mice immunized with these vaccines indicated little correlation between a vaccine serotype and protection against challenge with another strain of the homologous serotype. They concluded that agglutinogens were poorly predictive of protective antigens. Killed whole-cell vaccines were prepared from 342 clinical isolates of *P. aeruginosa*. Cross-protection studies indicated that 99% of the strains could be reduced to seven immunotypes. The immunotype schema of Fisher *et al.* soon led to preparation of a heptavalent LPS vaccine (Pseudogen™) and a human heptavalent hyperimmune serum globulin.[46]

The foregoing studies indicate that complex and defined vaccines containing LPS are highly protective in experimental infections and are serotype-specific immunogens. However, two major problems have prevented widespread use of LPS vaccines in man. First, immunogenic doses of LPS are toxic in some patient groups[47,48] and second, because LPS-induced immunity is serotype-specific,[49] a vaccine must contain at least several LPS chemotypes to afford broad protection against *P. aeruginosa* infection.

2.3. Defined LPS-based Vaccines of Low Toxicity

P. aeruginosa LPS can be detoxified by acid hydrolysis of the acid-labile bond between lipid A and the core polysaccharide region adjacent to the O-antigen.[50] Toxic lipid A is easily removed by solvent extraction. The resulting polysaccharide antigen is nontoxic and nonimmunogenic. Immunogenicity is restored by covalently coupling the polysaccharide to a suitable protein carrier.[51,52] Polysaccharide conjugate vaccines afford serotype-specific protection in a variety of animal models. The best-characterized conjugate vaccine was prepared by Cryz and colleagues[52-56] and is immunogenic and apparently safe in humans. Pier *et al.*[57-59] have described nontoxic, serotype-specific high-molecular weight polysaccharides (HMW-PS) isolated from slime and LPS of *P. aeruginosa*. On a weight basis, these polysaccharide preparations appear several hundred-fold less potent than conjugate vaccines.[60]

2.4. Cross-protective Vaccines

Many workers have attempted to prepare *P. aeruginosa* vaccines that are not serotype-specific. Candidate antigens for cross-protective vaccines have included outer-membrane protein,[61-63] mucoid exopolysaccharide,[64,65] flagella,[66-69] and enzymes such as protease,[70] elastase[71,72] and exotoxin A (ETA).[72,73] A candidate vaccine for induction of cross-reactive immunity to *P. aeruginosa* should meet several criteria: (1) The vaccine must be free of contaminating LPS. As little as 1 ng of LPS will induce homologous protection in mice[60] and repeated injection of higher doses can lead to nonspecific resistance to infection.[74,75] It is difficult to prepare cell-surface antigens such as outer membrane proteins entirely free of LPS.[62] (2) An antigen should induce passively protective antibody not only against the vaccine strain but against several challenge strains of unrelated LPS serotypes. Induction of active immunity by an antigen but failure to induce passively protective antibody suggests nonspecific resistance to infection. Ideally protection can be demonstrated by an appropriate monoclonal antibody. (3) The vaccine should be demonstrated to work in a model of infection, not just in a model of toxemia. For example, antisera to ETA should not only protect an animal against death induced by ETA challenge but should also demonstrate protective activity in infection alone or in combination with an appropriate antibiotic. Antisera to ETA[72] and elastase[71,72] fail this test.

In my opinion, flagella are the most promising non-LPS antigen vaccine candidates. About 90–95% of non-cystic fibrosis isolates of *P. aeruginosa* are mobile.[76,77] Motile strains of *P. aeruginosa* are more virulent in experimental infections than are nonmotile strains.[78–80] There are only two major flagella antigens, a and b.[76,81] Flagella type a can be subdivided into five antigen (a_0–a_4) subgroups[81,82]; however, considerable cross-protection exists among these a subgroups[69,83] Immunity is specific to the immunizing flagella antigen and independent of the O-antigen of the challenge strain.[67] This is an important observation because it is difficult to prepare flagella entirely free of contaminating LPS.[67,84] Several problems are associated with flagella vaccines. About 5–10% of clinical isolates lack a flagellum and are nonmotile. Antibody titers to flagella decline fairly rapidly following immunization[85]; in contrast with fairly persistent titers seen following LPS immunization.[86] Flagella vaccines have been shown to be effective in burned animal models; however, their activity has not yet been demonstrated in other models of infection such as peritonitis or pneumonia. It is not difficult to visualize how inhibition of motility can interfere with tissue invasion by *P. aeruginosa* from a colonized burn wound. It is difficult, though, to see the value of motility inhibition when *P. aeruginosa* is in the blood or a body cavity. A nonopsonic monoclonal antibody that inhibited the motility of *Proteus mirabilis* was recently demonstrated to be highly protective in a model of burn wound sepsis but inert in a model of peritonitis.[87] Fortunately, antisera to *P. aeruginosa* flagella have been shown to be opsonic,[69,83] so elimination of *P. aeruginosa* could result in part from antibody-mediated phagocytosis.

3. PASSIVE IMMUNOTHERAPY

Induction of active immunity with vaccines requires immunological competence. The very young, the elderly, and the patient with debility often respond poorly to vaccines. Furthermore, there is a several-day window following vaccination before protective immunity develops. It is well-established that immunity to *P. aeruginosa* infection requires complement,[88–91] phagocytes[90–92] (especially polymorphonuclear granulocytes, PMN) and opsonic antibody.[90,92] Complement is usually not limiting. PMN can be replaced by transfusion.[93,94] However this is still largely experimental, expensive, and potentially hazardous due to foreign PMN antigens and possible viral contamination.[95] Alternatively, lymphokines such as granulocyte–macrophage colony stimulating factor eventually may be employed to increase circulating

PMN.[96] Because of the ease of immunoglobulin administration, it is not surprising that a large number of investigators have attempted to prevent or treat established *P. aeruginosa* infections by passive immunotherapy.

3.1. Immune Serum Globulin

Immune serum globulin (ISG) has been available for four decades. It is prepared by Cohn[97] cold alcohol fractionation of human plasma. Plasma is pooled from 1000 or more donors to minimize lot-to-lot variation in antibody concentration. ISG contains specific immunoglobulin G (IgG) antibodies to *P. aeruginosa* LPS antigens.[98] In opsonophagocytic assays, ISG plus complement promotes ingestion and killing of *P. aeruginosa* by PMN.[92] ISG administered near the time of challenge with *P. aeruginosa* lowers mortality in burned[99] and normal mice.[100] ISG enhances the activity of several antibiotics in treatment of human[101] and experimental animal[102,103] infections; however, the antibiotics studied in these older reports, such as chloramphenicol, polymyxin B, and oxytetracycline seldom are used now to treat *P. aeruginosa* infections.

The results of two major clinical trials using ISG as an adjunct in burn therapy are equivocal. Stone and colleagues[104] treated patients every third day with intramuscular (IM) injections or intravenous (IV) infusion of approximately 60 mg ISG/kg body weight. They reported no difference in mortality or infection control in ISG-treated or control patients. Kefalides and colleagues[105] reported a 50% reduction in *P. aeruginosa* sepsis in Peruvian children with a 10–30% body-surface-area burn, who received 160 mg ISG/kg by the IM route on days 1, 3 and 5. Protection, however, was not seen in children with larger burns.

There are major drawbacks in the use of ISG for passive immunoprophylaxis. ISG prepared by Cohn cold-alcohol fractionation is anticomplementary. Severe complement-mediated adverse reactions are associated with IV infusion of ISG.[106] ISG is therefore given by the IM route. Following IM injection, varying amounts of ISG are degraded before absorption from the muscle mass occurs and 2–4 days are required before peak plasma levels of IgG are reached.[107] Pain and sterile abscess can develop at the site of injection. The limited amount of ISG that can be delivered to the muscle mass prompted numerous efforts to prepare IgG concentrates suitable for intravenous infusion.

3.2. Immune Serum Globulin for Intravenous Infusion

Human IgG derived from Cohn fraction II and prepared for IV infusion (IGIV) is currently available from several manufacturers. Anticomplementary activity is reduced or eliminated by three general methods: (1) enzymatic treatment with pepsin or plasmin; (2) chemical modification by reduction and alkylation or reduction and sulfonation; and (3) physical means such as low pH treatment or ion-exchange chromatography. IGIV prepared by enzymatic treatment or chemical modification often has less opsonic activity because of diminished function of the Fc region of IgG and a reduction in the concentration of IgG subclasses (especially IgG3).[108–110] The five IGIV preparations available in the United States are essentially native IgG preparations with approximately the same IgG subclass distribution as human plasma.[109–112]

Antibody to LPS antigens of the seven Fisher immunotypes are found in IGIV[98,113] as well as neutralizing antibody to ETA.[98] In opsonophagocytic assays IGIV promotes bacterial killing in the presence of complement.[98,114] In the absence of complement, little or no killing occurs.[115] Passive protection studies in normal mice,[98,113,116] mice compromised by corticosteroid,[117] and burned mice[118–120] indicate that IGIV is protective against most immunotypes of *P. aeruginosa*. However in granulocytopenic mice, IGIV prophylaxis at doses of 500 mg/kg body weight afforded little protection.[98,121] Studies in the author's laboratory demonstrated that high-dose IGIV therapy markedly enhanced the activity of tobramycin and azlocillin in therapy of cellulitis in neutropenic mice.[121] Neutropenia was induced by cyclophosphamide. Mice were challenged by contamination of a small dorsal surface wound with four immunotypes of *P. aeruginosa*. As seen in Table I adapted from ref. 121, monotherapy with antibiotic or IGIV was not particularly effective except in mice challenged with immunotype 3. In contrast, combination therapy appeared to be at least additive and in some cases synergistic. In the setting of a cancer treatment center, these four immunotypes have accounted for 75% of wound isolates and 76% of blood isolates.[122] Other studies in mice suggest that IGIV enhances β-lactam and aminoglycoside activity in therapy of established *Pseudomonas* burn-wound sepsis[119] and ciprofloxacin in therapy of established *P. aeruginosa* pneumonia.[123] High-dose IGIV (≥400 mg/kg) has been administered for prophylaxis of bacterial infections in patients with major burns,[124,125] chronic lymphocytic leukemia,[126,127] chronic sinopulmon-

TABLE I
IGIV and Antibiotic Therapy of Established *P. aeruginosa* Cellulitis in Neutropenic Mice

	No. mice dead/total (% dead) Fisher immunotype, challenge strain			
Treatment	1, 1369	2, ATCC 27313	3, ATCC 27314	7, ATCC 27318
Albumin[a] + saline	20/20 (100)	20/20 (100)	20/20 (100)	20/20 (100)
Albumin + antibiotic[b]	18/20 (90)	32/40 (80)	24/40 (60)[c]	16/20 (80)
IGIV[a] + saline	18/20 (90)	16/20 (80)	11/20 (55)[c]	18/20 (90)
IGIV + antibiotic	4/20 (20)[d]	21/40 (53)[c]	10/40 (25)[d]	11/20 (55)[c]

[a]Albumin or IGIV given at 500 mg/kg 16 hr post challenge.
[b]Antibiotic or saline given 16, 24, 32, 40, 48, 56, 64, and 72 hr post-challenge. Mice challenged with immunotypes 1 and 7 were treated with tobramycin at 4 and 8 mg/kg/dose, respectively. Mice challenged with immunotypes 2 and 3 were treated with azlocillin at 400 mg/kg/dose.
[c]$P<.05$. Treatment versus control.
[d]$P<.0001$. Treatment versus control.

ary disease,[128] and high-risk neonates.[129,130] These studies indicate IGIV administration is safe, and in some studies the incidence of serious infections was reduced.[126–130] However, IGIV therapy in these human studies was not specifically targeted towards *P. aeruginosa*, and its incidence was low or not reported.

3.3. Hyperimmune Immunoglobulin

Hyperimmune antibody to *P. aeruginosa* can be obtained in essentially two ways: Animals or humans can be immunized with an appropriate vaccine with the resulting immune sera collected for immunoglobulin purification, or alternatively, serum may be collected from people that have recovered from infection, or suffer chronic infection, or from the relatively few healthy donors who have naturally high levels of antibody to *P. aeruginosa* antigens. Animals can be immunized repeatedly with purified or complex vaccines and high-titered antisera can be obtained. Polyvalent immunoglobulins prepared from sera of immunized sheep[131] and horses[132] have been employed for prophylaxis of *P. aeruginosa* infection in humans. Caution must be exercised when using animal immunoglobulin because of the risk of serum sickness or immediate hypersensitivity reactions.[133] The use of *Pseudomonas* vaccines in healthy subjects to raise antibody poses an ethical problem. All vaccines have an inherent risk of potential toxicity especially if LPS is a component. Plasma donors are healthy adults. As such, they are at little risk of acquiring a *P. aeruginosa* infection. Thus, development of high levels of humoral antibody is of minimal benefit to the immunized plasma donor. Is use of a vaccine with at least some degree of potential toxicity justified in this population?

A *Pseudomonas* hyperimmune IgG, however obtained, should be formulated for intravenous infusion (PS-IGIV), so peak plasma levels of antibody are achieved immediately following administration. Proof that passive immunotherapy is efficacious in prophylaxis or therapy of established *P. aeruginosa* infection can come only from randomized, double-blind studies in an appropriate number of subjects. No PS-IGIV has yet met this test. However, the potential usefulness of a PS-IGIV can be tested in animal models of infection. Preclinical animal studies help suggest dosage regimens to employ in human studies. Because conventional IGIV has considerable protective activity in a variety of animal models, it is useful to compare the biological activity of an experimental PS-IGIV with that of IGIV preparations that ideally would be manufactured by the same method.

3.3.1. Immunoprophylaxis of Experimental Infections

The Parke-Davis PS-IGIV was prepared by immunizing plasma donors with the heptavalent LPS vaccine Pseudogen®.[46,134] Pollack[98] compared IgG antibody titers in the Parke-Davis PS-IGIV with those found in 27 lots of conventional or experimental IGIV. When compared with intact IGIV, anti-LPS titers in PS-IGIV ranged from 10-fold (immunotype 4) to 85-fold (immunotype 5) higher. In burned mice both IGIV and PS-IGIV were protective; however PS-IGIV was significantly more protective in granulocytopenic mice. Because the Parke-Davis vaccine was toxic in some patient groups,[47,48] it is not currently used for immunization of plasma donors.

Extracts of the 16 IATS serotypes of *P. aeruginosa* have been employed by Armour[135] and Sandoz[136,137] to immunize plasma donors. These complex vaccines contain LPS as an active immunogen.[41,42] Because the total LPS concentration in these complex 16-valent vaccines is fairly low compared with the heptavalent LPS Parke-Davis vaccine, they are reportedly less toxic. They are also less immunogenic than Pseudogen®. Holder and Neely[135] compared the Armour PS-IGIV with normal IGIV. Antibody levels to LPS were 2- to 4-fold higher in PS-IGIV. Against an IATS 6 strain in burned mice, PS-IGIV was about 10-fold more protective than normal IGIV. Armour PS-IGIV studies in humans have not been reported. The Sandoz 16-valent vaccine was used to immunize donors on days 0, 14 and 21.[136] On day 28, increases in anti-LPS titers ranged from 1.2-fold (IATS 16) to approximately 8-fold (IATS 6 and 7). Against 11 of 16 serotypes, titers rose less than four-fold over baseline. Following infusion of 15 g of Sandoz PS-IGIV into two volunteers, serum at 24-hr post-infusion was about 1.6-fold more protective against IATS 6 in passively immunized mice than baseline serum.[137] Efficacy studies of Sandoz PS-IGIV in humans have not been reported.

Cryz and colleagues have immunized volunteers with a novel octavalent vaccine.[55,56] The vaccine is prepared by acid hydrolysis of the LPS of eight serotypes of *P. aeruginosa*. The resulting nontoxic polysaccharide O-antigens were coupled to ETA. Conjugation destroyed the toxicity of ETA. The octavalent vaccine contains about 43% polysaccharide and 57% detoxified exotoxin A.[52-54] The vaccine was well-tolerated in 18 volunteers and led to mean increases in anti-LPS IgG titers from 2-fold (IATS 1) to 15-fold (IATS 10) at 28-days post-immunization.[55] Neutralizing antibody to ETA increased 30-fold. Immune serum was highly protective in experimental burn-wound sepsis. The results of a clinical trial are pending.[56]

In 1984 the author's laboratory described preparation of a PS-IGIV prepared from the plasma of normal, nonimmunized plasma donors.[138] Plasma samples from several thousand donors were screened by an enzyme-linked immunoassay (ELISA) for IgG antibody to LPS antigens of Fisher immunotypes 1, 2, 4, and 6. Plasma with ELISA titers ≥ 1:1,600 were generally passively protective in burned mice, whereas plasma with titers < 1:1,600 offered marginal or no protection. Plasma pools were prepared with titers of approximately 1:1600 against immunotypes 1, 2, 4, and 6 LPS. These four standards were used in ELISA on plasma of several thousand donors from multiple centers in the United States. Approximately 5% of the donor population had titers that met or exceeded the titer of the reference pools.

Several hundred liters of monovalent plasma enriched in IgG antibody to immunotypes 1, 2, 4, or 6 were collected, pooled, and fractionated into an intravenous IgG concentrate. Cutter PS-IGIV is commercially available in Germany as Psomaglobin® N. The mean ELISA titers of three lots of Cutter PS-IGIV were compared with mean titers of 15 lots of IGIV (Gamimune N). Results are shown in Table II. Mean IGIV titers were normalized to unity. For comparison, the mean ELISA titers of three lots of PS-IGIV prepared by Cryz *et al.* by immunizing donors with an octavalent conjugate vaccine (Aerugen Berna, Swiss Serum and Vaccine Institute) are also shown. These PS-IGIV titers are compared with the mean titers of two lots of IGIV (Sandoglobulin) normalized to unity. (Data in Table II are adapted from ref. 56 and 123.)

It is noteworthy that although Cutter PS-IGIV is screened only for high-titer plasma against immunotype 1, 2, 4, and 6, it is also enriched at least 3.4-fold in anti-LPS antibody against the other eight serotypes examined. This result implies that a plasma donor having naturally high levels of IgG antibody to one *P. aeruginosa* LPS serotype tends to have high antibody levels to multiple *P. aeruginosa* serotypes. It has also been shown that Cutter PS-IGIV contains approximately five-fold more neutralizing antibody than IGIV against ETA, a major virulence factor of *P. aeruginosa*.[139-142]

Cutter PS-IGIV has been characterized extensively in animal models of infection. In a murine model of burn wound sepsis, PS-IGIV prophylaxis was examined against 18 clinical isolates of *P. aeruginosa* including polyagglutinating strains.[143] Protection was evident against all clinical isolates and against

TABLE II
Mean-Fold Increase in Anti-LPS Titers of *Pseudomonas* IGIV (PS-IGIV) Compared with Conventional IGIV: Effect of Donor Immunization or Donor Selection on Product Titers

IATS serotype (Fisher Immunotype)	Immunized Ps-IGIV (3 lots) Sandogobulin (2 lots)	Selected PS-IGIV (3 lots) Gamimune N (15 lots)	Immunized Selected
1 (4)	6.8	3.4	2.00
2 (3)	2.2	5.9	0.37
3	3.9	7.6	0.51
4	5.9	4.3	1.37
5 (7)	2.4	5.7	0.42
6 (1)	10.0	10.7	0.93
7/8 (6)	NR[a]	8.2	—
9	NR	4.5	—
10 (5)	5.1	6.3	0.81
11 (2)	3.7	5.0	0.74
12	NR	4.1	—
15	NR	3.4	—

[a]NR is not reported.

16 of 18, the mean protective dose (ED_{50}) was ≤100 mg IgG/kg. Overall 88% (158 of 180) of control mice died. Mortality in mice treated with 56, 167 or 500 mg PS-IGIV/kg was 31%, 20% and 15% respectively. When compared with conventional IGIV in burn-wound sepsis, PS-IGIV was significantly more protective against five of seven immunotypes of *P. aeruginosa*.[138] Similarly, when compared with an IGIV enriched with 12% IgM and 12% IgA (Pentoglobin® Biotest), PS-IGIV was significantly more protective in burned mice against six of 10 challenge strains.[144] Burn-wound sepsis is a useful model for assessing immunoglobulin potency; during the past decade, however, the incidence of *Pseudomonas* burn infection has declined. Currently the most common serious *P. aeruginosa* infection is pneumonia.[4,145] A murine model of aspiration pneumonia was employed to compare the protective activity of Cutter PS-IGIV and IGIV.[123] The model is characterized in control mice by high mortality, a mean time to death of ≤2.0 days and a 60% incidence of bacteremia at 3-hr post-challenge. Mice were challenged with eight serotypes of *P. aeruginosa*. Overall mortality was 90% (117 of 130). Mortality in mice treated with 56, 167, or 500 mg IGIV/kg (N = 130/group) was 77%, 56%, and 38% respectively. In contrast, mortality in mice treated with these doses of PS-IGIV was 55%, 31%, and 11% respectively. Overall the ED_{50} (95% CL) of PS-IGIV was 90 mg IgG/kg (63-116) versus 328 mg IgG/kg (238-490) for IGIV (P < 0.0001). PS-IGIV was significantly more protective than IGIV against five of eight challenge strains. Against the other three strains both IGIV and PS-IGIV afforded ≥90% survival at 167 mg IgG/kg. Animal studies suggest that PS-IGIV prophylaxis against *P. aeruginosa* might be effective in the clinical setting. Whereas this is probably true, one drawback must be considered. Immunoglobulins prepared for IV infusion are fairly expensive. The incidence of serious nosocomial infections such as bacteremia or pneumonia varies greatly among hospitals and ranges from about two to 300 per 10,000 discharges.[4–8] Of these, 7–15% are due to *P. aeruginosa*.[1–5] Obviously wide-scale prophylaxis of *P. aeruginosa* infection would not be cost-effective, especially in this era of increasing containment of medical costs. There are, however, selected patients who might be considered as candidates for passive immunoprophylaxis. This population includes debilitated patients with respiratory tract, gastrointestinal tract, or burn-wound colonization with *P. aeruginosa*. Passive immunoprophylaxis would be ever more compelling if the colonized patient was neutropenic,[2,16,23] had hypogammaglobulinemia (<6.4 g IgG/L),[2,128,146,147] or if the colonizing strain exhibited multiple-antibiotic resistance.[148,149]

3.3.2. Therapy of Established Animal Infections

Immunoprophylaxis of *P. aeruginosa* infection is controversial because it is difficult to define the patient who might eventually develop infection. Immunotherapy of documented established infection seems reasonable because of the high mortality rate seen even with appropriate antimicrobial therapy.[4,150] To justify the use of PS-IGIV to treat serious *P. aeruginosa* infections in humans, preclinical studies in animals should address several issues. First, because antibiotics will remain the therapeutic mainstay for the foreseeable future, combination therapy with antibiotics plus PS-IGIV should confer a significant survival advantage over antibiotic therapy alone. Organ and body fluid culture should demonstrate a reduced bacterial burden with combination therapy. Combination therapy studies in larger animals such as dogs, sheep, and primates (which necessitates employment of far fewer animals than rodent studies), should lead to significant improvements in clinical parameters such as organ function, hemodynamic variables, and incidence of bacteremia. Second, the selected antibiotic(s) given alone should afford a degree of protection either in terms of prolonging survival or reducing cumulative mortality. This reflects the clinical situation where therapy with an appropriate antibiotic without doubt confers protection in an infected population. It has been my experience that the *in vitro* minimal inhibitory concentrations (MIC) of an antimicrobial is poorly predictive of its activity *in vivo*. For example, the MIC of ciprofloxacin against a strain each of immunotypes 1, 2, and 6 varied only two-fold and was 0.125, 0.250 and 0.250 μg per ml respectively.[143] In a model of burn-wound sepsis, the ED_{50} of ciprofloxacin against these three strains ranged from approximately 2.5 to 15.0 mg/kg/dose.[143] Third, treatment should be delayed until the infection is well-established. The timing will depend largely upon the experimental model employed. For example, in aspiration pneumonia in normal mice the mean time to death is usually <18 hr, whereas in burn wound sepsis it is usually ≥2 days. A useful guide is to begin therapy when the animal becomes bacteremic. Thus, in pneumonia, treatment might begin approximately 2 to 3 hr after challenge while in burns it would be appropriate to wait 16 to 24 hr post-challenge. The longer a potentially lethal infection is established, the poorer the result will be with antibiotic or immunoglobulin monotherapy. Therefore, if prophylaxis affords a similar level of success as post-challenge treatment, it can be assumed that treatment was begun too soon following challenge, and the infection was not well-established. Finally, as mentioned already, conventional IGIV enhances the activity of antibiotics in therapy of infection. To justify the cost of a hyperimmune globulin, it must afford a significant survival advantage over IGIV therapy. Activity against several *P. aeruginosa* serotypes should be examined.

Neeley and Holder[151] treated burned mice infected with four serotypes of *P. aeruginosa* with combinations of Armour PS-IGIV and antibiotics. Treatment began 18 hr post-infection. PS-IGIV was given at 2 mg/mouse and antibiotics (mezlocillin, pipercillin, ceftazidine, or tobramycin) were given twice daily for 2 days at clinically appropriate doses. The infections were often lethal, with survival ranging from zero to 30% depending on the challenge strain. Monotherapy with either PS-IGIV or an antibiotic usually led to improvement in survival at 5 days. In no case was combination therapy a significant improvement over monotherapy. The dosage of 2 mg/IgG/mouse is equivalent to 100 mg/kg in a 25-g mouse. Currently, conventional IGIV and other formulations of PS-IGIV are often employed in the clinical setting at 400–500 mg/kg. Amour PS-IGIV contains only 2- to 4-fold more anti-LPS antibody than conventional IGIV. An improved treatment result therefore may have been seen at IgG dosages of 8–10 mg/mouse.

Collins et al.[143] examined Cutter PS-IGIV and orally administered ciprofloxacin used against three strains of *P. aeruginosa* in a model of burn-wound sepsis. PS-IGIV was administered at 500 mg IgG/kg 16 hr after challenge. Ciprofloxacin was administered twice daily for 3 days at doses selected to yield approximately 50% survival. Data in Table III adapted from ref. 143 indicate that monotherapy with ciprofloxacin was significantly protective against the three strains. PS-IGIV plus ciprofloxacin was significantly more protective ($P < .01$) than ciprofloxacin monotherapy against immunotypes two and six. Overall, 47% of mice treated only with ciprofloxacin survived versus 80% receiving combination therapy ($P = .0002$).

Pennington and colleagues studied Cutter PS-IGIV in a model of pneumonia in normal[152,153] and neutropenic[154] guinea pigs. Survival was significantly improved in normal animals given 500 mg PS-IGIV/kg 2 hr post-challenge. Protection correlated with a marked increase in serum opsonic activity following PS-IGIV infusion and a significant decrease in lung bacterial burden 24 hr post-challenge. In contrast, PS-IGIV monotherapy was not protective in neutropenic guinea pigs. Tobramycin and ticarcillin alone offered 43% and 7% survival, respectively. When PS-IGIV was added to the tobramycin or ticarcillin treatment regimens, survival rose to 86% ($P < .05$) and 43% ($P = .08$) respectively. Overall, combination therapy was significantly more protective ($P = .0002$) than antibiotic monotherapy.

Cutter PS-IGIV activity in established pneumonia was compared with the activities of Cutter IGIV and an IGIV enriched with 12% IgM and 12% IgA (IgGMA Pentaglobin®, Biotest). When PsIGIV was compared with

TABLE III
Pseudomonas **IGIV and Oral Ciprofloxacin Therapy of Established Burn Wound Sepsis**

Treatment	No. mice dead/total (% dead)		
	1, 1369	2, ATCC 27313	6, ATCC 27317
Albumin + water	19/20 (95)	20/20 (100)	20/20 (100)
Albumin + ciprofloxacin	11/20^a (55)	12/20^a (60)	9/20^b (45)
PS-IGIV + water	12/20^a (60)	20/20 (100)	20/20 (100)
PS-IGIV + ciprofloxacin	7/20^b (35)	4/20^b (20)	1/20^b (5)

$^a P<.05$. Treatment versus control.
$^b P<.0001$. Treatment versus control.

Cutter IGIV, both IgG formulations were given at 500 mg/kg 5 hr postchallenge.[123] Ciprofloxacin at 10 mg/kg/dose was delivered in a 0.1 ml volume into the stomach via a gastric feeding needle at 5, 16, 24, 40, 48, 64, and 72 hr following challenge with Fisher immunotypes 3, 5, or 6 respectively. As seen in Table IV, 92% of control mice died within 7 days. Ciprofloxacin was significantly protective only against immunotype 5. IGIV alone was not protective. PS-IGIV was significantly protective against immunotypes 5 and 6. Combination therapy with IGIV and ciprofloxacin afforded significant protection to mice challenged with immunotypes 3 and 5, but combination therapy was superior to ciprofloxacin monotherapy only against immunotype 5. PS-IGIV plus ciprofloxacin therapy was highly protective against immunotypes 3, 5 and 6, and in each case combination therapy was significantly more protective than ciprofloxacin monotherapy. In the second study comparing PS-IGIV with Biotest IgM and IgA-enriched IGIV (IgGMA) against *P. aeruginosa* IATS 2, monotherapy with ciprofloxacin or IgGMA was not protective.[155] PS-IGIV alone was marginally protective ($P = .04$). Combination therapy with IgGMA plus ciprofloxacin was not protective, whereas PS-IGIV plus ciprofloxacin was highly protective ($P < 0.005$). At 16 hr following challenge, mice treated with PS-IGIV had 2000-fold fewer *P. aeruginosa* cells in the lungs than at 3 hr, whereas lungs of mice treated with IgGMA had a 27-fold increase in lung bacteria. At 100 mg IgG/kg, PS-IGIV significantly increased survival in mice challenged with ETA, whereas 400 mg IgGMA/kg was inactive. In the presence of complement and human PMN, PS-IGIV promoted >95% killing of five serotypes of *P. aeruginosa*, whereas killing promoted by IgGMA ranged from 34% to 70%. In this study, antitoxin activity, opsonic activity, and the ability to promote bacterial clearance from an infected organ correlated well with the ability of PS-IGIV to promote survival in infected mice.

TABLE IV
Pseudomonas **IGIV, Conventional IGIV and Oral Ciprofloxacin Therapy of Established Pneumonia**

Treatment	No. mice dead/total (% dead) Fisher immunotype, challenge strain		
	2, ATCC27313	5, ATCC 27316	6, A5
Albumin + water	18/20 (90)	18/20 (90)	19/20 (95)
Albumin + ciprofloxacin	13/20 (65)	8/20[a] (40)	16/20 (80)
PS-IGIV + water	12/19 (63)	4/20[b] (20)	9/20[a] (45)
IGIV + water	14/20 (70)	13/20 (65)	16/20 (80)
PS-IGIV + ciprofloxacin	6/30[b] (20)	2/29[b] (7)	12/29[b] (41)
IGIV + ciprofloxacin	12/30[b] (40)	7/29[b] (24)	24/30 (80)

[a]$P<.05$. Treatment versus control.
[b]$P<.0001$. Treatment versus control.

3.3.3. Human Studies

In a clinical study in New Delhi, children and adults with 5% to 65% full-thickness burns were treated within 72 hr of burning, with Wellcome PEV polyvalent vaccine and immune globulin prepared from plasma of donors immunized with PEV vaccine.[156] Overall, the incidence of *P. aeruginosa* bacteremia in patients who received immunotherapy was 2.3% (N = 176) versus 20% (N = 103) in control patients. Mortality in control patients was 30%. Mortality in patients receiving only immunoglobulin was 10% (N = 48), vaccine only 8% (N = 91), and immunoglobulin plus vaccine 11% (N = 37). The relevance of this apparently successful clinical study to Western burn care is questionable. Economic conditions in India mandate less rigorous treatment of burn patients including the use of less potent (less expensive) antibiotics and less patient isolation. This was reflected in the high incidence of infection in control patients, which considerably exceeds that seen in the West.[10,157] Cutter PS-IGIV has been examined in several small studies. Hunt et al.[158] treated 10 burned patients with *Pseudomonas* burn-wound sepsis, eight of whom had bacteremia. Following two infusions of 500 mg IgG/kg, baseline plasma levels rose from 1014 mg IgG/dl to 2205 mg IgG/dl. The *P. aeruginosa* isolates of nine patients were resistant to currently available antibiotics. Overall, in this small group only 40% of patients survived *P. aeruginosa* bacteremia. Kistler et al.[159] treated nine burned patients with PS-IGIV; five patients survived. The four patients who died had a mean burn index of 119, inhalation trauma, kidney failure, and polymicrobic sepsis. Van Wye and colleagues[160] administered Cutter PS-IGIV to 10 patients with moderately severe CF during hospitalization for pulmonary exacerbation. All patients were chronically colonized with antibiotic-resistant *P. aeruginosa*. In this small group of patients, a single dose of 500 mg IgG/kg was associated with greater and more prolonged improvement in lung function when compared with each patient's historical response to standard therapy. A significant improvement in serum opsonic activity against the autologous *P. aeruginosa* isolate was seen 24 hr after PS-IGIV infusion. The efficacy of PS-IGIV for therapy of documented *P. aeruginosa* pneumonia is now being evaluated in a multicenter clinical trial.

4. MONOCLONAL ANTIBODIES

4.1. Core Glycolipid Immunity

As previously discussed, immunization with smooth LPS vaccines results in O-antigen-specific active immunity and generation of passively protective serotype-specific antiserum. There are seven to 21 serotypes of *P. aeruginosa* depending upon the serotype system used.[43–45] A LPS vaccine would therefore have to contain at least several LPS antigens of common serotypes to provide broad protection. Mutants unable to synthesize O-antigen still retain lipid A and all or part of the core polysaccharide. Such mutants are termed rough, and are usually serum-sensitive and of minimal virulence. LPS of most gram-negative bacilli has the sugars heptose and 2-keto-3-deoxyoctonate acid immediately adjacent to lipid A.[162] In theory, an antibody reactive with these core sugars or lipid A should cross-react with like epitopes on LPS of heterologous bacteria. The inner core structure of *P. aeruginosa* LPS is chemically similar but not identical to the inner core of deep-rough mutants such as *E. coli* J5 and *Salmonella minnesota* Re 595.[162] Antibodies to LPS of these enteric deep-rough bacilli have been described that bind to LPS or to heat-treated cells of *P. aeruginosa*.[163-170] High levels of serum IgG (>10 µg/ml) and IgM (>30 µg/ml) to *E. coli* J5 LPS at the onset of *P. aeruginosa* sepsis correlated with enhanced survival.[171] Studies employing deep-rough mutant vaccines, antisera, or monoclonal antibody (MAb) to these antigens for immunotherapy of *P. aeruginosa* infections have yielded conflicting results. Ziegler and colleagues[172] immunized rabbits and humans with several doses of a boiled, whole-cell *E. coli* J5 vaccine. Both rabbit and human antiserum significantly reduced mortality from *P. aeruginosa* bacteremia in passively immunized neutropenic rabbits. Active immunization of rabbits with J5 vaccine led to even greater protection and was equal in protection to immunization with serotype-specific *P. aeruginosa* vaccine. Martinez and Callahan[173] treated neutropenic mice with human antiserum to *E. coli* J5 or a toxoid derived from ETA. Monotherapy with antiserum or toxoid alone was not protective; however combination therapy significantly protected against *P. aeruginosa* challenge. In a controlled clinical trial, human J5 antiserum or pre-immune serum was administered to 212 patients with documented gram-negative infection, 44 of whom had *P. aeruginosa* bacteremia.[174] Overall, J5 antiserum enhanced survival in the subset of patients with hypotension and profound shock. Survival in the subset of patients with *P. aeruginosa* infection that received J5 antiserum (N = 24) or preimmune serum (N = 20) was not reported. The reason for protection in the group given J5 antiserum is unclear. Baumgartner *et al.*[175] recently immunized humans with *E. coli* J5 vaccine according to the protocol of Ziegler *et al.*[172,174] A significant rise in IgG (3.25-fold) and IgM (3-fold) against *E. coli* J5 was noted; however, no increase in IgG or IgM was seen against *S. minnesota* Re 595 LPS or LPS of seven smooth enteric bacilli. In 1985 Teng *et al.*[176] reported development of a human IgM MAb reactive in immunoblot with lipid A of *E. coli* J5 LPS and *S. minnesota* Re 595 LPS. The MAb also reacted with purified LPS of a variety of smooth gram-negative bacilli including *P. aeruginosa*. As little as 2 µg MAb/mouse increased the LD_{50} of *P. aeruginosa* 40-fold in a model of bacteremic peritonitis. Similarly, the LD_{50} of strains of *E. coli* and *K. pneumoniae* was increased 15- to 18-fold. This human IgM MAb now termed HA-IA was recently studied in a septic population of 543 patients.[177] In the 37% who were shown to have gram-negative bacteremia, HA-IA therapy significantly lowered mortality ($P = .014$). No effect was observed in the 343 patients who did not have gram-negative bacteremia. The incidence of *Pseudomonas* sepsis was 9.2% in the 105 patients treated with HA-IA and 18.6% in the 95 control patients. Outcome in the subset of patients with *Pseudomonas* sepsis was not reported. In contrast to the above reports, others have shown cross-reactive immunity affords little or no protection against *P. aeruginosa*. Ng et al.[178] immunized rabbits with Re mutants of *S. minnesota* and *S. typhi*. Both antigens stimulated antibody to Re LPS detected by indirect hemagglutination and immunodiffusion. The antisera afforded no protection to mice challenged with ≤5 LD_{50} of *P. aeruginosa*, *E. coli*, *S. typhimurium*, or *K. pneumoniae*. Pennington and Menkes[179] immunized guinea pigs with *E. coli* J5 vaccine. Immunization induced a four-fold rise in serum antibody to the J5 antigen. Actively immunized animals were not significantly protected against intratracheal challenge with *E. coli*, *K. pneumoniae*, or two serotypes of *P. aeruginosa*. Also, sera from immunized animals were not opsonic. In contrast, immunization with *P. aeruginosa* LPS afforded significant protection against homologous challenge. Cryz et al.[180] immunized mice with *E. coli* J5 LPS, *S. typhimurium* Re mutant LPS and smooth *P. aeruginosa* LPS. In burned mice challenged with five serotypes of *P. aeruginosa*, the two enteric rough LPS vaccines were nearly devoid of protective effects, although the *S. typhimurium* Re LPS vaccine was protective against one of five *P. aeruginosa* challenge strains. On the other hand, homologous LPS conferred serotype-specific protection against all five serotypes. Dunn et al.[163] studied a murine IgG1 MAb to *E. coli* J5 that cross-reacted with LPS and heat-treated cells of *P. aeruginosa*. When given to mice by the IV route at 2 mg/kg, the MAb increased the LD_{50} of *K. pneumoniae* and *E. coli* 0:111 by six-fold but was inactive against *P. aeruginosa* challenge. Whereas J5 antiserum has been shown by Ziegler et al. to be efficacious in gram-negative sepsis, a recent controlled clinical study indicated that a J5-IGIV preparation from sera of J5-vaccine-immunized donors was not superior to conventional IGIV in reversing gram-negative septic shock or in lowering mortality.[181]

4.2. Immunotherapy with *P. aeruginosa*-Specific Monoclonal Antibodies

MAb have been prepared against a variety of *P. aeruginosa* cell-surface-associated antigens including outer-membrane proteins F,[182–185] H2,[182,185] I[185,186] and ferripyochelin-binding protein,[187] pili,[188,189] flagella,[190,191] mucoid exopolysaccharide,[65,192] O-antigen-deficient LPS,[193] and smooth LPS,[182,194–202] and also against exoproducts including alkaline phosphatase,[203] elastase,[204] ETA,[205,206] and exotoxin S (exo-S).[207] In addition, MAb have been described against nitrosating enzyme,[208] heat shock proteins,[209] aminoglycoside-resistance factor,[210] and cephalosporinase.[211] MAb against some of these antigens have been studied in protection assays.

4.2.1. Mucoid Exopolysaccharide

Pier et al.[65] administered an opsonic murine IgG MAb to mice 2 hr before intratracheal challenge with a mucoid strain of *P. aeruginosa* enmeshed in agar beads. Seven days following challenge, the lungs of 86% of mice treated with the opsonic MAb were sterile versus only 14% of lungs of mice treated with a nonopsonic MAb reactive with mucoid exopolysaccharide. An opsonic MAb of human origin, if broadly cross-reactive with mucoid clinical strains of *P. aeruginosa*, could interfere with *P. aeruginosa* colonization of lungs of young patients with CF.

4.2.2. Outer Membrane Proteins

Two murine MAb, an IgG1 (MA2-10) against porin protein F and an IgG of unspecified subclass (MA1-6) against lipoprotein H2, were given to mice prior to ocular wounding and topical challenge with *P. aeruginosa*. Each MAb minimized ocular disease in infected mice. In contrast, a murine IgG2a (MA4-4) against porin F was less effective, and IgG1 against lipoprotein I was inactive.[185] Protection in this eye infection model may have resulted from the MAb opsonic activity or by interfering with microbial attachment to the scarified cornea. The anti-porin F MAb (MA4-4) was protective in murine models of peritonitis and burn-wound sepsis.[183] Direct comparisons between MAb against outer membrane protein and smooth LPS in models of murine peritonitis,[194] murine burn wound sepsis,[194] and guinea pig pneumonia[196] indicate that anti-outer-membrane protein MAb are several hundred-fold less protective than anti-LPS MAb. Because outer membrane proteins are highly conserved in *P. aeruginosa*, MAb against these antigens remain an attractive target for the development of broadly cross-reactive immunotherapeutics.

4.2.3. Flagella

MAb against flagella antigens a[190] and b[190,191] recently have been described. An anti-a MAb, combined with an anti-b MAb, bound to 98.4% (N = 257) of motile clinical isolates of *P. aeruginosa*.[190] The MAb were highly protective in a model of burn-wound sepsis when given up to 7 hr following challenge.[190] The potency of these MAb appears comparable to anti-LPS MAb. The anti-flagella MAb were weakly opsonic, and their protection likely relies upon inhibition of bacterial motility. It remains to be seen if anti-flagella MAb protect in other models of infection such as peritonitis and pneumonia.

4.2.4. Polysaccharide Core of P. aeruginosa LPS

Terashima and colleagues[193] have described a human IgM MAb (MH-4H7) that binds to an outer-core polysaccharide epitope of 72% (N = 81) of strains of Homma serotypes A, F, G, H, K, and M. MH-4H7 did not bind to strains of serotypes B, E, and I. In a peritonitis model in normal mice, MH-4H7 increased the LD_{50} of selected strains of serotypes A, F, H, and K by 3- to 8-fold. No protection was evident against serotype M. Protection was variable against serotype G and ranged from a 1.3- to 180-fold increase in LD_{50}. Complement-dependent opsonic killing of serotypes A and G was noted. MH-4H7 was significantly protective against two serotype G strains in burned and neutropenic mice. Other investigators have described MAb cross-reactive with *P. aeruginosa* core polysaccharides and lipid A of heterologous serotypes, however, protection studies have not been reported.[212–217]

4.2.5. O-antigen

Numerous investigators have prepared murine and human MAb to O-antigens of *P. aeruginosa*. When tested for efficacy *in vivo*, these MAb tend to be serotype-specific and protective at low doses, and to enhance the activity of antimicrobial agents in therapy of established infection.[218] There are, however, reports of MAb that cross-react in serologic assay with two or more *P. aeruginosa* serotypes. Seeking such cross-reactive MAb is a worthwhile task, for if protective, their inclusion in a therapeutic "cocktail" will reduce the total number of MAb required to provide broad coverage against *P. aeruginosa* serotypes. For example, Zweerink *et al.*[199] described a human IgM MAb derived from Epstein–Barr virus (EBV) transformed B-cells. In immunoassay this MAb, 9H10, reacted with LPS of IATS serotypes 2, 5, 7/8, 10, and 16. The MAb was protective in neutropenic mice against IATS 2 and 7/8 but not against IATS 5. Similarly, Lang *et al.*[201] prepared a human IgM derived from an EBV-transformed cell line fused with a human myeloma cell line. This MAb, 2-8AH79, reacted in immunoassay with O-polysaccharide of Fisher immunotypes 1, 3, 4, and 6. In a model of burn wound sepsis, however, 2-8AH79 was protective only against immunotypes 3 and 4.

Barclay *et al.*[195] prepared a panel of 18 murine MAb reactive in ELISA with a cell wall extract of IATS 1. In a murine model of peritonitis, at least one MAb each of isotypes IgG1, IgG2, IgG2b, IgG3, and IgM was highly protective with a PD_{50} of ≤0.009 μg MAb/mouse. These investigators found no clear relationship between potency in the mouse protection test and ELISA reactivity or immunoglobulin isotype. Pier *et al.*[219] studied human anti-LPS MAb of IgG2, IgM, and IgA isotypes. All three MAb were potent in an opsonophagocytic assay against their homologous serotype of *P. aeruginosa*. The opsonic activity of the IgG2 MAb was markedly enhanced by complement. The activity of the IgA MAb was indifferent to complement, while the opsonic activity of the IgM MAb was absolutely dependent on complement. The three MAb were equally protective in neutropenic mice, although when complement was depleted by cobra venom factor, IgM was inactive.

Several groups have prepared human MAb that could be suitable for formulation of a therapeutic MAb "cocktail." Suzuki et al.[198] described two IgG MAb and an IgM MAb obtained from EBV-transformed B-cells. In a murine model of peritonitis, these three MAb were protective against IATS serotypes 1, 3, and 6 and dosages ≤3.1 μg MAb/mouse. Sawada et al.[220–222] prepared five human IgG2 MAb from tonsillar B-cells fused with a murine myeloma. In a murine model of peritonitis, these five MAb were protective at ≤4.3 μg IgG/mouse against homologous challenge strains of Homma serotypes A, E, G, B, and I. These five serotypes are equivalent to IATS 3, 11, 6, (2, 5 and 16), and 1, respectively, and account for about 80% of clinical isolates of P. aeruginosa. Zweerink et al.[199,223,224] prepared four passively protective IgM MAb from EBV-transformed B-cells. Three of the MAb reacted with homologous LPS serotypes of IATS 1, 10, and 11. The other MAb was reactive against IATS 2 and 7/8. When given 2 hr before challenge, these four MAb were protective at ≤2 μg/mouse in a model of peritonitis in neutropenic animals.[199] Survival in MAb-treated mice correlated with rapid elimination of P. aeruginosa from the peritoneal cavity or inhibition of microbial proliferation. In a model of pneumonia in neutropenic mice, MAb RM5 was highly protective against homologous IATS 11.[224] Protection in pneumonia required higher doses of MAb than were required for protection in peritonitis.[199,224] Survival in mice treated 2 hr before aerosol challenge with 0, 2.5, 10, or 40 μg IgM/mouse was 7%, 35%, 55%, and 93%, respectively.[224] Survival in MAb-treated mice correlated with a reduced incidence of bacteremia and a lower microbial burden within the lung. This study indicates that sufficient IgM MAb can diffuse into the infected lung to promote opsonic clearance of P. aeruginosa. A human IgM MAb, ICI, reactive with IATS 2 and 5 LPS, was prepared from EBV-derived B-cells.[220–225] Guinea pigs were treated IV with MAb ICI 2 hr after intratracheal challenge with P. aeruginosa IATS 2.[200] MAb ICI therapy of established pneumonia significantly enhanced survival; none of 31 controls survived versus 18 of 47 ICI-treated animals. Survival correlated with a decreased incidence of bacteremia. Examination of bronchoalveolar lavage fluid by immunofluorescent staining indicated that bacteria within the lung were coated with human IgM. MAb ICI is part of a panel of human MAb that have been formulated into a MAb "cocktail."[226] The preparation contains five IgM reactive with IATS serotypes 1, 2/5, 6, 8, and 11 plus an IgG1 that neutralizes the enzymatic activity of ETA. The safety, pharmacokinetics, and functional activity of these MAb has been studied in humans.[226] Each of the five IgM MAb are potent complement-dependent opsonins against homologous serotypes, and each is protective in a model of burn-wound sepsis at doses ranging from 0.04 to 0.40 mg/kg.[227] The IgM MAb enhance the activity of ciprofloxacin treatment in murine models of established burn-wound sepsis, aspiration pneumonia, and cellulitis in neutropenic mice.[228]

4.3. Safety and Efficacy Considerations for Monoclonal Antibody Therapy

A number of safety concerns must be addressed when considering using human or murine Monoclonal Antibody (MAb) for immunotherapy. A few examples of real problems and potential problems follow: Significant levels of cytokines IL-1, IL-6, and TNF have been found in ascites fluid from mice injected with various hybridomas.[229] If not removed during MAb purification, these cytokines could induce local or systemic inflammation in the MAb recipient. The use of murine hybridomas or human B-cell–murine myeloma hybridomas could lead to contamination of MAb by murine retroviruses. Some of these viruses can infect human cells in tissue culture.[230] The use of pooled human AB serum in culture of human lymphocytes led to a multicenter outbreak of hepatitis A.[231] Ideally, hybridomas should be cultured in serum-free medium. A murine IgM MAb reactive with *S. minnesota* Re 595 LPS and *E. coli* J5 LPS also bound strongly to DNA-histone.[232] The implications of infusing a large dose of antinuclear antibody are not known. Because murine immunoglobulin is immunogenic in humans, it seems reasonable that MAb for immunotherapy of *P. aeruginosa* infection should be of human origin. In addition, it is obvious that MAb intended for human use must be free of extraneous macromolecules such as nonantibody hybridoma-derived proteins and oncogenic DNA. Furthermore, the MAb should be produced and processed in such a manner that no structural changes occur that could affect safety or efficacy.

It is clear that MAb against O-antigens of gram-negative bacteria are highly protective. As previously discussed, the literature is replete with conflicting reports of efficacy of MAb and antisera directed against other antigens such as LPS core polysaccharide and outer-membrane proteins. Chong and Huston[74] have shown that pretreatment of mice with as little as 1 ng of LPS protects against heterologous *E. coli* challenge, and 100 ng of LPS is protective against *P. aeruginosa*. This observation and similar observations by others[60,75,233] should prompt all investigators to examine their MAb preparations for LPS contamination in the *Limulus* amebocyte lysate assay before beginning preclinical studies in animals.

REFERENCES

1. Bennett, J. V., 1974, Nosocomial infections due to *Pseudomonas*, *J. Infect. Dis.* **130**:S4–S7.
2. Tapper, M. L., and Armstrong, D., 1974, Bacteremia due to *Pseudomonas aeruginosa* complicating neoplastic disease: A progress report, *J. Infect. Dis.* **130**:S14–23.

3. Baltch, A. A., and Smith, R. P., 1985, Combinations of antibiotics against *Pseudomonas aeruginosa*, *Am. J. Med.* **79**:8–16.
4. Bisbe, J., Gatell, J. M., Puig, J., Mallolas, J., Martinez, J. A., Jimenez de Anta, M. T., and Soriano, E., 1988, *Pseudomonas aeruginosa* bacteremia: Univariate and multivarate analyses of factors influencing the prognosis in 133 episodes, *Rev. Infect. Dis.* **10**:629–635.
5. Kato, M., de la Vega, S. L., and Mohar, A., 1990, Infections in patients with cancer in Mexico, *Rev. Infect. Dis.* **12**:960–961.
6. May, J. R., Herrick, N. C., and Thompson, D., 1972, Bacterial infection in cystic fibrosis, *Arch. Dis. Child.* **47**:903–913.
7. Mearns, M. B., Hunt, G. H., and Rushworth, R., 1972, Bacterial flora of the respiratory tract in patients with cystic fibrosis, *Arch. Dis. Child.* **47**:902–907.
8. Bryan, C. S., and Reynolds, K. L., 1984, Bacteremic nosocomial pneumonia. Analysis of 172 episodes from a single metropolitan area, *Am. Rev. Respir. Dis.* **135**:426–432.
9. Craig, C. P., and Connelly, S., 1984, Effect of intensive care unit nosocomial pneumonia on duration of stay and mortality, *Infect. Control* **12**:233–238.
10. McManus, A. T., Mason, A. D., Jr., McManus, W. F., and Pruitt, B. A., Jr., 1985, Twenty-five year review of *Pseudomonas aeruginosa* bacteremia in a burn center, *Eur. J. Clin. Microbiol.* **4**:219–223.
11. Eickhoff, T. C., and Ehret, J. M., 1976, In vitro comparison of cefoxitin, cefamandole, cephalexin and cephalothin, *Antimicrob. Agents Chemother.* **9**:994–999.
12. Reimer, L. G., Stratton, C. W., and Reller, L. B., 1981, Minimum inhibitory and bactericidal concentrations of 44 antimicrobial agents against three standard control strains in broth with and without human serum, *Antimicrob. Agents Chemother.* **19**:1050–1055.
13. Digranes, A., Dibb, W. L., and Østervold, B., 1984, In vitro comparison of the activity to five β-lactam antibiotics and gentamicin against 493 clinical, bacterial isolates: A Norwegian study, *Curr. Ther. Res.* **35**:610–617.
14. Parry, M. F., Folta, D., Nossek, H., Anderson, M., Azzarello, L., Holmes, D., Jacob, R., McElree, S., Sabato, S., Tatton, B., and Welch, B., 1985, Comparative activity of ciprofloxacin and other new agents against 1454 clinical isolates at a community hospital, *Curr. Ther. Res.* **38**:755–761.
15. Satta, G., Cornaglia, G., Foddis, G., and Pompei, R., 1988, Evaluation of ceftriaxone and other antibiotics against *Escherichia coli*, *Pseudomonas aeruginosa*, and *Streptococcus pneumoniae* under in vitro conditions simulating those of serious infections, *Antimicrob. Agents Chemother.* **32**:552–560.
16. Schimpff, S. C., Greene, W. H., Young, V. M., and Wiernik, P. H., 1974, Significance of *Pseudomonas aeruginosa* in the patient with leukemia or lymphoma, *J. Infect. Dis.* **130**:S24–S31.
17. Mathisen, G. E., Meyer, R. D., Thompson, J. M., and Finegold, S. M., 1982, Clinical evaluation of moxalactam, *Antimicrob. Agents Chemother.* **21**:780–786.
18. Bayer, A. S., Hirano, L., and Yih, J., 1988, Development of β-lactam resistance and increased quinoline MICs during therapy of experimental *Pseudomonas aeruginosa* endocarditis, *Antimicrob. Agents Chemother.* **32**:231–235.
19. Milatovic, D., and Bravery, I., 1987, Development of resistance during antibiotic therapy, *Eur. J. Clin. Microbiol.* **6**:234–244.
20. LeBel, M., Bergeron, M. G., Vallee, F., Fiset, C., Chasse, G., Bigonesse, P., and Rivard, G., 1986, Pharmacokinetics and pharmacodynamics of ciprofloxacin in cystic fibrosis patients, *Antimicrob. Agents Chemother.* **30**:260–266.
21. Shooter, R. A., Walker, K. A., Williams, V. R., Horgan, G. M., Parker, M. T., Asheshov, E. H., and Bullimore, J., 1966, Faecal carriage of *Pseudomonas aeruginosa* in hospital patients. Possible spread from patient to patient, *Lancet* **2**:1331–1334.
22. Bauernfiend, A., Emminger, G., Hörl, G., Lorbeer, B., Przyklenk, B., and Weisslein-Pfister, C., 1987, Selective pressure of antistaphylococcal chemotherapeutics in favor of *Pseudomonas aeruginosa* in cystic fibrosis, *Infection* **15**:469–470.

23. Griffith, S. J., Nathan, C., Selander, R. K., Chamberlin, W., Gordon, S., Kabins, S., and Weinstein, R. A., 1989, The epidemiology of *Pseudomonas aeruginosa* in oncology patients in a general hospital, *J. Infect. Dis.* **160**:1030–1036.
24. Bodey, G. P., Bolivar, R., Fainstein, V., and Jadeja, L., 1983, Infections caused by *Pseudomonas aeruginosa*, *Rev. Infect. Dis.* **5**:279–313.
25. Grogan, J. B., 1966, *Pseudomonas aeruginosa* carriage in patients, *J. Trauma* **6**:639–643.
26. Schimpff, S. C., Moody, M., and Young, V. M., 1970, Relationship of colonization with *Pseudomonas aeruginosa* to development of *Pseudomonas* bacteremia in cancer patients, *Antimicrob. Agents Chemother.* **10**:240–244.
27. Janda, J. M., and Bottone, E. J., 1981, *Pseudomonas aeruginosa* enzyme profiling: Predictor of potential invasiveness and use as an epidemiological tool, *J. Clin. Microbiol.* **14**:55–60.
28. Cash, H. A., Straus, D. C., and Bass, J. A., 1983, *Pseudomonas aeruginosa* exoproducts as pulmonary virulence factors, *Can. J. Microbiol.* **29**:448–456.
29. Nicas, T. I., and Iglewski, B. H., 1985, The contribution of exoproducts of virulence of *Pseudomonas aeruginosa*, *Can. J. Microbiol.* **31**:387–392.
30. Gessard, C., 1982, Sur les colorations bleue et verte des linges a pansements, *Compt. Rend. Acad. Sci.* **94**:536–568.
31. Curtin, J. A., Petersdorf, R. J., and Bennett, I. L., Jr., 1961, *Pseudomonas* bacteremia: Review of ninety-one cases, *Ann. Intern. Med.* **54**:1077–1107.
32. Davis, S. D., Iannette, A., and Wedgwood, R. J., 1971, Antibiotics for *Pseudomonas aeruginosa* sepsis: Inadequate proof of efficacy, *J. Infect. Dis.* **124**:104–106.
33. Baltch, A. L., and Griffin, P. E., 1977, *Pseudomonas aeruginosa*: A clinical study of 75 patients, *Am. J. Med. Sci.* **247**:119–129.
34. Baltch, A. L., Hammer, M., Smith, R. P., and Stuphen, N., 1979, *Pseudomonas aeruginosa* bacteremia. Susceptibility of 100 blood culture isolates to given antimicrobial agents and its clinical significance, *J. Lab. Clin. Med.* **94**:201–214.
35. Millican, C., Evans, G., and Markley, K., 1966, Susceptibility of burned mice to *Pseudomonas aeruginosa* and protection by vaccination, *Ann. Surg.* **163**:603–610.
36. Markley, K., and Smallman, E., 1968, Protection by vaccination against *Pseudomonas* infection after thermal injury, *J. Bacteriol.* **96**:867–874.
37. Jones, R. J., 1968, Protection against *Pseudomonas aeruginosa* infection by immunization with fractions of culture filtrates of *P. aeruginosa*, *Br. J. Exp. Pathol.* **49**:411–420.
38. Jones, R. J., 1972, Specificity of early protective responses induced by *Pseudomonas* vaccines, *J. Hyg.* **70**:343–351.
39. Miller, J. M., Spilsbury, J. F., Jones, R. J., Roe, E. A., and Lowbury, E. J. L., 1976, A new polyvalent *Pseudomonas* vaccine, *J. Med. Microbiol.* **10**:19–27.
40. Jones, R. J., Roe, E. A., and Gupta, J. L., 1978, Low mortality in burned patients in a *Pseudomonas* vaccine trial, *Lancet* **ii**:401–403.
41. MacIntyre, S., McVeigh, T., and Owen, P., 1986, Immunochemical and biochemical analysis of the polyvalent *Pseudomonas aeruginosa* vaccine PEV, *Infect. Immun.* **51**:675–686.
42. MacIntyre, S., Lucken, R., and Owen, P., 1986, Smooth lipopolysaccharide is the major protective antigen for mice in the surface extract from IATS serotype 6 contributing to the polyvalent *Pseudomonas aeruginosa* vaccine PEV, *Infect. Immun.* **52**:76–84.
43. Brokopp, C. D., Gomez-Lus, R., and Farmer, J. J., III, 1977, Serological typing of *Pseudomonas aeruginosa*: Use of commercial antisera and live antigens, *J. Clin. Microbiol.* **5**:640–649.
44. Fisher, M. W., Devlin, H. B., and Gnabasik, F. J., 1969, New immunotype schema for *Pseudomonas aeruginosa* based on protective antigens, *J. Bacteriol.* **98**:835–836.
45. Verder, E., and Evans, J. A., 1961, A proposed antigenic schema for the identification of strains of *Pseudomonas aeruginosa*, *J. Infect. Dis.* **109**:183–193.
46. Hanessian, S., Regan, W., Watson, D., and Haskell, T. H., 1971, Isolation and characterization of antigenic components of a new heptavalent *Pseudomonas* vaccine, *Nature* **229**:209–210.

47. Young, L. S., Meyer, R. D., and Armstrong, D., 1973, *Pseudomonas aeruginosa* vaccine in cancer patients, *Ann. Intern. Med.* **79**:518–527.
48. Pennington, J. E., 1974, Preliminary investigation of *Pseudomonas aeruginosa* vaccine in patients with leukemia and cystic fibrosis, *J. Infect. Dis.* **130**:S159–S162.
49. Harvath, L., and Andersen, B. R., 1976, Evaluation of type-specific and non-type specific *Pseudomonas* vaccine for treatment of *Pseudomonas* sepsis during granulocytopenia, *Infect. Immun.* **13**:1139–1143.
50. Drewry, D. J., Symes, K. C., Gray, G. W., and Wilkinson, S. G., 1975, Studies of polysaccharide fractions from the lipopolysaccharide of *Pseudomonas aeruginosa* N.C.T.C. 1999, *Biochem J.* **149**:93–106.
51. Tsay, G. C., and Collins, M. S., 1984, Preparation and characterization of a nontoxic polysaccharide-protein conjugate that induces active immunity and passively protective antibody against *Pseudomonas aeruginosa* immunotype 1 in mice, *Infect. Immun.* **45**:217–221.
52. Cryz, S. J., Jr., Fürer, E., Sadoff, J. C., and Germanier, R., 1986, *Pseudomonas aeruginosa* immunotype 5 polysaccharide-toxin A conjugate vaccine, *Infect. Immun.* **52**:161–165.
53. Cryz, S. J., Jr., Fürer, E., Cross, A. S., Wegmann, A., Germanier, R., and Sadoff, J. C., 1987, Safety and immunogenicity of a *Pseudomonas aeruginosa* O-polysaccharide-toxin A conjugate vaccine in humans, *J. Clin. Invest.* **80**:51–56.
54. Cryz, S. J., Jr., Fürer, E., Sadoff, J. C., and Germanier, R., 1987, A polyvalent *Pseudomonas aeruginosa* O-polysaccharide-toxin A conjugate vaccine, *Antibiot. Chemother.* **39**:249–255.
55. Cryz, S. J., Sadoff, J. C., Cross, A. S., and Fürer, E., 1989, Safety and immunogenicity of a polyvalent *Pseudomonas aeruginosa* O-polysaccharide-toxin A vaccine in humans, *Antibiot. Chemother.* **42**:177–183.
56. Cryz, S. J., Jr., Fürer, E., Sadoff, J. C., Fredking, T., Que, J. U., and Cross, A. S., 1991, Production and characterization of a human hyperimmune intravenous immunoglobulin against *Pseudomonas aeruginosa* and *Klebsiella* species, *J. Infect. Dis.* **163**:1055–1061.
57. Pier, G. B., Sidberry, H. F., Zolyomi, S., and Sadoff, J. C., 1978, Isolation and characterization of a high-molecular weight polysaccharide from the slime of *Pseudomonas aeruginosa*, *Infect. Immun.* **22**:908–918.
58. Pier, G. B., Sidberry, H. F., and Sadoff, J. C., 1981, High-molecular weight polysaccharide antigen from *Pseudomonas aeruginosa* immunotype 2, *Infect. Immun.* **34**:461–468.
59. Pier, G. B., and Thomas, D. M., 1983, Characterization of the human immune response to a polysaccharide vaccine from *Pseudomonas aeruginosa*, *J. Infect. Dis.* **148**:206–213.
60. Cryz, S. J., Jr., Fürer, E., and Germanier, R., 1984, Protection against fatal *Pseudomonas aeruginosa* burn wound sepsis by immunization with lipopolysaccharide and high molecular weight polysaccharide, *Infect. Immun.* **43**:795–799.
61. Lam, J. S., Mutharia, L. M., Hancock, R. E. W., Holby, N., Lam, K., Baek, L., and Costerton, J. W., 1983, Immunogenicity of *Pseudomonas aeruginosa* outer membrane antigens examined by crossed immunoelectrophoresis, *Infect. Immun.* **42**:88–98.
62. Matthews-Greer, J. M., and Gilleland, H. E., Jr., 1987, Outer membrane protein F (porin) preparation of *Pseudomonas aeruginosa* as a protective vaccine against heterologous immunotype strains in a burned mouse model, *J. Infect. Dis.* **155**:1281–1291.
63. Gilleland, H. E., Jr., and Matthews-Greer, J. M., 1987, Perspectives on the potential for successful development of outer membrane protein vaccines, *Eur. J. Clin. Microbiol.* **6**:231–233.
64. Garner, C. V., DesJardins, D., and Pier, G. B., 1990, Immunogenic properties of *Pseudomonas aeruginosa* mucoid exopolysaccharide, *Infect. Immun.* **58**:1835–1842.
65. Pier, G. B., Small, G. J., and Warren, H. B., 1990, Protection against mucoid *Pseudomonas aeruginosa* in rodent models of endobronchial infection, *Science* **249**:537–540.
66. Montie, T. C., Drake, D., Sellin, H., Slater, O., and Edmonds, S., 1987, Motility, virulence and protection with a flagella vaccine against *Pseudomonas aeruginosa* infection, *Antibiot. Chemother.* **39**:233–248.

67. Holder, I. A., Wheeler, R., and Montie, T. C., 1982, Flagellar preparations from *Pseudomonas aeruginosa*: Animal protection studies, *Infect. Immun.* **35**:276–280.
68. Holder, I. A., and Naglich, J. G., 1986, Experimental studies of the pathogenesis of infections due to *Pseudomonas aeruginosa*: Immunization using divalent flagella preparations, *J. Trauma* **26**:118–122.
69. Rotering, H., and Dorner, F., 1989, Studies on a *Pseudomonas aeruginosa* flagella vaccine, *Antibiot. Chemother.* **42**:218–228.
70. Sezen, I. Y., Scharmann, W., and Blobel, H., 1975, Effects of an antiserum prepared against purified protease of *Pseudomonas aeruginosa*, *Zentralbl. Bakteriol. Hyg. I. Abt. Orig.* **231**: 126–132.
71. Cryz, S. J., Jr., Fürer, E., and Germanier, R., 1983, Passive protection against *Pseudomonas aeruginosa* infection in an experimental leukopenic mouse model, *Infect. Immun.* **40**: 659–664.
72. Cryz, S. J., Jr., Fürer, E., and Germanier, R., 1983, Protection against *Pseudomonas aeruginosa* infection in a murine burn wound sepsis model by passive transfer of antitoxin A, antielastase and antilipopolysaccharide, *Infect. Immun.* **39**:1072–1079.
73. Lydick, E., McLean, A. A., Woodhour, A. F., and Callahan, L. T., III., 1985, Responses of adult volunteers to a *Pseudomonas aeruginosa* exotoxoid-A vaccine, *J. Infect. Dis.* **151**:375.
74. Chong, K. T., and Huston, M., 1987, Implications of endotoxin contamination in the evaluation of antibodies to lipopolysaccharide in a murine model of gram-negative sepsis, *J. Infect. Dis.* **156**:713–719.
75. Marx, A., Meitert, E., Salageanu, A., Olinescu, A., Savulian, C., Sima, F., and Chersulick, E., 1987, Specific and nonspecific protection of mice by *Pseudomonas aeruginosa* lipopolysaccharides, *Zentralbl. Bakteriol. Hyg. A.* **264**:154–162.
76. Lányi, B., 1970, Serological properties of *Pseudomonas aeruginosa* II. Type-specific thermolabile (flagellar) antigens, *Acta Microbiol. Acad. Hung.* **17**:35–48.
77. Ansorg, R. A., Knoche, M. E., Spries, A. F., and Kraus, C. J., 1984, Differentiation of the major flagellar antigens of *Pseudomonas aeruginosa* by the slide coagglutination technique, *J. Clin. Microbiol.* **20**:84–88.
78. McManus, A. T., Moody, E. E., and Mason, A. D., 1980, Bacterial motility: A component in experimental *Pseudomonas aeruginosa* burn wound sepsis, *Burns* **6**:235–239.
79. Craven, R. A., and Montie, T. C., 1981, Motility and chemotaxis of three strains of *Pseudomonas aeruginosa* used for virulence studies, *Can. J. Microbiol.* **27**:458–460.
80. Drake, D., and Montie, T. C., 1988, Flagella, motility and invasive virulence of *Pseudomonas aeruginosa*, *J. Gen. Microbiol.* **134**:43–52.
81. Allison, J. S., Dawson, M., Drake, D., and Montie, T. C., 1985, Electrophoretic separation and molecular weight characterization of *Pseudomonas aeruginosa* H-antigen flagillins, *Infect. Immun.* **49**:770–774.
82. Ansorg, R., 1978, Flagellaspezifisches H-antigenschema von *Pseudomonas aeruginosa*, *Zentralbl. Bakteriol. Mikrobiol. Hyg. [A]* **242**:228–238.
83. Anderson, T. R., and Montie, T. C., 1987, Opsonphagocytosis of *Pseudomonas aeruginosa* treated with antiflagellar serum, *Infect. Immun.* **55**:3204–3206.
84. Montie, T. C., Craven, R. C., and Holder, I. A., 1982, Flagellar preparations from *Pseudomonas aeruginosa*: Isolation and characterization, *Infect. Immun.* **35**:281–288.
85. Ansorg, R., Schmitt, W., and Schwerk, V., 1978, Antikörperbildung gegen somatische und flagelläre Antigene von *Pseudomonas aeruginosa*, *Med. Microbiol. Immunol.* **165**:181–189.
86. Moody, M. R., Kessel, R. W. I., Young, V. M., and Fiset, P., 1978, Role of nonagglutinating antibody in the protracted immunity of vaccinated mice to *Pseudomonas aeruginosa* infection, *Infect. Immun.* **21**:905–913.
87. Harmon, R. C., Rutherford, R. L., Wu, H. M., and Collins, M. S., 1989, Monoclonal antibody-mediated protection and neutralization of motility in experimental *Proteus mirabilis* infection, *Infect. Immun.* **57**:1936–1941.

88. Heidbrink, P. J., Toews, G. B., Gross, G. N., and Pierce, A. K., 1982, Mechanisms of complement-mediated clearance of bacteria from the murine lung, *Am. Rev. Respir. Dis.* **125:**517–520.
89. Cerquetti, M. C., Sordelli, D. O., Bellanti, J. A., and Hooke, A. M., 1986, Lung defenses against *Pseudomonas aeruginosa* in C5-deficient mice with different genetic backgrounds, *Infect. Immun.* **52:**853–857.
90. Young, L. S., and Armstrong, D., 1972, Human immunity to *Pseudomonas aeruginosa* I. In-vitro interaction of bacteria, polymorphonuclear leukocytes, and serum factors, *J. Infect. Dis.* **126:**257–276.
91. Bjornson, A. B., and Michael, J. G., 1971, Contribution of humoral and cellular factors to the resistance of experimental infection by *Pseudomonas aeruginosa* in mice I. Interaction between immunoglobulins, heat labile serum factors, and phagocytic cells in the killing of bacteria, *Infect. Immun.* **4:**462–467.
92. Bjornson, A. B., and Michael, J. G., 1972, Contribution of humoral and cellular factors to the resistance to experimental infection by *Pseudomonas aeruginosa* in mice, II. Opsonic, agglutinative and protective capacities of immunoglobulin G anti-*Pseudomonas* antibodies, *Infect. Immun.* **5:**775–782.
93. Epstein, R. B., Wayman, F. J., Bennett, B. T., and Anderson, B. R., 1974, *Pseudomonas* septicemia in neutropenic dogs I. Treatment with granulocyte transfusions, *Transfusion* **14:**51–57.
94. Strauss, R. G., 1978, Therapeutic neutrophil transfusions: Are controlled studies no longer appropriate? *Am. J. Med.* **65:**1001–1006.
95. Winston, D. J., Ho, W. G., Howell, C. L., Miller, M. J., Mickey, R., Martin, W. J., Lin, C. -H., and Gale, R. P., 1980, Cytomegalovirus infections associated with leukocyte transfusions, *Ann. Intern. Med.* **93:**671–675.
96. Tanaka, T., Okamura, S., Okada, K., Suga, A., Shimono, N., Ohhara, N., Yoshio, H., Sawae, Y., and Niho, Y., 1989, Protective effect of recombinant murine granulocyte-macrophage colony-stimulating factor against *Pseudomonas aeruginosa* infection in leukopenic mice, *Infect. Immun.* **57:**1792–1799.
97. Cohn, E. J., Strong, L. E., Hughes, W. C., Jr., Mulford, D. J., Ashworth, J. N., Melin, M., and Taylor, H. L., 1946, Preparation and properties of serum and plasma proteins IV. A system for the separation into fractions and lipoprotein components of biological tissue and fluids, *J. Am. Chem. Soc.* **68:**459–475.
98. Pollack, M., 1983, Antibody activity against *Pseudomonas aeruginosa* in immune globulins prepared for intravenous use in humans, *J. Infect. Dis.* **147:**1090–1098.
99. Rosenthal, S. M., 1967, Local and systemic therapy of *Pseudomonas* septicemia in burned mice, *Ann. Surg.* **165:**97–103.
100. Fisher, M. W., and Manning, M. C., 1958, Studies on the immunotherapy of bacterial infections: I. The comparative effectiveness of human γ-globulin against various bacterial species in mice, *J. Immunol.* **81:**29–31.
101. Waisbren, B. A., 1957, The treatment of bacterial infections with the combination of antibiotics and gamma globulin, *Antibiot. Chemother.* **7:**322–333.
102. Fisher, M. W., 1957, Synergism between human gamma globulin and chloramphenicol in the treatment of experimental bacterial infections, *Antibiot. Chemother.* **7:**315–321.
103. Milican, R. C., Rust, J., and Rosenthal, S. M., 1957, Gamma globulin factors protective against infections from *Pseudomonas* and other organisms, *Science* **126:**509–511.
104. Stone, H. H., Graber, C. D., Martin, J. D., Jr., and Kolb, L., 1965, Evaluation of gamma globulin for prophylaxis against burn sepsis, *Surgery* **58:**810–814.
105. Kefalides, N. A., Arana, J. A., Bazan, A., Bocanegra, M., Stastry, P., Velarde, N., and Rosenthal, S. M., 1962, Role of infection in mortality from severe burns: Evaluation of plasma, gamma-globulin, albumin and saline-solution therapy in a group of Peruvian children, *N. Engl. J. Med.* **267:**317–323.

106. Barandun, S., Kistler, P., Jeunet, F., and Isliker, H., 1962, Intravenous administration of human γ-globulin, *Vox Sang.* **7:**157–174.
107. Smith, G. N., Griffiths, B., Mollison, D., and Mollison, P. L., 1972, Uptake of IgG after intramuscular and subcutaneous injection, *Lancet* **2:**1208–1212.
108. Ceska, M., 1981, Binding of protein A to some human gamma-globulins used intravenously, *Vox Sang.* **40:**395–402.
109. Skvaril, F., and Gardi, A., 1988, Difference among available immunoglobulin preparations for intravenous use, *Pediatr. Infect. Dis. J.* **7:**S43–S48.
110. Steele, R. W., and Steele, R. W., 1989, Functional capacity of immunoglobulin G preparations and the F(ab')$_2$ split product, *J. Clin. Microbiol.* **27:**640–643.
111. Lundblad, J. L., Mitra, G., Sternberg, M. M., and Schroeder, D. D., 1986, Comparative studies of impurities in intravenous immunoglobulin preparations, *Rev. Infect. Dis.* **8:**S382–S390.
112. Greenbaum, B. H., 1990, Differences in immunoglobulin preparations for intravenous use: A comparison of six products, *J. Pediatr. Hematol. Oncol.* **12:**490–496.
113. Davis, S. D., 1975, Efficacy of modified human immun serum globulin in the treatment of experimental murine infections with seven immunotypes of *Pseudomonas aeruginosa*, *J. Infect. Dis.* **131:**717–721.
114. Hill, H. R., and Bathras, J. M., 1986, Protective and opsonic activities of a native pH 4.25 intravenous immunoglobulin G preparation against common bacterial pathogens, *Rev. Infect. Dis.* **8:**S396–S400.
115. Hill, H. R., Augustine, N. H., and Shigeoka, A. O., 1984, Comparative opsonic activity of intravenous gamma globulin preparations for common bacterial pathogens, *Am. J. Med.* **76:**61–66.
116. Tomioka, H., Iwamura, Y., Suzuki, Y., Ohtomo, S., and Hashimoto, Y., 1980, Protective effects of S-sulfonated human gamma globulin against experimental infections in mice, *Infect. Immun.* **30:**329–336.
117. Jupa-Marcinkowski, V., Mynard, M. C., Danve, B., and Schmitz, P. I. M., 1985, The influence of immunoglobulin on the development of *Pseudomonas aeruginosa* infection in an immunocompromised mouse model, *J. Biol. Stand.* **13:**235–242.
118. Collins, M. S., and Roby, R. E., 1983, Anti-*Pseudomonas aeruginosa* activity of an intravenous human IgG preparation in burned mice, *J. Trauma* **23:**530–534.
119. Collins, M. S., and Dorsey, J. H., 1984, Comparative anti-*Pseudomonas aeruginosa* activity of chemically modified and native immunoglobulin G (human) and potentiation of antibiotic protection against *Pseudomonas aeruginosa* and group B *Streptococcus in vivo*, *Am. J. Med.* **76:**155–160.
120. Holder, I. A., and Naglich, J. G., 1984, Experimental studies of the pathogenesis of infections due to *Pseudomonas aeruginosa*: Treatment with intravenous immunoglobulin. *Am. J. Med.* **76:**161–167.
121. Collins, M. S., Tsay, G. C., Hector, R. F., Roby, R. E., and Dorsey, J. H., 1986, Immunoglobulin G: Potentiation of tobramycin and azlocillin in the treatment of *Pseudomonas aeruginosa* sepsis in neutropenic mice and neutralization of exotoxin A *in vivo*, *Rev. Infect. Dis.* **8:**S420–S425.
122. Moody, M. R., Young, V. M., Kemton, D. M., and Vermeulen, G. D., 1972, *Pseudomonas aeruginosa* in a center for cancer research. I. Distribution of intraspecies types from human and environmental sources, *J. Infect. Dis.* **125:**95–101.
123. Collins, M. S., Edwards, A., Roby, R. E., Mehton, N. S., and Ladehoff, D., 1989, *Pseudomonas* immune globulin improves survival in experimental *Pseudomonas aeruginosa* bacteremic pneumonia, *Antibiot. Chemother.* **42:**184–192.
124. Munster, A. M., Moran, K. T., Thupari, J., Allo, M., and Wunchurch, R. A., 1987, Prophylactic intravenous immunoglobulin replacement in high-risk burn patients, *J. Burn Care Rehabil.* **8:**376–380.

125. Waymack, J. P., Jenkins, M. E., Alexander, J. W., Warden, G. D., Miller, A. C., Carey, M., Ogle, C. K., and Kopcha, R. G., 1989, A prospective trial of prophylactic intravenous immune globulin for the prevention of infections in severely burned patients, *Burns* **15:** 71–76.
126. Cooperative Group for the Study of Immunoglobulin in Chronic Lymphocytic Leukemia, 1988, Intravenous immunoglobulin for the prevention of infection in chronic lymphocytic leukemia: A randomized, controlled clinical trial, *N. Engl. J. Med.* **319:**902–907.
127. Griffiths, H. Brennan, V., Lea, J., Bunch, C., Lee, M., and Chapel, H., 1989, Crossover study of immunoglobulin replacement therapy in patients with low-grade B-cell tumors, *Blood* **73:**366–368.
128. Rolfman, C. M., Lederman, H. M., Lavi, S., Stein, L. D., Levison, H., and Gelfand, E. W., 1985, Benefit of intravenous IgG replacement in hypogammaglobulinemic patients with chronic sinopulmonary disease, *Am. J. Med.* **79:**171–174.
129. Chirico, G., Rondini, G., Plebani, A., Chiara, A., Massa, M., and Ugazio, A. G., 1987, Intravenous gammaglobulin therapy for prophylaxis of infection in high-risk neonates, *J. Pediatr.* **110:**437–441.
130. Clapp, D. W., Kliegman, R. M., Baley, J. E., Shenker, N., Kyllonen, K., Fanaroff, A. A., and Berger, M., 1989, Use of intravenously administered immune globulin to prevent nosocomial sepsis in low birth weight infants: Report of a pilot study, *J. Pediatr.* **115:** 973–978.
131. Sakiel, S., Schiller, B., Buchowicz, J., and Kotkowska-Tomanek, E., 1983, Anti-*Pseudomonas* immunoglobulin: III. Preliminary clinical evaluation, *Arch. Immunol. Ther. Exp.* **31:**517–521.
132. Meitert, T., Meitert, E., Szegli, G., and Peligrad, I., 1982, Therapeutic *Pseudomonas aeruginosa* antisera: Preparation, control and administration, *Arch. Roum. Pathol. Exp. Microbiol.* **41:**115–121.
133. Bielory, L., Kemeny, D. M., Richards, D., and Lessof, M. H., 1990, IgG subclass antibody production in human serum sickness, *J. Allergy Clin. Immunol.* **85:**573–577.
134. Jones, C. E., Alexander, J. W., and Fisher, M., 1973, Clinical evaluation of *Pseudomonas* hyperimmune globulin, *J. Surg. Res.* **14:**87–96.
135. Holder, I. A., and Neely, A. N., 1987, Experimental studies of the pathogenesis of infections due to *Pseudomonas aeruginosa*: Post-sepsis treatment using *Pseudomonas* hyperimmune globulin and antibiotics alone and in combination, *Serodiag. Immunother.* **1:**185–192.
136. Martindale, J. J., Ganzinger, V., Steinmüller, W., Millendorfer, F. A., Kollaritsch, H., and Wiedermann, G., 1988, Tolerability and immunogenicity of a polyvalent *Pseudomonas aeruginosa* extract vaccine in human volunteers, *Zentralbl. Bakteriol. Hyg. A* **268:**376–385.
137. Martindale, J. J., Ganzinger, V., Steinmüller, W., Gaundera, E., Millendorfer, A., and Bachmayer, H., 1989, Pharmacokinetics of anti-*Pseudomonas* hyperimmunoglobulin after single intravenous administration in health subjects, *Serodiag. Immunother. Infect. Dis.* **3:** 93–99.
138. Collins, M. S., and Roby, R. E., 1984, Protective activity of an intravenous immune globulin (human) enriched in antibody against lipopolysaccharide antigens of *Pseudomonas aeruginosa*, *Am. J. Med.* **76:**168–174.
139. Liu, P. V., Yoshii, S., and Hsieh, H., 1973, Exotoxins of *Pseudomonas aeruginosa*. II. Concentration, purification and characterization of exotoxin A, *J. Infect. Dis.* **128:**514–519.
140. Pollack, M., Callahan, L. T., III., and Taylor, N. S., 1976, Neutralizing antibody to *Pseudomonas aeruginosa* exotoxin in human sera: Evidence for *in vivo* toxin production during infections, *Infect. Immun.* **14:**942–947.
141. Pollack, M., Taylor, N. S., and Callahan, L. T., III, 1977, Exotoxin production by clinical isolates of *Pseudomonas aeruginosa*, *Infect. Immun.* **15:**776–780.
142. Bjorn, M. J., Vasil, M. L., Sadoff, J. C., and Iglewski, B. H., 1977, Incidence of exotoxin production by *Pseudomonas* species, *Infect. Immun.* **16:**362–366.
143. Collins, M. S., Tsay, G. C., Hector, R. E., Roby, R. E., and Dorsey, J. H., 1987, Therapy of

experimental *Pseudomonas* burn wound sepsis with ciprofloxacin and *Pseudomonas* immune globulin, *Antibiot. Chemother.* **39**:222–232.
144. Collins, M. S., Hector, R. E., Edwards, A. A., Ladehoff, D. K., and Dorsey, J. H., 1987, Prophylaxis of gram-negative and gram-positive infections in rodents with three intravenous immunoglobulins and therapy of experimental polymicrobial burn wound sepsis with *Pseudomonas* immunoglobulin and ciprofloxacin, *Infection* **15**:60–68.
145. Salata, R. A., Lederman, M. M., Shlaes, D. M., Jacobs, M. R., Eckstein, E., Tweardy, D., Toossi, Z., Chmielewski, R., Marino, J., King, C. H., Graham, R. C., and Ellner, J. J., 1987, Diagnosis of nosocomial pneumonia in intubated, intensive care unit patients, *Am. Rev. Respir. Dis.* **135**:426–432.
146. Chapel, H. M., and Bunch, C., 1987, Mechanisms of infection in chronic lymphocytic leukemia, *Semin. Hematol.* **24**:291–296.
147. Rolfman, C. M., Levison, H., and Gefland, E. W., 1987, High-dose versus low-dose intravenous immunoglobulin in hypogammaglobulinaemia and chronic lung disease, *Lancet* **1**:1075–1077.
148. Wingard, J. R., Dick, J., Charache, P., and Saral, R., 1986, Antibiotic-resistant bacteria in surveillance stool cultures of patients with prolonged neutropenia, *Antimicrob. Agents Chemother.* **30**:435–439.
149. Dick, J. D., Shull, V., Karp, J. E., and Valentine, J., 1988, Bacterial and host factors affecting *Pseudomonas aeruginosa* colonization versus bacteremia in granulocytopenic patients, *Eur. J. Clin. Oncol.* **24**:S47–S54.
150. Hilf, M., Yu, V. L., Sharp, J., Zuravleff, J. J., Korvick, J. A., and Muder, R. R., 1989, Antibiotic therapy for *Pseudomonas aeruginosa* bacteremia: Outcome correlations in a prospective study of 200 patients, *Am. J. Med.* **87**:540–546.
151. Neely, A. N., and Holder, I. A., 1987, Use of passive immunotherapy in the treatment of experimental *Pseudomonas aeruginosa* infections in burns, *Antibiot. Chemother.* **39**:26–40.
152. Pennington, J. E., Pier, G. B., and Small, G. J., 1986, Efficacy of intravenous immune globulin for treatment of *Pseudomonas aeruginosa* pneumonia, *J. Crit. Care* **1**:4–10.
153. Pennington, J. E., Small, G. J., Lostrom, M. E., and Pier, G. B., 1986, Polyclonal and monoclonal antibody therapy for experimental *Pseudomonas aeruginosa* pneumonia, *Infect. Immun.* **54**:239–244.
154. Pennington, J. E., and Small, G. J., 1987, Passive immune therapy for experimental *Pseudomonas aeruginosa* pneumonia in the neutropenic host, *J. Infect. Dis.* **155**:973–978.
155. Collins, M. S., Mehton, N. S., Edwards, A. A., and Ladehoff, D. K., 1989, Der therapieeffekt von immunoglobulin bei der experimentellen bakteriellen pneumonie durch *Pseudomonas aeruginosa* korreliert mit der *in vitro* opsonin-aktivität und der *in vivo* neutralisation von exotoxin A, *Intensivmed* **26**:97–101.
156. Jones, R. J., Rae, E. A., and Gupta, J. L., 1980, Controlled trial of *Pseudomonas* immunoglobulin and vaccine in burn patients, *Lancet* **ii**:1263–1265.
157. Jones, R. J., 1979, Antibody responses of burned patients immunized with a polyvalent *Pseudomonas* vaccine, *J. Hyg.* **82**:453–462.
158. Hunt, J. L., and Purdue, G. F., 1988, A clinical trial of IV tetravalent hyperimmune *Pseudomonas* globulin G in burned patients, *J. Trauma* **28**:146–151.
159. Kistler, D., Piert, M., and Hettich, R., 1989, Use of *Pseudomonas* hyper-immunoglobulin to treat septic shock in burn cases, *J. Burn Care Rehabil.* **10**:321–326.
160. Van Wye, J. E., Collins, M. S., Baylor, M., Pennington, J. E., Hsu, Y. P., Sampanvejsopa, V., and Moss, R. B., 1990, *Pseudomonas* hyperimmune globulin passive immunotherapy for pulmonary exacerbations in cystic fibrosis, *Pediatr. Pulmonol.* **9**:7–18.
161. Liu, P. V., and Wang, S., 1990, Three new major somatic antigens of *Pseudomonas aeruginosa*, *J. Clin. Microbiol.* **28**:922–925.
162. Wilkinson, S. G., 1983, Composition and structure of lipopolysaccharides from *Pseudomonas aeruginosa*, *Rev. Infect. Dis.* **5**:S941–S949.

163. Dunn, D. L., Ewald, D. C., Chandan, N., and Cerra, F. B., 1986, Immunotherapy of gram-negative bacterial sepsis: A single murine monoclonal antibody provides cross-genera protection, *Arch. Surg.* **121:**58–62.
164. Aldridge, M. C., Chadwick, S. J. D., Cheslyn-Curtis, S., Rapson, N., and Dudley, H. A. F., 1987, Antibody to endotoxin core glycolipid reverses reticuloendothelial system depression in an animal model of severe sepsis and surgical injury, *J. Trauma* **27:**1166–1172.
165. Baumgartner, J. D., O'Brien, T. X., Kirkland, T. N., Glauser, M. P., and Ziegler, E. J., 1987, Demonstration of cross-reactive antibodies to smooth gram-negative bacteria in antiserum to *Escherichia coli* J5, *J. Infect. Dis.* **156:**136–143.
166. Bogard, W. C., Jr., Dunn, D. L., Abernethy, K., Kilgarriff, C., and Kung, P. C., 1987, Isolation and characterization of murine monoclonal antibodies specific for gram-negative bacterial lipopolysaccharide: Association of cross-genus reactivity with lipid A specificity, *Infect. Immun.* **55:**899–908.
167. Pollack, M., Raubitschek, A. A., and Larrick, J. W., 1987, Human monoclonal antibodies that recognize conserved epitopes in the core-lipid A region of lipopolysaccharides, *J. Clin. Invest.* **79:**1421–1430.
168. Appelmelk, B. J., Verweij-van Vught, A. M. J. J., Maaskant, J. J., Schouten, W. F., De Jonge, A. J. R., Thijs, L. G., and Maclaren, D. M., 1988, Production and characterization of mouse monoclonal antibodies reacting with the lipopolysaccharide core region of gram-negative bacilli, *J. Med. Microbiol.* **26:**107–114.
169. Aydintug, M. K., Inzana, T. J., Letonja, T., Davis, W. C., and Corbeil, L. B., 1989, Cross-reactivity of monoclonal antibodies to *Escherichia coli* J5 with heterologous gram-negative bacteria and extracted lipopolysaccharides, *J. Infect. Dis.* **160:**846–857.
170. Priest, B. P., Brinson, D. N., Schroeder, D. A., and Dunn, D. L., 1989, Treatment of experimental gram-negative bacterial sepsis with murine monoclonal antibodies directed against lipopolysaccharide, *Surgery* **106:**147–155.
171. Pollack, M., Huang, A. I., Prescott, R. K., Young, L. S., Hunter, K. W., Cruess, D. F., and Tsai, C. M., 1983, Enhanced survival in *Pseudomonas aeruginosa* septicemia associated with high levels of circulating antibody to *Escherichia coli* endotoxin core, *J. Clin. Invest.* **72:**1874–1881.
172. Ziegler, E. J., McCutchan, J. A., Douglas, H., and Braude, H., 1975, Prevention of lethal *Pseudomonas* bacteremia with epimerase-deficient *E. coli* antiserum, *Trans. Assoc. Am. Physicians* **88:**101–108.
173. Martinez, D., and Callahan, L. T., III, 1985, Prophylaxis of *Pseudomonas aeruginosa* infections in leukopenic mice by a combination of active and passive immunization, *Eur. J. Clin. Microbiol.* **4:**186–189.
174. Ziegler, E. J., McCutchan, A., Fierer, J., Glauser, M. P., Sadoff, J. C., Douglas, H., and Braude, A. I., 1982, Treatment of gram-negative bacteremia and shock with human antiserum to a mutant *Escherichia coli*, *N. Engl. J. Med.* **307:**1225–1230.
175. Baumgartner, J. D., Heumann, D., Calandra, T., and Glauser, M. P., 1991, Antibodies to lipopolysaccharides after immunization of humans with the rough mutant of *Escherichia coli* J5, *J. Infect. Dis.* **163:**769–772.
176. Teng, N. N. H., Kaplan, H. S., Hebert, J. M., Moore, C., Douglas, H., Wunderlich, A., and Braude, A. I., 1985, Protection against gram-negative bacteremia and endotoxemia with human monoclonal IgM antibodies, *Proc. Natl. Acad. Sci. USA* **82:**1790–1794.
177. Ziegler, E. J., Fisher, C. J., Jr., Sprung, C. L., Straube, R. C., Sadoff, J. C., Foulke, G. E., Wortel, C. H., Fink, M. P., Dellinger, R. P., Teng, N. N. H., Allen, E., Berger, H. J., Knatterud, G. L., LoBuglio, A. F., Smith, C. R., and the HA-1A Sepsis Study Group, 1991, Treatment of gram-negative bacteremia and septic shock with HA-1A human monoclonal antibody against endotoxin, *N. Engl. J. Med.* **324:**429–436.
178. Ng, A-K., Chen, C-L. H., Chang, C-M., and Nowotany, A., 1976, Relationship of structure to function in bacterial endotoxins: Serologically cross-reactive components and their

effect on protection of mice against some gram-negative infections, *J. Gen. Microbiol.* **94:** 107–116.
179. Pennington, J. E., and Menkes, E., 1981, Type-specific versus cross-protective vaccination for gram negative bacterial pneumonia, *J. Infect. Dis.* **144:**599–603.
180. Cryz, S. J., Jr., Merdow, P. M., Fürer, E., and Germancer, R., 1985, Protection against fatal *Pseudomonas aeruginosa* sepsis by immunization with smooth and rough lipopolysaccharides, *Eur. J. Clin. Microbiol.* **4:**180–185.
181. Calandra, T., Glauser, M. P., Schellekens, J., Verhoef, J., and the Swiss-Dutch J5 Study Group, 1988, Treatment of gram-negative septic shock with human IgG antibody to *Escherichia coli* J5: A prospective, double-blind, randomized trial, *J. Infect. Dis.* **158:**312–319.
182. Hancock, R. E. W., Wieczorek, A. A., Mutharia, L. M., and Poole, K., 1982, Monoclonal antibodies against *Pseudomonas aeruginosa* outer membrane antigens: Isolation and characterization, *Infect. Immun.* **37:**166–171.
183. Hancock, R. E. W., Mutharia, L. M., and Mouat, E. C. A., 1985, Immunotherapeutic potential of monoclonal antibodies against *Pseudomonas aeruginosa* protein F, *Eur. J. Clin. Microbiol.* **4:**224–227.
184. Battershill, J. L., Speert, D. P., and Hancock, R. E. W., 1987, Use of monoclonal antibodies to protein F of *Pseudomonas aeruginosa* as opsonins for phagocytosis by macrophages, *Infect. Immun.* **55:**2531–2533.
185. Moon, M. M, Hazlett, L. D., Hancock, R. E. W., Berk, R. S., and Barrett, R., 1988, Monoclonal antibodies provide protection against ocular *Pseudomonas aeruginosa* infection, *Invest. Opthalmol. Vis. Sci.* **29:**1277–1284.
186. Finke, M., Muth, G., Reichhelm, T., Thoma, M., Duchêne, M., Hungerer, K.-D., Domdey, H., and vonSpecht, B.-U., 1991, Protection of immunosuppressed mice against infection with *Pseudomonas aeruginosa* by recombinant *P. aeruginosa* lipoprotein I and lipoprotein I-specific monoclonal antibodies, *Infect. Immun.* **59:**1251–1254.
187. Sokol, P. A., and Woods, D. E., 1986, Monoclonal antibodies to *Pseudomonas aeruginosa* ferripyochelin-binding protein, *Infect. Immun.* **53:**621–627.
188. Saiman, L. Sadoff, J., and Prince, A., 1989, Cross-reactivity of *Pseudomonas aeruginosa* antipilin monoclonal antibodies with heterogenous strains of *P. aeruginosa* and *Pseudomonas cepacia*, *Infect. Immun.* **57:**2764–2770.
189. Doig, P., Sastry, P. A., Hodges, R. S., Lee, K. K., Paranchych, W., and Irvin, R. I., 1990, Inhibition of pilus-mediated adhesion of *Pseudomonas aeruginosa* to human buccal epithelial cells by monoclonal antibodies directed against pili, *Infect. Immun.* **58:**124–130.
190. Rosok, M. J., Stebbins, M. R., Connelly, K., Lostrom, M. E., and Siadak, A. W., 1990, Generation and characterization of murine antiflagellum monoclonal antibodies that are protective against lethal challenge with *Pseudomonas aeruginosa*, *Infect. Immun.* **58:**3819–3828.
191. Ochi, H., Ohtsuka, H., Yokuta, S. I., Uerzumi, I., Terashima, M., Irie, K., and Noguchi, H., 1991, Inhibitory activity on bacterial motility and *in vivo* protective activity of human monoclonal antibodies against flagella of *Pseudomonas aeruginosa*, *Infect. Immun.* **59:** 550–554.
192. Irvin, R. T., and Ceri, H., 1985, Immunochemical examination of the *Pseudomonas aeruginosa* glycocalyx: A monoclonal antibody which recognizes L-guluronic acid residues of alginic acid, *Can. J. Microbiol.* **31:**268–275.
193. Terashima, M., Uezumi, I., Tomio, T., Kato, M., Irie, K., Okuda, T., Yokota, S., and Noguchi, H., 1991, A protective human monoclonal antibody directed to the outer core region of *Pseudomonas aeruginosa* lipopolysaccharide, *Infect. Immun.* **59:**1–6.
194. Sawada, S., Suzuki, M., Kawamura, T., Fujinaga, S., Masuho, Y., and Tomibe, K., 1984, Protection against infection with *Pseudomonas aeruginosa* by passive transfer of monoclonal antibodies to lipopolysaccharides and outer membrane proteins, *J. Infect. Dis.* **150:** 570–576.

195. Barclay, G. R., Yap, P. L., McClelland, D. B. L., Jones, R. J., Roe, E. A., McCann, M. C., Micklem, L. R., and James, K., 1986, Characterization of mouse monoclonal antibodies produced by immunization with a single serotype component of a polyvalent *Pseudomonas aeruginosa* vaccine, *J. Med. Microbiol.* **21:**87–90.
196. Pennington, J. E., Small, G. J., Lostrom, M. E., and Pier, G. B., 1986, Polyclonal and monoclonal antibody therapy for experimental *Pseudomonas aeruginosa* pneumonia, *Infect. Immun.* **54:**239–244.
197. Stoll, B. J., Pollock, M., Young, L. S., Koles, N., Gascon, R., and Pier, G. B., 1986, Functionally active monoclonal antibody that recognizes an epitope on the O side chain of *Pseudomonas aeruginosa* immunotype-1 lipopolysaccharide, *Infect. Immun.* **53:**656–662.
198. Suzuki, H., Okubo, Y., Moriyami, M., Susaki, M., Matsumoto, Y., and Hozumi, T., 1987, Human monoclonal antibodies to *Pseudomonas aeruginosa*, *Microbiol. Immunol.* **31:**959–966.
199. Zweerink, H. J., Gammon, M. C., Hutchison, C. F., Jackson, J. J., Lombardo, D., Miner, K. M., Puckett, J. M., Sewell, T. J., and Sigal, N. H., 1988, Human monoclonal antibodies that protect mice against challenge with *Pseudomonas aeruginosa*, *Infect. Immun.* **56:**1873–1879.
200. Hector, R. F., Collins, M. S., and Pennington, J. E., 1989, Treatment of experimental *Pseudomonas aeruginosa* pneumonia with a human IgM monoclonal antibody, *J. Infect. Dis.* **160:**483–489.
201. Lang, A. B., Fürer, E., Larrick, J. W., and Cryz, S. J., Jr., 1989, Isolation and characterization of a human monoclonal antibody that recognizes epitopes shared by *Pseudomonas aeruginosa* immunotype 1, 3, 4 and 6 lipopolysaccharides, *Infect. Immun.* **57:**3851–3855.
202. Yoshida, K., Kimura, F., Uchida, K., Kawaharajo, K., Koizumi, N., Nakajima, S., and Nagaoka, K., 1989, Production and some properties of monoclonal antibodies against serotype strains of *Pseudomonas aeruginosa*, *J. Pharmacobiol-Dyn.* **12:**398–404.
203. Husson, M. O., Mielcarek, C., Gavini, F., Caron, C., Izard, D., and Leclerc, H., 1989, Isolation and characterization of monoclonal antibodies against alkaline phosphatese of *Pseudomonas aeruginosa*, *J. Clin. Microbiol.* **27:**1115–1118.
204. Lagacé, J., and Fréchette, M., 1991, Four epitopes of *Pseudomonas aeruginosa* elastase defined by monoclonal antibodies, *Infect. Immun.* **59:**712–715.
205. Galloway, D. R., Hedstrom, R. C., and Pavlovskis, O. R., 1984, Production and characterization of monoclonal antibodies to exotoxin A from *Pseudomonas aeruginosa*, *Infect. Immun.* **44:**262–267.
206. Chia, J. K. S., Pollack, M., Avigar, D., and Steinbach, S., 1986, Functionally distinct monoclonal antibodies reactive with enzymatically active and binding domains of *Pseudomonas aeruginosa* toxin A, *Infect. Immun.* **52:**756–762.
207. Woods, D. E., and Que, J. V., 1987, Purification of *Pseudomonas aeruginosa* exoenzyme S, *Infect. Immun.* **55:**579–586.
208. Venezia, N. D., Calmels, S., and Bartsch, H., 1991, Production of polyclonal and monoclonal antibodies for specific detection of nitrosation-proficient denifrifying bacteria in biological fluids, *Biochem. Biophys. Res. Commun.* **176:**262–268.
209. Allan, B., Linseman, M., MacDonald, L. A., Lam, J. S., and Kropinski, A. M., 1988, Heat shock response of *Pseudomonas aeruginosa*, *J. Bacteriol.* **170:**3668–3674.
210. Norris, S. A., and Sciortino, C. V., 1988, Monoclonal antibody to an aminoglycoside-resistance factor from *Pseudomonas aeruginosa*, *J. Infect. Dis.* **158:**1324–1328.
211. Murakami, K., and Yoshida, T., 1985, Monoclonal antibodies against species-specific cephalosporinase of *Pseudomonas aeruginosa*, *Eur. J. Biochem.* **146:**693–697.
212. Sawada, S., Kawamura, T., Masuho, Y., and Tomibe, K., 1985, A new common polysaccharide antigen of strains of *Pseudomonas aeruginosa* detected with a monoclonal antibody, *J. Infect. Dis.* **152:**1290–1299.
213. Lam, M. Y. C., McGroarty, E. J., Kropinski, A. M., MacDonald, L. A., Pedersen, S. S., Høiby, N., and Lam, J. S., 1989, Occurrence of a common lipopolysaccharide antigen in standard and clinical strains of *Pseudomonas aeruginosa*, *J. Clin. Microbiol.* **27:**962–967.

214. Rivera, M., and McGroarty, E. J., 1989, Analysis of a common-antigen lipopolysaccharide from *Pseudomonas aeruginosa*, *J. Bacteriol.* **171:**2244–2248.
215. Yokota, S., Ochi, H., Ohtsuka, H., Kato, M., and Noguchi, H., 1989, Heterogeneity of the L-rhamnose residue in the outer core of *Pseudomonas aeruginosa* lipopolysaccharide, characterized by using human monoclonal antibodies, *Infect. Immun.* **57:**1691–1696.
216. Yokota, S., Ochi, H., Uezumi, I., Ohtsuka, H., Irie, K., and Noguchi, H., 1990, N-acetyl-L-galactosaminuronic acid as an epitope common to the O-polysaccharides of *Pseudomonas aeruginosa* A and H (Homma) recognized by a protective human monoclonal antibody, *Eur. J. Biochem.* **192:**109–113.
217. Yokota, S. I., Kaya, S., Araki, Y., Ito, E., Kawamura, T., and Sawada, S., 1990, Occurrence of D-rhamnan as the common antigen reactive against monoclonal antibody E87 in *Pseudomonas aeruginosa* IFO 3080 and other strains, *J. Bacteriol.* **172:**6162–6164.
218. Collins, H. H., Cross, A. S., Dobek, A., Opal, S. M., McClain, J. B., and Sadoff, J. C., 1989, Oral ciprofloxacin and a monoclonal antibody to lipopolysaccharide protect leukopenic rats from lethal infection with *Pseudomonas aeruginosa*, *J. Infect. Dis.* **159:**1073–1082.
219. Pier, G. B., Thomas, D., Small, G., Siadak, A., and Zweerink, H., 1989, In vitro and in vivo activity of polyclonal and monoclonal human immunoglobulins G, M, and A against *Pseudomonas aeruginosa* lipopolysaccharide, *Infect. Immun.* **57:**174–179.
220. Sawada, S., Kawamura, T., Masuho, Y., and Tomibe, K., 1985, Characterization of a human monoclonal antibody to lipopolysaccharides of *Pseudomonas aeruginosa* serotype 5: A possible candidate as an immunotherapeutic agent for infections with *P. aeruginosa*, *J. Infect. Dis.* **152:**965–970.
221. Sawada, S., Kawamura, T., and Masuho, Y., 1987, Immunoprotective human monoclonal antibodies against five major serotypes of *Pseudomonas aeruginosa*, *J. Gen. Microbiol.* **133:**3581–3590.
222. Sawada, S., Kawamura, T., Masuho, Y., Iyobe, S., and Hashimoto, H., 1989, Protection against experimental *Pseudomonas* infection with O antigen-specific human monoclonal antibodies, *Antibiot. Chemother.* **42:**210–217.
223. Zweerink, H. J., Gammon, M. C., Hutchinson, C. F., Jackson, J. J., Pier, G. B., Puckett, J. M., Sewell, T. A., and Sigal, N. H., 1988, X-linked immunodeficient mice as a model for testing the protective efficacy of monoclonal antibodies against *Pseudomonas aeruginosa*, *Infect. Immun.* **56:**1209–1214.
224. Zweerink, H. J., Detolla, L. J., Gammon, M. C., Hutchinson, C. F., Puckett, J. M., and Sigal, N. H., 1990, A human monoclonal antibody that protects mice against *Pseudomonas*-induced pneumonia, *J. Infect. Dis.* **162:**254–257.
225. Collins, M. S., Edwards, A. A., Ladehoff, D., and Mehton, N. S., 1989, Activity of anti-lipopolysaccharide human IgM monoclonal antibodies in the treatment of *Pseudomonas aeruginosa–Staphylococcus aureus* polymicrobic cellulitis, *Serodiag. Immunother. Infect. Dis.* **3:**225–230.
226. Saravolatz, L. D., Markowitz, N., Collins, M. S., Bogdanoff, D., and Pennington, J. E., 1991, Safety, pharmacokinetics and functional activity of human anti-*Pseudomonas aeruginosa* monoclonal antibodies in septic and non-septic patients, *J. Infect. Dis.*, in press.
227. Collins, M. S., Ladehoff, D. K., Mehton, N. S., and Noonan, J. S., 1990, Opsonic and protective activity of five human IgM monoclonal antibodies reactive with lipopolysaccharide antigen of *Pseudomonas aeruginosa*, *FEMS Microbiol. Immunol.* **64:**263–268.
228. Collins, M. S., Ladehoff, D., and Mehton, N. S., 1991, Therapy of established experimental *Pseudomonas aeruginosa* infections with oral ciprofloxacin and five human monoclonal antibodies against lipopolysaccharide antigens, *Antibiot. Chemother.*, in press.
229. Gearing, A. J. H., Leung, H., Bird, C. R., and Thorpe, R., 1989, Presence of the inflammatory cytokines IL-1, TNF and IL-6 in preparations of monoclonal antibodies, *Hybridoma* **8:**361–367.
230. Bartal, A. H., Feit, C., Erlandson, R., and Hirshaut, Y., 1982, The presence of viral particles

in hybridoma clones secreting monoclonal antibodies, *N. Engl. J. Med.* **306:**1423.
231. Weisfuse, I. B., Graham, D. J., Will, M., Parkinson, D., Snydman, D. R., Atkins, M., Karron, R. A., Feinstone, S., Rayner, A. A., Fisher, R. I., Mills, B. J., Dutcher, J. P., Weiss, G. R., Glover, A., Kuritsky, J. N., and Hadler, S. C., 1990, An outbreak of hepatitis A among cancer patients treated with interleukin-2 and lymphokine-activated killer cells, *J. Infect. Dis.* **161:** 647–652.
232. Sumazaki, R., Fujita, T., Kabashima, T., Nishikaku, F., Koyama, A., Shibaski, M., and Takita, H., 1986, Monoclonal antibody against bacterial lipopolysaccharide cross-reacts with DNA-histone, *Clin. Exp. Immunol.* **66:**103–110.
233. Woods, J. P., Black, J. R., Barrit, D. S., Connell, T. D., and Cannon, J. G., 1987, Resistance to meningococcemia apparently conferred by anti-H.8 monoclonal antibody is due to contaminating endotoxin and not to specific immunoprotection, *Infect. Immun.* **55:**1927–1928.

The State of the Art in the Development of *Pseudomonas aeruginosa* Vaccines

STANLEY J. CRYZ, JR.

1. CLINICAL SIGNIFICANCE

Pseudomonas aeruginosa continues to be a leading cause of life-threatening infections among various compromised patient populations (Table I). Dramatic advances in the fields of cancer chemotherapy, bone marrow transplantation, and the care of critically ill patients has greatly increased the numbers of hospitalized individuals at high risk for acquiring a serious *P. aeruginosa* infection. *P. aeruginosa* is now the second most common bacterial nosocomial pathogen, accounting for more than 11% of all isolates reported to the Centers for Disease Control.[1]

P. aeruginosa bacteremia and pneumonia are among the most difficult bacterial infections to prevent or treat in a hospital environment. The mortality rate for such infections can exceed 50%, and is usually the highest for any bacterial pathogen.[2,3] Both the debilitated condition of the infected patient and a high frequency of multiple antibiotic resistance contribute to this finding. In one study, fully 35% of *P. aeruginosa* clinical isolates were resistant to one or more commonly used aminoglycoside antibiotics.[4] A particularly vexing problem to deal with is the emergence of resistant variants during therapy with newer generation β-lactam and aminoglycoside antibiotics. This

---

STANLEY J. CRYZ, JR. • Swiss Serum and Vaccine Institute, CH-3001 Berne, Switzerland.

Pseudomonas aeruginosa as an Opportunistic Pathogen, edited by Mario Campa *et al.* Plenum Press, New York, 1993.

TABLE I
Patient Populations at Risk for Acquiring a *P. aeruginosa* Infection

Cystic fibrosis
Burned
Cancer, especially hematological malignancies
Patients receiving immunosuppressive therapy
Surgical and medical intensive care unit patients
Diabetics
Catheterized patients
Intravenous drug abusers

is often associated with a fatal outcome.[5–7] An expanding population of high-risk patients combined with the modest success of current therapeutic agents to treat serious *P. aeruginosa* infections has led to renewed interest in the development of vaccines, polyclonal immunoglobulins, and human monoclonal antibodies as adjuncts to conventional therapy.

2. HUMAN IMMUNITY TO *P. AERUGINOSA*

Immunity to *P. aeruginosa* appears to be dependent upon two mechanisms: the eradication of the invading organisms by phagocytic cells, and the neutralization of potent toxins and enzymes by antibodies. *P. aeruginosa* isolates that cause invasive disease are almost uniformly resistant to the bactericidal activity of normal human serum.[8,9] Resistance is conferred by the presence of complete, smooth lipopolysaccharide (LPS).[10] Phagocytosis and subsequent killing occur only in the presence of opsonic antibody.[8,10] Studies by Pollack and Young[11] and Cross *et al.*[12] have found that individuals who survived an episode of *P. aeruginosa* septicemia possessed significantly higher serum antibody levels to LPS and exotoxin A (ETA). These two types of antibodies appear to mediate their protective effect by independent and additive mechanisms. Therefore, survival was highest in patients who had elevated levels of antibody to both antigens.

Two LPS-based vaccines (*Pseudogen*®, Parke Davis; and *PEV*, Burroughs Wellcome) or globulins prepared from individuals immunized with these vaccines and have been evaluated clinically in various high-risk patient populations. These studies are described in Table II and have been reviewed extensively elsewhere[8]. Results from these trials can be summarized briefly as follows. In burned patients, active or passive immunization significantly reduced morbidity and mortality due to *P. aeruginosa*.[13,14] Interpretation of these findings is complicated by the fact that the trials were neither double-

TABLE II
Summary of Clinical Trials Performed with P. aeruginosa LPS-Based Vaccines and Anti-LPS Immune Globulin

Vaccine and patient population	Study design	Total no. of patients	Summary
Pseudogen®[a]			
Burned	Historical controls	357	14.7% mortality in controls due to P. aeruginosa versus 3.1% in vaccines; no deaths due to P. aeruginosa in patients who received vaccine plus immunoglobulin.
Acute leukemia, pediatric	Randomized	58	5 vaccines and 3 controls had infections with P. aeruginosa associated with fatal outcome.
Adults, cancer and intensive care unit patients post-removal of tumors	Randomized	361	Significant ($p<.01$) reduction in P. aeruginosa-associated deaths: 31 controls versus 13 vaccinees; no protection against bacteremia; low antibody titers; high rate of reactions.
Adults, intensive care unit	Randomized	99	P. aeruginosa primary cause of death in 5 controls versus 1 vaccinee; low antibody titers.
Trauma, intensive care unit	Randomized, double-blind, saline placebo	124	8 deaths associated with P. aeruginosa in vaccine group (3 thought primary and 5 contributing cause) versus 3 in control group (1 primary, 2 contributing).
Adult & pediatric leukemias	Randomized	44	1 non-fatal P. aeruginosa infection in vaccinees versus 2 P. aeruginosa infections in controls, 1 of which was fatal.
Colonized cystic fibrosis patients	Non-randomized; no control group	12	No clinical improvement in spite of vigorous immune response.
PEV[b]			
Burned	Alternate enrollment	146	8 cases of P. aeruginosa bacteremia in control group; 6 considered to be primary cause of death; no mortalities in vaccinated group.
Burned	Alternate enrollment	279	Patients treated with vaccine, immunoglobulin, or combined regimen had significantly fewer P. aeruginosa blood isolates (2.3%) compared with controls (20%); no P. aeruginosa-specific mortality rates given; small quantity (1.5 ml and 0.6 ml) of P. aeruginosa globulin highly effective.
Noncolonized cystic fibrosis patients	Randomized	34	No clinical benefit noted; vaccinated group had slightly reduced pulmonary function; immune response and serological data not reported in detail.

[a] Pseudogen® is a heptavalent, purified LPS vaccine produced by Parke Davis.
[b] PEV produced by Burroughs Wellcome, contains extracts from 16 serotypes of P. aeruginosa. LPS appears to be the primary active ingredient.

blind nor placebo-controlled (historical control groups were used). In addition, topical antimicrobials, a common treatment regimen for burned patients, were not employed in one study.[14]

Vaccination of cancer patients who had either solid or hematological malignancies provided, at best, a modest level of protection against *P. aeruginosa*.[15–17] This was most likely attributable to the poor immunogenicity of the vaccine (*Pseudogen*®) in immunosuppressed patients. Only a transient rise in anti-LPS levels was noted in most vaccinees. Two studies involving active immunization of intensive-care-unit patients with *Pseudogen*® yielded conflicting results.[18] In one instance, vaccination reduced the number of deaths where *P. aeruginosa* was deemed to be the primary cause. In a second study, vaccination afforded no protection.

Immunization of 12 cystic fibrosis (CF) patients who were colonized with *P. aeruginosa* induced a vigorous serum anti-LPS antibody response.[17] However, there was no improvement in their clinical statuses. The *PEV* vaccine was administered to 17 noncolonized CF children (mean age 7.2 years), while 17 age-matched CF children served as non-vaccinated controls[19]. After 3 years of surveillance, there were no differences between the groups as gauged by either the rate of colonization or overall clinical status. There was some evidence that pulmonary function deteriorated more rapidly in the vaccinated group subsequent to infection. Several aspects of this study are noteworthy. First, detailed immunological response data were not presented. The serum antibody response was determined for only a portion of the 16 vaccine antigens. The immune responses to "some serotypes were poor."[19] Second, the authors suggested that the ELISA assay used to measure serum antibody levels may not have detected protective antibodies. Third, although all isolates were serotyped (74% were nonmucoid), the serotype distribution was not stated. In light of the variable immune response to the individual vaccine antigens, it would be of considerable interest to compare the serotypes of the strains isolated versus the magnitude of the immune response to the respective serotypes.

Most strains of *P. aeruginosa* that colonize the lungs of CF patients produce copious amounts of alginate, a random polymer of mannuronic and guluronic acids. Pier *et al*.[20] have reported that older (≥12 years) noncolonized CF patients had significantly higher levels of opsonic antibody specific for alginate than either colonized age-matched or younger CF patients. Such opsonic anti-alginate antibodies were postulated to play a critical role in the prevention of *P. aeruginosa* pulmonary colonization.

The foregoing studies indicate that elevated levels of anti-LPS and anti-ETA antibodies may provide protection against fatal *P. aeruginosa* sepsis, especially in immunocompetent patient populations. In addition, anti-alginate antibody with proper functional attributes may prevent *P. aeruginosa* from colonizing the lungs of CF patients.

3. DEVELOPMENT AND CLINICAL EVALUATION OF IMMUNOLOGICAL AGENTS AGAINST P. AERUGINOSA

3.1. Background

As noted, both immunocompetent and immunocompromised patient populations are at risk for acquiring a fatal *P. aeruginosa* infection. CF, diabetic, and burned patients may be candidates for active vaccination because they are able to mount a rapid, vigorous humoral immune response. In contrast, immunocompromised patients who respond poorly to vaccination would receive only a marginal benefit. Perhaps the largest-risk group are patients in the intensive care unit, where it has been shown that 10% of individuals who remain on-unit more than 72 hours develop bacteremia.[21] Whereas a substantial proportion of these patients are immunocompetent, the time interval between vaccination and the onset of the risk period may be insufficient to allow for the mounting of a protective immune response. These patients may benefit more from passive immunotherapy. Therefore, human polyclonal and monoclonal preparations have been developed.

3.2. *P. aeruginosa* Vaccines

P. aeruginosa vaccines clinically evaluated to date are listed in Table III.

3.2.1. Pseudogen®

Studies with this vaccine, which is composed of purified LPS, are described in section 2. Due to a combination of moderate immunogenicity and a high rate of adverse reactions, trials with this vaccine have been discontinued.

3.2.2. PEV

This whole-cell extract vaccine has been evaluated in burned and in CF patients (see section 2). In addition, it has been used to immunize plasma donors to produce a hyperimmune globulin.[22] This vaccine is no longer being produced.

3.2.3. Ribosomal Vaccines

Ribosomal vaccines have been prepared by Lieberman and colleagues.[23] Phase I safety and immunogenicity studies in humans are reported to be underway, but no results have been published.

TABLE III
P. aeruginosa Vaccines that Have Been or Are Undergoing Clinical Evaluation

Vaccine	Description	Phase of study	Comments
Pseudogen®	Heptavalent LPS	Completed efficacy studies in burned, cancer, ICU, and CF patients.	Moderately immunogenic; evidence of protection in burned patients; modest efficacy in cancer and ICU patients; no longer being evaluated.
PEV	16-valent extract vaccine; LPS primary active ingredient	Tested for efficacy in burned and CF patients.	Moderately immunogenic; afforded protection in burned patients; ineffective in CF patients; no longer being evaluated.
HMW-PS	Polysaccharide ($M_r > 100{,}000$); serologically identical to O-PS of LPS	Two serotypes completed Phase I testing.	Safe and immunogenic in healthy adults.
Flagella	Purified flagella, free of LPS	Used to immunize plasma donors.	Appears to be immunogenic and safe; multiple doses required.
Alginate	Highly purified *P. aeruginosa* alginate	Phase I	Poorly immunogenic in healthy adults.
O-PS-toxin A	Octavalent, O-PS coupled to ETA	Completed Phase II study in healthy adults. Undergoing Phase II study in CF patients. Undergoing Phase I study in adult and pediatric bone marrow transplant patients.	Safe and immunogenic in all populations studied.
Alginate-toxin A conjugate	Reduced-molecular-weight alginate coupled to ETA	Completed Phase I trials in healthy adults.	Safe and immunogenic.

3.2.4. Flagella Vaccines

Five monovalent flagella vaccines have been prepared and used to immunize plasma donors.[24] Five intravenous immune gamma globulin (IVIG) preparations were made, which contained high ELISA antibody titers to the homologous antigen. These IVIG preparations were able to facilitate the killing of flagellated strains of *P. aeruginosa* by phagocytic cells. However, the potency of these experimental preparations was not compared with normal, commercial IVIG. Furthermore, the ability of anti-flagella IVIG to prevent fatal experimental *P. aeruginosa* infections was not documented.

3.2.5. High-Molecular-Weight Polysaccharide

Pier and co-workers have described the isolation and purification of high-molecular-weight polysaccharide (HMW-PS) from several serotypes of *P. aeruginosa*. HMW-PS appears to be serologically identical to the O-polysaccharide (O-PS) moiety of LPS. In small-scale Phase I studies, HMW-PS isolated from *P. aeruginosa* immunotypes 1 and 2 was found to be safe upon parenteral administration to human volunteers.[25,26] Most vaccinees responded with a significant rise in both binding and opsonic antibodies.

3.2.6. Alginate or Mucoid Exopolysaccharide

Pier *et al.*[27] have purified mucoid exopolysaccharide (MEP) from several mucoid *P. aeruginosa* CF isolates. Different MEP appear to contain both a shared (common) and a serospecific epitope. Anti-MEP antibodies induced in rabbits by immunization have been shown to mediate phagocytic killing of *P. aeruginosa*.[28] Interestingly, anti-MEP antibody present in normal human serum did not promote phagocytic killing of mucoid *P. aeruginosa*.[27] Therefore, the bulk of "naturally-acquired" antibodies to MEP may be nonprotective.

Phase I studies of MEP have been performed in healthy adults.[29] Unfortunately, only a meager antibody response was engendered (G.B. Pier, personal communication). MEP of a higher molecular weight is now undergoing Phase I testing.

3.2.7. Alginate Conjugates

In an attempt to increase the immunogenicity of the native alginate, small molecular weight alginate (<500,000) has been covalently coupled to either native ETA and to a nontoxic ETA-deletion mutant. In both instances, the conjugates were far more effective at eliciting opsonic anti-alginate antibody than was native alginate. The native ETA-alginate conjugate vaccine has been found to be safe and immunogenic in healthy adult volunteers.

3.2.8. O-PS-Toxin A Conjugate Vaccine

To produce a vaccine capable of engendering both an anti-LPS and an anti-ETA antibody response, serologically reactive O-PS from *P. aeruginosa* LPS has been covalently coupled to ETA in a manner that irreversibly detoxifies ETA, yet preserves the immunogenicity of both vaccine moieties.[30,31] An octavalent conjugate vaccine has been produced and evaluated in Phase I and II studies.[32] This vaccine is well-tolerated and induces high levels of opsonic and ETA-neutralizing antibodies in most subjects. Passively transferred human anticonjugate immunoglobulin G (IgG) protects mice against fatal *P. aeruginosa* sepsis.

Several studies are now underway to gauge the safety and immunogenicity of this conjugate vaccine in high-risk patient populations. Schaad[33] and co-workers have immunized young (1-18 years of age) CF patients with no history of infection or colonization with *P. aeruginosa* who possessed low-serum-antibody levels to LPS and ETA. Vaccination engendered a significant rise in anti-LPS and anti-ETA antibodies, which was long-lived. The vaccinees have remained uncolonized and in good health after 8 months of observation.

Gottlieb *et al.*[34] have initiated Phase I studies with this vaccine in allogeneic bone marrow transplant (BMT) patients. Immunization of either the donor or the recipient alone 1 week prior to BMT did not evoke a significant rise in antibody levels. In contrast, immunization of both donor and recipient stimulated a substantial antibody rise that persisted for 3 months post-transplantation, the time during which patients are most susceptible to acquiring a serious infection due to their severely immunosuppressed state.

4. PASSIVE IMMUNOTHERAPY

Collins *et al.*[35] have prepared a hyperimmune IVIG against *P. aeruginosa* through a screening program designed to identify plasma donors with elevated antibody levels to LPS. Several lots of this product have been produced and contain ≥3-fold higher levels of anti-LPS antibody to 12 serotypes of *P. aeruginosa*. Several studies are in progress to evaluate the clinical efficacy of this IVIG. Twenty-six burned patients were randomized to receive the IVIG (250 mg/kg body weight on days 0, 3, 5, 7, 10, and 13) or standard care.[36] The incidence of *P. aeruginosa* infections of all types was comparable in both groups. However, septicemia developed in only two of six infected patients who received IVIG compared with five of seven controls. One patient in the control group succumbed to septic shock. In two additional studies, patients diagnosed with *P. aeruginosa* pneumonia or septicemia received 400 mg/kg body weight of IVIG on the first day of therapy and

100-200 mg/kg on the following day. In the first study,[37] 10 patients received IVIG while 10 patients who had previously received normal globulin served as historical controls. Although, mortality rates were not stated, the group that received the *P. aeruginosa* IVIG was believed to fare better clinically based upon a reduced need for antibiotics and fewer days of fever. In the second trial,[36] 30 patients were randomized to receive the IVIG or conventional therapy. Overall mortality was 20% in the control group, whereas there were no deaths in the treatment group. However, none of the deaths in the control group was attributable to *P. aeruginosa*. Although promising, the above studies must be interpreted with caution due to the small numbers of patients evaluated and the fact that they were not performed in a double-blind, placebo-controlled manner.

Several hundred plasma donors have been simultaneously immunized with the octavalent *P. aeruginosa* O-PS–toxin A vaccine and a polyvalent *Klebsiella* capsular polysaccharide vaccine.[38] Their plasma has been processed into a hyperimmune IVIG. When compared with a commercial IVIG, the hyperimmune product had substantially (3- to 20-fold) higher levels of IgG antibodies to all eight *P. aeruginosa* vaccine serotypes and to ETA. Opsonic antibody titers were 3- to >100-fold higher depending upon the serotype. The hyperimmune product also neutralized 20 times more ETA than the commercial IVIG. Similarly, on a weight basis, the hyperimmune product provided significantly higher levels of protection against experimental *P. aeruginosa* sepsis when passively transferred to mice.

A multi-center, randomized, double-blind, placebo-controlled trial to evaluate this product is scheduled to begin in late 1990 under the auspices of the Veterans Administration Cooperative Studies Program and the U.S. Army. The IVIG will be administered to patients upon entry onto the intensive care unit. These patients will show no overt sign of infection, and are expected to remain more than 48 hr. The trial is expected to run for 3 years and 4,500 patients will be enrolled. The trial design and number of patients will allow several clinical endpoints to be evaluated including incidence of infection, severity of occurring infection, time to onset of infection, and mortality.

4.1. Human Monoclonal Antibodies against *P. aeruginosa*

Whereas the production of polyclonal human hyperimmune IVIG preparations against *P. aeruginosa* is feasible, there are several drawbacks. Screening programs are tedious and costly, and less than 1% of screened donors have acceptable levels of antibody titers. In addition, maintenance of the "donor pool" is often difficult due to logistical considerations. Vaccination programs have the advantage of rapidly expanding the donor pool as 70–80% of vaccinees were found to have acceptable levels of antibody (author's unpublished observations). However, a constant supply of vaccine is needed and immunized donors need to be screened regularly to endure that adequate antibody levels are maintained.

To circumvent these problems, several laboratories have reported the isolation of lymphoblastoid or hybridoma cell lines secreting human monoclonal antibodies (MAb) to *P. aeruginosa* LPS. Sawada et al.[40] have fused human tonsilar lymphocytes to a mouse myeloma and obtained cell lines secreting IgG antibody to five serotypes of *P. aeruginosa* (Fisher immunotypes [IT] 1–4 and Habs serotype 3). These serotypes account for roughly 50–70% of *P. aeruginosa* blood isolates. These MAb are opsonic and protect against experimental *P. aeruginosa* sepsis.

Zweerink et al.[41] have produced several lymphoblastoid cell lines (LCL) secreting IgM Mab recognizing *P. aeruginosa* IT-2 through IT-7 by Epstein-Barr-virus (EBV) transformation of peripheral blood lymphocytes (PBL) from CF patients. Three of these lines produced MAb specific for IT-2, 4, and 5, which were protective. Another line produced a MAb that recognized IT-3, 6, and 7 LPS, but afforded protection only against an IT-3 and IT-6 challenge. These four cell lines would cover approximately 60–65% of all *P. aeruginosa* blood isolates. However, LCL have a limited life span and produce relatively low levels of MAb. The authors have reported that these LCL have been fused with myeloma cell lines to produce hybridomas, but no data was given.

In our laboratory, we have developed a system to rapidly isolate LCL secreting MAb to *P. aeruginosa* LPS and to produce stable hybridomas from these lines.[42,43] Briefly, volunteers were immunized with the octavalent *P. aeruginosa* vaccine described earlier. PBL expressing anti–*P. aeruginosa* LPS antibody on their cell surfaces were enriched for and transformed with EBV. LCL stably secreting satisfactory levels of antibody were used with F3B6 heteromyeloma cell line and stable hybridomas isolated. Nine MAb were isolated that consistently secreted high levels of IgM specific for *P. aeruginosa* IT-1 through IT-7 and Habs 3 and 4 were isolated. These MAb were protective against fatal experimental *P. aeruginosa* sepsis in a serospecific manner. These nine MAb would cover greater than 90% of *P. aeruginosa* bacteremic isolates. Phase I safety and pharmacokinetic studies are planned for the near future.

REFERENCES

1. Horan, T. C., White, J. W., Jarvis, W. R., Emori, T. G., Culver, D. H., Munn, V. P., Thornsberry, C., Olson, D. R., and Hughes, J. M., 1986, Nosocomial infection surveillance, 1984, *M.M.W.R.* **35**:17SS–29SS.
2. Lechi, A., Arosio, E., Pancera, P., Anesi, P., Zannini, G., Todeschini, G., and Cetto, G., 1984, *Pseudomonas* septicemia. A review of 60 cases observed in a university hospital, *J. Hosp. Infect.* **5**:29–37.

3. Bryan, C. S., Reynolds, K. L., and Brenner, E. R., 1983, Analysis of 1,186 episodes of gram-negative bacteremia in non-university hospitals: The effects of antimicrobial therapy, *Rev. Infect. Dis.* **5**:629–638.
4. Cross, A. S., Opal, S., and Kopecko, D., 1983, Progressive increase in antibiotic resistance of gram-negative bacterial isolates. Walter Reed Hospital, 1976-1980: Specific analysis of gentamicin, tobramycin, and amikacin resistance, *Arch. Intern. Med.* **143**:2075–2080.
5. Jimenez-Lucho, V. E., Saravolatz, L. D., Medeiros, A. A., and Pohlod, D., 1986, Failure of therapy in *Pseudomonas* endocarditis: Selection of resistant mutants, *J. Infect. Dis.* **154**:64–68.
6. Sanders, C. C., and Sanders, W. E., Jr., 1985, Microbial resistance to newer generation β-lactam antibiotics: Clinical and laboratory implications, *J. Infect. Dis.* **151**:399–406.
7. Foord, R. D., Butcher, M. E., and Williams, A. H., 1987, The emergence of resistance of *Pseudomonas aeruginosa* in patients treated with ceftazidine, *Scand J. Infect. Dis.* **19**:143.
8. Cryz, S. J., Jr., 1984, *Pseudomonas aeruginosa* infections, in: *Bacterial vaccines*, (R. Germanier, ed.), Academic Press, Orlando, FL, pp. 317–351.
9. Young, L. S., and Armstrong, D., 1972, Human immunity to *Pseudomonas aeruginosa*. I. In-vitro interaction of bacteria, polymorphonuclear leukocytes, and serum factors, *J. Infect. Dis.* **126**:257–276.
10. Cryz, S. J., Jr., Pitt, T. L., Fürer, E., and Germanier, R., 1984, Role of lipopolysaccharide in virulence of *Pseudomonas aeruginosa*, *Infect. Immun.* **44**:508–513.
11. Pollack, M. S., and Young, L. S., 1979, Protective activity of antibodies to exotoxin A and lipopolysaccharide at the onset of *Pseudomonas aeruginosa* septicemia in man, *J. Clin. Invest.* **63**:276–286.
12. Cross, A. S., Sadoff, J. C., Iglewski, B. H., and Sokol, P. A., 1980, Evidence for the role of toxin A in the pathogenesis of infection with *Pseudomonas aeruginosa* in humans, *J. Infect. Dis.* **142**:538–546.
13. Alexander, J. W., and Fisher, M. W., 1974, Immunization against *Pseudomonas* in infection after thermal injury, *J. Infect. Dis.* **130**:S152–S158.
14. Jones, R. J., Rowe, E. A., and Gupta, J. L., 1980, Controlled trial of *Pseudomonas* immunoglobulin and vaccine in burn patients, *Lancet* **1**:1263–1265.
15. Young, L. S., Meyer, R. D., and Armstrong, D., 1973, *Pseudomonas aeruginosa* vaccine in cancer patients, *Ann. Intern. Med.* **79**:518–527.
16. Haghbin, M., Armstrong, D., and Murphy, M. L., 1973, Controlled prospective trial of *Pseudomonas aeruginosa* vaccine in children with acute leukemia, *Cancer* **32**:761–766.
17. Pennington, J. E., 1974, Preliminary investigations of *Pseudomonas aeruginosa* vaccine in patients with leukemia and cystic fibrosis, *J. Infect. Dis.* **130**:S159–S162.
18. Polk, H. C., Jr., Borden, S., and Aldrete, J. A., 1973, Prevention of *Pseudomonas* respiratory infection in a surgical intensive care unit, *Ann. Surg.* **177**:607–615.
19. Langford, D. T., and Hiller, J., 1984, Prospective, controlled study of a polyvalent *Pseudomonas* vaccine in cystic fibrosis—three year results, *Arch. Dis. Child.* **59**:1131–1134.
20. Pier, G. B., Saunders, J. M., Ames, P., Edwards, M. S., Auerlach, H., Goldfarb J, Speert, D. P., and Hurrvitch, S., 1987, Opsonophagocytic killing antibody to *Pseudomonas aeruginosa* mucoid exopolysaccharide in older noncolonized patients with cystic fibrosis, *N. Engl. J. Med.* **317**:793–798.
21. Maki, D. B., 1989, Risk factors for nosocomial infection in intensive care: "Devices vs nature" and goals for the next decade, *Arch. Intern. Med.* **149**:30–35.
22. Holder, I. A., and Neely, A. N., 1987, Experimental studies of the pathogenesis of infections due to *Pseudomonas aeruginosa*: Passive intravenous immunotherapy using *Pseudomonas* immunoglobulins, *Serodiag. Immunother.* **1**:153–162.
23. Lieberman, M. M., 1989, *Pseudomonas aeruginosa* ribosomal vaccine. A comparison of the immunogenicity of vaccines from two different serotypes, in: *Pseudomonas aeruginosa Infection*, Antibiotics Chemotherapy Vol. 42 (N. Hoiby, S. S. Pederson, G. H. Shand, G. Döring, and I. A. Holder, eds.), Karger, Basel, Switzerland, pp. 193–203.

24. Rotering, H., and Dorner, F., 1989, Studies on a *Pseudomonas aeruginosa* flagella vaccine, in: *Pseudomonas aeruginosa Infection*, Antibiotics Chemotherapy Vol. 42 (N. Hoiby, S. S. Pederson, G. H. Shand, G. Döring, and I. A., Holder, eds.), Karger, Basel, Switzerland, pp. 218–228.
25. Pier, G. B., and Bennett, S. E., 1986, Structural analysis and immunogenicity of *Pseudomonas aeruginosa* immunotype 2 high molecular weight polysaccharide, *J. Clin. Invest.* **77:**491–495.
26. Pier, G. B., 1982, Safety and immunogenicity of high molecular weight polysaccharide vaccine from immunotype 1 *Pseudomonas aeruginosa*, *J. Clin. Invest.* **69:**303–308.
27. Pier, G. B., Matthews, W. J., and Eardly, D. D., 1983, Immunochemical characterization of the mucoid exopolysaccharide of *Pseudomonas aeruginosa*, *J. Infect. Dis.* **147:**494–503.
28. Ames, P., DesJardins, D., and G. B. Pier, 1985, Opsonophagocytic killing activity of rabbit antibody to *Pseudomonas aeruginosa* mucoid exoploysaccharide, *Infect. Immun.* **49:**281–285.
29. Pier, G. B., 1989, Immunologic properties of *Pseudomonas aeruginosa* mucoid exopolysaccharide (alginate), in: *Pseudomonas aeruginosa Infection*, Antibiotics Chemotherapy Vol. 42 (N. Hoiby, S. S. Pederson, G. H. Shand, G. Döring, and I. A., Holder, eds.), Karger, Basel, Switzerland, pp. 80–87.
30. Cryz, S. J., Jr., Lang, A. B., Sadoff, J. C., Germanier, R., and Fürer, E., 1987, Vaccine potential of *Pseudomonas aeruginosa* O-polysaccharide-toxin A conjugates, *Infect. Immun.* **55:**1547–1551.
31. Cryz, S. J., Jr., Fürer, E., Cross, A. S., Wegmann, A., Germanier, R., and Sadoff, J. C., 1987, Safety and immunogenicity of *Pseudomonas aeruginosa* O-polysaccharide–toxin A conjugate vaccine in humans, *J. Clin. Invest.* **80:**51–56.
32. Cryz, S. J., Jr., Sadoff, J. C., Cross, A. S., and Fürer, E., 1989, Safety and immunogenicity of a polyvalent *Pseudomonas aeruginosa* O-polysaccharide–toxin A vaccine in humans, in: *Pseudomonas aeruginosa Infection*, Antibiotics Chemotherapy Vol. 42 (N. Hoiby, S. S. Pederson, G. H. Shand, G. Döring, and I. A. Holder, eds.), Karger, Basel, Switzerland, pp. 177–183.
33. Schaad, V. B., Lang, A. B., Wedgwood, J., Ruedeberg, A., Que, J. U., Fürer, E., and Cryz, S. J., Jr., Society and immunogenicity of *Pseudomonas aeruginosa* conjugate vaccine in cystic fibrosis, *Lancet* **338:**1236–1237.
34. Gottlieb, D. J., Cryz, S. J., Jr., Fürer, E., Que, J. U., Prentice, H. G., Duncombe, A. S., and Brenner, M. K., 1990, Immunity against *Pseudomonas aeruginosa* adaptively transferred to bone marrow transplant recipients, *Blood* **76:**2470–2475.
35. Collins, M. S., Edwards, A., Robey, R. E., Mehton, N. S., and Ladehoff, D., 1989, *Pseudomonas* immune globulin therapy improves survival in experimental *Pseudomonas aeruginosa* bacteremic pneumonia, in: *Pseudomonas aeruginosa Infection*, Antibiotics Chemotherapy Vol. 42 (N. Hoiby, S. S. Pederson, G. H. Shand, G. Döring, and I. A., Holder, eds.), Karger, Basel, Switzerland, pp.184–192.
36. Stuttman, R., Petrovici, V., and Hartert, M., 1987, Prophylactic *Pseudomonas* immunoglobulin in burn patients, *Infection* **15:**S71–S74.
37. Böhm, D., 1987, Clinical experience in a surgical intensive care unit with a *Pseudomonas* immunoglobulin in ventilated patients suffering from *Pseudomonas* pneumonia, *Infection* **15:** S64–S66.
38. Class, I., Junginger, W., and Klöss, T., 1987, *Pseudomonas* immunoglobulin in surgical intensive care patients on mechanical ventilation, *Infection* **15:**S67–S70.
39. Granström, M., Wretlind, B., Markham, B., and Cryz, S. J., Jr., 1988, Enzyme-linked immunosorbent assay to evaluate the immunogenicity of a polyvalent *Klebsiella* capsular polysaccharide vaccine in humans, *J. Clin. Microbiol.* **26:**2257–2261.
40. Sawada, S., Kawamura, T., and Masuho, Y., 1987, Immunoprotective human monoclonal antibodies against five major serotypes of *Pseudomonas aeruginosa*, *J. Gen. Microbiol.* **133:** 3581–3590.
41. Zweerink, H. J., Gammon, M. C., Hutchinson, C. F., Jackson, J.J., Lombardo, D., Miner,

K. M., Puckett, J. M., Sewell, T. J., and Sigal, N. H., 1988, Human monoclonal antibodies that protect mice against challenge with *Pseudomonas aeruginosa*, *Infect. Immun.* **56**:1873–1879.
42. Lang, A. B., Fürer, E., Senyk, G., Larrick, J. W., and Cryz, S. J., Jr., 1990, Systemic generation of antigen specific human monoclonal antibodies with therapeutic activities using active immunization, *Hum. Antibodies Hybridomas* **1**:96–103.
43. Lang, A. B., Bruderer, U., Fürer, E., Larrick, J. W., and Cryz, S. J., Jr., 1990, Immunoprotective capacities of human murine monoclonal antibodies recognizing serotype specific and common determinants of gram-negative bacteria, in: *Therapeutic Monoclonal Antibodies* (C. A. K. Borrebaeck and J. W. Larrick, eds.), Stockton Press, New York, pp.223–234.

19

Perspectives for the Control of Chronic *Pseudomonas aeruginosa* Lung Infections of Cystic Fibrosis Patients

DONALD E. WOODS

1. INTRODUCTION

Although *Pseudomonas aeruginosa* plays a prominent role in bacillary pneumonia in acutely ill individuals, most of the patients who develop nonbacteremic *P. aeruginosa* pneumonia have pre-existing chronic pulmonary disease of other severe medical disorders.[1,2] This is particularly evident in person with cystic fibrosis (CF). The great majority of CF individuals become colonized with *P. aeruginosa* and poor clinical status is associated with increased numbers of this organism in the sputum.[3]

Most *P. aeruginosa* strains involved in CF lung infections are highly resistant to the great majority of the more commonly used antibiotics and chemotherapeutic agents.[4] This organism poses additional problems by virtue of its ubiquity in the environment; it has been shown to persist in environments where other potential pathogens are unable to survive.[5,6] Further, pulmonary infection with *P. aeruginosa* is accompanied by severe

---

DONALD E. WOODS • Department of Microbiology and Infectious Diseases, University of Calgary Health Sciences Centre, Calgary, Alberta, Canada T2N 4N1.

Pseudomonas aeruginosa as an Opportunistic Pathogen, edited by Mario Campa *et al.* Plenum Press, New York, 1993.

tissue damage as evidenced by histopathological descriptions of lungs from fatal cases of *P. aeruginosa* pneumonia.

The pulmonary histopathology of *P. aeruginosa* infections in CF is dominated by bronchial changes. These include epithelial metaplasia with loss of cilia, predominance of mucus versus serous acini in hyperplastic bronchial glands, goblet cell hyperplasia, acute and chronic inflammatory infiltrates, bronchiectasis, and mucopurulent plugging of the airways.[7] Chronic organized alveolar inflammatory exudate is present in the lungs of patients examined after the first 2 years of age.[7]

Clearly, pulmonary infection with *P. aeruginosa* may be accompanied by severe tissue damage. *P. aeruginosa* produces a variety of exoproducts that have been implicated in lung injury, including exotoxin A (ETA), proteases, phospholipase C (PLC), and exoenzyme S (exo-S). Evidence for the involvement of these exoproducts in lung injury comes from studies in animal models, immunological studies in patients, histopathological examination of lung tissue from patients infected with *P. aeruginosa*, and phenotypic comparisons of strains isolated from different infection sites including lung isolates of *P. aeruginosa*.

2. ANIMAL STUDIES

The chronic rat lung infection model has been used by a number of investigators to assess the role of *P. aeruginosa* exoproducts in lung disease due to this organism. The observations made from the rat model concerning the role of *P. aeruginosa* virulence factors in chronic lung infections are consistent with those seen in chronic *P. aeruginosa* lung infections in CF patients. Similarities are seen between the pathological descriptions of chronically infected rat lungs and lung tissue examined at autopsy from patients dying of *P. aeruginosa* lung infections.[8] Additional similarities exist between the animal model and chronically infected CF patients; both develop higher titers of antibody to *P. aeruginosa* antigens including lipopolysaccharide (LPS), ETA, proteases, exo-S, and alginate without clearing the organisms from their lungs. Further, both groups may develop circulating immune complexes containing any or all of the above antigens.[9,10]

Recently, we have demonstrated that the sequence of events during *P. aeruginosa* lung infection in CF patients, predicted by epidemiological studies, is correct.[11] Infection by nonmucoid *P. aeruginosa* isolates, producing significant levels of recognized virulence determinants, is followed by conversion of these nonmucoid organisms to mucoid isolates, producing lower levels of virulence determinants. We employed the chronic rat lung infection model to induce the *in vivo* conversion to the mucoid phenotype by *P. aeruginosa* strain PAO. At 6 months following initial inoculation, *P. aeruginosa* PAO organisms isolated from homogenates of infected rat lung tissue demonstrated the mucoid phenotype on primary isolation medium. The exopolysaccharide responsible for the phenotype was confirmed as alginate by nuclear magnetic resonance (NMR) spectral analysis. Reversion to the nonmucoid phenotype was noted following two passages of the mucoid lung isolates *in vitro*. Comparison of *in vitro* production of specific virulence factors revealed significant decreases ($P<.01$) in the levels of ETA, exo-S, phospholipase C, and pyochelin produced by the mucoid *P. aeruginosa* PAO rat lung isolates, which then reverted to parental levels of production following reversion of the bacteria to the nonmucoid phenotype. LPS of the mucoid PAO lung isolates failed to react with a serotype B-specific monoclonal antibody in contrast to the original PAO organisms and the revertant PAO organisms. Restriction digestion of chromosomal DNA and Southern hybridization with *P. aeruginosa* virulence-factor-specific probes demonstrated that conversion to the mucoid phenotype was associated with rearrangement of chromosomal DNA upstream of the ETA gene. Analysis of organisms that had reverted to the nonmucoid phenotype by *in vitro* passage revealed hybridization patterns identical to those of the original PAO organism. These studies indicate that *in vivo* conversion to the mucoid phenotype by *P. aeruginosa* is not unique to the CF lung environment, but is simply associated with chronic *P. aeruginosa* infection states. Further, this conversion to the mucoid phenotype may be associated with rearrangement of *P. aeruginosa* chromosomal DNA, and this genetic rearrangement is associated with qualitative or quantitative coordinate changes in specific extracellular virulence factors as well as LPS serotype. We are currently defining the mechanism of the rearrangement and its effect on the conversion to the mucoid phenotype. Results from these studies further strengthen our belief in the utility of the chronic rat lung infection model as a tool to investigate chronic *P. aeruginosa* lung infections.

In a series of studies aimed at defining the role of *P. aeruginosa* exoproducts in chronic lung infections, we employed a genetic approach, using isogenic mutants deficient in single virulence properties. Each mutant strain was tested in the rat model of chronic *P. aeruginosa* lung infection and the infection compared with that caused the parental strains. We concluded that *P. aeruginosa* virulence is multifactorial, and that strains lacking either elastase, ETA, or exo-S are less virulent in the chronic rat lung infection model.[12-14]

Additional studies to examine the role of exoproducts in lung infections have involved direct instillation of purified *P. aeruginosa* exoproducts into the lungs of experimental animals. Cash *et al.*[15] reported that intratracheal administration of ETA and protease, alone or in combination, resulted in histopathological changes that closely resembled those seen in the lungs of infected rats. Gray and Kreger[16] instilled 10–100 μg of *P. aeruginosa* elastase into rabbit lungs and reported hemorrhage as well as necrosis of certain cell types. More recently, we have demonstrated that intratracheal administration of purified exo-S[17] elicits extensive, grossly observable rat lung damage by 2 hr post-injection. Light and electron microscopic characterization of the lesions reveals: (1) injury and necrosis of bronchial epithelium, type I pneumocytes and capillary endothelial cells from 1 h post-injection: (2) associated hemorrhage, fibrinous exudation, and released type II cell lamellar bodies in alveolar lumina from one to 24 hr post-injection; and (3) collapse of alveolar septal connective tissue and damage to pulmonary arterioles and venules.[18]

3. REGULATION OF VIRULENCE

Further evidence that *P. aeruginosa* exoproducts may play a role in lung injury during lung infection was provided by our studies on the regulatory effect of iron on these products.[12] Yields of ETA, elastase, and alkaline protease are inversely proportional to the iron concentration in the medium.[19] Mutants have been isolated that are resistant to the regulation of either ETA or elastase by iron, indicating that iron regulates these exoproducts independently.[20] When *P. aeruginosa* strain PAO was grown in low-iron medium, it was more virulent than it was when it was grown in high-iron medium. However, the virulence of strain Fe18, a mutant resistant to the effect of iron on yields of ETA, was unaffected. These studies suggest that the regulation of extracellular virulence factors by iron is important in the determination of *P. aeruginosa* virulence. More importantly, these data demonstrate that lung injury due to *P. aeruginosa* can be decreased markedly by the suppression of exoproduct release, further demonstrating the importance of these determinants of pathogenicity in chronic *P. aeruginosa* lung disease.

We also demonstrated that the host environment surrounding *P. aeruginosa* markedly affects the levels of exoproducts released.[21] We compared the phenotypes of a number of *P. aeruginosa* strains obtained from a variety of clinical sources that included burn wounds, skin wounds, urine, CF patient sputum, acute pneumonia sputum, and blood. These clinical isolates were examined for quantitative levels of total protease, elastase, phospholipase C, ETA and exo-S produced *in vitro* under defined conditions. Exoproduct levels varied significantly, depending on the site of strain isolation, and confirmed previous observations that the virulence of *P. aeruginosa* is multifactorial. However, the results indicate that certain exoproducts may play a more important role in certain types of infection. In particular, proteolytic activity and exo-S are significant pathogenic determinants in pulmonary infections due to *P. aeruginosa*.[21]

4. DIRECT VERSUS INDIRECT LUNG INJURY

Direct lung injury by *P. aeruginosa* exoproducts seems to be responsible for a substantial portion of the total lung injury during infection by this organism. Additionally, indirect lung injury due to the over-exuberant host response to

P. aeruginosa exoproducts must also be taken into consideration when examining total lung injury during *P. aeruginosa* infection. The continuous presence of *P. aeruginosa* and its exoproducts serves to maintain a chronic inflammatory response, with an accumulation of polymorphonuclear leukocytes (PMN) and the release of endogenous proteases. The deleterious effects of these proteases on the lungs are normally inhibited by the anti-proteolytic activity found in bronchial mucus secretions. The best-characterized of these inhibitors is the bronchial mucus inhibitor (BMI), which is thought to protect the respiratory tract from the proteolytic activity of PMN elastase and cathepsin G.[22] Another inhibitor that protects lungs from the actions of PMN elastase is α-1-proteinase inhibitor.[23] During active infection with *P. aeruginosa*, however, the proteinase inhibitors may be inactivated by *P. aeruginosa* elastase.

Moskowitz and Heinrich[24] demonstrated that α-1-proteinase inhibitor was inactivated by *P. aeruginosa* culture supernatants. More recently, Morihara *et al.*[25] showed that *P. aeruginosa* elastase inactivates α-1-proteinase inhibitor by splitting the peptide bond between Pro[357] and Met[358], leading to changes near the active site. Johnson *et al.*[26] found that *P. aeruginosa* elastase could rapidly destroy the ability of BMI to inhibit PMN elastase and cathepsin G. Thus, the action of *P. aeruginosa* elastase on respiratory protease inhibitors could lead to significant indirect lung injury during infection by *P. aeruginosa*.

Studies in my laboratory have attempted to differentiate direct lung injury due to *P. aeruginosa* exoproducts released during chronic *P. aeruginosa* lung infections, from indirect lung injury due to host immune responses. Our initial aim was to examine the possibility that intervention with alternate-day steroid therapy (anti-inflammatory regimen, methylprednisolone, 1 mg/kg) could suppress the formation of circulating immune complexes in rats chronically infected with *P. aeruginosa*.[27] We were surprised that not only does alternate-day steroid therapy suppress the formation of circulating immune complexes, but this treatment regimen also leads to bacterial clearance from the lungs of experimental animals. We have taken our studies with steroids further and have looked at the direct effect of steroids on *P. aeruginosa in vitro*.[27] We found that 10 ng/ml methylprednisolone completely blocks the secretion of a variety of *P. aeruginosa* exoproducts including protease, ETA and exo-S. Further, we have extended these studies to demonstrate that antibiotics such as ciprofloxacin, tobramycin, and ceftazidime can also significantly suppress the release of *P. aeruginosa* exoproducts.[28,29]

5. EFFECTS OF ANTIBIOTICS ON VIRULENCE

We examined the effects of subinhibitory concentrations of ciprofloxacin, tobramycin, and ceftazidime on *P. aeruginosa* exoenzyme expression *in vitro* and *in vivo* in the chronic rat lung infection model.[28] ETA, exo-S, PLC, elastase and total protease activities were suppressed by antibiotics at concentrations as low as 1/20 of the minimum inhibitory concentration (MIC) over a 24-hr period. When *P. aeruginosa* strain DG1 broth cultures were exposed to antibiotic levels equal to 1/10 of the MIC continuously for 10 days, exoenzyme S activity was reduced in all treatment groups. Elastase activity was reduced only by ciprofloxacin and tobramycin treatment. This suppressive effect of the antibiotics persisted throughout the 10 days and was not influenced by the increase in MIC of ciprofloxacin detected during the course of the experiment. Rats chronically infected with *P. aeruginosa* were treated with subinhibitory doses of antibiotics and compared with untreated controls. Bacterial numbers were identical in lung homogenates from each of the four study groups. However, the lungs from antibiotic-treated rats had significantly less histological damage than those from control rats ($P<.001$). The protective effect was greatest for ciprofloxacin and tobramycin. Further, *P. aeruginosa* isolates from ciprofloxacin- and tobramycin-treated rats demonstrated significantly less exo-S and elastase activity than isolates from untreated rats ($P<.001$). Isolates from ceftazidime-treated lungs expressed less exo-S activity ($P<.001$); however, they expressed an equivalent amount of elastase activity as isolates from controls. Thus, the suppression of *P. aeruginosa* exoenzymes can arrest progressive lung injury during chronic *P. aeruginosa* lung infections.

In a separate comparative study of different *P. aeruginosa* strains, we evaluated the effects of subinhibitory antibiotic treatment upon *P. aeruginosa* exoenzyme expression and lung injury *in vivo*.[28] One hundred and twenty-eight animals were separated into two groups of 64 animals. One group was inoculated with *P. aeruginosa* DG1, the other with *P. aeruginosa* 3740. Each group was divided into four subgroups of 16 animals on the basis of 10-day antibiotic treatment with ciprofloxacin, tobramycin, and ceftazidime, or untreated controls. *P. aeruginosa* DG1 is nonmucoid and expresses significant yields of exo-S and elastase. *P. aeruginosa* 3740 is a mucoid organism isolated from the sputum of a CF patient and demonstrates only modest elastase activity (10% of DG1 levels). Lung bacterial counts were similar in treatment and control groups. Lungs from antibiotic-treated rats demonstrated fewer histological changes than those from untreated animals ($P<.001$). No detectable decrease in elastase or mucoid phenotype was observed in 3740 lung isolates from antibiotic-treated animals. These studies provide further evidence that antibiotic protection against lung injury by *P. aeruginosa* may involve modulation of virulence factors.

In one study done in collaboration with Dr. P. A. Sokol, we examined the effects of subinhibitory concentrations of tetracycline on surface expression of *P. aeruginosa* ferripyochelin binding protein (FBP) and *P. aeruginosa* virulence in the chronic rat lung infection model.[30] Rats were inoculated with *P. aeruginosa* DG1; one-half of the inoculated animals served as untreated

CONTROL OF LUNG INFECTIONS OF CF PATIENTS 403

controls, while the other half received daily injections of 15 mg/kg tetracycline. Using indirect immunofluorescence and immuno-electron microscopy, FBP was shown to be surface-exposed in bacteria isolated from control animals. No FBP was detectable, however, on the surface of bacterial isolated from the lungs of animals treated with tetracycline. The numbers of bacteria recovered from the lungs of infected animals did not differ between control and tetracycline-treated groups, although the degree of pathology observed in tetracycline-treated animals was significantly lower than in untreated controls ($P = .002$, one-way ANOVA). Subinhibitory doses of tetracycline reduced proteolytic activity *in vitro*. These results suggest that exposure to subinhibitory concentrations of tetracycline can repress FBP surface expression as well as proteolytic activity in *P. aeruginosa*, leading to a significant decrease in lung injury during infections with this organism.

6. PATIENT STUDIES

We have demonstrated that up-regulation of *P. aeruginosa* virulence is clearly associated with exacerbations of lung disease in CF patients; and conversely, down-regulation of *P. aeruginosa* virulence is associated with recovery from these exacerbations. A single CF patient was studied retrospectively to determine the relationship between clinical status and anti–exo-S antibody levels as well as the levels of exo-S produced *in vitro* by the patient's colonizing *P. aeruginosa* strain.[27] As shown in Fig. 1, over a 5-year period, diminished clinical status, as indicated by a decrease in Shwachman score, was preceded on each occasion by a change in the exo-S phenotype of the *P. aeruginosa* strain colonizing the airways of this patient. Fig. 1 also shows that rises in anti–exo-S antibody titers overlap the points at which the patient was experiencing exacerbations in pulmonary symptoms (decreased Shwachman score). From this longitudinal study of a single patient, it is apparent that increases in anti–exo-S antibody levels were preceded by a change (up-regulation) in the exo-S phenotype of the colonizing *P. aeruginosa* strain. Thus while the increases in anti–exo-S antibody levels overlap points of diminished clinical status, the observation that these increases are preceded by a possible increase in exo-S production by the colonizing *P. aeruginosa* strain, argues for a role of the direct action of *P. aeruginosa* toxins in the pathogenesis of lung injury in CF patients.

We are preparing a manuscript detailing the results of retrospective and prospective studies examining the influence of variations in the levels of *P. aeruginosa* exoenzymes on the clinical course of CF patients. Partial representations of the data obtained from these studies are presented in Figs. 2 and 3 in which *in vitro* levels were determined of elastase and exo-S produced by the strains colonizing the airways of CF patients. As shown in Fig. 2, *P. aeruginosa* strains from our strain bank originally obtained from patients seen at routine

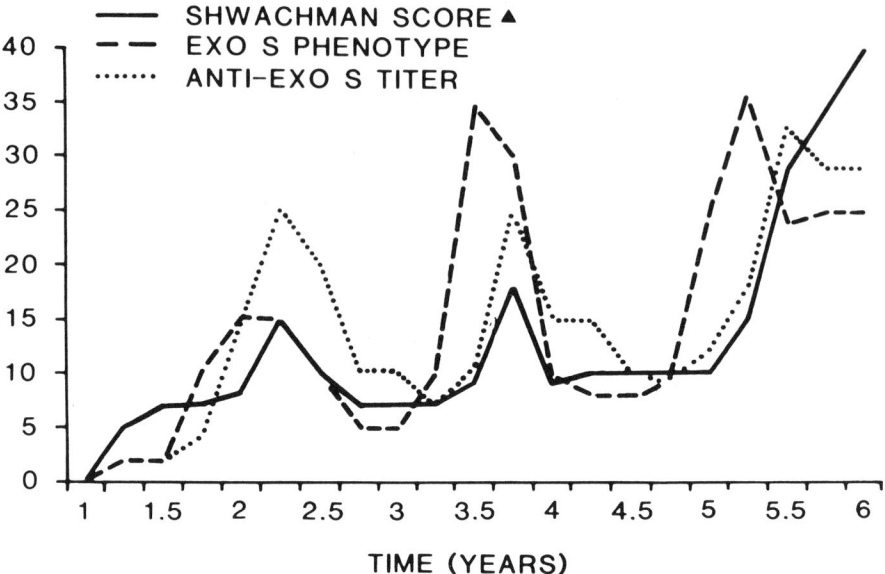

FIGURE 1. Retrospective study of a single CF patient over a 5-year period. Correlation of clinical status (Shwachman scores) with serum anti–exo-S phenotype of colonizing *P. aeruginosa* strain. Reproduced with permission from ref. 27.

clinic visits were analyzed for exoenzyme levels and these levels were compared with those produced by strains originally isolated from hospitalized patients classified as seriously ill. These data show that: (1) patients seen at routine clinic visits are predictably healthier than hospitalized patients, as indicated by Shwachman scores; (2) this improved clinical status is correlated with the production of significantly lower levels of elastase and exo-S by the colonizing *P. aeruginosa* strains; and (3) nonmucoid *P. aeruginosa* strains produce higher levels of elastase and exo-S than do mucoid *P. aeruginosa* strains isolated from the same patient.

We have repeated the study in a prospective fashion: We analyzed *P. aeruginosa* strains isolated from CF patients for *in vitro* production of elastase and exo-S; however, strains from the same patient were analyzed for exoenzyme levels at the time of the patient's entry into the hospital and at the time of the patient's discharge. The strains were determined to be the same by genotyping of chromosomal DNA using the upstream ETA probe that we have used in a number of our studies. The data are shown in Fig. 3 and reveal

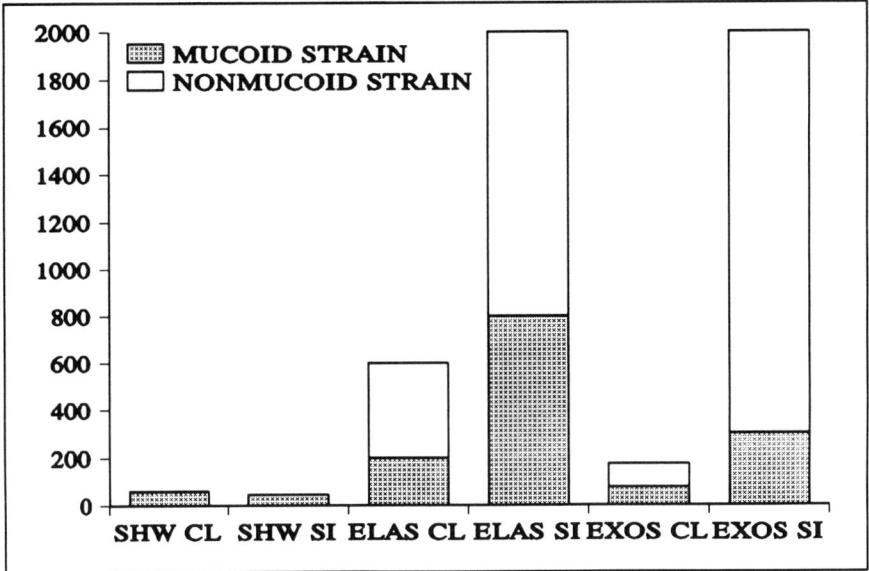

FIGURE 2. Retrospective study of CF patients. SHW (Shwachman scores), CL (Clinic), SI (Seriously Ill), ELAS (Elastase), EXOS (Exoenzyme S).

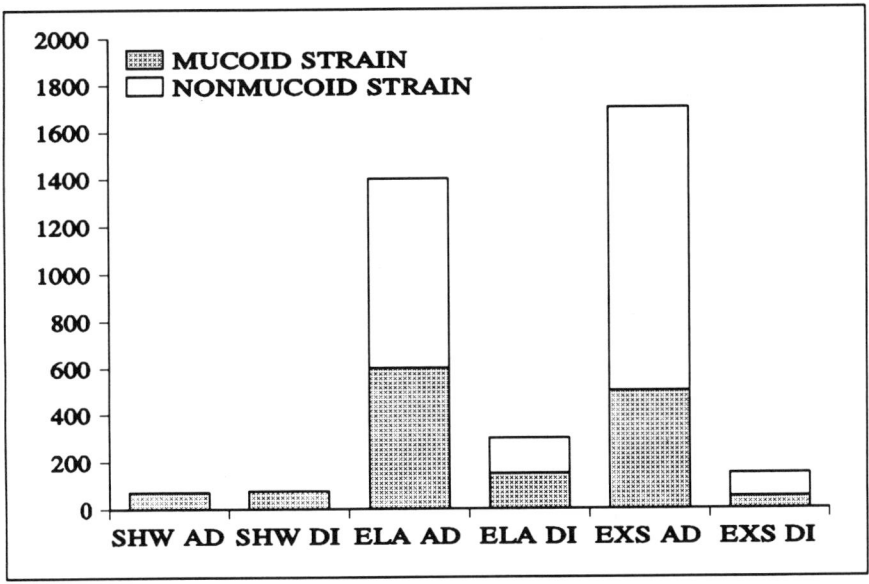

FIGURE 3. Prospective study of CF patients SHW (Schwachman scores), AD (Admission), DI (Discharge), ELA (Elastase), EXS (Exoenzyme S).

that improvement in clinical status can be correlated with down-regulation in the production of elastase and exo-S.

7. ROLE OF *P. AERUGINOSA* IN EXACERBATIONS OF LUNG DISEASE

A number of theories have been offered to explain the occurrence of exacerbations of respiratory disease in CF patients. For example, Marks[31] noted that the respiratory-virus season is often heralded by an increase in the frequency of pulmonary exacerbations in CF patients. Associations have been made between these periodic viral infections and deterioration of lung function[32] or mortality of the patient.[33] Wright et al.,[34] while investigating the effectiveness of amantadine-HCL as an antiviral drug, observed that a substantial proportion of exacerbations were associated with viral influenza A infections. These findings have been supported by other studies, which determined that 20–29% of exacerbations were correlated with viral infections.[35,36] Furthermore, a synergistic relationship has been suggested to exist between viral lung infection and subsequent bacterial colonization.[33] Using the rat model of chronic *P. aeruginosa* lung infection, we have obtained preliminary evidence that superinfection of animals infected with *P. aeruginosa* with respiratory syncytial virus (RSV) significantly alters the histopathological findings from those seen with *P. aeruginosa* infection alone. Table I illustrates the significant increase in the mean pathological index associated with combined RSV and *P. aeruginosa* infections compared with infections with either organism alone.

Evidence from this study and the published literature indicate a possible relationship between viral infection and exacerbations of lung disease in CF. Based on *in vitro* studies in which we have examined the interaction between *P. aeruginosa* and interferon-2-alpha, we hypothesize that it may not be the virus itself, but the host's immune response to the virus that triggers the onset

TABLE I
Mean Pathological Indices of Chronically Infected Rats

Treatment group (N = 5)	Mean pathological index[a]
Pseudomonas aeruginosa[b] only	54.9 ± 4.8[c]
Respiratory syncytial virus only[d]	10.3 ± 2.7
Pseudomonas aeruginosa + respiratory syncytial virus[e]	88.6 ± 9.9

[a]Calculated as previously described.[12]
[b]*P. aeruginosa* strain DG1 inoculated in agar beads as described.[8]
[c]Mean ± S.D.
[d]3.4×10^4 PFU/ml inoculated intratracheally.
[e]Respiratory syncytial virus inoculated into rats inoculated 90 days earlier with *P. aeruginosa* strain DG1 in agar beads.

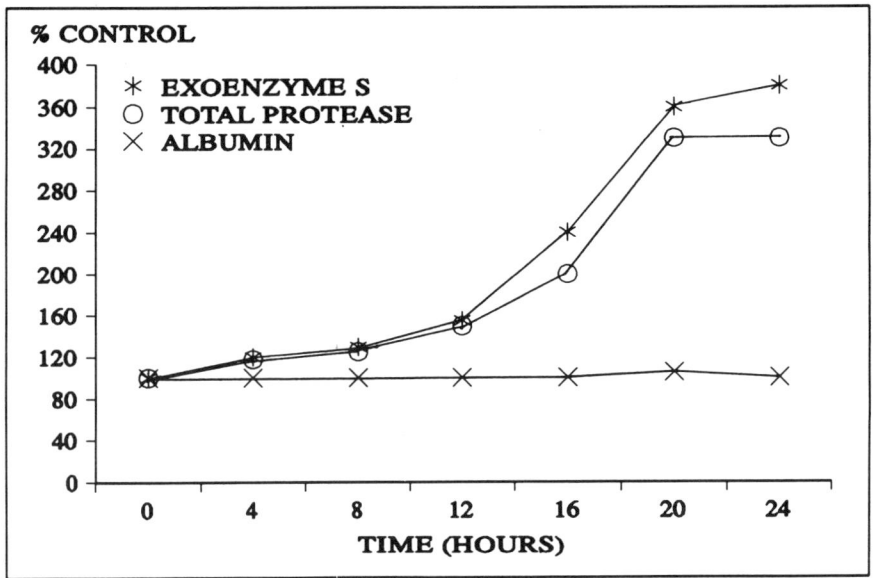

FIGURE 4. Effects of interferon-2-alpha on *Pseudomonas aeruginosa* exoenzyme production; 10-ml cultures of *P. aeruginosa* strain DG1 were incubated with 10^5 IU interferon-2-alpha for 24 hr at 32°C (Schering, Inc.) and the supernatant fluid analyzed for exo-S and total protease activity.

of exacerbations. In response to viral infections the host produces interferon; we have obtained evidence (Fig. 4) that interferon-2-alpha, when incubated with *P. aeruginosa*, leads to a significant increase in the production of exo-S and in total protease activity, both of which are significant pathogenic determinants in chronic *P. aeruginosa* lung infections.

Based on the results from the *in vitro* interferon studies, we examined bronchoalveolar lavage fluid from animals treated as described in Table I, for the presence of interferon. Data presented in the Table II indicate that interferon is indeed produced in response to RSV infection. We are pursuing this line of inquiry, investigating those parameters associated with the apparent effects of viral superinfections on exacerbations of chronic *P. aeruginosa* infections of the lung.

8. CONCLUSION

To summarize: (1) We know that *P. aeruginosa* exoproducts play a significant role in the progressive pathology seen in chronic lung infections due to this organism; (2) CF patients tend to harbor *P. aeruginosa* strains for long periods of time; (3) these colonizing *P. aeruginosa* strains undergo remarkable

TABLE II
Interferon Induction in Chronically Infected Rats

Treatment group (N = 5)	PFU MHV-A59[a]
Pseudomonas aeruginosa[b] only	245 ± 23[c]
Respiratory syncytial virus only[d]	232 ± 25
Pseudomonas aeruginosa + respiratory syncytial virus[e]	141 ± 15
MEM control	297 ± 5
Interferon control[f]	144 ± 13

[a] Interferon was assayed by incubating confluent monolayers of L-2 cells overnight with a 1:5 dilution in minimal essential medium (MEM) of bronchoalveolar lavage fluid from treated rats. The cells were washed extensively and challenged with 300 plaque-forming units (PFU) of mouse hepatitis virus strain A59. The decrease in the number of PFU is an indirect indicator of the amount of interferon present in the samples.
[b] *P. aeruginosa* strain DG1 inoculated in agar beads as described.[8]
[c] Mean ± S.D.
[d] 3.4×10^4 PFU/ml inoculated intratracheally.
[e] Respiratory syncytial virus inoculated into rats inoculated 90 days earlier with *P. aeruginosa* strain DG1 in agar beads.
[f] Human interferon-2-alpha (10^4 IU).

phenotypic changes during this time, including changes in the expression of exoproducts, and these phenotypic variations correlate with exacerbations of lung disease in CF patients. Thus, *P. aeruginosa* has an enormous adaptive capacity that allows it to persist in the respiratory tracts of CF patients. Further, it has been recognized that the majority of CF patients possess significant levels of circulating antibodies to a variety of cellular and extracellular antigens associated with this organism. Thus, we feel that neither active nor passive immunization against *P. aeruginosa* is a rational therapeutic approach to control infectious lung injury in CF patients.

A variety of agents, including antibiotics, steroids and interferon, have been shown to affect the expression of *P. aeruginosa* exoproducts. An important question, and one we are attempting to answer, is: What are the environmental factors that influence up-regulation of virulence in *P. aeruginosa* strains colonizing the airways of CF patients which lead to exacerbations of their lung disease? Although the answer may include any number of factors, we have begun to examine some of these in detail. By understanding the ability of *P. aeruginosa* to regulate colonization, persistence, and expression of virulence in the lungs of CF patients, we hope to learn how to down-regulate virulence and/or adaptive mechanisms, and thus help control infectious lung injury caused by *P. aeruginosa* in CF patients.

ACKNOWLEDGMENTS. This work was supported by the Canadian Cystic Fibrosis Foundation.

REFERENCES

1. Reynolds, H. Y., Disant'agnese, P.A., Dailey, S., and Markarian, B., 1972, *Pseudomonas aeruginosa*: A prototype of hospital-based infection. *Radiology* **105**:555–562.
2. Tillotson, J. R., and Lerner, A. M., 1968, Characteristics of non bacteremic *Pseudomonas* pneumonia. *Ann. Intern. Med.* **68**:295–307.
3. Hanissian, A. S., Templeton, G., Chandler, R. W., and Robinson, H., 1974, Quantitative bacteriology of sputum in cystic fibrosis: A prospective study. *Cystic Fibrosis Club Abstr.* #18, 15th Annual Meeting.
4. Duncan, I. B. R., 1974, Susceptibility of 1,500 isolates of *Pseudomonas aeruginosa* to gentamicin, carbenicillin, colistin and polymyxin B. *Antimicrob. Agents Chemother.* **5**:9–15.
5. Farmer, J. J., III. 1976, *Pseudomonas* in the hospital. *Hosp. Practice.* **10**:63–70.
6. Young, V. (ed), 1977, *Pseudomonas aeruginosa: Ecological Aspects of Patient Colonization*, Raven Press, New York, p. 137.
7. Bedrossian, C. W. M., Greenberg, S. D., Singer, D. B., Hansen, J. J., and Rosenberg, H. S., 1976, The lung in cystic fibrosis: A quantitative sutdy including prevalence of pathologic findings among different age groups. *Human Pathol.* **7**:195–204.
8. Cash, H. A., Woods, D. E., McCullough, B., Johanson, W. G., and Bass, J. A., 1979, A rat model of chronic respiratory infection with *Pseudomonas aeruginosa*. *Am. Rev. Respir. Dis.* **119**: 453–459.
9. Woods, D. E., and Bryan, L. E., 1985, Studies on the ability of alginate to act as a protective immunogen against *Pseudomonas aeruginosa* infection in animals. *J. Infect. Dis.* **151**:581–588.
10. McFarlane, H., Holzel, A., Brenchley, P., Allan, J. D., Wallwork, J. C., Singer, B. E., and Wolsley, B., 1975, Immune complexes in cystic fibrosis. *Br. Med. J.* **1**:423–428.
11. Woods, D. E., Sokol, P. A., Bryan, L. E., Storey, D. G., Mattingley, S. J., Vogel, H. J., and Ceri, H., *In vivo* regulation of virulence in *Pseudomonas aeruginosa* associated with genetic rearrangement. *J. Infect. Dis.* in press.
12. Woods, D. E., Cryz, S. J., Friedman, R. L., and Iglewski, B. H., 1982, Contribution of toxin A and elastase to virulence of *Pseudomonas aeruginosa* in chronic lung infections of rats. *Infect. Immun.* **36**:1223–1228.
13. Sokol, P. A., and Woods, D. E., 1984, Relationship of iron and extracellular virulence factors to *Pseudomonas aeruginosa* lung infections. *J. Med. Microbiol.* **18**:125–133.
14. Woods, D. E., and Sokol, P. A., 1985, Use of transposon mutants to assess the role of exoenzyme S in chronic pulmonary disease due to *Pseudomonas aeruginosa*. *Eur. J. Clin. Microbiol.* **4**:163–169.
15. Cash, H. A., Straus, D. C., and Bass, J. A., 1982, *Pseudomonas aeruginosa* exoproducts as pulmonary virulence factors. *Can. J. Microbiol.* **29**:448–456.
16. Gray, L., and Kreger, A., 1979, Microscopic characterization of rabbit lung damage produced by *Pseudomonas aeruginosa* proteases. *Infect. Immun.* **23**:150–159.
17. Woods, D. E., and Que, J. U., 1987, Purification of *Pseudomonas aeruginosa* exoenzyme S. *Infect. Immun.* **55**:579–586.
18. Woods, D. E., Hwang, W. S., Shahrabadi, M. S., and Que, J. U., 1988, Alternation of pulmonary structure by *Pseudomonas aeruginosa* exoenzyme S. *J. Med. Microbiol.* **26**:133–141.
19. Bjorn, M. J., Pavloskis, O. R., Thompson, M. R., and Iglewski, B. H., 1979, Production of exoenzyme S during *Pseudomonas aeruginosa* infections of burned mice. *Infect. Immun.* **24**: 837–842.
20. Sokol, P. A., Cox, C. D., and Iglewski, B. H., 1982, *Pseudomonas aeruginosa* mutants altered in their sensitivity to the effect of iron on toxin A or elastase yields. *J. Bacteriol.* **151**:783–787.
21. Woods, D. E., Shaffer, M. S., Rabin, H. R., Campbell, G. D., and Sokol, P. A., 1986, Phenotypic comparison of *Pseudomonas aeruginosa* strains isolated from a variety of clinical sites, *J. Clin. Microbiol.* **24**:260–264.

22. Haveman, K., and Janoff, A. (eds.), 1978, *Neurtal proteases of human polymorphonuclear leukocytes*, Urban and Schwarzenberg, Munich, p. 195.
23. Heimburger, N., 1971, *Proc. Int. Res. Conf. on Proteinase Inhibitors*, Berlin, p. 1.
24. Moskowitz, R. W., and Heinrich, G., 1971, Bacterial inactivation of human serum alpha-1 antitrypsin, *J. Lab. Clin. Med.* **77:**777.
25. Morihara, K., Tsuzuki, H., Harada, M., and Iwata, T., 1984, Purification of human plasma α_1-proteinase inhibitor and its inactivation by *Pseudomonas aeruginosa* elastase, *J. Biochem.* **95:** 795–804.
26. Johnson, D. A., Carter-Hamm, B., and Dralle, W. M., 1982, Inactivation of human bronchial mucosal proteinase inhibitor by *Pseudomonas aeruginosa* elastase, *Am. Rev. Respir. Dis.* **126:** 1070–1073.
27. Woods, D. E., To, M., and Sokol, P. A., 1989, *Pseudomonas aeruginosa* exoenzyme S as pathogenic determinant in respiratory infections, *Antibiot. Chemother.* **42:**27–35.
28. Grimwood, K., To, M., Rabin, H. R., and Woods, D. E., 1989, Inhibition of *Pseudomonas aeruginosa* exoenzyme expression by subinhibitory antibiotic concentrations, *Antimicrob. Agents Chemother.* **33:**41–47.
29. Grimwood, K., To, M., Rabin, H. R., and Woods, D. E., 1989, Subinhibitory antibiotics reduce *Pseudomonas aeruginosa* tissue injury in the rat lung model, *J. Antimicrob. Chemother.* **24:**937–945.
30. LeVatte, M. A., Woods, D. E., Shahrabadi, M. S., Semple, R., and Sokol, P. A., 1990, Subinhibitory concentrations of tetracycline inhibit surface expression of the *Pseudomonas aeruginosa* ferripyochelin binding protein *in vivo*, *J. Antimicrob. Chemother.* **26:**215–225.
31. Marks, M. I., 1984, Respiratory viruses in cystic fibrosis, *N. Engl. J. Med.* **311:**1695–1696.
32. Want, E. E. L., Prober, C. G., Manson, B., Corey, M., and Levison, H., 1984, Association of respiratory viral infections with pulmonary deterioration in patients with cystic fibrosis, *N. Engl. J. Med.* **311:**1653–1658.
33. Abman, S. J., Ogle, J. W., Butler-Simon, N., Rumack, C. M., and Accurso, F. J., 1988, Role of respiratory syncytial virus in early hospitalizations for respiratory distress of young infants with cystic fibrosis, *J. Pediatr.* **113:**826–830.
34. Wright, P. F., Khaw, K. T., Oxman, M. N., and Shwachman, H., 1976, Evaluation of the safety of amantadine HCL and the role of respiratory viral infections in children with cystic fibrosis, *J. Infect. Dis.* **134:**144–149.
35. Efthimious, J., Hodson, M. E., Taylor, P., Taylor, A. G., and Batten, J. C., 1984, Importance of viruses and *Legionella pneumophila* in respiratory exacerbations of young adults with cystic fibrosis, *Thorax* **39:**150–154.
36. Peterson, N. T., Hoiby, M., Mordhorst, C. H., Lind, K., Flensborg, E. W., and Bruun, B., 1981, Respiratory infections in cystic fibrosis patients caused by virus, *Chlamydia* and *Mycoplasma*: Possible synergism with *Pseudomonas aeruginosa*. *Acta Pediatr. Scand.* **70:** 623–628.

Index

Abrin, 79
Acquired resistance to *Pseudomonas aeruginosa*, 297–311
　bacterial antibody in, 303–304
　complement in, 304
　in cystic fibrosis patients, 305–310
　　antibody isotype in, 308–310
　　complement in, 310
　　naturally acquired resistance, 306
　　vaccine-induced immunity, 306–308
　exotoxin A antibody, 299–300
　naturally acquired immunity, 299–300
　T-cell immunity, 304–305
　vaccine-induced immunity, 300–303
Active immunity, 298, 353
Adaptability of *Pseudomonas aeruginosa*, 2–3, 145, 397
Age and resistance, corneal studies, 199–200
AIDS patients, and *Pseudomonas aeruginosa*-caused diseases, 239
Alginate
　and attachment of *Pseudomonas aeruginosa*, 23, 26–27, 208–209
　immunological aspects, 298–299
　vaccines, 389
Amikacin, 332
Aminoglycosides, 331-338
　action against *Pseudomonas aeruginosa*, 332, 334
　amikacin, 332
　burn injuries, 276
　in combination therapy, 332
　cytoplasmic membrane penetration, 335–336

Aminoglycosides (*Cont.*)
　efficacy of, 331–334
　endocarditis, 227
　gentamicin, 332
　outer membrane permeation, 334–335
　plasmid-mediated resistance, 336
　resistance to *Pseudomonas aeruginosa*, 336–338
　skin infections, 226
　tobramycin, 332
Amyloid P, and protease control, 139
Animal models, 118
　burned mouse model, 109, 112, 174, 278
　corneal infection studies, 109, 188–199
　for immunotherapy, 359–363
　neutropenic rabbit model, 109
　for pulmonary infections, 109, 398–400
Anthrax, 80
Antibiotics
　aminoglycodisases, 331–338
　for cystic fibrosis patients, 258, 401–403
　effect on elastase, 150
　and increased incidence of *Pseudomonas aeruginosa*, 6, 7, 12, 223
　beta-lactams, 322–331
　and production of phenazine pigments, 48
　and protease control, 139
　quinolones, 338–342
　resistance of *Pseudomonas aeruginosa* to, 59–60, 108, 109, 150, 276–277, 349–350
　　adaptive resistance, 337–338
　　causes of, 321–322, 337
　　non-enzymatic resistance, 337
　See also specific drugs

411

Anti-inflammatory therapy, cystic fibrosis patients, 258–259
Aplacillin, 323
Aprotinin, and protease control, 139
Attachment of *Pseudomonas aeruginosa*, 19–36, 208–209
  adherence in pathogenesis, 20–21
  adhesin-receptor interactions, 23
  alginate, role of, 23, 26–27, 208–209
  capsule, structure and function of, 23–27
  corneal attachment, 20–21
  and cystic fibrosis, 249–250
  elastase, role in, 149
  and epithelial cell type, 21–22
  and exoenzyme S, 28, 32–33, 114–115
  host factors in, 209
  and human respiratory cells, 21, 149
  inflammation, role in, 249
  pili
    and burn injuries, 283–284
    and exoenzyme S receptors, 32–33
    pilin-pilin interactions, 30–31
    role of, 20–21, 23, 31–32
    structural organization of, 33
    structural variability in, 30
    structure of, 29
    synthesis and assembly of, 29
  tracheal epithelial cell attachment, 20
Azthreonam, 324

Bacteremia, 224–226
  clinical presentation, 225
  dermatologic manifestations, 225
  epidemiology, 224–225
  prognosis of, 226
  routes of transmission, 224–225
  treatment of, 225–226
Bacteria, effects of pyo on, 48
Bathroom, as *Pseudomonas aeruginosa* habitat, 3–4, 11
Binding techniques, 89
Bone/joint infections, 230
  addict-associated infections, 230
  epidemiology, 230
  osteochondritis, 230
Brain abscess, 231–232
  causes of, 231–232
  treatment of, 232
Burn injuries, 275–290
  antimicrobial treatment, 276–277
  burned mouse model, 109, 112, 174, 278
  host susceptivity factors, 286–290
  immunotherapy, 277, 363, 390–391

Burn injuries (*Cont.*)
  mortality and infection, 275–276
  ocular infections, 234
  phenazine pigments at burn site, 52
  post-burn immunosuppression syndrome, 286
  and *Pseudomonas aeruginosa*, 7, 108, 174, 232
  virulence-related factors, 277–285
    burn-wound infection, 286–290
    exotoxin A, 278–281
    flagella, 284–285
    motility, 284
    pili and adherence, 283–284
    proteolytic enzymes, 281–283

Carbapenems, 323, 329
Carbenicillin, 323
Catheterization, and incidence of *Pseudomonas aeruginosa*, 2, 7, 9, 20, 229
Cefoperazone, 323
Cefotaxime, 323
Cefpirome, 323
Cefsulodin, 323–324
Ceftazidime
  meningitis, 231
  study of, 401–403
Ceftriaxone, 323
Cell-mediated immunity, 298
Central nervous system infections
  brain abscess, 231–232
  meningitis, 231
Cephalosporins, 323–324, 328, 329
  azthreonam, 324
  cefoperazone, 323
  cefotaxime, 323
  cefpirome, 323
  cefsulodin, 323–324
  ceftriaxone, 323
Chimeric toxins, 98–99; binding to cells, 99
Cholera, 80
Chromatography, detection of phenazine, 46–47
Ciliary beating, effects of pyo on, 51–52, 208
Ciprofloxacin, study of, 401–403
Colony forming units, 11
Complement
  in acquired resistance to *Pseudomonas aeruginosa*, 304, 310
  in corneal resistance, 199
  in phagocytosis of *Pseudomonas aeruginosa*, 166–167, 210

Connective tissue, proteases' effects, 132–133
Corneal infections
  adherence of *Pseudomonas aeruginosa*, 20–21
  cause of, 188
  studies of, 188–200
    age in resistance, 199–200
    complement in corneal resistance, 199
    humoral response studies, 197–199
    immunization studies, 200
    mouse model, 188–190
    resistance/susceptibility studies, 190–199
Cystic fibrosis, 245–260
  acquired resistance to *Pseudomonas aeruginosa*, 308–310
    antibody isotype in, 308–310
    complement in, 310
    naturally acquired resistance, 306
    vaccine-induced immunity, 306–308
  bacterial infections of respiratory tract, 246
  and chronic *Pseudomonas aeruginosa* infections, 19, 26, 108, 184–185, 258
  events in lung infection, 398–400
  genetic factors, 184, 245
  host defenses
    adhesins and receptors, 249–250
    humoral immune response, 253–254
    inflammatory response, 248–249
    microenvironmental factors, 254
    neutrophil enzyme effect, 257–258
    regulatory system, 255–256
    surface enlargement strategy, 256–257
    virulence, exoproducts in, 250–253
  immunization against *Pseudomonas aeruginosa*, 306–308, 386
  prevention of
    disinfection and hygiene, 260
    vaccination, 259–260
  risk of *Pseudomonas aeruginosa*
    dental treatment, 248
    and fragmented immunoglobulins, 174
    hospital acquisition, 247–248
    immunoglobulin subclass distribution, 175
    intestinal colonization, 248
    nonopsonic antibody, 174–175
    phagocytic receptor expression, 175–176
    proteolytic activity in bronchial secretions, 175
    sibling contagion, 247
  treatment of *Pseudomonas aeruginosa*
    antibiotics, 258
    anti-inflammatory therapy, 258–259
Cytokine secretion, effects of pyo on, 50–51

Deletion analysis, genetic study of, 82–83
Dental equipment
  as *Pseudomonas aeruginosa* habitat, 4, 248, 260
  Pseudomonas aeruginosa risk and cystic fibrosis patients, 248
Dialysis infections, 237
  clinical features, 237
  general considerations, 237
Diphtheria, 80; endocytic uptake of toxins, 89–93
Disinfection, as prevention method, 260
Drug abuse
  and bone/joint infections, 230
  and endocarditis, 226, 227

Ear infections
  external otitis, 235
  malignant external otitis, 235–236
  mastoiditis, 237
  otitis media, 236–237
Ecology of *Pseudomonas aeruginosa*, 2–6
  adaptability of organism, 2–3
  in healthy humans, 6
  inanimate environments for, 3–6
Ecthyma gangrenosum, 225, 233
Elastase, 115–119, 145–159
  and adherence, 149
  biological effects of, 147, 149
  chemical activity, 146–147
  effect on phagocytosis, 170, 171
  and environmental conditions
    antibiotic effects, 150
    comparison of strains from different sources, 150
    culture conditions, 150
    duration of culture, 151–152
    media composition, 150–151
  genetic regulation of, 116–117
  and lung damage, 147, 149
  molecular studies
    elastase-deficient mutants, 152–154
    elastase genes, types of, 154–155
    processing of elastase, 155–156
    secretion of elastase, 157–158
  from mucoid and nonmucoid strains, 146–147
  and pathogenesis, 117–119
  proteins digested by, 146
  secretion factors, 116
  structure of, 115–116
  and virulence, 149
Endocarditis
  clinical presentation, 227

Endocarditis (*Cont.*)
  epidemiology, 226–227
  treatment of, 227
Endophthalmitis, 234–235
  causes of, 234
  clinical features, 235
Endoscopy, and *Pseudomonas aeruginosa* infection, 239
Epidemiology of *Pseudomonas aeruginosa*, 7–12
  incidence of infections, 7
  routes of transmission, 7–12
    endogenous routes, 12
    hospital personnel, 8–11
    investigation techniques, 8
    sink drain organisms, 11–12
Escherichia coli, 80
Exoenzyme S, 60, 113–115
  and attachment of *Pseudomonas aeruginosa*, 28, 32–33, 114–115
  and pathogenesis, 114
  purification problems, 113–114
  secretion factors, 115
  as toxin, 28
Exoproducts, 62, 110–113, 398
  effects on phagocytic cells, 170–171, 211
  elastase, 115–119
  exoenzyme S, 60, 113–115
  exotoxin A, 79, 110–114
  and infection process, 109
  phospholipases, 119–120
  See also individual topics
Exotoxin A, 79, 110–114
  antibody and acquired resistance, 299–300
  and burn injuries, 278–281
  and cystic fibrosis patients, 253
  effect on phagocytosis, 171
  and immunization, 113, 390
  molecular structure of, 110–111
  probe for, 8
  receptor-mediated endocytosis, 112
  structure-function relationship, 81–83
  synthesis of: *see* Toxin A synthesis
  virulence factors, 60, 110–111, 112–113
External otitis, 235
  cause of, 235
  clinical manifestations, 235
  treatment of, 235
Eye: *see* Ocular infections

Fecal contamination, with *Pseudomonas aeruginosa*, 6, 12
Fibronectin, in phagocytosis of *Pseudomonas aeruginosa*, 167

Flagella
  anti-flagella serum, 285, 303, 353, 389
  monoclonal antibodies against, 366
  as virulence factor, 284–285
Foramidocillin, 323

Gastric acidity, and increased incidence of *Pseudomonas aeruginosa*, 6, 12
Gastrointestinal infections
  general considerations, 237–238
  perirectal disease, 238–239
  typhlitis, 238
Genetic studies
  corneal infections, 188–200
  systemic infections, 185
  T-cell immunity, 185–188
Gentamicin, 332
Glycocalyx, and attachment of *Pseudomonas aeruginosa*, 208
Green nail syndrome, 232; characteristics of, 232

Hand disinfection, 11
High-molecular weight polysaccharide vaccines, 389
Hospital transmission
  endogenous infection routes, 12
  hospital personnel, 8–11
  incidence of infections, 7
  investigation methods, 8
  prevention of, 11–12
  sink drain transmission, 11
Hot tubs, infection related to use, 233
Humoral response
  corneal infections, 197–199
  cystic fibrosis patients, 253–254
Hyperimmune immunoglobulin, 356–363
  animal studies, 359–363
  experimental infection studies, 356–359
  human studies, 363

Imipenem, 323
Immune system, 207–216
  active and passive immunity, 298
  cell-mediated immunity, 298
  and cystic fibrosis: *see* Cystic fibrosis, host defenses
  immune responses, types of, 184
  immunosuppression and *Pseudomonas aeruginosa*, 213–216
  infection process of *Pseudomonas aeruginosa*, events in, 208–212
  proteases' effects, 135–139

Immune system (*Cont.*)
  T-cell immunity, 212–213, 214; genetic studies, 185–188
  See also Acquired resistance to *Pseudomonas aeruginosa*
Immunization, 300–303, 383–390
  alginate vaccines, 389
  anti-flagella serum, 285, 303, 353, 389
  antigens eliciting immunity, 300–303
  clinical trials, summary of, 385
  complex vaccines, 350, 351
  cross-protective vaccines, 352–353
  and cystic fibrosis patients, 306–308, 386
  defined vaccines, 350, 351–352
  and exotoxin A, 113
  high-molecular weight polysaccharide vaccines, 389
  intravenous IgG strategy, 307
  mucoid exopolysaccharide vaccines, 389
  O-PS-toxin A conjugate vaccine, 390
  PEV, 384, 386, 387, 388
  Pseudogen, 384, 386, 387
  ribosomal vaccines, 387
  studies of, 200, 259–260
  supplementation of vaccines, 308
  vaccination, nature of, 300
Immunocompromised patients
  common types of, 59, 109, 383, 384
  and *Pseudomonas aeruginosa*, 2, 6, 7, 59, 108–109, 223, 252–253
Immunoglobulins
  fragmented, in cystic fibrosis, 174
  in phagocytosis of *Pseudomonas aeruginosa*, 167
Immunotherapy, 353–369, 390–392
  burn injuries, 277, 363, 390–391
  hyperimmune immunoglobulin, 356–363
    animal studies, 359–363
    experimental infection studies, 356–359
    human studies, 363
  immune serum globulin, 354
  intravenous IgG strategy, 307, 354–356
  monoclonal antibodies, 363–369, 391–392
    core glycolipid immunity, 363–365
    efficacy of, 369
    Pseudomonas aeruginosa specific MAb, 365–369
    safety factors, 369
Infection process, events in, 208–212, 398–400
Inflammatory responses
  and attachment of *Pseudomonas aeruginosa*, 249

Inflammatory responses (*Cont.*)
  nature of, 209–210
  proteases' effects, 138
Intestinal colonization, in cystic fibrosis patients, 248
Iron, and toxin A synthesis, 62–64, 400

Keratitis, 188, 234
  clinical presentation, 234
  epidemiology, 234
  treatment of, 234

Beta-lactamase, 328–329
Beta-lactams, 322–331
  anti-pseudomonal drugs, 322–324
  aplacillin, 323
  carbapenems, 323, 329
  carbenicillin, 323
  cephalosporins, 323–324, 328, 329
  efficacy of, 324–330
  foramidocillin, 323
  imipenem, 323
  beta-lactamase, 328–329
  outer membrane permeability, 324–328
  penicillin-binding proteins, 324, 329–330
  resistance of *Pseudomonas aeruginosa* to, 323, 330–331
  respiratory infections, 228–229
  skin infections, 226
  ticarcillin, 323
Laminin, proteases' effects, 133–134
Leukemia, and risk of *Pseudomonas aeruginosa*, 173
Leukocidin, effect on phagocytosis, 170

Macrophages, in phagocytosis, 164, 167–168, 169, 210
Mafenide acetate, burn injuries, 277
Malignant external otitis, 235–236
  clinical presentation, 236
  diagnosis of, 236
  pathogenesis, 235
  prognosis of, 236
  risk factors, 235
  treatment of, 236
Mammalian cell susceptibility, 81–100
  acidic compartments, role of, 86
  binding event, 88–89
  chimeric toxins, 98–99
  endocytic uptake of *Pseudomonas aeruginosa*, 89–93
  ETA compared to viral infections, 87–88

Mammalian cell susceptibility (*Cont.*)
  LM fibroblasts
    activation/escape of *Pseudomonas aeruginosa* toxin, 93–97
    isolation of receptor for *Pseudomonas aeruginosa* toxin, 97–98
  OVCAR cells, resistance to *Pseudomonas aeruginosa* toxins, 98
  process in cell invasion, 87–88
  receptor-mediated endocytosis, 83–86
  temperature dependence, 86–87
Mastoiditis, 237
Meningitis, 231
  clinical presentation, 231
  epidemiology, 231
  routes of infection, 231
  treatment of, 231
Mitochondrial respiration, effects of pyo on, 49
Modeccin, 80
Mono ADP ribosyltransferases, 61
Monoclonal antibodies, 363–369, 391–392
  against flagella, 366
  core glycolipid immunity, 363–365
  efficacy of, 369
  laboratory production of, 392
  limitations of studies, 391–392
  mucoid exopolysaccharide, 366
  O-antigen, 367–369
  outer membrane proteins, 366
  polysaccharide core of *Pseudomonas aeruginosa* LPS, 367
  Pseudomonas aeruginosa-specific MAb, 365–369
  safety factors, 369
Mononuclear phagocytes, and phagocytosis, 164
Morphological technique, 89
Mucoid exopolysaccharide, effect on phagocytosis, 172
Mucoid exopolysaccharide vaccines, 389
Mucoid *Pseudomonas aeruginosa* strains, 3, 19; attachment of organism, 23, 26–27

National Nosocomial Infections Surveillance System, 7
Neonatal infections, 236–237
Neutropenia, and risk of *Pseudomonas aeruginosa*, 173
Neutrophil inhibitor, effect on phagocytosis, 171
Neutrophils
  and cystic fibrosis patients, 256

Neutrophils (*Cont.*)
  effects of pyo on, 49–50
  neutrophil elastase, 257–258
  neutrophil enzyme effect, 257–258
  and phagocytosis, 164, 166, 167, 169
Nonmucoid *Pseudomonas aeruginosa*, 4, 5, 19; adherence of, 21

O-antigens, monoclonal antibody studies, 367–369
Ocular infections
  corneal infections, studies of, 188–200
  endophthalmitis, 234–235
  general considerations, 233–234
  keratitis, 234
Opportunistic infection, *Pseudomonas aeruginosa* as, 2, 6, 7, 108–109, 169–170; See also Immunocompromised patient
Osteochondritis, 230
  cause of, 230
  treatment of, 230
Otitis media, 236–237
OVCAR cells, resistance to *Pseudomonas aeruginosa* toxins, 98
Oxyradicals
  effects of pyo on, 48
  in phagocytic killing of *Pseudomonas aeruginosa*, 168

PA103, 66, 68, 113
PAO1, 8, 11, 66, 68, 154
PAO1-PRI, 66
PAO-E64, 153
Passive immunity, 298, 300; see also Immunotherapy
Penicillin
  burn injuries, 276–277
  in combination therapy, 332
  endocarditis, 227
Penicillin-binding proteins, 324, 329–330
Perirectal disease, 238–239
  characteristics of, 239
  treatment of, 239
Pertussis, 80
PEV, 384, 386, 387, 388
Phagocyte-derived antibiotics, 169
Phagocytosis, 163–176
  human phagocytic receptors, 165
  mononuclear phagocytes, 164, 210
  nonopsonic phagocytosis, 166
  opsonic phagocytosis, 165–166, 210
  polymorphonuclear leukocytes, 164

Phagocytosis (*Cont.*)
  process of, 164–165, 210–211
  role of phagocytic cells in infection, 163
  zipper hypothesis of, 165
Phagocytosis of *Pseudomonas aeruginosa*, 166–176
  and disease states
    burns, 174
    cystic fibrosis, 174–176
    neutropenia, 173
  killing of *Pseudomonas aeruginosa*
    mechanisms in, 169
    nonoxidative microbicidal mechanisms, 169
    oxidative microbicidal mechanisms, 168–169
  nonopsonic phagocytosis
    bacterial factors in, 168
    macrophages in, 167–168
    phagocytic receptors, 168
  opsonic phagocytosis
    complement in, 166–167
    fibronectin in, 167
    immunoglobulin in, 167
  and *Pseudomonas aeruginosa* products
    cytotoxins, 170–171, 211
    elastase, 171
    exotoxin A, 171
    mucoid exopolysaccharide, 172
    pyocyanine, 173
    slime glycolipoprotein, 172–173
  and strain of *Pseudomonas aeruginosa*, 168
Phenazine pigments
  chemical classification of, 44
  detection methods, 46–47
  effects
    on bacteria, 48
    on cell proliferation and cytokine secretion, 50–51
    ciliary beating, 51–52
    mitochondrial respiration, 49
    neutrophil function, 49–50
    vascular reactivity, 52
  in infections, 43–54
  intratracheal instillation, effects of, 52
  purification and synthesis of, 46
  regulation of production, 47–48
  role in chronic *Pseudomonas aeruginosa* infection, 53
  at sites of infection, 52–53
  structure/chemical properties of, 44–46
Phosphate deficiency, and production of phenazine pigments, 48

Phospholipases, 119–120
  genetic regulation of, 119–120
  and pathogenesis, 120
Photoaffinity labeling, 83
Pili: *see* Attachment of *Pseudomonas aeruginosa*
Plant interactions, with *Pseudomonas aeruginosa*, 6
Polluted water, as *Pseudomonas aeruginosa* habitat, 3–4
Polymyxin B, 350
Premature infants, ocular infections, 234
Prevention of *Pseudomonas aeruginosa*
  disinfection and hygiene, 260
  in sink drains, 11–12
  See also Immunization; Immunotherapy
Proteases, 129–140, 209, 251
  and burn injuries, 281–283, 286–290
  effects on immune system, 135–139, 214
  extracellular release *in vivo*, 131–132
  inhibitors of, 139
  molecules degraded by, 209
  and pathogenesis, 131–132
  secretion, control of, 130–131
  tissue damage from, 132–134
  types of, 130, 209
Pseudogen, 384, 386, 387
Pseudomonas aeruginosa
  acquired resistance to, 297–311
  attachment of *Pseudomonas aeruginosa*, 19–36
  in burn infections, 275–290
  as chronic disease, 2
  and cystic fibrosis, 245–260
  early descriptions of, 1–2, 60
  ecology of, 2–6
  epidemiology of, 7–12, 108
  exotoxins, 107–121
  genetic studies, 185–200
  and immune system, 207–216
  immunization against, 300–303, 383–390
  immunotherapy, 353–369, 390–392
  infection, events in, 208–212
  mammalian cell susceptibility, 81–100
  as opportunistic infection, 2, 59, 108–109, 169–170
  phagocytosis, 163–176
  phenazine pigments in infections, 43–54
  proteases and pathogenesis, 129–140
  rise in incidence of infections, 223
  toxin A synthesis, 60–74
  toxins with similar features to, 79–80
  See also specific topics

Pseudomonas aeruginosa-caused diseases, 297–298
  and AIDS patients, 239
  bacteremia, 224–226
  bone/joint infections, 230
  brain abscess, 231–232
  dialysis infections, 237
  endocarditis, 226–227
  endophthalmitis, 234–235
  external otitis, 235
  keratitis, 234
  malignant external otitis, 235–236
  mastoiditis, 237
  meningitis, 231
  neonatal infections, 236–237
  otitis media, 236–237
  perirectal disease, 238–239
  post-endoscopic infections, 239
  respiratory infections, 227–229
  skin infections, 232–233
  typhlitis, 238
  urinary tract infections, 229
  wound infections, 232
Pseudomonas aeruginosa cellulitis, 233
Pseudomonas aeruginosa pneumonia, 228, 239
  clinical presentation, 228
  radiologic studies, 228
  treatment of, 228–229
Pseudomonas aeruginosa pyoderma, 233;
  characteristics of, 233
Pulmonary infections
  and adherence of *Pseudomonas aeruginosa*, 20
  in cystic fibrosis patients, 19, 108
  and phenazine pigments, 52–53
Pyocyanine
  antibiotic effect of, 208
  effect on phagocytosis, 173, 211–212
  and inflammatory response, 210
  and *Pseudomonas aeruginosa* colonization, 208
Pyo-fluorescein agar, detection of phenazine, 46

Quinolones, 338–342
  assays of uptake, 341
  ciprofloxin, 338
  efficacy of, 338
  resistance of *Pseudomonas aeruginosa* to, 341–342
  uptake across outer membrane, 338–340

Receptor-mediated endocytosis, 83–87, 112

Receptor-mediated endocytosis (*Cont.*)
  acidic agents, role of, 86, 93
  intracellular routing patterns, 84–86
  temperature dependence, 86–87
  and viral infections, 88
Resistance to *Pseudomonas aeruginosa*
  and autosomal genes, 193
  corneal infection studies, 190–199
  mechanisms in, 384
  OVCAR cell line, 98
  See also Acquired resistance to *Pseudomonas aeruginosa*
Respiratory enzymes, effects of pyo on, 49
Respiratory infections, 227–229
  antibiotics, effects of, 401–403
  clinical presentation, 228
  direct lung injury, 400–401
  epidemiology, 227–228
  events in lung infection, 398–400
  exacerbations and *Pseudomonas aeruginosa*, 406–407
  indirect lung injury, 401
  radiologic studies, 228
  treatment of, 228–229
  virulence, regulation of, 400
  See also Cystic fibrosis
Respiratory system
  attachment of *Pseudomonas aeruginosa*, 21, 149
  elastase, effects on lungs, 147, 149
  proteases' effects, 132
Rhamnolipids, 208
Ribosomal vaccines, 387
Ricin, 80
Routes of transmission, 7–12
  hospital personnel, 8–11
  investigation techniques, 8

Shigella, 80
Silver nitrate, burn injuries, 277
Sink drains
  prevention of *Pseudomonas aeruginosa* contamination, 11–12, 260
  as *Pseudomonas aeruginosa* habitat, 4
  transmission of *Pseudomonas aeruginosa* from, 9, 11–12
Skin infections, 6, 232–233
  ecthyma gangrenosum, 225, 233
  features of disseminated *Pseudomonas aeruginosa*, 225
  general considerations, 232
  green nail syndrome, 232
  Pseudomonas aeruginosa cellulitis, 233

Skin infections (Cont.)
  Pseudomonas aeruginosa pyoderma, 233
  toeweb infection, 233
  vesicular lesions, 225
  water-associated infections, 233
Slime glycolipoprotein, effect on phagocytosis, 172–173
Structure-function relationships, of Pseudomonas aeruginosa, 81–83
Surgical treatment, endocarditis, 227
Swimming pools, as Pseudomonas aeruginosa habitat, 4
Systemic infections, genetic studies, 185

T-cell immunity
  genetic studies, 185–188
  Pseudomonas aeruginosa, effects on, 212–213, 214
Temperature dependence, receptor-mediated endocytosis, 86–87
Ticarcillin, 323
Tobramycin, 332; study of, 401–403
Toeweb infection, 233
  characteristics of, 233
Toxin A synthesis, 60–74
  environmental factors in, 61–64; iron, effects of, 62–64, 400
  genetic regulation of, 64–73, 111
    activator in, 64–66
    cross-reactive epitope, 111
    gene products in toxin A synthesis, 72–73
    mutational analysis of genes, 68–69
    regB gene in toxin A synthesis, 68

Toxin A synthesis (Cont.)
  genetic regulation of (Cont.)
    toxA gene in, 64–66
    toxR gene in toxin A expression, 69–71
    toxR gene in toxin A synthesis, 66–67
    toxR gene transcriptional analysis, 67
  historical view, 60–61
  See also Exotoxin A
Tracheal epithelial cells, adherence of Pseudomonas aeruginosa, 20
Typhlitis, 238
  clinical presentation, 238
  treatment of, 238
Typing methods, for Pseudomonas aeruginosa, 8

Unlabeled antibody technique, 88–89
Urinary tract infections, 229
  clinical presentation, 229
  epidemiology, 229
  treatment of, 229

Vaccination: see Immunization
Vascular reactivity, effects of pyo on, 52
Viral infections
  adenovirus, 88
  compared to Pseudomonas aeruginosa invasion, 87–88
  and receptor-mediated endocytosis, 88

Water sources, of Pseudomonas aeruginosa, 3–4, 7
Wound infections, 232; and use of antibiotics, 232